Practical Clinical Andrology

Carlo Bettocchi • Gian Maria Busetto
Giuseppe Carrieri • Luigi Cormio
Editors

Practical Clinical Andrology

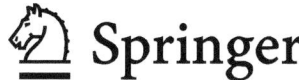 Springer

Editors
Carlo Bettocchi
Andrology and Male Genitalia
Reconstructive Surgery Unit
University of Foggia, Policlinico
"Riuniti" Foggia
Foggia, Italy

Giuseppe Carrieri
Department of Urology
University of Foggia, Policlinico
"Riuniti" Foggia
Foggia, Italy

Gian Maria Busetto
Department of Urology
University of Foggia, Policlinico
"Riuniti" Foggia
Foggia, Italy

Luigi Cormio
Department of Urology and Andrology
University of Foggia, "L. Bonomo"
Teaching Hospital Andria
Andria, Italy

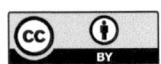

DBI S.r.l.

ISBN 978-3-031-11700-8   ISBN 978-3-031-11701-5   (eBook)
https://doi.org/10.1007/978-3-031-11701-5

This Springer imprint is published by the registered company Springer Nature Switzerland AG
The registered company address is: Gewerbestrasse 11, 6330 Cham, Switzerland

Preface

We are proud and honored to introduce the first edition of *Practical Clinical Andrology*.

As you know, nowadays andrological matters represent a remarkable issue in everyday practice.

The spectrum of andrological diseases is wide: erectile dysfunction, infertility and ejaculation disorders, penile curvature, oncologic disease and sexual problems related to this condition, gender dysphoria, and the so-called andrological emergencies, such as priapism and testicular torsion.

Their prevalence is relevant since erectile dysfunction reaches 52% in male patients between 40 and 70 years old and infertility affects 15% couples who try to conceive. Each of these subjects has been fully described, beginning from etiology and physiopathology coming to diagnostic pathway and to therapeutic strategies.

The aim of this work is to provide a complete and detailed overview of each andrological field evaluating both clinical and surgical aspects. Every chapter has been written and reviewed by some of the most recognized in this field with large experience. Pictures, videoclips, and interactive platforms give this book a modern and innovative look, in order to provide a more efficient learning process.

This book, published Open Access, would be helpful both to young urologists who want to expand their andrological skills and to andrologists in their everyday practice.

We highly hope this work may be useful and valuable in your practice and we look forward to hearing your feedback.

Foggia, Italy   Carlo Bettocchi
Foggia, Italy   Gian Maria Busetto
Foggia, Italy   Giuseppe Carrieri
Andria, Italy   Luigi Cormio

Contents

Contributors

Ashok Agarwal American Center for Reproductive Medicine, Cleveland Clinic, Cleveland, OH, USA

Fabio Michele Ambruoso Department of Emergency and Organ Transplantation-Urology, Andrology and Kidney Transplantation Unit, University of Bari, Bari, Italy

Federico Belladelli Division of Experimental Oncology/Unit of Urology, URI-Urological Research Institute, IRCCS Ospedale San Raffaele, Milan, Italy
University Vita-Salute San Raffaele, Milan, Italy

Carlo Bettocchi Andrology and Male Genitalia Reconstructive Surgery Unit, University of Foggia, Policlinico "Riuniti" Foggia, Foggia, Italy

Stefano Bettocchi Department of Medical and Surgical Sciences, Institute of Obstetrics and Gynecology, University of Foggia, Foggia, Italy

Nicola Bianchi Endocrinology Unit, Medical Department, Azienda Usl, Bologna Maggiore-Bellaria Hospital, Bologna, Italy

Gian Maria Busetto Department of Urology, University of Foggia, Policlinico Riuniti, Foggia, Italy

Omer Onur Cakir Department of Urology, University College London Hospitals NHS Trust, London, UK

Marco Capece Department of Neurosciences, Reproductive Sciences and Odontostomatology, University of Naples Federico II, Naples, Italy

Paolo Capogrosso Department of Urology and Andrology, Ospedale di Circolo and Macchi Foundation, Varese, Italy

Carlotta Cocchetti Andrology, Women's Endocrinology and Gender Incongruence Unit, Careggi University Hospital, Florence, Italy

Giuseppe Carrieri Department of Urology and Organ Transplantation, University of Foggia, Foggia, Italy

Fabio Castiglione Department of Urology, University College London Hospitals NHS Trust, London, UK

Luigi Cirillo Department of Neurosciences, Science of Reproduction and Odontostomatology, University of Naples Federico II, Naples, Italy

Sergio Concetti Urology Unit, Surgical Department, Azienda Usl, Bologna Maggiore-Bellaria Hospital, Bologna, Italy

Luigi Cormio Department of Urology and Andrology, University of Foggia, "L. Bonomo" Teaching Hospital Andria, Andria, Italy

Giovanni Corona Endocrinology Unit, Medical Department, Azienda Usl, Bologna Maggiore-Bellaria Hospital, Bologna, Italy

Domenico Costantino Family Law at the Department of Law, University of Bari, Bari, Italy

Fabio Crocerossa Department of Urology, Magna Graecia University of Catanzaro, Catanzaro, Italy

Carlo D'Alterio Department of Neurosciences, Reproductive Sciences and Odontostomatology, University of Naples Federico II, Naples, Italy

Nicola D'Altilia Department of Urology and Renal Transplantation, Policlinico Riuniti di Foggia, University of Foggia, Foggia, Italy

Alessandra Daphne Fisher Andrology, Women's Endocrinology and Gender Incongruence Unit, Careggi University Hospital, Florence, Italy

Angelo di Giovanni Department of Neurosciences, Reproductive Sciences and Odontostomatology, University of Naples Federico II, Naples, Italy

Mauro Dicuio Urology Unit, Surgical Department, Azienda Usl, Bologna Maggiore-Bellaria Hospital, Bologna, Italy
Department of Urology, Sahlgrenska University Hospital, Goteborg, Sweden

Stefano Eleuteri Faculty of Medicine and Psychology, Sapienza University of Rome, Rome, Italy

Ugo Falagario Department of Urology and Organ Transplantation, University of Foggia, Foggia, Italy

Giuseppe Fallara Division of Experimental Oncology/Unit of Urology, URI-Urological Research Institute, IRCCS Ospedale San Raffaele, Milan, Italy
University Vita-Salute San Raffaele, Milan, Italy

Ginevra Farnetani Department of Experimental and Clinical Biomedical Sciences "Mario Serio", Centre of Excellence DeNothe, University of Florence, Florence, Italy

Fabiana Divina Fascilla Obstetrics and Gynecologic Unit, Department of Obstetrics and Gynecology, "Di Venere" General Hospital, Bari, Italy

Marco Finati Department of Urology and Organ Transplantation, University of Foggia, Foggia, Italy

Ferdinando Fusco Department of Woman, Child and General and Specialized Surgery, Urology Unit, University of Campania 'Luigi Vanvitelli', Naples, Italy

Carlo Foresta Unit of Andrology and Reproductive Medicine & Centre for Male Gamete Cryopreservation, Department of Medicine, University of Padova, Padova, Italy

Antonio Franco Department of Urology, S. Andrea Hospital, Rome, Italy

Giorgio Franco Department of Urology, Policlinico Umberto I, Rome, Italy

Roberta Galizia Department of Dynamic, Clinical and Health Psychology, Sapienza University of Rome, Rome, Italy

Valentina Giorgelli Group of Psychiatric Neuroscience, Department of Basic Medical Sciences, Neuroscience and Sense Organs, University of Bari Aldo Moro, Bari, Italy

Giuseppe Grande Unit of Andrology and Reproductive Medicine & Centre for Male Gamete Cryopreservation, Department of Medicine, University of Padova, Padova, Italy

Alessandra Graziottin Department of Obstetrics and Gynecology, University of Verona, Verona, Italy

Center of Gynecology and Medical Sexology, H. San Raffaele Resnati, Milan, Italy

Alessandra Graziottin Foundation for the Cure and Care of Pain in Women NPO, Milan, Italy

Francesca Greco Department of Medical and Surgical Sciences, Institute of Obstetrics and Gynecology, University of Foggia, Foggia, Italy

Murat Gül Department of Urology, Selcuk University School of Medicine, Konya, Turkey

Emmanuele A. Jannini Chair of Endocrinology and Medical Sexology, Department of Systems Medicine, University of Rome Tor Vergata, Rome, Italy

Csilla Krausz Department of Experimental and Clinical Biomedical Sciences "Mario Serio", Centre of Excellence DeNothe, University of Florence, Florence, Italy

Elisabetta Lavorato "Azienda Ospedaliera Universitaria Policlinico di Bari"—Psychiatry Unit, Bari, Italy

Luigi Napolitano Department of Neurosciences, Science of Reproduction and Odontostomatology, University of Naples Federico II, Naples, Italy

Mario Maggi Endocrinology Unit, Department of Experimental and Clinical Biomedical Sciences "Mario Serio", Careggi Hospital, University of Florence, Florence, Italy

Elisa Maseroli Andrology, Women's Endocrinology and Gender Incongruence Unit, Careggi University Hospital, Florence, Italy

Maria Matteo Department of Medical and Surgical Sciences, University of Foggia, Foggia, Italy

Phisiopathology and Assisted Reproductive Unit, University Hospital of Foggia, Foggia, Italy

Nicola Mondaini Department of Urology, Magna Graecia University of Catanzaro, Catanzaro, Italy

Maria Grazia Morena Department of Medical and Surgical Sciences, Institute of Obstetrics and Gynecology, University of Foggia, Foggia, Italy

Ferdinando Murgia Gynecologic Oncology Unit, Department of Obstetrics and Gynecology, "F. Miulli" General Regional Hospital, Bari, Italy

Luigi Nappi Department of Medical and Surgical Sciences, Institute of Obstetrics and Gynecology, University of Foggia, Foggia, Italy

Tea Palieri Department of Medical and Surgical Sciences, Institute of Obstetrics and Gynecology, University of Foggia, Foggia, Italy

Alessandro Palmieri Department of Neurosciences, Reproductive Sciences and Odontostomatology, University of Naples Federico II, Naples, Italy

Fabrizio Palumbo Department of Urology, Di Venere Hospital, Bari, Italy

Ambra Pisante Department of Medical and Surgical Sciences, Institute of Obstetrics and Gynecology, University of Foggia, Foggia, Italy

Edoardo Pozzi Division of Experimental Oncology/Unit of Urology, URI-Urological Research Institute, IRCCS Ospedale San Raffaele, Milan, Italy

University Vita-Salute San Raffaele, Milan, Italy

Alessandro Procacci Department of Urology, Di Venere Hospital, Bari, Italy

Flavia Proietti Department of Urology, Policlinico Umberto I, Rome, Italy

Olga Prontera Endocrinology Unit, Medical Department, Azienda Usl, Bologna Maggiore-Bellaria Hospital, Bologna, Italy

Antonio Rampino Group of Psychiatric Neuroscience, Department of Basic Medical Sciences, Neuroscience and Sense Organs, University of Bari Aldo Moro, Bari, Italy

Marco Recchia Department of Urology and Organ Transplantation, University of Foggia, Foggia, Italy

Anna Ricapito Department of Urology and Organ Transplantation, "Policlinico Riuniti", University of Foggia, Foggia, Italy

Ramadan Saleh Department of Dermatology, Venereology and Andrology, Faculty of Medicine, Sohag University, Sohag, Egypt

Ajyal IVF Center, Ajyal Hospital, Sohag, Egypt

Andrea Salonia Division of Experimental Oncology/Unit of Urology, URI-Urological Research Institute, IRCCS Ospedale San Raffaele, Milan, Italy
University Vita-Salute San Raffaele, Milan, Italy

Francesco Sebastiani Department of Urology, Di Venere Hospital, Bari, Italy

Gennaro Selvaggi Department of Plastic and Reconstructive Surgery, Institute of Clinical Sciences, The Sahlgrenska Academy, Sahlgrenska University Hospital, University of Gothenburg, Gothenburg, Sweden

Alessandra Sforza Endocrinology Unit, Medical Department, Azienda Usl, Bologna Maggiore-Bellaria Hospital, Bologna, Italy

Chiara Simonelli Department of Dynamic, Clinical and Health Psychology, Sapienza University of Rome, Rome, Italy

Felice Sorrentino Department of Medical and Surgical Sciences, Institute of Obstetrics and Gynecology, University of Foggia, Foggia, Italy

Marco Spilotros Department of Emergency and Organ Transplantation-Urology, Andrology and Kidney Transplantation Unit, University of Bari, Bari, Italy

Carlo Trombetta Urology Clinic, Trieste, Italy

Linda Vignozzi Andrology, Women's Endocrinology and Gender Incongruence Unit, Department of Experimental and Clinical Biomedical Sciences "Mario Serio", University of Florence, Florence, Italy

Vincenzo Mirone Department of Neurosciences, Science of Reproduction and Odontostomatology, University of Naples Federico II, Naples, Italy

Laura Vona Department of Medical and Surgical Sciences, Institute of Obstetrics and Gynecology, University of Foggia, Foggia, Italy

Francesco Maria Zullo Department of Medical and Surgical Sciences, Institute of Obstetrics and Gynecology, University of Foggia, Foggia, Italy

Introduction: *History of Sexual Medicine*

Emmanuele A. Jannini

1.1   Introduction

Life, biologically speaking and limited to creatures who do not clone themselves, always arises from a sexual act. Although in an age of medically assisted reproduction, this paradigm may have innovative exceptions, it is still evident that the fundamental biological function, primeval, constitutive, and constitutional is precisely sex. Everything comes from sex that gives birth to everything is living and not cloned. The sexual function is therefore, without a shadow of a doubt, the earliest and most important of all biological functions. In other words, the first brick of the building of physiology and therefore of physiopathology, and consequently of medicine itself, is precisely sex. However, sexual medicine is a field of science still too frequently ignored by academic medicine [1].

Andrology and sexual medicine have had closer relations than those, more recent and not always easy, between gynecology and sexual medicine. For this reason, it is useful, before addressing its history, to establish priorities, not just semantics. The precedence of Andrology over the Medicine of Sexuality has a trivially alphabetical reason and a more profoundly historical one: the landing of Andrology (especially in its original major competence, that of Male Reproductive Medicine) in the port of Medicine and Science has far preceded Sexology and for a long time even included it, especially if not exclusively in its male declination. The opposite precedence (sexual medicine first and then Andrology) instead has logic on its side, once it has admitted, the fundamental concept that Sexology is a chapter of internal medicine and therefore susceptible (and the fruits are very visible and incontrovertible by now for about 30 years and beyond) of scientific exploration. In our species, in fact, sex precedes reproduction, unless this is, as we said before, medically assisted, as well as precedes any other biological, psychic, behavioral, and social human function. The obvious need to specify the sexological content derives from the observation that the etymology *andros*—inevitably refers to the male. The (re)discovery of the female component, of the sexuality of the woman, of the couple as an entity object of scientific, diagnostic, and therapeutic competence requires the constant citation of sexology, in its various exceptions of Sexual Medicine, Medical Sexology, Clinical Sexology, and Psychosexology, each of which with more or less defined connotations and contents [2].

E. A. Jannini (✉)
Chair of Endocrinology and Medical Sexology,
Department of Systems Medicine, University of
Rome Tor Vergata, Rome, Italy

© The Author(s) 2023
C. Bettocchi et al. (eds.), *Practical Clinical Andrology*,
https://doi.org/10.1007/978-3-031-11701-5_1

1.2   Andrologists, Sexual Physicians, Medical Sexologists, Sexologists, and Psychosexologists

Traditionally, the andrologist had first defined himself as a physiopathologist and doctor of male reproduction, over time discovering the need to recognize sexuality, and not just the reproductive act, as an object of clinical interest. The reasons for this delay are not only the daughters of cultural heritage unwilling to recognize that sex and reproduction in the human species do not necessarily coincide, but also rather in the enormous cultural delay that sexology had, and in some ways still has, towards reproductive pathophysiology. The use of the Galilean method, humus and irreplaceable culture medium for andrology and sexual medicine, has not been considered as indispensable by generations of so-called, more or less self-defined, sexologists. Nor can it be blamed on these alone. The Italian medical schools where the word "sexology" or "sex" or "sexual dysfunction" appear in the students' curriculum are still very few: even today it is possible to graduate in medicine and surgery without having received formal lessons and clinical training on some of the most widespread and most dramatically impacting human pathologies on the quality of life of the population: sexual dysfunctions.

It is surprising, but it is also true, that similar shortcomings are recorded in the field of psychological academic training. The only exam in sexology (Psychology and Psychopathology of Sexual Behavior) has traditionally been a complementary exam and, after the reform has eliminated, the term of complementary exam, there are not many faculties or schools of psychology that have structurally activated it. The same courageous attempt by a single university in Italy, that of L'Aquila, to offer a specialist degree course with a focus on Sexology has been tempered by the obligation to unify courses due to a lack of staff: so, sexology has returned to being a Cinderella. This has allowed the proliferation of private schools that issue sexologist qualifications without any legal value and not always with a decent teaching staff. If one looks at the curriculum of professors teaching in these schools, which have proliferated thanks to the inaction of public academic training, it is very, very rare to find international scientific publications. This clearly denounces how far Italian (and not only Italian) sexology still has to go.

But some positive signs are beginning to be seen: second-level university masters, which issue non-professional qualifications in medical sexology or medicine of sexuality (the third-level master is not yet active in Italy for any subject), are officially recognized from the state as a postgraduate training, they begin to spread throughout the country and already a university, in the course of medicine and surgery in English, offers its students an official and compulsory course in Endocrinology and Sexology. It happens in Rome, Tor Vergata. Finally, very recently, the two Universities of Rome, Tor Vergata and Sapienza, joined in a shared 2 years Master course of Clinical Psychosexology in the Faculty of Psychology, providing an unique didactical product.

It is clear that public recognition of the figure of the sexologist, being a doctor (sexual physician) or a psychologist (clinical psychosexologists), is increasingly indispensable. A recognition that starts from the definition of the trainer, who can only be university, identified on the basis of a true, proven, scientific activity dedicated to this fundamental subject. The same specialization schools that already did it must increasingly feel the responsibility of training specialists capable of intercepting the healthcare needs of the population in question. It is quite clear that such a professional figure will soon become one of the most important supports for the quality of life of patients and couples [3].

1.3   Development of the Sexual Medicine

Medical sexology and the medicine of sexuality are born in psychiatric land. In fact, the first great scholars to deal with the function—and dysfunction—of human sexuality were psychiatrists. Among these, Richard Freiherr von Krafft-Ebing must be remembered, who wrote the *Psychopathia Sexualis* (psychopathy of sex), or Magnus Hirschfeld, who published the first scientific journal in 1908, *Zeitschrift für Sexualwissenschaft* (*Journal for Sexual Research*) [4]. This early period was also the *belle époque* of the great psychodynamic theories and research of Sigmund Freud and of his psychoanalysis and of the *Berliner Institut für Sexualwissenschaft* (Institute for Sexual Research), destroyed in 1933 by Nazi sexophobia [5].

Unfortunately, and not only for this last reason, the psychiatric paternity did not last long. These, in fact, have become increasingly disinterested in male and female sexual dysfunctions, such as, for example, erectile dysfunction, ejaculatory dysfunction, vaginismus, hypoactive sexual desire disorder, anorgasmia, etc. Likely, this decline in interest resulted in the highly controversial classification of sexual dysfunctions published in the fifth edition of the *Diagnostic and Statistical Manual of Mental Disorders (DSM-5)*, published by the American Psychiatric Association (APA) [6].

Sexology in its infancy was thus abandoned in the orphanage of science, transforming itself into psychosexology and letting the psychologist become the only adoptive parent. Thus, there have been many psychologists who have ignored medical-scientific methods for promoting an opinion-based psychosexology based on improvization and presumption. For example, Virginia Johnson herself, wife of gynecologist Bill Masters, despite the undeniable merit of being the true thinking mind of the famous couple, was not a graduate [7]. This self-referential arrogance of some (certainly not all) psychosexologists has led to the non-recognition of sexology as a science not only by the biomedical and psychiatric milieu, but also by academic psychology itself.

It could be said that the date of birth of sexual medicine goes back to the commercialization of the first oral treatment of erectile dysfunction, the type 5 phosphodiesterase inhibitor [8]. In the following two to three decades, studies on animal sexual behavior, psycho-neuro-endocrinological research, imaging of the human brain during the appetitive phase, arousal, coitus, ejaculation, and orgasm flourished, which have shown that sexual function is linked to the same neurobiological substrate involving the Psychiatric Sciences. Despite this, the birth of Medical Sexology—or

Sexual Medicine—also took place, thanks to experts with training in genitourinary surgery and not psychosexology. It was, in fact, especially urologists who were among the first to understand the possibility of grafting the branch of sexology on the medical trunk. Both the urology with the prostheses and the pharmaceutical industry with successful drugs such as hormones, type 5 phosphodiesterase inhibitors, dapoxetine, and other remedies, have made a formidable contribution to this progress [9].

But another important step was needed for the full growth of the Sexual Medicine. The biopsychosocial model (BPSm) is an integrative perspective which has been found tremendously important for overcoming the traditional risk of the psychological reductionism ("it is all in your mind") as well the more recent medical reductionism ("just take a pill to fix it"). The BPSm aims of being a multifaceted and comprehensive model able to interpret human sexual behavior and its risk factors, symptoms, and diseases from the social (history, society, and education), psychological (intrapsychic and relational), and biological (medical) perspective. Certainly, the BPSm is written in the first chapters of the "statute" of Sexual Medicine. However, this model, fundamental for the research, the clinical efforts, the education, the *Weltanschauung* itself of the field of sexual medicine, is far of misinterpretations, limits, and biases [10].

Some claim to apply BPSm concepts to their work in Sexual Medicine, but they lack robust historical, cultural, and sociological foundations. Others are experts in surgical practices and do not know the rudiments of psychology and psychosexology. Finally, others are competent in the cultural interpretation of sexual behavior, but are unable to diagnose and set up treatments for male, female, and third sex sexual dysfunctions. The BPSm was mistakenly conceived as an umbrella under which to shelter from the rain of one's "holistic" ignorance.

In reality, the historical evolution of Sexual Medicine has increasingly highlighted the need not only for integration and dialogue between the different scientific cultures that compose it, but also—and above all—for each one of those parts of the background to be enriched that are missing

[11]. There is also another important criticism to be made against the BPSm: words, terms, definitions, when used too frequently and inappropriately, wear out and lose their meaning. For this reason, the BPSm needs to be recovered, refounded, and filled with new scientific contents.

The enrichment of the historical model of bio-psycho-sociologism comes to us from systems medicine, one of the most powerful and effective contemporary approaches to interpret the genesis of diseases and also of general health itself. Systems medicine is an interdisciplinary field of study that looks at the systems of the human body as part of an integrated whole, incorporating biochemical, physiological, and environment interactions. Systems medicine draws on systems science and systems biology, and considers complex interactions within the human body in light of a subject's genomics, behavior, and environment. It encompasses systems which are traditionally outside the radar of BPSm such as politics, economy, crisis, pollution, energy and demographic choices, pandemics, and so on, describing the various systems that make up the complex reality that characterizes our world [12].

The historical evolution of Sexual Medicine passes precisely through Systems Medicine (SM = SM) to create a new model of integration of reality that proceeds through the understanding of the various systems that generate sexual health and the risks of losing it [13]. The most obvious term for it is Systems Sexology (Fig. 1.1), which is candidate for being the final, evolved paradigm of Sexual Medicine.

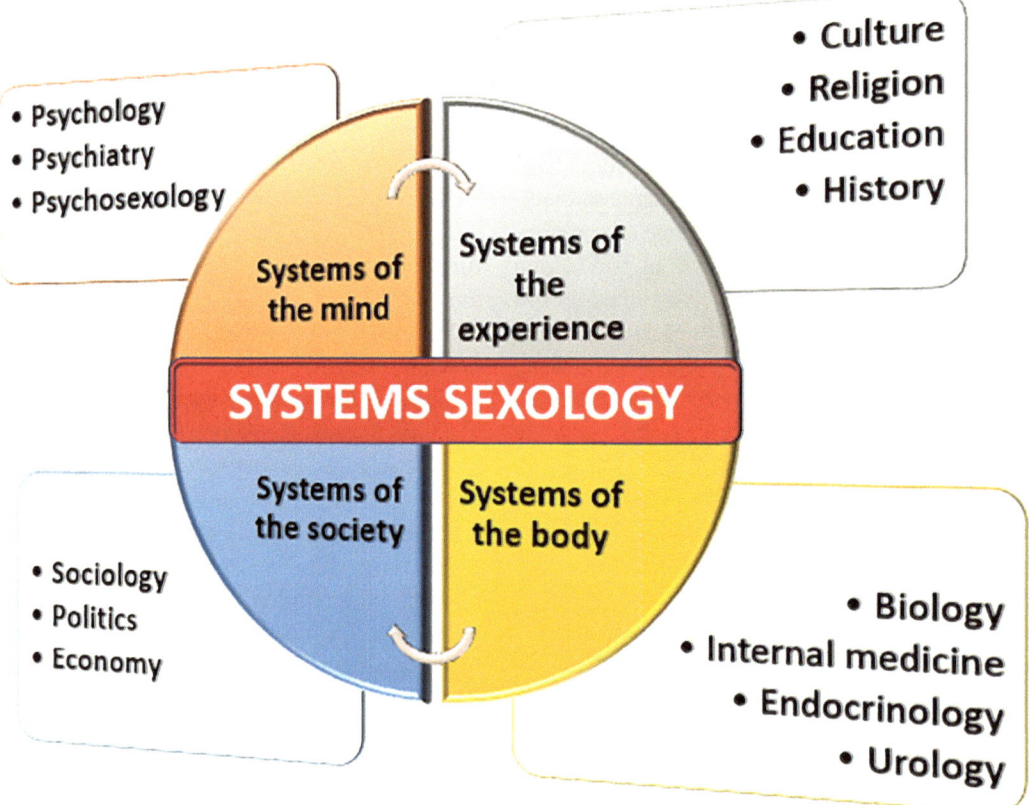

Fig. 1.1 Evolution of sexual medicine. After the era of psychological and medical reductionisms, Sexual Medicine evolved in the more mature Bio-Psycho-Social model, having a further evolution in the more complex, integrated, and efficient model of Systems Sexology to interpretate human sexual behavior and related dysfunctions

1.4 The Role of the Scientific Societies and Journals: The International Society of Sexual Medicine

The history of sexual medicine is not only matter of the evolution of the model; the field, in fact, grows and strengthens, thanks to two powerful fertilizers: scientific societies and scientific journals.

The International Society of Sexual Medicine (ISSM) is the universal scientific home and temple for all researchers, practitioners, and caregivers dealing with Sexual Medicine. This Society has as mission "To be the most respected and trusted source of information, education and professional development on human sexual health through the delivery of world-class publications, research findings, online and in person opportunities for knowledge exchange, world-wide." The ISSM has set itself the goal of disseminating knowledge and raising global awareness on sexual health issues, ensuring that the latest and most modern evidence-based scientific studies in the field of sexual medicine reach both male and female sexual health professionals, and also patients, in a global, inclusive and universal vision. The composition of the actual governance is very interesting and well representing the cul-

tural and geographical universality of the ISSM. The president is a Danish psychiatrist, Annamaria Giraldi, and the president-elect is a Canadian urologist, Gerald Brock (Table 1.1). The other members are from Brazil, USA, Korea, Lebanon, Switzerland, China, and Japan [14].

A core of the ISSM is its Publication Committee, the Pubcom, which has as mission to oversee the development and production of ISSM's publications, including the journals and any other newsletters, guidelines, or documents, to provide direction to editors and the staff concerning format, schedule, market, and distribution, increasing the scientific strength and reputation of all the ISSM publications. Within the activities of the Society, the journals (*Sexual Medicine Reviews*, *Journal of Sexual Medicine*, *Sexual Medicine Open Access*, and the *Video Journal of Prosthetic Surgery*) are in fact probably within the most important.

Sexual Medicine Reviews (SMR) has an Impact Factor of 4.836 (2020) and published evidence-based, primarily systematic, in-depth reviews of the highest caliber on multidisciplinary clinical, or translational topics in Sexual Medicine with the aim to represent the diversity of subjects in basic science and clinical practice that define sexual health, sexual function, sexual dysfunction, and sexual medicine,

Table 1.1 The President of the International Society of Sexual Medicine. Note the gender prevalence (the first woman elected president is the last one in this list)

Name	Years	Country
Vaclav Michal (Honorary)	1978–1986	Czechoslovakia
Adrian Zorgniotti	1986–1988	U.S.A.
Gorm Wagner	1988–1994	Denmark
Robert J. Krane	1994–1998	U.S.A.
Ronald W. Lewis	1998–2000	U.S.A.
Sidney Glina	2000–2002	Brazil
Jacques Buvat	2002–2004	France
P. Ganesan Adaikan	2004–2006	Singapore
Ira D. Sharlip	2006–2008	U.S.A.
John Dean	2008–2010	United Kingdom
Edgardo F. Becher	2010–2012	Argentina
Chris G. McMahon	2012–2014	Australia
Wayne J.G. Hellstrom	2014–2016	U.S.A.
Luca Incrocci	2016–2018	Netherlands
Luiz Otavio Torres	2018–2020	Brazil
Annamaria Giraldi	2020–2022	Denmark

targeting the sexual investigator, practitioner, and trainee. The current Editor-in-Chief is the Irwin Goldstein.

The Journal of Sexual Medicine (JSM), being the oldest Journal of the ISSM and of the International Society for the Study of Women's Sexual Health, has an impact factor 3.802 (2020) obtained by publishing multidisciplinary basic science and clinical research to define and understand the scientific basis of male, female, and couples' sexual function and dysfunction. The JSM provides healthcare professionals in sexual medicine with essential educational content and promotes the exchange of scientific information generated from experimental and clinical research. The JSM includes basic science and clinical research studies in the psychologic and biologic aspects of male, female, and couples' sexual function and dysfunction, and highlights new observations and research, results with innovative treatments and all other topics relevant to clinical sexual medicine. The objective of the JSM is to serve as an interdisciplinary forum to integrate the exchange among disciplines concerned with the whole field of human sexuality. The journal accomplishes this objective by publishing original articles, as well as other scientific and educational documents that support the mission of the International Society for Sexual Medicine. The current Editor-in-Chief is John P. Mulhall.

Sexual Medicine—a Gold Open Access publication—(SMOA) displays an impact factor of 2.491 (2020) and publishes multidisciplinary clinical, basic, and epidemiological research to define and understand the basis of sexual function and dysfunction in diverse populations. SMOA welcomes manuscripts on basic anatomy and physiology pertaining to human sexuality, pharmacology, clinical management of sexual dysfunction, epidemiological studies in sexuality, psychosexual and interpersonal dimensions of human sexuality, clinical trials, and other articles of interest to clinicians and researchers interested in human sexuality. The open access format of the journal ensures that accepted manuscripts will be rapidly published and fully accessible by interested healthcare professionals worldwide. SMOA emphasis on papers relevant to specific populations distinguishes it from the JSM, which will continue to publish manuscripts on issues of general interest to sexual medicine practitioners worldwide, and SMR, which publishes systematic reviews of controversial topics in sexual medicine. The journal considers all types of original clinical and basic research papers, including studies conducted with human subjects and experimental models, as well as high-quality clinical, epidemiological, and healthcare policy papers related to sexual function and dysfunction. SMOA particularly focuses on papers of regional or specialty interest, although any manuscript dealing with sexuality research is also be considered. Specific interest is in the following areas of content: Education, Epidemiology, Basic Science, Psychology, Outcomes Assessment, Anatomy/Physiology, Intersex and Gender Identity Disorders, Sexual Orientation, Ejaculatory Disorders, Women's Sexual Health, Men's Sexual Health, Couples Sexual Dysfunctions, Pharmacotherapy, Peyronie's Disease, Pain, Erectile Dysfunction, Premature Ejaculation, Hypoactive Sexual Desire Disorder, Dyspareunia, Pharmacotherapy for Sexual Dysfunction, Surgical Management of Sexual Dysfunction, Endocrinology, and Oncology. The current Editor-in-Chief is Alan Shindel.

Finally, the *Video Journal of Prosthetic Urology* (VJPU) was created by the ISSM to serve as a forum for sexual medicine to allow its members to exchange notable ideas via the visual medium. The members are scattered across the globe being prosthetic urology, a tiny subspecialty of sexual medicine. A specific goal of the VJPU is to facilitate the transmission of surgical technique knowledge regarding the implantation of surgical devices related to sexual medicine. Its editorial team welcomes video submission of anything felt needs illustrating in the field of sexual medicine. Diverse videos, as how to make a surgical video, robot-assisted vasovasostomy, repair of penile injuries, and communication skills development in sexual medicine are currently published. The Editor-in-Chief is currently Rafael Carrion.

A number of other scientific journals contributed directly or indirectly to the development of the history of Sexual Medicine. *The International Journal of Impotence Research* (IJIR) addresses sexual medicine for all sexes and genders as an interdisciplinary field. This publishes work from basic science researchers, urologists, obstetricians and gynecologists, endocrinologists, cardiologists, family practitioners, internists, neurologists, psychiatrists, psychologists, radiologists, and other physical and mental health care professionals. It also includes work from gender and sexuality researchers, sex therapists, and others with scholarly expertise in human sexuality and sexual well-being. The editor-in-chief is Ege can Serefoglu (TR), and the journal displays a 2020 impact factor of 2.896.

A number of other important journals should be mentioned for their contribution to the history of Sexual Medicine, although they mainly center their scientific interest in psychosexology, not always with a strong impact factor. Table 1.2 is a list of these journals.

Last but not least, the historically neglected, although fundamental part of Sexual Medicine, i.e., the medicine of female sexual behavior, received finally deep scientific attention and full research and clinical development in the International Society for the Study of the Women Sexual Health (ISSWSH), which is a multidisciplinary, academic, and scientific organization whose purposes are to provide opportunities for communication among scholars, researchers, and practitioners about women's sexual function and sexual experience, to support the highest standards of ethics and professionalism in research, education, and clinical practice of women's sexuality, and to provide the public with accurate information about women's sexuality and sexual health. Noel N. Kim (USA) is the current president.

Table 1.2 List of scientific journals dealing directly or indirectly with sexual medicine. Note that a number of these journals display a low, if any, impact factor. It should be noted that several of peer-reviewed, well-established generalist journals, as well of endocrinology, gynecology, urology, psychology, and psychiatry, published articles of Sexual Medicine

Advances in Sexual Medicine
AIDS and Behavior
AIDS Education and Prevention
American Journal of Sexuality Education
Andrologia
Andrology
Archives of Sexual Behavior
Asian Journal of Andrology
Biology of Sex Differences
British Journal of Sexual Medicine
Canadian Journal of Human Sexuality
Culture, Health & Sexuality
GLQ: A Journal of Lesbian and Gay Studies
Indian Journal of Health, Sexuality & Culture
Indian Journal of Sexually Transmitted Diseases and AIDS
International Journal of Impotence Research
International Journal of Sexual Health
International Journal of Advanced Studies in Sexology
Integrative Medicine In Nephrology And Andrology
International Journal of STD and AIDS
International Journal of Transgender Health
Journal of Bisexuality
Journal of Child Sexual Abuse
Journal of Counseling Sexology & Sexual Wellness
Journal of Gay & Lesbian Mental Health
Journal of Gay and Lesbian Social Services
Journal of GLBT Family Studies
Journal of Homosexuality
Journal of Lesbian Studies
Journal of LGBT Youth
Journal of Sex & Marital Therapy
Journal of Sex Education and Therapy
Journal of Sex Research
Journal of Sexual Aggression
Journal of Sexual Medicine
Journal of Social Work and Human Sexuality
Journal of the History of Sexuality
Law & Sexuality
Porn Studies
Psychology & Sexuality
Research Journal of Sexology Sciences
Scandinavian Journal Sexology
Sexes
Sex Roles

(continued)

Table 1.2 (continued)

Sexología y Sociedad
Sexologies: European Journal of Sexual Health (Revue Européenne de Santé Sexuelle)
Sexual Abuse
Sexual Addiction and Compulsivity
Sexual and Relationship Therapy
Sexual Development
Sexual Medicine Open Access
Sexual Medicine Reviews
Sexualities
Sexuality & Culture
Sexuality and Disability
Sexuality Research and Social Policy
Sexually Transmitted Diseases
Sexually Transmitted Infections
Sexuologie
Studies in Gender and Sexuality
Trends in Urology Gynaecology and Sexual Health
Video Journal of Prosthetic Urology
World Journal of Men's Health
Zeitschrift für Sexualforschung

## 1.5	The European Contribution to the History of Sexual Medicine: The European Society of Sexual Medicine and the European Academy of Andrology

The ISSM has a number of affiliated societies, such as the International Society for the Study of the Women's Sexual Health, and the Asia-Pacific (APSM), the Middle-East (MESSM), the South-Asian (SASSM), the Latin-American (SLAM), and the North America (SMSNA) Societies of Sexual Medicine. Within those, it is peculiarly brilliant – for number of affiliated members and scientific production - the European Society for Sexual Medicine (ESSM), currently ruled by Carlo Bettocchi (Table 1.3).

The ESSM supports scientists in the field of Sexual Medicine to translate fundamental research findings to clinical use, to develop and adopt new medicines, technologies, and methods for the treatment of sexual dysfunctions and for the improvement of human sexual health. ESSM supports the scientists in the field of Sexual Medicine through research grants, travel fellow-

ships, personal awards, and studentships. Moreover, by providing access to the best scientific papers, the newsletter *ESSMTODAY*, the literature review section, cases that matter, and many other opportunities, ESSM is providing continuously the essential scientific update that is needed in order to pursue its main purpose, to promote research and exchange of knowledge about the clinical entity of sexual dysfunction throughout Europe.

The ESSM means Education and Science in Sexual Medicine. In the last years, ESSM has established several educational programs and developed criteria for certification in Sexual Medicine and in Sexology. In fact, one of the main merits of the ESSM is the education in Sexual Medicine, which is ruled by the Multidisciplinary Committee of Sexual Medicine (MJCSM). The MJCSM was set up by the European Union of Medical Specialists (UEMS), the oldest medical organization in Europe which celebrated its 60th anniversary in 2018 through 43 Specialist Sections and their European Boards, addressing training in their respective Specialty and incorporating representatives from academia (Societies, Colleges, and Universities). The MJCSM is built on the representatives of the UEMS boards of Endocrinology, Dermatology, Urology, Obstetrics and Gynecology, and Psychiatry having as main objective to guarantee the highest standards of care in the field of Sexual Medicine in the countries of the European Union and associated European countries, by ensuring that the training in sexual medicine is raised to the optimal level. This is achieved by making recommendations on the standards required for the training of physicians who practice Sexual Medicine and on the maintenance of such standards, establishing criteria to which the training centers of Sexual Medicine should conform, setting up a system for assessment of training in Sexual Medicine, promoting Continuous Professional Development in Sexual Medicine, and facilitating the exchange of trainees between training centers of the various countries of the Union and associated countries to ensure a better harmonization and quality of training. The MJCSM and the ESSM strongly collaborate in

Table 1.3 Milestones of the European Society of Sexual Medicine

Year	Milestone
1995	The European Society of Impotence Research (ESIR) was born and the first Congress was held in Porto Carras, Greece. Our journey began into medical knowledge, research, and innovation across Europe
1997	The second Congress was held in Madrid. The third Congress was held in Barcelona in 2000, after the tremendous earthquake that hit Turkey in 1999, where the Congress should have been held
2001	The name of the Society changed into European Society for Sexual and Impotence Research (ESSIR) in order to embrace more deeply the broad field of sexual medicine, both male and female
2003	Changing again its name into the actual European Society for Sexual Medicine (ESSM). Characterizing once again its need to improve and spread the research into sexual medicine, a field which is continuously developing across the world, bringing sexual awareness to light more and more not only in the medical field but also among people
2005	The tenth anniversary of ESSM, a society which is always stronger and more deeply rooted across Europe, with 13 National Societies affiliated to ESSM and about 1400 members
2009	ESSM became stronger and now it harbors 25 National Affiliated Societies
2012	First examination to become a Fellow of the European Committee of Sexual Medicine (FECSM)
2013	First examination to become a European Federation of Sexology (EFS) & ESSM Certified Psycho-Sexologist (ECPS)
2015	Celebrating the 20th anniversary of ESSM
2020	Celebrating the 25th anniversary of ESSM

order to provide adequate qualification to medical doctors in Sexual Medicine since 2012. Thanks to this collaboration, the MJCSM issues the only available certification for sexual medicine: The Fellow of the European Committee of Sexual Medicine (FECSM), a mark of excellence obtained by a large number of doctors, not only from Europe, after a serious exam [15]. In order to help candidates prepare for the MJCSM exam, the ESSM arranges preparation courses. The courses offer a focused overview of Sexual Medicine aimed directly at increasing the chance of success in passing the exam. Lectures are delivered by renowned experts, and the course is highly recommended for anyone who aims for FECSM certification.

Another important historical step was reached by the ESSM with the ESSM School of Sexual Medicine and Advanced Course which is run with the support of the European Society with the ISSM and the European Federation of Sexology (see later). Participants did have the opportunity to learn the essentials of sexuality that are necessary for effective clinical practice, even for those whose usual practice is exclusively with one gender. Similarly, the Society runs the ESSM Surgical Academy to offer various training units for surgeons to improve their knowledge, technical and communicative skills, and master novel operation techniques in genital surgery, according to high European standards of education, prior to performing them on patients.

As I mentioned earlier, the historical link between Andrology and Sexual Medicine is very strong. In fact, the European Academy of Andrology (EAA) also gave an important contribution to the earlier development of Sexual Medicine. The EAA was founded in 1992 in Castle Elmau (Germany) by a group of 15 distinguished andrologists from 10 European countries, who met on the occasion of the seventh European Workshop on Molecular and Cellular Endocrinology of the Testis. The EAA is a nonprofit organization promoting research and education in andrology and public awareness in the area of male health, currently ruled by Csilla Krausz (IT). The EAA has a worldwide scope in terms of membership, research, and influence but retains a clear focus upon Europe. A main feature of the Academy is the accreditation of high-quality andrology training centers, which are located mainly in Europe and also in America and the Middle East. The EAA is devoted to the development of andrological sciences and to disseminate knowledge in this field. To accomplish these tasks, the Academy organizes biennially the European Congress of Andrology (ECA). Furthermore, the Academy organizes Schools and Educational Courses to cover the entire range of the educational Curriculum built also in collaboration with the European Urological Association (EAU) Section of Andrological Urology (ESAU). One of the primary missions of the EAA Certified centers is to organize educational courses. Each Center is supposed to organize at least one Educational Course every 5 years. Training of the attendees of the Centers will be concluded by an examination administered by the EAA. The examination will test the candidate's proficiency in clinical andrology and its related fields (seminology, endocrinology, microbiology, imaging, morphology, urology, gynecology, immunology, and psychology) judged by international referees. Upon successful completion of the examination, the candidate will be awarded a certificate, or mark of excellence, of *Clinical Andrologist* from the EAA. Finally, *Andrology* is the official journal of the Academy since January 2013. This is a joint publication of the EAA and the American Society of Andrology (ASA) and replaces the old International Journal of Andrology and the Journal of Andrology, which were closed after merging in 2012. The growing impact factor is 3.842, and it is currently ruled by Marie Claude Hofmann (ASA) and Aleksander Giwercman (Deputy Editor, EAA).

The mentioned ESAU is a section of the EAU and seeks to reach a clearer perspective of what andrology has to offer and increase knowledge through investigation. ESAU promotes every aspect of clinical andrology, such as basic and clinical research, education, and training. The section facilitates interaction and close collaboration with the EAA. It takes a new direction towards active participation in ongoing European Educational Programs, and a major goal is to realize a common European Educational Program in Andrology. The current chairman is Nikolaos Sofikitis (GR).

1.6 The Psychosexological Societies in the Field of Sexual Medicine and Other Journals Which Contributed to Its Development

Two sexological societies, born in the psychological and psychosexological environment, contributed to the history of the Sexual Medicine from their perspective.

The World Association for Sexual Health (WAS) is an international organization representing sexological societies and psychosexologists worldwide. Founded in 1978 in Rome, Italy, the main goal of WAS is to promote sexual health for all through psychosexological science. The WAS previously named World Association for Sexology but changed its name in order to stress that sexology is a tool for achieving sexual health. In 2010, the WAS instituted September 4 as the *World Sexual Health Day* in an effort to increase social awareness about the role that sexuality plays in human health, and to promote the fact that sexual health is only attainable through sexual rights. Elna Rudolph (ZA) is the current president of the WAS Executive Committee. The official journal of the WAS is the *International Journal of Sexual Health*, previously established in 1988 under the title *Journal of Psychology & Human Sexuality*. It has an Impact Factor of 1.944 (2020) and is ruled by Eli Coleman.

The European Federation of Sexology (EFS) has over 30 active societies or professional associations of psychosexology and individual members, mainly from Europe. In 1988, under the impulse of an Italian psychiatrist, Willy Pasini, the EFS was founded as a regional society of WAS, with the aims to be the link between the different associations working in the field of sexology in Europe, to encourage the development of teaching in sexology, arouse sexological research plans, incite the organization of scientific congress in sexology, and contribute with societies which have the same objectives. The EFS is currently under the presidency of Mehmet Sungur (TR).

1.7   Forecast and Conclusion

Sexual Medicine will be all the stronger in the future; the more it will be able to rely on evidence and not on opinion, the more it will be based on research, even basic and translational, and not only on clinical experience, although very important, the more it will consider as qualifying objective criteria such as scientific production and the Hirsh index and not the power games of small factions, the more it will give strength to inclusive logics and not to cultural separations and barriers, thus overcoming the diabolical temptation to remain within the enclosure of a single gender, of a single nation, of a single educational background. Very positive signs in this sense are clearly observed, even if there is still some way to go in the direction of the full maturity of the field.

In fact, here I demonstrated that the history of Sexual Medicine coincides strictly with its scientific production, well represented by the Societies and Journals. Examining this amazing vitality seems evident that the field appears as one of the most vital areas of medicine, young and rich in scientific, academic, and clinical satisfactions for its students, fellows, and practitioners who are becoming more and more numerous in every part of the world. And this will significantly increase the sexual health of our patients, of all genders and sexual orientations, also thanks to the book you are about to read!

References

1. Jannini EA, Reisman Y. Medicine without sexual medicine is not medicine: an MJCSM and ESSM petition on sexual health to the political and university authorities. J Sex Med. 2019;16(6):943–5. https://doi.org/10.1016/j.jsxm.2019.04.001.

2. Education and treatment in human sexuality: the training of health professionals. Report of a WHO meeting. World Health Organ Tech Rep Ser. 1975;(572):5–33. PMID: 809930.

3. Pinchera A, Jannini EA, Lenzi A. Research and academic education in medical sexology. J Endocrinol Investig. 2003;26(3 Suppl):13–4.

4. Hirschfeld M, editor. Journal for sexual research. Leipzig: George H. Wigand's Verlag; 1908.

5. Three FS. Essays on the theory of sexuality (Drei Abhandlungen zur Sexualtheorie). 1905. Trans. Strachey J. New York: Basic Books; 1962.

6. American Psychiatric Association (ed) Diagnostic and statistical manual of mental disorders. 5th ed. Washington, DC.

7. Masters WH, Johnson V. Human sexual response. Toronto/New York: Bantam Books; 1966.

8. Goldstein I, Lue TF, Padma-Nathan H, Rosen RC, Steers WD, Wicker PA. Oral sildenafil in the treatment of erectile dysfunction. Sildenafil Study Group. N Engl J Med. 1998;338(20):1397–404. https://doi.org/10.1056/NEJM199805143382001.

9. Jannini EA, Eardley I, Sand M, Hackett G. Clinical and basic science research in sexual medicine must rely, in part, on pharmaceutical funding? J Sex Med. 2010;7(7):2331–7. https://doi.org/10.1111/j.1743-6109.2010.01898.x.

10. Nimbi FM, Galizia R, Rossi R, Limoncin E, Ciocca G, Fontanesi L, Jannini EA, Simonelli C, Tambelli R. The biopsychosocial model and the sex-positive approach: an integrative perspective for sexology and general health care. Sex Res Soc Policy. 2021; https://doi.org/10.1007/s13178-021-00647-x.

11. Jannini EA, Lenzi A. Introduction to the integrated model: medical, surgical and psychological therapies for the couple. J Endocrinol Investig. 2003;26(3 Suppl):128–31. PMID: 12834039.

12. Federoff HJ, Gostin LO. Evolving from reductionism to holism: is there a future for systems medicine? JAMA. 2009;302(9):994–6. https://doi.org/10.1001/jama.2009.1264. PMID 19724047.

13. Jannini EA. SM = SM: the interface of systems medicine and sexual medicine for facing non-communicable diseases in a gender-dependent manner. Sex Med Rev. 2017;5(3):349–64. https://doi.org/10.1016/j.sxmr.2017.04.002.

14. Lewis RW. Comprehensive history of the International Society for Sexual Medicine. Sex Med Rev. 2021;9(4):517–41. https://doi.org/10.1016/j.sxmr.2021.03.004.

15. Serefoglu EC, Reisman Y, Bitzer J, Vignozzi L, Jannini EA. The only available certification for sexual medicine: the Fellow of the European Committee Sexual Medicine (FECSM). Int J Impot Res. 2021; https://doi.org/10.1038/s41443-021-00506-8.

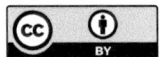

Sexuality and Sexual Orientation in the Twenty-First Century

2

Chiara Simonelli, Roberta Galizia, and Stefano Eleuteri

Learning Outcomes

By the end of this chapter, you will be able to:

- Recognize the different components of sexual identity (biological sex, gender identity, gender role, and sexual orientation).
- Have a knowledge of the factors that can determine sexual orientation.
- Know the main tools used to assess sexual orientation.
- Know the incidence of different sexual orientations.
- Know the contemporary issues on sexual orientation in clinical and research fields.
- Explain the rationale and benefits of moving to an integrated and sex-positive approach throughout the healthcare setting.

C. Simonelli (✉) · R. Galizia
Department of Dynamic, Clinical and Health Psychology, Sapienza University of Rome, Rome, Italy
e-mail: chiara.simonelli@uniroma1.it; roberta.galizia@uniroma1.it

S. Eleuteri
Faculty of Medicine and Psychology, Sapienza University of Rome, Rome, Italy
e-mail: stefano.eleuteri@uniroma1.it

2.1 Definitions and Conceptualizations: Sexual Identity, Gender Identity, Gender Role, and Sexual Orientation

The relationships between sexual orientation and gender, gender and sex, masculinity and femininity have over time been the subject of discussion in the field of feminist theory and, more recently, in the field of gender studies [1, 2].

Current theories of sexology, which are placed within a sociological, biological, psychological, and social perspective, consider sexual orientation a component of sexual identity. The latter, in fact, is a multidimensional construct, an "umbrella" term consisting not only of sexual orientation, but also of three other different and independent components: biological sex, gender identity, and gender role [3, 4].

Often the term "sexual orientation" is used interchangeably with the term "gender identity" [5]. It is therefore necessary to begin by giving a definition of each component in order to promote a correct use of these and to avoid that a series of convictions, beliefs, and stereotypes related to the sphere of psychosexuality are reiterated.

Biological sex refers to a person's femininity or masculinity [3, 4]. It is determined by five biological factors which are the sex chromosomes (XX or XY), the presence of male or female

© The Author(s) 2023
C. Bettocchi et al. (eds.), *Practical Clinical Andrology*,
https://doi.org/10.1007/978-3-031-11701-5_2

gonads, the hormones, the internal reproductive systems, and the external sexual organs.

The term *gender identity* is the subjective perception belonging to the female, male, ambivalent gender, or neither [6]. Gender identity is based on psychological characteristics which, starting from biological sex, within a specific culture of belonging, are encouraged in one sexual identity and discouraged in the other. Gender identity may or may not correspond to biological sex [7]. In other words, a person with male/female biological sex can perceive and self-identify as female or as neither female nor male.

Sexual orientation, on the other hand, refers to erotic and/or emotional attraction to a person of different sex (heterosexual), people of the same sex (homosexual), or both (bisexual). However, if until recently the prevailing scientific position considered sexual orientation as a stable trait, fixed and resistant over time, today the new theoretical perspectives suggest that sexual orientation can be flexible [5]. This means that some people may experience different sexual orientations throughout their life. In this sense, some authors such as Diamond [8] and Baumeister [9] have spoken respectively of sexual fluidity and erotic plasticity. Sexual orientation, therefore, can be thought of as a continuum that cannot always find its place in the categories usually considered and known (heterosexual, homosexual, and bisexual). However, even with respect to these categories that are mainly referred to, in some scientific research or in the clinical setting, there is often confusion, exchanging bisexual people with homosexual people [5]. The term bisexuality generally refers to attraction to more than one gender and can include several expressions [10], such as people who are attracted to both men/males and women/females, people who are mainly attracted to a gender but who recognize that it is not exclusive, people who feel their sexuality is fluid and constantly evolving, and people who are attracted to another person regardless of gender or sex. Not all people attracted to more than one gender describe themselves as bisexual. Asexuality is also considered a sexual orientation by some experts. It refers to low or absent sexual attraction and sexual behav-

iors. Asexual people can feel both romantic or aromantic attraction to others [11].

Asexuality is considered separate from sexual desire disorders (HSDD) as, usually, asexual people do not report distress and have a lifelong lack of sexual attraction.

In light of this, sexual orientation is a multidimensional construct, consisting of a multiplicity of aspects [5], such as self-identification, sexual behavior, erotic attraction, sexual fantasies, affective involvement, and the current relational status. Each person therefore develops a personal organization of erotic and affective attractions, fantasies, and sexual activities.

Sexual orientation, therefore, differs from gender identity: the first refers to the attraction that a person has towards another person and the second refers to the perception of oneself as female, male, or other [5].

Finally, the term *gender role*, introduced by Money and Tucker [12], indicates the set of verbal and non-verbal behaviors that express to themselves and to others the gender to which people feel they belong. This role is mostly the result of social habits that the person has learned. People can conform to these "cultural rules" or not to communicate to themselves and to others their adherence or not to the female or male sexual stereotype [3]. On the basis of socio-cultural norms, people are expected to behave in line with biological sex; that is, that males behave or say things "like males" and females "like females" [13]. In this way, the gender role is the result of external conditioning, which derives from how the gender identity is constructed [14, 15].

In general, sexual orientation, gender identity, and gender role coincide. The relationships between these components can be expressed in different ways, such as: (a) people with gender identity in accordance with chromosomal and phenotypic sex and with heterosexual, homosexual, or bisexual orientation; (b) people with gender identity in disagreement with chromosomal sex but in accordance with the phenotypic one and with heterosexual, homosexual, or bisexual orientation (for example, androgen insensitivity syndrome and adrenogenital syndrome); (c) people with gender identity in accordance with chromosomal sex but in disagreement with phenotypic sex and with heterosexual, homosexual, or bisexual orientation (for example, Turner syndrome and Klinefelter syndrome); and (d) people with gender identity in disagreement with chromosomal sex, with phenotypic sex and with heterosexual, homosexual, or bisexual orientation (for example, gender dysphoria).

In light of the above, it is important to specify that these definitions are not to be considered and used as static labels, predefined categories that stigmatize the person as a whole. An integrated, inclusive, and non-judgmental approach to sexuality is essential to fully recognize and understand the different manifestations of human sexuality.

2.2 Determining Factors of Sexual Orientation

The issue of the origin of sexual orientation, especially homosexual, has been the subject of study by scientists for more than a century. The interest of the scholars was to understand which factors determined homosexual attraction. In other words, the question was as follows: "are people born or become homosexuals?" Today, the emerging scientific perspective considers sexual orientation as a multidimensional phenomenon influenced by a complex interaction between genetic, neuroanatomical, neuroendocrinological, and environmental factors.

Several studies have shown that human sexual orientation has a genetic basis, that certain areas of the brain and neuroendocrine processes appear to differ in homosexual and heterosexual men.

The first contemporary family-genetic study on sexual orientation [16] using a more sophisticated methodology highlighted the presence of familiarity in male homosexuality: 20% of the siblings of homosexual males were homosexuals against 4% of the siblings of heterosexual males. However, it is not possible to distinguish genetic from environmental factors from family studies; for this reason, several studies have conducted research on twins and adoptions. In this regard, a study conducted by Bailey and Pillard [17]

showed that 52% of identical twins of homosexual males were also homosexual. There are different results on non-identical twins: only 22% of non-identical twins of homosexual males were homosexual and only 11% of adoptive siblings of homosexual males were homosexual. On a sample of homosexual women, Bailey et al. [18] found similar results (48% for identical twins, 16% for non-identical twins, and 6% for adoptive sisters), concluding that variations of sexual orientation can be influenced from 30% to 70% by genetic factors.

A limited number of studies have attempted to detect the presence of specific genes that contribute to the variation in sexual orientation. A genetic linkage of male homosexuality to markers on the X chromosome emerged from a study [19]. It seems that the terminal portion of Xq28 could code for homosexuality. However, it is difficult to establish any direct gene products [20].

Neuroscientific studies have also shown some differences in brain morphology between heterosexual men and homosexual men involving the interstitial nuclei of the anterior hypothalamus, which are larger in heterosexual men, and the anterior commissure, which is larger in homosexual men [21, 22]. However, these findings deserve further investigation.

Some studies have also shown the existence of endocrine and biochemical influences, and their development markers (such as the ratio between the length of the second and fourth toes, influenced by prenatal exposure to androgens) in the development of sexual orientation. However, even these results have not always found scientific confirmation [5, 23].

In addition to neuroanatomic and neuroendocrine differences, there appear to be differences in some cognitive abilities, mainly in spatial abilities. Gladue et al. [24] found that homosexual men, like heterosexual women, exhibited worse spatial ability than heterosexual men. Homosexual women had similar results to heterosexual women. These data, although they require further in-depth studies, suggest a possible correlation between biological and neuropsychological factors and the development of sexual orientation.

Overall, the factors that determine sexual orientation remain unclear although the scientific community has recognized the multifactorial nature of this sexual component [25].

Moreover, so far, most of the studies have examined in isolation the multiple biopsychosocial factors that influence sexual orientation. Studies that integrate biological, psychological, and socio-relational factors could deepen the idea that not all people develop sexual orientation according to an identical path.

2.3 The Assessment of Sexual Orientation

Increasingly, in the field of scientific research, scholars are recognizing the importance of introducing sexual orientation as a variable in their research. While the problems related to the measurement and evaluation of other socio-demographic variables, such as race and ethnicity, have been debated for a long time, there is certainly still much to be done with regard to the measurement of sexual orientation [26]. To date, researchers interested in measuring sexual orientation have a number of tools at their disposal, such as the Kinsey Scale [27], the Klein Scale [28], the Shively and DeCecco Scale [29], and the Sell Assessment [30]. However, none of these measures are totally without limitations.

The scale of measurement of sexual orientation most influential and used over these years is the one proposed by Kinsey et al. [27]. Kinsey et al. had proposed a seven-point bipolar scale ranging from "exclusively heterosexuality" to "exclusively homosexuality" (Table 2.1). This scale has a number of limitations. A limit of the Kinsey scale is that it groups into the same categories people who are significantly different from each other based on different aspects or dimensions of sexuality [31, 32]. A second problem with this scale is that it forces the combination of the psychological and behavioral components of sexual orientation and restricts individuals to make trade-offs between homosexuality and heterosexuality.

Table 2.1 The Kinsey scale (1948)

0 Exclusively heterosexual—Person who makes no physical contacts which result in erotic arousal or orgasm, and makes no psychic responses to a person of his/her own sex
1 Predominantly heterosexual/only incidentally homosexual—Person who has only incidental homosexual contacts which have involved physical or psychic response, or incidental psychic response without physical contact
2 Predominantly heterosexual but more than incidentally homosexual—Person who has more than incidental homosexual experience, and/or if he/she responds rather definitely to homosexual stimuli
3 Equally heterosexual and homosexual—Person who is about equally homosexual and heterosexual in his/her overt experience and/or the his/her psychic reactions
4 Predominantly homosexual but more than incidentally heterosexual—Person who has more overt activity and/or psychic reactions in the homosexual, while still maintaining a fair amount of heterosexual activity and/or responding rather definitive to heterosexual contact
5 Predominantly homosexual/only incidentally heterosexual—Person who is almost entirely homosexual in his/her overt activities and/or reactions
6 Exclusively homosexual—Person who is exclusively homosexual, both in regard to his/her overt experience and in regard to his/her psychic reactions

A solution to this problem was identified by Klein et al. [28] who, to avoid the loss of important information on the various components of sexual orientation, developed a scale that measures and evaluates the various dimensions of sexual orientation separately. The measure developed by Klein et al. takes the name of Klein Sexual Orientation Grid (KSOG) and evaluates sexual orientation on seven dimensions: sexual attraction, sexual behavior, sexual fantasies, emotional preference, social preference, self-identification, and heterosexual/homosexual lifestyle (Tables 2.2, 2.3, and 2.4). However, even this tool has limitations as the multi-dimensional assessment makes the tool less practical for researchers. Furthermore, each dimension of the scale has not been thoroughly studied; this tool also forces people to choose between heterosexuality and homosexuality.

Shively and DeCecco [29] developed a five-point scale on which heterosexuality and homo-

Table 2.2 Klein Sexual Orientation Grid (KSOG; 1985)

Variable	Past	Present	Ideal
A. Sexual attraction. To whom are you sexually attracted?			
B. Sexual behavior. With whom have you had sex?			
C. Sexual fantasies. About whom are your sexual fantasies?			
D. Emotional preference. To whom do you feel more drawn or close to emotionally?			
E. Social preference. With which gender do you socialize?			
F. Lifestyle preference. In which community do you like to spend your time? In which do you feel most confortable?			
G. Self-identification. How do you label or identify yourself?			

Table 2.3 Scale for measuring variables A, B, C, D, E of the KSOG

1	2	3	4	5	6	7
Other sex only	Other sex mostly	Other sex somewhat more	Both sexes equally	Same sex somewhat more	Same sex mostly	Same sex only

Table 2.4 Scale for measuring variables F and G of the KSOG

1	2	3	4	5	6	7
Heterosexual only	Heterosexual mostly	Heterosexual somewhat more	Heterosexual/ Homosexual equally	Homosexual somewhat more	Homosexual mostly	Homosexual only

Table 2.5 Shively and DeCecco scale (heterosexuality)

1	2	3	4	5
Not at all heterosexual		Somewhat heterosexual		Very heterosexual

Table 2.6 Shively and DeCecco scale (homosexuality)

1	2	3	4	5
Not at all homosexual		Somewhat homosexual		Very homosexual

sexuality are measured independently (Tables 2.5 and 2.6). This scale evaluates two dimensions of sexual orientation: physical and emotional preference. However, the Shively and DeCecco scale has limitations as its psychometric properties have not been thoroughly studied and the dimensions of physical and emotional preference may be reductive and not always appropriate [26].

The Sell Assessment of Sexual Orientation [30] was developed starting from the limits of the instruments for measuring sexual orientation described above. In fact, the Sell Assessment measures and evaluates sexual orientation on a continuum, takes into account various dimensions of sexual orientation, and considers homo-

sexuality and heterosexuality separately. The Sell Assessment consists of 12 questions, six of which assess sexual attractions, four assess sexual behavior, and two assess sexual orientation identity (see the six questions measuring sexual attractions in Table 2.7). The limit of this measuring instrument concerns its psychometric properties, largely under-examined [30, 33].

Despite the numerous research and theories on sexual orientation, there is still no widely accepted consensus on how the construct of sexual orientation should be defined and measured [5, 26]. Since there is no more recommendable measure than another, further research on measuring sexual orientation would be useful.

Table 2.7 The Sell assessment of sexual orientation (Sell, 1996): sexual attractions questions

1. During the past year, how many different men were you sexually attracted to (choose one answer):
a. None
b. 1
c. 2
d. 3–5
e. 6–10
f. 11–49
g. 50–99
h. 100 or more

2. During the past year, on average, how often were you sexually attracted to a man (choose one answer):
a. Never
b. Less than 1 time per month
c. 1–3 times per month
d. 1 time per week
e. 2–3 times per week
f. 4–6 times per week
g. Daily

3. During the past year, the most I was sexually attracted to a man was (choose one answer):
a. Not at all sexually attracted
b. Slightly sexually attracted
c. Mildly sexually attracted
d. Moderately sexually attracted
e. Significantly sexually attracted
f. Very sexually attracted
g. Extremely sexually attracted

4. During the past year, how many different women were you sexually attracted to (choose one answer):
a. None
b. 1
c. 2
d. 3–5
e. 6–10
f. 11–49
g. 50–99
h. 100 or more

5. During the past year, on average, how often were you sexually attracted to a woman (choose one answer):
a. Never
b. Less than 1 time per month
c. 1–3 times per month
d. 1 time per week
e. 2–3 times per week
f. 4–6 times per week
g. Daily

6. During the past year, the most I was sexually attracted to a woman was (choose one answer):
a. Not at all sexually attracted
b. Slightly sexually attracted
c. Mildly sexually attracted
d. Moderately sexually attracted
e. Significantly sexually attracted
f. Very sexually attracted
g. Extremely sexually attracted

2.4 Incidence in Sexual Orientation

Research conducted by Rahman et al. [34] assessed the incidence of heterosexuality, bisexuality, and homosexuality of women and men in 28 countries using data from 191,088 participants from a 2005 British Broadcasting Corporation (BBC) Internet survey. Sexual orientation was assessed in terms of self-reported sexual identity and degree of self-reported same-sex attraction. The percentage of men who defined themselves as heterosexual (90.0%) was higher than the percentage who reported being predominantly not attracted to men (82.6%). Similarly, the percentage of women who defined themselves as heterosexual (90.7%) was higher than the percentage who reported being predominantly not attracted to women (66.2%). These data are interesting because they show that among both men and women who define themselves as heterosexual there is a percentage of people who are moderately or predominantly attracted to the same sex. These data could mean that not only some people may not want to disclose their sexual orientation to third parties but also that sexual orientation can be defined in different ways. In addition, the average rates of male and female heterosexual identity (90.0% and 90.7%) do not appear to differ between nations. According to the data collected by the National Survey of Sexual Health and Behavior [35], men (4.2%) more than women (0.9%) seem to define themselves as homosexuals, while women (3.6%) more than men (2.6%) seem to define themselves as bisexuals. Interestingly, between nations, there does not appear to be a variability in terms of the incidence of sexual orientation, and this may mean that other non-social factors can influence the development of sexual orientation [34]. Researchers tend to consider sexual behavior more than sexual self-identification, using the term men who have sex with men (MSM): this fact could explain the difficulty of precisely defining sexual orientation and, consequently, establishing a precise percentage of the incidence of sexual orientations.

2.5 Contemporary Issues on Sexual Orientation in Clinical and Research Fields

Homosexual orientation is no longer listed as a disorder in the *Diagnostic and Statistical Manual of Sexual Disorders (DSM)* since 1973 [36–38]. Over the years, scientific research has accumulated a series of data that have shown that same-sex attraction is not associated with worse psychological functioning than someone who is attracted to the other sex [39, 40]. Furthermore, some differences between heterosexual people and homosexual people with respect to self-esteem were not highlighted [41–43]. However, researches conducted in Western countries have found a consistent pattern of lower rates of depression and anxiety among heterosexual people compared to people with other sexual orientations [44, 45], as well as higher rates of substance use [44] and suicide [44, 46]. Furthermore, within the same LGBQ community, a recent meta-analysis [47] found that bisexual people show higher or equivalent rates of anxiety and depression than lesbian/gay people. These data appear to be associated with experiences of discrimination and minority stress [40]. In fact, although on the one hand, there has been a sociocultural and scientific progress with respect to the various forms of sexual identity, and on the other hand, people belonging to the LGBQ community are still victims of stigma, heterosexism, violence, and discrimination [48–53]. One out of eight lesbian and bisexual people and four out of ten gay men in the United States are discriminated against because of their sexual orientation [49]. The consequences of discrimination are numerous: people who are victims of it tend to have difficulties in accepting their sexual orientation and developing their identity in a free and serene way [40]. Episodes of discrimination and aggression can increase stress levels to the point of leading the victim to internalize social stereotypes, to fear future aggression and discrimination, to experience confusion, guilt, and anger [40]. In some cases, discrimination can also come from the LGBQ community itself: some bisexual people, in fact, report feeling excluded due to their sexual orientation often considered unclear [52–54]. For this reason, some bisexual people avoid opening up to their sexual orientation due to the dual discrimination that comes from both members of the same LGBQ community and from heterosexual people [55]. These social pressures often lead many extremely religious LGBQ people to seek methods to alter their sexual orientation and conform to heterosexuality [56]. Some people even report seeking these methods because they are victims of threats of rejection by family or religious organizations [57]. These methods that attempt to alter same-sex attraction are called "Sexual Orientation Change Efforts (SOCE)." These include conversion, reparative, or reorientation practices [58, 59]. SOCE start, in fact, from the consideration that homosexuality is pathological and, for this reason, it must be "treated." However, scientific studies have come to the conclusion that these practices are ineffective and often harmful to people [40, 59]. Negative consequences associated with SOCE include depression, suicidal tendency, decreased self-esteem, internalized homophobia, sexual dysfunction, and problematic interpersonal relationships [57, 60–62]. Given the potential negative consequences of SOCE and given that these practices are not in line with current ethical standards of the APA ("do no harm" is the fundamental guideline that guides most professional organizations), associations such as the American Academy of Pediatrics, the American Psychological Association, the American Psychiatric Association, the National Association of Social Workers, the American Medical Association, the American Counseling Association, American Psychoanalytic Association, and the National Association of School Psychologists have adopted policies against SOCE.

The fact that stereotypes about sexual orientation are still present today in those who practice the health professions [63, 64], to the point of pushing the client not to reveal his/her sexual orientation to his/her professional [40], is evidence of the impact that the beliefs and perceptions of healthcare professionals can have on clients.

Heteronormativity is not only widespread in the clinical setting but also in research through theories, questionnaires, and interviews [65]. It is therefore necessary that health professionals and sexual health researchers recognize the prejudices that still today revolve around sexual orientation and the various components of sexual identity and to disseminate research on sexual orientation in an honest, precise, and evidence-based way in order to reduce discrimination and the resulting psychological consequences.

2.6   Conclusions: Toward a Sex-Positive Approach

As we saw in the previous paragraphs, although there has been general socio-cultural progress in terms of human sexuality, society as a whole is still strongly conditioned by a sex-negative culture. In this regard, Bullough [66] reported that societies could be of two types: sex-negative or sex-positive. The former encourages sexual asceticism, the idea that sex is risky and problematic, the prejudices associated with specific sexual practices, sexism, and homophobia [67]. The latter, on the other hand, encourages the pleasurable aspects linked to sexuality and not necessarily linked to procreation. A sex-positive approach recognizes and embraces differences relating to sexuality by taking into account various sexual identities, orientations, and practices. In this sense, the sex-positive approach is in line with what is maintained by the World Health Organization according to which every person is unique and sexuality is a complex phenomenon influenced by the interaction of biological, psychological, social, and relational factors. Therefore, sexuality, as a multidimensional phenomenon, deserves to be freely expressed respecting its facets. It is therefore necessary that all sexual health professionals and researchers who deal with sexual health become familiar with the heteronormative history of sexual orientation and all the consequences attached to it in order to avoid re-proposing and reiterating prejudices, stereotypes, and discrimination. Constant commitment and collaboration between different health professionals remains an important goal to be achieved in order to reduce discrimination against sexual minorities, the emotional consequences, and monetary costs on health services that can result. By moving from a sexually negative perspective to a sexually positive approach, sexual health experts should evaluate the emerging health problems associated with minority status and stress and take action by promoting positive, uncritical, and mindful information about sexuality.

References

1. Grewal I, Kaplan C. Global identities: theorizing transnational studies of sexuality. GLQ. 2001;7(4):663–79.
2. Nagoshi JL, Nagoshi CT, Brzuzy S. Gender and sexual identity: transcending feminist and queer theory. New York: Springer; 2013.
3. Diamond M. Sex and gender are different: sexual identity and gender identity are different. Clin Child Psychol Psychiatry. 2002;7(3):320–34.
4. Vignozzi L, Tripodi F. Sexuality in the developmental age. In: Kirana PS, Tripodi F, Reisman Y, Porst H, editors. The EFS and ESSM syllabus of clinical sexology. Medix; 2013. p. 162–91.
5. Rossi R, Dean J. Sexual Orientation. In: Tripodi F, Reisman Y, Porst H, editors. Kirana PS. The EFS and ESSM syllabus of clinical sexology, Medix; 2013. p. 278–301.
6. Pfeffer CA. Queering families: the postmodern partnerships of cisgender women and transgender men. Oxford University Press; 2017.
7. Castañeda NN, Pfeffer CA. Gender identities. In: Risman B, Froyum C, Scarborough W, editors. Handbook of the sociology of gender. Handbooks of sociology and social research. Cham: Springer; 2018. p. 119–30.
8. Diamond LM. Sexual fluidity. Harvard University Press; 2008.
9. Baumeister RF. Gender and erotic plasticity: sociocultural influences on the sex drive. Sex Relation Ther. 2004;19(2):133–9.
10. Bowes-Catton H. Resisting the binary: discourses of identity and diversity in bisexual politics 1988–1996. Lesbian Gay Psychol Rev. 2007;8(1):58–70.
11. Prause N, Graham CA. Asexuality: classification and characterization. Arch Sex Behav. 2007;36(3):341–56.
12. Money J, Tucker P. Sexual signatures on being a man or a woman. Little Brown & Co.; 1975.
13. Szymanowicz A, Furnham A. Gender and gender role differences in self-and other-estimates of multiple intelligences. J Soc Psychol. 2013;153(4):399–423.
14. Galambos NL. Gender and gender role development in adolescence. In: Lerner RM, Steinberg L, editors.

Handbook of adolescent psychology. Wiley; 2004. p. 233–62.
15. Calvo-Salguero A, García-Martínez JMÁ, Monteoliva A. Differences between and within genders in gender role orientation according to age and level of education. Sex Roles. 2008;58(7):535–48.
16. Pillard RC, Weinrich JD. Evidence of familial nature of male homosexuality. Arch Gen Psychiatry. 1986;43(8):808–12.
17. Bailey JM, Pillard RC. A genetic study of male sexual orientation. Arch Gen Psychiatry. 1991;48(12):1089–96.
18. Bailey JM, Pillard RC, Neale MC, Agyei Y. Heritable factors influence sexual orientation in women. Arch Gen psychiatry. 1993;50(3):217–23.
19. Hamer DH, Hu S, Magnuson VL, Hu N, Pattatucci AM. A linkage between DNA markers on the X chromosome and male sexual orientation. Science. 1993;261(5119):321–7.
20. Vito MP. Factors influencing homosexuality in men: a term paper. 2020.
21. LeVay S. A difference in hypothalamic structure between heterosexual and homosexual men. Science. 1991;253(5023):1034–7.
22. Byne W, Tobet S, Mattiace LA, Lasco MS, Kemether E, Edgar MA, et al. The interstitial nuclei of the human anterior hypothalamus: an investigation of variation with sex, sexual orientation, and HIV status. Horm Behav. 2001;40(2):86–92.
23. Gladue BA. The biopsychology of sexual orientation. Curr Dir Psychol Sci. 1994;3(5):150–4.
24. Gladue BA, Beatty WW, Larson J, Staton RD. Sexual orientation and spatial ability in men and women. Psychobiology. 1990;18(1):101–8.
25. Jannini FA, Blanchard R, Camperio Ciani A, Bancroftù J. Male homosexuality: nature or culture? J Sex Med. 2010;7(10):3245–53.
26. Sell RL. Defining and measuring sexual orientation for research. In: Meyer IH, Northridge ME, editors. The health of sexual minorities. Boston: Springer; 2007. p. 355–74.
27. Kinsey AC, Pomeroy WB, Martin CE. Sexual behavior in the human male. Philadelphia/London: B. Saunders Company; 1948. p. 47.
28. Klein F, Sepekoff B, Wolf TJ. Sexual orientation: a multi-variable dynamic process. J Homosex. 1985;11(1–2):35–49.
29. Shively MG, De Cecco JP. Components of sexual identity. J Homosex. 1977;3(1):41–8.
30. Sell RL. The Sell assessment of sexual orientation: background and scoring. J Gay Lesbian Bisex Identity. 1996;1(4):295–310.
31. Weinrich JD, Snyder PJ, Pillard RC, Grant I, Jacobson DL, Robinson SR, et al. A factor analysis of the Klein Sexual Orientation Grid in two disparate samples. Arch Sex Behav. 1993;22(2):157–68.
32. Weinberg MS, Williams CJ, Pryor DW. Dual attraction: understanding bisexuality. Oxford University Press; 1995.

33. Gonsiorek JC, Sell RL, Weinrich JD. Definition and measurement of sexual orientation. Suicide Life Threat Behav. 1995;25:40–51.

34. Rahman Q, Xu Y, Lippa RA, Vasey PL. Prevalence of sexual orientation across 28 nations and its association with gender equality, economic development, and individualism. Arch Sex Behav. 2020;49(2):595–606.

35. Herbenick D, Reece M, Schick V, Sanders SA, Dodge B, Fortenberry JD. Sexual behaviors, relationships, and perceived health status among adult women in the United States: results from a national probability sample. J Sex Med. 2010;7(5):277–90.

36. American Psychiatric Association. Mental disorders: diagnostic and statistical manual. 1st ed. Washington, DC: American Psychiatric Association; 1952.

37. American Psychiatric Association. Diagnostic and statistical manual of mental disorders. 2nd ed. Washington, DC: American Psychiatric Association; 1968.

38. Drescher J, Merlino JP. American psychiatry and homosexuality: an oral history. Routledge; 2007.

39. Rothblum ED. Introduction to the special section: mental health of lesbians and gay men. J Consult Clin Psychol. 1994;62(2):211.

40. Przeworski A, Peterson E, Piedra A. A systematic review of the efficacy, harmful effects, and ethical issues related to sexual orientation change efforts. Clin Psychol Sci Pract. 2021;28(1):81.

41. Coyle A. A study of psychological well-being among gay men using the GHQ-30. Br J Clin Psychol. 1993;32(2):218–20.

42. Herek GM. Gay people and government security clearances: a social science perspective. Am Psychol. 1990;45(9):1035–42.

43. Savin-Williams RC. Gay and lesbian youth: expressions of identity. Hemisphere Publishing Corp; 1990.

44. Gilman SE, Cochran SD, Mays VM, Hughes M, Ostrow D, Kessler RC. Risk of psychiatric disorders among individuals reporting same-sex sexual partners in the National Comorbidity Survey. Am J Public Health. 2001;91(6):933.

45. Mays VM, Cochran SD, Roeder MR. Depressive distress and prevalence of common problems among homosexually active African American women in the United States. J Psychol Hum Sex. 2004;15(2–3):27–46.

46. Rotheram-Borus MJ, Hunter J, Rosario M. Suicidal behavior and gay-related stress among gay and bisexual male adolescents. J Adolesc Res. 1994;9(4):498–508.

47. Ross LE, Salway T, Tarasoff LA, MacKay JM, Hawkins BW, Fehr CP. Prevalence of depression and anxiety among bisexual people compared to gay, lesbian, and heterosexual individuals: a systematic review and meta-analysis. J Sex Res. 2018;55(4–5):435–56.

48. Herek GM (1991) Stigma, prejudice, and violence against lesbians and gay men. In: Gonsiorek J, Weinrich J. (eds). Homosexuality: research implications for public policy. Newbury Park, CA: Sage, pp. 60–80.

49. Herek GM. Sexual stigma and sexual prejudice in the United States: a conceptual framework. In: Hope DA, editor. Contemporary perspectives on lesbian, gay, and bisexual identities. Nebraska symposium on motivation, vol. 54. New York: Springer; 2009. p. 65–111.

50. Mays VM, Cochran SD. Mental health correlates of perceived discrimination among lesbian, gay, and bisexual adults in the United States. Am J Public Health. 2001;91(11):1869–76.

51. Meyer IH. Prejudice, social stress, and mental health in lesbian, gay, and bisexual populations: conceptual issues and research evidence. Psychol Bull. 2003;129(5):674.

52. Eleuteri S, Rossi R, Simonelli C. Comment aborder le travail clinique avec les clients bisexuels âgés et leurs partenaires? Sexologies. 2019;28(3):114–9.

53. Silvaggi M, Eleuteri S, Colombo M, Fava V, Malandrino C, Simone S, et al. Attitudes towards the sexual rights of LGB people: factors involved in recognition and denial. Sexologies. 2019;28(3):e72–81.

54. Herek GM. Heterosexuals' attitudes toward bisexual men and women in the United States. J Sex Res. 2002;39(4):264–74.

55. Balsam KF, Mohr JJ. Adaptation to sexual orientation stigma: a comparison of bisexual and lesbian/gay adults. J Counsel Psychol. 2007;54(3):306–19.

56. Maccio EM. Influence of family, religion, and social conformity on client participation in sexual reorientation therapy. J Homosex. 2010;57(3):441–58.

57. Shidlo A, Schroeder M. Changing sexual orientation: a consumers' report. Prof Psychol Res Pr. 2002;33(3):249.

58. Nicolosi J. Reparative therapy of male homosexuality: a new clinical approach. Jason Aronson; 1997.

59. Haldeman DC. Therapeutic antidotes: helping gay and bisexual men recover from conversion therapies. J Gay Lesbian Psychother. 2002;5(3–4):117–30.

60. Flentje A, Heck NC, Cochran BN. Experiences of ex-ex-gay individuals in sexual reorientation therapy: reasons for seeking treatment, perceived helpfulness and harmfulness of treatment, and post-treatment identification. J Homosex. 2014;61(9):1242–68.

61. Jacobsen J, Wright R. Mental health implications in Mormon women's experiences with same-sex attraction: a qualitative study. Counsel Psychol. 2014;42(5):664–96.

62. Dehlin JP, Galliher RV, Bradshaw WS, Hyde DC, Crowell KA. Sexual orientation change efforts among current or former LDS church members. J Counsel Psychol. 2015;62(2):95.

63. Garnets L, Hancock KA, Cochran SD, Goodchilds J, Peplau LA. Issues in psychotherapy with lesbians and gay men: a survey of psychologists. Am Psychol. 1991;46(9):964.

64. Liddle BJ. Therapist sexual orientation, gender, and counseling practices as they relate to ratings on help-

fulness by gay and lesbian clients. J Counsel Psychol. 1996;43(4):394.

65. Gingold HG, Hancock KA, Cerbone AR. A word about words: stigma, sexual orientation/identity, and the "heterosexist default". NYS Psychol. 2006;8(4):20–4.

66. Bullough VL. Sexual variance in society and history. Wiley; 1976.

67. Glickman C. The language of sex positivity. Electronic J Hum Sex. 2000;3:1–5.

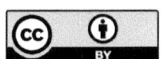

Erectile Dysfunction: From Pathophysiology to Clinical Assessment

3

Vincenzo Mirone, Ferdinando Fusco, Luigi Cirillo, and Luigi Napolitano

3.1 Penile Erection

Penile erection is a complex phenomenon characterized by the equilibrium of the neurological, vascular, hormonal, and muscular compartments [1]. In normal condition, penile erection requires coordinated involvement of intact central and peripheral nervous systems, corpora cavernosa, and spongiosa, normal arterial blood supply, and venous drainage [2].

Generally, erection is associated with several psychological and physical changes: heightened sexual arousal, full testicular assent and swelling, dilatation of the urethral bulb, an increase in glans and coronal size, cutaneous flush over the epigastrium, chest, and buttocks, nipple erection, tachycardia and elevation in blood pressure, hyperventilation, and generalized myotonia [3].

3.1.1 Anatomy

We can divide the penis into three parts: root (radix), body (shaft), and glans [4].

The root is the proximal part of the penis located in the urogenital triangle. It consists of two muscles (ischiocavernosus and bulbospongiosus) and the crura and the bulb of penis which represent proximal expansions of the erectile tissues.

The body of penis is enveloped in skin and in three fasciae (dartos, buck, and tunica albuginea) [5].

The body of the penis contains three erectile tissues: the two corpora cavernosa and the corpus spongiosum. Corpora cavernosa consists of bundles of smooth muscle fibers, collagenous extracellular matrix, endothelial cell-lined sinuses, helicine arteries, and nerve terminals. Penis anatomy is represented in Fig. 3.1.

Each corpus cavernosum is wrapped by the tunica albuginea. The tunica albuginea is a membrane that covers and protects the corpora cavernosa. It consists of an inner and an outer fascial layer, the first circular and the second longitudinal. The corpora cavernosa lies in the dorsal part of the penis, while the corpus spongiosum lies in the ventral groove between them.

The corpus spongiosum houses the urethra. It has a proximal dilation that projects into the root of penis.

The glans is the most distal part of the penis. It is a sensitive structure at the end of the body of

V. Mirone · L. Cirillo (✉) · L. Napolitano
Department of Neurosciences, Science of Reproduction and Odontostomatology, University of Naples Federico II, Naples, Italy
e-mail: mirone@unina.it

F. Fusco
Department of Woman, Child and General and Specialized Surgery, Urology Unit, University of Campania 'Luigi Vanvitelli', Naples, Italy

© The Author(s) 2023
C. Bettocchi et al. (eds.), *Practical Clinical Andrology*,
https://doi.org/10.1007/978-3-031-11701-5_3

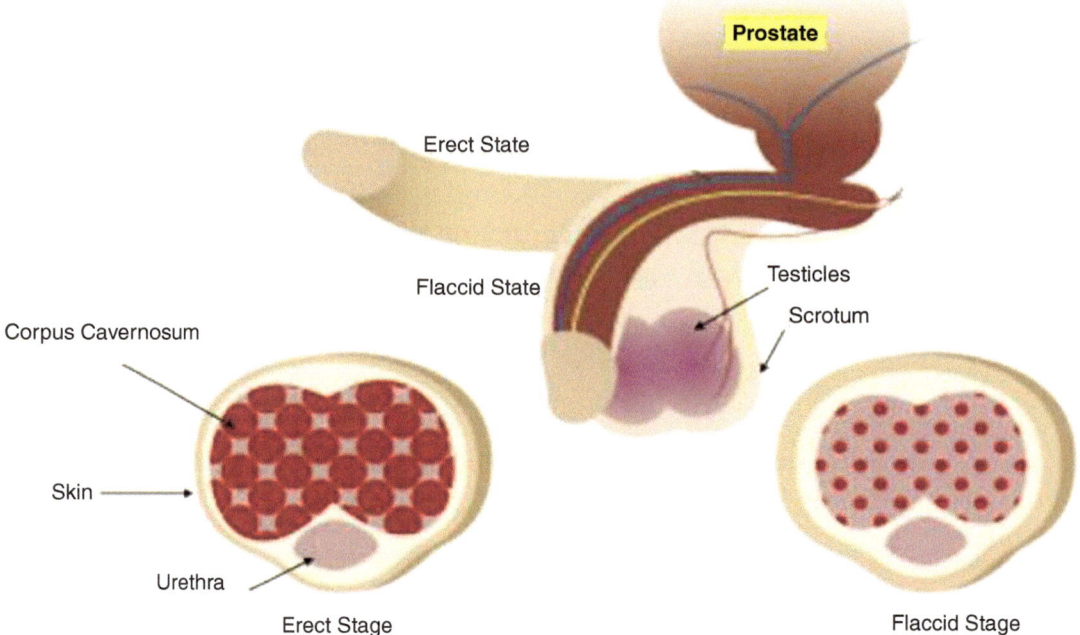

Fig. 3.1 Simple anatomy of the male reproductive system

penis which gets its shape from the bulbous expansion of the corpus spongiosum.

The glans is covered by a fold of skin that covers called prepuce [6].

3.1.2 Innervation

The penis is characterized by autonomic (sympathetic and parasympathetic) and somatic (sensory and motor) innervation system. The autonomic system regulates the neurovascular events occurring during erection and detumescence. The somatic system is responsible for sensation and the contraction of the bulbocavernosus and ischiocavernosus muscles. From the neurons in the spinal cord and peripheral ganglia, the sympathetic and parasympathetic nerves merge form the cavernous nerves, which enter the corpora cavernosa and corpus spongiosum to affect the neurovascular events during erection and detumescence [6].

From peripheral nerve fiber, the impulses reach the spinal erection centers and while some

follow the ascending tract (resulting in sensory perception), others activate the autonomic nuclei to induce penile erection. The sympathetic system originates from T10-T12, and the chain ganglia cells projecting to the penis are located in the sacral and caudal ganglia. The parasympathetic system arising from neurons in the intermediolateral cell columns of S2-S4 is carried by cavernous nerves from the peri-prostatic nerve plexus. In S2-S4, it has been described the Onuf's nucleus, identified as the center of somatomotor penile innervation. Onuf's nucleus is a particular group of neurons located in the ventral part the anterior horn of the sacral spinal cord. It is involved in many functions as the maintenance of micturition and defecatory continence, as well as muscular contraction during orgasm. It contains motor neurons and is the origin of the pudendal nerve.

The Onuf's nucleus regulates external sphincter muscles of the anus and urethra. In this connection, the ischiocavernosus and bulbocavernosus muscles are involved into in penile erection and ejaculation [7].

3.1.3 Vasculature

The penis receives arterial supply from three sources originated by internal pudendal arteries: dorsal arteries of the penis, deep arteries of the penis, and bulbourethral artery [8]. The first supply the fibrous tissue surrounding the corpora cavernosa, corpus spongiosum, spongy urethra, and penile skin [4]. The second supply the erectile tissue of the penis, while the arteries of the bulb of the penis supply the bulbous part of the corpus spongiosum, urethra, and bulbourethral gland. The penile skin is supplied by superficial and deep branches of the external pudendal arteries.

The venous system is characterized by the deep dorsal vein of the penis which receives blood from the cavernous spaces. The superficial dorsal vein which drains blood from the skin and subcutaneous tissue of the penis. Regarding the lymphatic system, the penis skin and all the perineum drain into superficial inguinal nodes. The intermediate and proximal parts of the urethra and cavernous bodies drain into the internal iliac lymph nodes, and the distal spongy urethra and glans penis drain to the deep inguinal nodes.

3.1.4 Erectile Process

The erectile process involves specifically the cavernous smooth musculature and the smooth muscles of the arteriolar and arterial walls [1]. In the flaccid state, there is a tonically contraction of these structures. The relaxing of smooth muscle resulting in increase of intracavernosal pressure that leads to compression of the subtunical venules against the tunica albuginea [9]. This reduces venous drainage from the corpora cavernosa and increases pressure within the corpora. Three types of erection have been described: nocturnal, that follows the rapid eye movement sleep periods; reflexogenic due to genital stimulations; and the central or psychogenic related to many stimulations trigger points (imaginative, visual, auditory, olfactory, gustatory, tactile, etc.) Many central transmitters are involved in the erectile control such as dopamine, acetylcholine, nitric

oxide (NO), oxytocin, and adrenocorticotropin/α-melanocyte-stimulating hormone which have a facilitatory role, serotonin with either facilitatory or inhibitory, and enkephalins with inhibitory role [10]. According to several studies, it is know that the central supraspinal systems controlling sexual arousal are localized in the limbic system (e.g., olfactory nuclei, medial preoptic area, nucleus accumbens, amygdala, and hippocampus) and hypothalamus (paraventricular and ventromedial nuclei). In particular, amygdala, medial preoptic area (MPOA), paraventricular nucleus (PVN), the periaqueductal gray, and ventral tegmentum have been described as the most important structures involved in the central control of the male sexual response [11].

Erection is mediated by a spinal reflex, which involves different central and peripheral neural and/or humoral mechanisms [12]. This reflex is initiated by recruitment of penile autonomic and somatic afferents, and it is regulated by supraspinal influences related to visual, olfactory, and imaginary stimuli. Erection is regulated by a balance between pro- and anti-erectile mediators. Acetylcholine is the most important neurotransmitter for ganglionic transmission, vascular smooth muscle relaxation, and release of NO from endothelial cells. Nitric oxide (NO) is a potent relaxant of peripheral vascular smooth muscle, and its action is mediated by cGMP. It is synthesized from endothelium via eNOS and by nitrergic nerves via nNOS. It is produced from endogenous L-arginine by NO synthase (NOS) located in the sinusoidal endothelial cells and by the NANC activated by electrical or chemical stimulation [9]. NO pathway is reported in Fig. 3.2.

Nitric oxide through the activation of guanylate cyclase stimulates the production of cGMP. cGMP activates the potassium channels and inhibits calcium entry into the cell. When intracellular calcium concentration is low, light chains of myosin are dephosphorylated and this induces corporal smooth muscle relaxation. Smooth muscle contraction and relaxation is regulated by sarcoplasmic free Ca^{2+}. Norepinephrine and prostaglandin F2a activate receptors on smooth muscle cells to increase inositol triphosphate and

Fig. 3.2 Physiology of erection

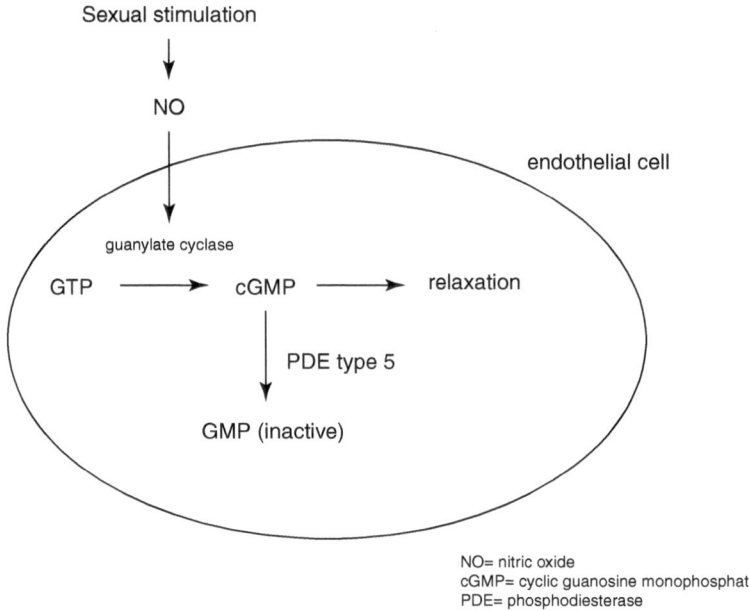

Sexual stimulation

NO

endothelial cell

guanylate cyclase

GTP $\longrightarrow$ cGMP $\longrightarrow$ relaxation

PDE type 5

GMP (inactive)

NO= nitric oxide
cGMP= cyclic guanosine monophosphate
PDE= phosphodiesterase

diacylglycerol. This resulting in the release of calcium from intracellular stores and influx from extracellular space. The interaction between Ca^{2+} and calmodulin exposes sites of interaction with myosin light-chain kinase with phosphorylation of myosin light chains and exits in muscle contraction. Relaxation of the muscle is related to a decrease of free Ca^{2+} in the sarcoplasma. Calmodulin dissociates from myosin light-chain kinase and inactivates it. NO, cyclic GMP (cGMP), and cAMP are inhibitory pathways through phosphorylation. Cyclic AMP (cAMP) and cGMP are the second messengers involved in smooth muscle relaxation. They activate cAMP- and cGMP-dependent protein kinases, through several mechanisms due to calcium influx and muscle relaxing [1].

NO is involved in the initiation of erection through activation of nNOS, and in attainment of erection through PI3K/Akt-dependent phosphorylation of eNOS [13].

The penile erectile tissue plays a primary role in the erectile process. In the flaccid state, the penile tissue is moderately contracted with a low flow of blood for nutritive purposes. This is also evidenced by the cold weathers in which blood PO_2 decreases and tissue contraction raises [14].

All this changes when the sexual stimulation comes on. As a consequence of the sexual stimulation, the neurotransmitters release results in the relaxation of this smooth muscles and the following events take place:

– Dilatation of the arterioles and arteries by increased blood flow
– Trapping of the incoming blood by the expanding sinusoids
– Compression of the subtunical venular plexuses between the tunica albuginea and the peripheral sinusoids, reducing the venous outflow
– Stretching of the tunica to its capacity, which occludes the emissary veins between the inner circular and the outer longitudinal layers and further decreases the venous outflow to a minimum
– An increase in PO_2 (to about 90 mmHg) and intracavernous pressure (around 100 mmHg), which raises the penis from the dependent position to the erect state (the full-erection phase)
– A further pressure increase (to several hundred millimeters of mercury) with contraction of the ischiocavernosus muscles (rigid-erection phase)

3.2   Pathophysiology of Erectile Dysfunction

Erectile dysfunction (ED) is defined as the persistent inability to attain and/or maintain penile erection sufficient to permit satisfactory sexual performance [15].

Erectile dysfunction may affect physical and physiological health and has a strong impact on quality of life and relationships. It is recognized as a possible early sign of coronary artery and peripheral vascular disease. Therefore, physicians should ask male patients about sexual health in order to identify potential life-threatening underlying conditions such as cardiovascular disease [16, 17]. ED is known to have psychological as well as organic causes. Nonorganic erectile dysfunction is also known as psychogenic or adrenaline-mediated erectile dysfunction (noradrenaline-mediated or sympathetic-mediated erectile dysfunction). It has not been well studied but is an important factor to consider when evaluating and managing men with this condition [18].

Stress, depression, and anxiety are generally defined as heightened anxiety related to the inability to achieve and maintain an erection before or during sexual relations, and are commonly associated with psychogenic erectile dysfunction [19].

Erectile dysfunction possibly generates from any process that impairs either the neural or the vascular pathways that contribute to erection. Neurogenic erectile dysfunction is caused by a deficit in nerve signaling to the corpora cavernosa [20]. Such deficits can be secondary to, for example, spinal cord injury, multiple sclerosis, Parkinson's disease, lumbar disc disease, traumatic brain injury, radical pelvic surgery (radical prostatectomy, radical cystectomy, and abdominoperineal resection), and diabetes. Upper motor neuron lesions (above spinal nerve T10) do not result in local changes in the penis but can inhibit the central nervous system (CNS)-mediated control of the erection. By contrast, sacral lesions (S2–S4 are typically responsible for reflexogenic erections) cause functional and structural alterations owing to the decreased innervation [21].

The functional change resulting from such injuries is the reduction in NO load that is available to the smooth muscle. The structural changes center on apoptosis of the smooth muscle and endothelial cells of the blood vessels, as well as upregulation of fibrogenetic cytokines that lead to collagenization of the smooth muscle. These changes result in veno-occlusive dysfunction (venous leak). Vascular disease and endothelial dysfunction lead to erectile dysfunction through reduced blood inflow, arterial insufficiency, or arterial stenosis. Vasculogenic erectile dysfunction is by far the most common etiology of organic erectile dysfunction [22]. Many men assume that erectile dysfunction is a natural consequence of aging. But, despite age stands as an independent risk factor for ED, about one-third of 70-year-old men report no erectile difficulties. Thus, physicians should not automatically assume that erectile dysfunction is anyway attributable to aging.

Risk factors for developing erectile dysfunction include tobacco use, obesity, sedentary lifestyle, and chronic alcohol use. These factors are believed to make hormonal changes that could easily lead to lower testosterone levels and result in impaired endothelial function [23–25].

Several studies have suggested that chronic inflammation and circulating inflammatory markers affect systemic endothelial function [26]. Chronic inflammation may, therefore, represent a link between ED and cardio vascular diseases (CVD). ED onset and severity are associated with increased expression of markers of inflammation. Markers and mediators such as C-reactive protein (CRP), intercellular adhesion molecule 1, interleukin (IL)-6, IL-10, and IL-1B, and tumor necrosis factor alpha (TNF-α) were found to be expressed at higher levels in patients with ED. In addition, endothelial and prothrombotic factors such as von Willebrand factor (vWF), tissue plasminogen activator (tPA), plasminogen activator inhibitor 1 (PAI-1), and fibrinogen are also expressed at higher levels in ED patients [27, 28]. Androgens play an important role in both penile and vascular health, with cellular targets located in both endothelial and smooth muscle cells [29–32].

Androgens promote endothelial cell survival, inhibit proliferation and intimal migration of vascular smooth muscle cells, and reduce endothelial expression of pro-inflammatory markers [33]. Within the penis, low androgen levels are associated with apoptosis of endothelial and smooth muscle cells as well as with pathologic structural remodeling [34]. Besides, both hypo- and hyperthyroidism can lead to erectile impairment. Also, people diagnosed with hypertension, mellitus diabetes, dyslipidemia, and depression have an increased risk of developing erectile dysfunction. The metabolic syndrome also known as syndrome X and insulin resistance syndrome is the term that consists of a cluster of disease states abdominal obesity, atherogenic dyslipidemia, raised blood pressure, insulin resistance ± glucose intolerance, proinflammatory state, and prothrombotic state. Coronary artery diseases and ED share similar risk factors such as hypertension, diabetes mellitus, smoking, and hypercholesterolemia, and many of these factors are part of MetS [35].

MetS may cause ED through multiple mechanisms. All components of MetS are frequently found in the obese population. Abdominal obesity promotes insulin resistance that is associated with hyperinsulinemia and hyperglycemia [36]. It may also lead to an abnormal lipid profile, hypertension, and vascular inflammation, all of which promote the development of atherosclerosis. Endothelial dysfunction leads to a decrease in vascular nitric oxide levels, with resulting impaired vasodilation; the increase in free radical concentration also leads to atherosclerotic damage. In light of these common pathways, MetS could be a strong risk factor for ED as well as ED might be a harbinger of cardiovascular diseases [18, 37]. Some drugs and medicines, for example, α-blockers, benzodiazepines, β-blockers, clonidine, digoxin, histamine H2-receptor blockers, ketoconazole, methyldopa, monoamine oxidase inhibitors, phenobarbital, phenytoin, selective serotonin reuptake inhibitors, spironolactone, thiazide diuretics, and tricyclic antidepressants can cause erectile dysfunction although the exact mechanisms are not always known [15]. The most common iatrogenic cause of erectile dysfunction is radical pelvic surgery [22]. Generally, the damage that occurs during these procedures is primarily neurogenic in nature (cavernous nerve injury) but accessory pudendal artery injury can also contribute. Pelvic fractures can also cause erectile dysfunction in a similar manner, owing to nerve distraction injury and arterial trauma [22]. Finally, patients with erectile dysfunction are more likely to also have premature ejaculation, lower urinary tract symptoms associated with benign prostatic hypertrophy (BPH), and overactive bladder compared with the general male population [38].

3.3   Diagnosis

The basic work-up of a male patient seeking medical care for erectile dysfunction needs to include an evaluation of all the risk factors mentioned. Physician should investigate medical and sexual history and physically examinate the lower genitourinary tract, the penis, and testicles. Then, hormonal blood levels should be examined (i.e., testosterone, prolactin, LH, and FSH).

Given the personal and social implications of sexual dysfunction, assessing sexual history is not an easy task. Hence, expert-guided, validated, and standardized sexual inventories, structured interviews, and self-reported questionnaires, can help both inexperienced and seasoned clinicians to address sexual health and related conditions. The severity of erectile dysfunction is often described as mild, moderate, or severe according to the five-item International Index of Erectile Function (IIEF5) questionnaire, with a score of 1–7 indicating severe, 8–11 moderate, 12–16 mild–moderate, 17–21 mild, and 22–25 no erectile dysfunction. The EDITS questionnaire evaluates the erectile dysfunction treatment outcomes. The physical examination of patients includes evaluation of the chest (including heart rhythm, breathing, and signs of gynecomastia (enlargement of the breasts)), penis, prostate and testes, and the distribution of body hair. Small testes and prostate, depending on patient age, mammary glands growth could imply an underlying hypogonadism. Increased pulse rate (tachycardia) might suggest hyperthyroidism, whereas reduced pulse rate (bradycardia) might be evident in men with heart block (arrhythmia), hypothyroidism or in those who use certain drugs (for example, βblockers). Diminished or absent pulses in the various arteries examined could be indicative of impaired blood flow caused by atherosclerosis. The evaluation of the penis in the flaccid condition might show the presence of Peyronie's disease (involving palpable fibrous plaques), phimosis, or frenulum breve that can all contribute to erectile dysfunction.

Few biochemical and hormonal parameters are of extreme importance as well as levels of cholesterol, triglycerides, fasting glucose, and glycosylated hemoglobin (HbA1c) are key determinants of cardiovascular and metabolic risk stratification [22].

US is the imaging method of choice for initial evaluation of the penis because it can assess anatomy and dynamic blood flow. There are three principal US modalities to evaluate the penis. The first is gray-scale or B-mode US that evaluates the penile anatomy and nonvascular abnormalities, such as plaques, fibrosis, tunica albuginea defects, masses, and fluid collections. The second color Doppler US, allows simultaneous display of moving blood superimposed on a gray-scale image. It is used for the assessment of vascular flow and its direction. The third modality, spectral Doppler US, displays blood flow velocity over time as a waveform, so it is a graphic representation of the flow. It allows evaluation of the speed and direction of the flow.

The main role of imaging is to differentiate vascular from nonvascular causes. Currently, Doppler US is used to investigate arterial or venous defects in patients suffering from ED with no response to PDE-5. ED is also a consequence of pelvic surgery (prostate, bladder, and rectal cancer surgery), and it may also be consequence of vascular or neural injuries [39, 40]. Doppler US is also used to confirm organic damage before penile prostheses [41].

Rigiscan has represented an important tool in the differentiation between psychogenic ED and organic ED. It is a non-invasive diagnostic instrument that assesses male nocturnal penile tumescence and rigidity by making repetitive measurements of radial rigidity at the base and tip of the penis. Rigiscan has proved to be the preferential choice in distinguishing psychogenic ED from organic ED. It has more advantages over penile color-doppler US [42].

References

1. Dean RC, Lue TF. Physiology of penile erection and pathophysiology of erectile dysfunction. Urol Clin North Am. 2005;32(4):379–95, v.
2. Bhasin S, Enzlin P, Coviello A, Basson R. Sexual dysfunction in men and women with endocrine disorders. Lancet. 2007;369(9561):597–611.
3. Kandeel FR, Koussa VK, Swerdloff RS. Male sexual function and its disorders: physiology, pathophysiology, clinical investigation, and treatment. Endocr Rev. 2001;22(3):342–88.
4. Sam P, LaGrange CA. Anatomy, abdomen and pelvis, penis. In: StatPearls. Treasure Island, FL: StatPearls Publishing; 2022. http://www.ncbi.nlm.nih.gov/books/NBK482236/.
5. Cavayero CT, McIntosh GV. Penile prosthesis implantation. In: StatPearls. Treasure Island, FL: StatPearls Publishing; 2022. http://www.ncbi.nlm.nih.gov/books/NBK563292/.
6. El-Sakka AI, Lue TF. Physiology of penile erection. ScientificWorldJournal. 2004;4(Suppl 1):128–34.
7. Schellino R, Boido M, Vercelli A. The dual nature of Onuf's nucleus: neuroanatomical features and peculiarities, in health and disease. Front Neuroanat. 2020;14:572013.
8. Vascularization of the male penis—PubMed. 2022. https://pubmed.ncbi.nlm.nih.gov/15631359/.
9. Kalsi J, Muneer A. Erectile dysfunction—an update of current practice and future strategies. J Clin Urol. 2013;6(4):210–9.
10. Andersson K-E. Mechanisms of penile erection and basis for pharmacological treatment of erectile dysfunction. Pharmacol Rev. 2011;63(4):811–59.
11. Myers B, Dolgas CM, Kasckow J, Cullinan WE, Herman JP. Central stress-integrative circuits: forebrain glutamatergic and GABAergic projections to the dorsomedial hypothalamus, medial preoptic area, and bed nucleus of the stria terminalis. Brain Struct Funct. 2014;219(4):1287–303.
12. Melis MR, Argiolas A. Erectile function and sexual behavior: a review of the role of nitric oxide in the central nervous system. Biomolecules. 2021;11(12):1866.
13. Hurt KJ, Musicki B, Palese MA, Crone JK, Becker RE, Moriarity JL, et al. Akt-dependent phosphorylation of endothelial nitric-oxide synthase mediates penile erection. Proc Natl Acad Sci U S A. 2002;99(6):4061–6.
14. Padmanabhan P, McCullough AR. Penile oxygen saturation in the flaccid and erect penis in men

with and without erectile dysfunction. J Androl. 2007;28(2):223–8.

15. Romano L, Granata L, Fusco F, Napolitano L, Cerbone R, Priadko K, et al. Sexual dysfunction in patients with chronic gastrointestinal and liver diseases: a neglected issue. Sex Med Rev. 2021;S2050-0521(21)00039-1.

16. Salonia A, Bettocchi C, Boeri L, Capogrosso P, Carvalho J, Cilesiz NC, et al. European Association of Urology guidelines on sexual and reproductive health-2021 update: male sexual dysfunction. Eur Urol. 2021;80(3):333–57.

17. Creta M, Sagnelli C, Celentano G, Napolitano L, La Rocca R, Capece M, et al. SARS-CoV-2 infection affects the lower urinary tract and male genital system: a systematic review. J Med Virol. 2021;93(5):3133–42.

18. Mirone V, Napolitano L, D'Emmanuele di Villa Bianca R, Mitidieri E, Sorrentino R, Vanelli A, et al. A new original nutraceutical formulation ameliorates the effect of Tadalafil on clinical score and cGMP accumulation. Arch Ital Urol Androl. 2021;93(2):221–6.

19. McCabe MP, Althof SE. A systematic review of the psychosocial outcomes associated with erectile dysfunction: does the impact of erectile dysfunction extend beyond a man's inability to have sex? J Sex Med. 2014;11(2):347–63.

20. Shridharani AN, Brant WO. The treatment of erectile dysfunction in patients with neurogenic disease. Transl Androl Urol. 2016;5(1):88–101.

21. Krassioukov A, Elliott S. Neural control and physiology of sexual function: effect of spinal cord injury. Top Spinal Cord Inj Rehabil. 2017;23(1):1–10.

22. Yafi FA, Jenkins L, Albersen M, Corona G, Isidori AM, Goldfarb S, et al. Erectile dysfunction. Nat Rev Dis Primer. 2016;2:16003.

23. Moreau KL, Hildreth KL, Meditz AL, Deane KD, Kohrt WM. Endothelial function is impaired across the stages of the menopause transition in healthy women. J Clin Endocrinol Metab. 2012;97(12):4692–700.

24. Fusco F, Verze P, Capece M, Napolitano L. Suppression of spermatogenesis by exogenous testosterone. Curr Pharm Des. 2021;27(24):2750–3.

25. Barone B, Napolitano L, Abate M, Cirillo L, Reccia P, Passaro F, et al. The role of testosterone in the elderly: what do we know? Int J Mol Sci. 2022;23(7):3535.

26. Huang AL, Vita JA. Effects of systemic inflammation on endothelium-dependent vasodilation. Trends Cardiovasc Med. 2006;16(1):15–20.

27. Kany S, Vollrath JT, Relja B. Cytokines in inflammatory disease. Int J Mol Sci. 2019;20(23):E6008.

28. Sanchez E, Pastuszak AW, Khera M. Erectile dysfunction, metabolic syndrome, and cardiovascular risks: facts and controversies. Transl Androl Urol. 2017;6(1):28–36.

29. Traish AM. Androgens play a pivotal role in maintaining penile tissue architecture and erection: a review. J Androl. 2009;30(4):363–9.

30. Napolitano L, Barone B, Crocetto F, Capece M, La Rocca R. The COVID-19 pandemic: is it a wolf consuming fertility? Int J Fertil Steril. 2020;14(2):159–60.

31. Napolitano L, Barone B, Morra S, Celentano G, La Rocca R, Capece M, et al. Hypogonadism in patients with Prader Willi syndrome: a narrative review. Int J Mol Sci. 2021;22(4):1993.

32. Capece M, Creta M, Calogero A, La Rocca R, Napolitano L, Barone B, et al. Does physical activity regulate prostate carcinogenesis and prostate cancer outcomes? A narrative review. Int J Environ Res Public Health. 2020;17(4):E1441.

33. Cai J-J, Wen J, Jiang W-H, Lin J, Hong Y, Zhu Y-S. Androgen actions on endothelium functions and cardiovascular diseases. J Geriatr Cardiol JGC. 2016;13(2):183–96.

34. Mirone V, Imbimbo C, Fusco F, Verze P, Creta M, Tajana G. Androgens and morphologic remodeling at penile and cardiovascular levels: a common piece in complicated puzzles? Eur Urol. 2009;56(2):309–16.

35. Martín-Timón I, Sevillano-Collantes C, Segura-Galindo A, Del Cañizo-Gómez FJ. Type 2 diabetes and cardiovascular disease: have all risk factors the same strength? World J Diabetes. 2014;5(4):444–70.

36. Kahn BB, Flier JS. Obesity and insulin resistance. J Clin Invest. 2000;106(4):473–81.

37. Besiroglu H, Otunctemur A, Ozbek E. The relationship between metabolic syndrome, its components, and erectile dysfunction: a systematic review and a meta-analysis of observational studies. J Sex Med. 2015;12(6):1309–18.

38. Irwin GM. Erectile dysfunction. Prim Care. 2019;46(2):249–55.

39. Creta M, Celentano G, Napolitano L, La Rocca R, Capece M, Califano G, et al. Inhibition of androgen signalling improves the outcomes of therapies for bladder cancer: results from a systematic review of preclinical and clinical evidence and meta-analysis of clinical studies. Diagnostics (Basel). 2021;11(2):351.

40. Crocetto F, Arcaniolo D, Napolitano L, Barone B, La Rocca R, Capece M, et al. Impact of sexual activity on the risk of male genital tumors: a systematic review of the literature. Int J Environ Res Public Health. 2021;18(16):8500.

41. Varela CG, Yeguas LAM, Rodríguez IC, Vila MDD. Penile Doppler ultrasound for erectile dysfunction: technique and interpretation. AJR Am J Roentgenol. 2020;214(5):1112–21.

42. Liu T, Xu Z, Guan Y, Yuan M. Comparison of RigiScan and penile color duplex ultrasound in evaluation of erectile dysfunction. Ann Palliat Med. 2020;9(5):2988–92.

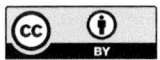

Erectile Dysfunction: Medical Therapy and Rehabilitation

4

Alessandro Palmieri, Marco Capece, Angelo di Giovanni, and Carlo D'Alterio

4.1 Introduction

Medical treatment for erectile dysfunction (ED) has dramatically evolved in the last decades. However, to set realistic expectations with the patient, a correct counselling is fundamental. Every kind of medical treatment must be discussed with the patient regarding risk factors, prognostic factors, treatment alternatives, correct drug use, and adverse reactions [1].

The advent of oral phosphodiesterase 5 inhibitors (PDE-5Is) has been a revolutionary change in the management of ED, since those drugs have high efficacy, ease of use, good tolerability, and low to moderate adverse reactions. Oral PDE-5Is were considered a first-line treatment choices, whereas at the present time, other medical and physical therapies may be used in the first instance for selected patients. Those include vacuum devices, intraurethral agents, intracavernosal injection therapy, extracorporeal shock wave therapy, and hormonal treatment.

4.1.1 Oral Pharmacotherapy: PDE-5Is

Phosphodiesterase 5 inhibitor (PDE-5I) drugs are the most common drugs for the management of erectile dysfunction.

The four molecules synthesized and approved by the European Medicines Agency (EMA) are as follows:

- Sildenafil citrate, the first drug approved for the management of erectile dysfunction in 1998 by the FDA
- Vardenafil approved in 2003
- Tadalafil also approved by the FDA in 2003
- Avanafil approved in 2012

However, they are not initiators of erection and an adequate sexual stimulation is required [2].

PDE5-Is are actually effective in about 65% of patients; the effectiveness of this type of drug is defined as the patient's ability to undertake sufficient sexual intercourse [3].

The choice of the molecule must be personalized; adequate counselling is essential in order to investigate patients' comorbidities, the frequency of intercourses, and expectations [4].

A. Palmieri (✉) · M. Capece · A. di Giovanni
C. D'Alterio
Department of Neurosciences, Reproductive Sciences and Odontostomatology, University of Naples Federico II, Naples, Italy
e-mail: info@alessandropalmieri.it

© The Author(s) 2023
C. Bettocchi et al. (eds.), *Practical Clinical Andrology*,
https://doi.org/10.1007/978-3-031-11701-5_4

4.1.1.1 Pharmacokinetic and Pharmacodynamic Features

The endothelial cells of the corpora cavernosa release nitric oxide (NO), which activates guanylate cyclase, further enhancing the synthesis of cyclic guanosine monophosphate (cGMP).

cGMP is an intracellular second messenger molecule that causes relaxation and vasodilatory effect in smooth muscle cells. It is degraded and inactivated by the enzyme phosphodiesterases. At least 11 different subtypes are currently known.

In the human corpus cavernosum, there are a greater percentage of PDE-2, PDE-3, PDE-4, and PDE-5. The latter phosphodiesterase is the most widely expressed form within the corpus cavernosum. The drugs used for erectile dysfunction are competitive inhibitors of PDE-5; therefore, they enhance the releasing effect of nitric oxide. Inhibiting the activity of the enzyme responsible for the degradation of GMPc, they allow an accumulation of the cyclic nucleotide in response to nitrergic stimulation. The end result is calcium sequestration from the cytoplasm to the endoplasmic reticulum with arteriolar and trabecular smooth muscle relaxation and venous vasoconstriction [5].

Sildenafil

Sildenafil was the first erectile dysfunction drug that hits the world market in 1998 [6]. His discovery was accidental; in fact, originally, the drug was to be used for the treatment of hypertension and angina pectoris. The drug did not prove effective for this purpose, but patients reported unexpected penile erections [7].

Sildenafil takes effect 30–60 min after its administration with a half-life of 4–8 h [8]. Its action can last up to 12 h after the drug intake. Its effectiveness is reduced after a large meal or with the ingestion of fatty foods [9].

The dosages available on the market are 25 mg, 50 mg, 75 mg, and 100 mg.

A placebo-controlled study evaluated the improvement of erection in 465 patients using different dosages of sildenafil. After 24 weeks of treatment in the dose-response study, improved erections are reported in 56%, 77%, and 84% of the men taking 25, 50, and 100 mg of sildenafil, respectively [10].

The most common side effects are headache (16%), flushing (10%), and dyspepsia (7%). Other side effects include nasal congestion, diarrhoea, and changes in vision [7].

Vardenafil

Vardenafil was introduced in 2003. It is effective 30 min after the intake. Most patients report satisfactory erections within 15 min [11].

It is available in the market in doses of 5 mg, 10 mg, and 20 mg. The starting dose is 10 mg, and it can be modified according to the patient's response [12]. A 10 mg orodispersible dose was also recently introduced to the market.

The absorption of vardenafil is reduced after a fatty meal [9].

The most frequent side effects include facial flushing and nasal congestion (9–11%) [13].

After 12 weeks of treatment with vardenafil, a placebo control study showed a statistically significant improvement in erections in 66%, 76%, and 80% of patients taking 5 mg, 10 mg, and 20 mg formulation, respectively [14].

Tadalafil

Tadalafil was approved in the United States in November 2003 [15]. It has particular pharmacokinetic properties. Absorption does not appear to be influenced by the intake of fatty meals or alcohol [16]. The peak of the serum concentration is reached about 2 h after the ingestion differently from sildenafil, vardenafil, and avanafil that require 1 h. In addition, the half-life of the molecule ($t\frac{1}{2}$) is around 17.5 h [17, 18]. Therefore, a chronic administration of tadalafil enhances erectile function up to 36 h and may restore a more physiological sexual intercourse [19, 20]. However, tadalafil's prolonged half-life has higher risk of long-lasting adverse effects than other PDE5-Is. Indeed up to 30% of men taking tadalafil report side effects lasting longer than 1–2 h [21].

Avanafil

Avanafil is the latest d approved. It was launched on the market in 2013 [22]. The available formulations are 50 mg, 100 mg, and 200 mg, and the recommended starting dose is 100 mg [17].

Avanafil is rapidly absorbed and quickly eliminated after an oral administration.

Avanafil has the highest selectivity for phosphodiesterase 5 among PDE5-Is, thus side effects are minimized. Adverse effects are generally consistent with the known pharmacology of PDE5-Is, and the most commonly reported adverse events are headaches, flushing, backpain, nausea, muscle cramps, and fatigue. Besides most of this events are mild and self-resolving [18].

The active ingredient is effective 15 min after the intake. The absorption of avanafil is reduced from fatty meals, and its duration is approximately 6 h [23].

Hellstrom et al. showed successful attempts within 15 min in 64%, 67%, and 71% after avanafil dosages of 50 mg, 100 mg, and 200 mg, respectively [23].

Patients suffering from chronic renal failure or hepatic insufficiency do not require a dosage modification [24].

4.1.1.2 The Right Molecule for the Right Patient

The choice of the best PDE-5Is is not supported by any double or triple blind study that compares the effectiveness of the different drugs.

This choice depends on the patient's characteristics such as frequency of intercourse (occasional or regular use with 3 weekly or more intercourse), treatment expectations tolerability, and side effects.

In a recent meta-analysis, *Chen* et al demonstrated that patients affected by ED seeking for an immediate efficacy should start with Sildenafil 50 mg while the others could benefit of Tadalafil 10 mg that has higher tolerability [25].

4.1.1.3 Pharmacological Interactions

The association of NO-donor drugs and PDE-5Is can lead to a cGMP accumulation. Such condition can result in hypotension and cardiogenic shock. Therefore, the intake of nitrates is an absolute contraindication for PDE-5I administration [26].

Considering the pharmacokinetic characteristic, patients treated with PDE5-Is experiencing chest pain must delay any nitro-glycerine intake up to 12, 24, and 48 h for avanafil, sildenafil/vardenafil, and tadalafil, respectively [21].

4.1.1.4 Cardiovascular Safety

The use of PDE-5I has not shown negative side effects on the cardiovascular system; in fact, there is no increase in the rate of myocardial infarction in patients assuming those drugs.

Chronic or on-demand use is well tolerated with a similar safety profile for the various molecules [27, 28].

All molecules that inhibit phosphodiesterase 5 are contraindicated in the following situations:

- Patients with resting hypotension (blood pressure <90/50 mmHg)
- Patients who have suffered a myocardial infarction, stroke, or life-threatening arrhythmias over the past 6 months
- Patients with hypertension (blood pressure >170/100 mmHg)
- Patients with angina during sexual intercourse
- Patients with unstable angina
- Patients with congestive heart failure

4.1.1.5 Non-responders

Some patients do not respond adequately to oral PDE-5Is; this mainly happens for two reasons:

1. Incorrect use of the drug
2. Lack of actual efficacy of the prescribed molecule

Regarding the incorrect use, patients must be informed about the correct intake procedure.

McCullough suggests carrying out the PDE-5Is treatment for at least 6/8 weeks before establishing its ineffectiveness [29]. The most frequent causes of incorrect use are as follows:

1. Failure to use an adequate dosage.
2. Lack of or inadequate sexual stimulation.

3. Search for intercourse ignoring the right timing of the drug. In fact, there is a period of time between the intake and the pharmacological action in which the drug will be ineffective. Moreover, some patients require a longer time for the drug to start acting [30, 31].

Furthermore, the absorption of the drug can be delayed by the intake of fatty foods or a large meal.

The clinician is always required to verify that the patient has taken an official drug. Unfortunately, a black market has increased over the last decades; thus, the efficacy and safety of unauthorized and uncontrolled tablets cannot be guaranteed.

In addition to that, *Marchal Escalona* et al. recently reported that a polyformism of the PDE5A gene encoding the PDE-5 enzyme may affect the efficacy of the drugs. Thus, there may be variability in the clinical response of the clinical response in subjects using PDE5i [32].

4.1.1.6 On-Demand Vs Daily Treatment

Recently, there has been a great interest in daily PDE5I administration as a new and innovative approach to manage erectile dysfunction. The advantage of daily intake for the management of erectile dysfunction is the complete separation of drug use from sexual activity, eliminating the unpleasant effect indicated by patients as "I feel drugs control my sex life" or "I wish they would. my erections came more spontaneously" [33]. The main goal of ED therapy is to achieve an improvement in erectile function; however, this improvement is not the only factor for sexual satisfaction. In fact, self-confidence and spontaneity of erection may play an important role in increasing the general satisfaction of patients [34]. In this regard, a study observed that patients who started ED treatment with tadalafil once a day (OaD) reported greater improvement in self-esteem and sexual spontaneity than patients who started treatment with sildenafil on-demand. On the other hand, there were no significant differences between the two regarding the improvement of IIEF-EF, of orgasmic function, of the

domains of general satisfaction, and of the EDITS score [35].

Regarding tolerability, it is important to emphasize that chronic administration of tadalafil does not appear to result in up-regulation of PDE5 in human penile tissue, an effect which has been observed in rat penile tissue continuously exposed to high doses of sildenafil [36, 37]. This means that the phenomenon of tachyphylaxis occurs against sildenafil and over time, the drug loses its effectiveness since more PDE5 enzymes are produced and the concentration of the drug is no longer sufficient to ensure its inhibition. On the other hand, tadalafil does not seem to show a loss of its efficacy over time due to tachyphylaxis. An additional benefit of tadalafil OaD is that overall drug exposure can be reduced in men who engage sexual intercourse more than twice a week, and side effects can be minimized in men who have difficulty tolerating higher doses of PDE5I [33, 38].

The SURE multicenter study was one of the first trials to investigate the usefulness of chronic tadalafil dosing: 4262 men with ED were treated with 20 mg of tadalafil three times per week or 20 mg on-demand in a 12-day cross-over project [39]. The results of this study showed that over 60% of men in both arms of the study reported normalization of erectile function. Over 70% of men in both groups reported being able to successfully penetrate and complete intercourse. There were no differences in the success rate between routine and on-demand dosing for any efficacy parameter. There was a substantial difference in the timing of intercourse between the treatment arms: within 4 h of taking the drug, 53% of the on-demand arm attempted intercourse while only 29% of the OaD arm attempted intercourse within this time limit. This suggests a greater flexibility in the OaD group. Although efficacy data showed no differences, the three times weekly dosing regimen for tadalafil was preferred by only 43% of enrolled patients; therefore, on-demand therapy was preferred by most men. Anyway, in the SURE study, it is evident that routine dosing may be a good option too.

The impact of daily tadalafil dosage on female partner satisfaction with sexual activity has also been a topic of recent interest and research. A partner preference study on sildenafil on-demand versus tadalafil OaD indicated that 79% of female partners preferred tadalafil OaD, citing a more relaxed approach to sexual intimacy and greater flexibility with respect to the timing of intercourse. Based on this, it can be inferred that such flexibility would be attractive to many patients' partners [40].

However, it has to be stated that in some studies, side effects were more common at higher doses of tadalafil, but this dose-response relationship was not confirmed in all studies. In general, the incidence of these side effects decreases over time with chronic therapy [38].

4.1.1.7 PDE5-I in Penile Rehabilitation

The advent of PDE-5I drugs has also introduced an innovation in the treatment of ED following radical prostatectomy (RP) and other major pelvic surgeries. It should be emphasized that ED is poorly responsive to PDE5Is in patients who underwent radical prostatectomy. However, these drugs are considered first-line therapy in patients who have undergone nerve sparing (NS) surgery regardless of the surgical technique used [41, 42]; their effectiveness has been demonstrated, and they have therefore entered the therapeutic protocols according to the European Association of Urology guidelines [43].

The use of sildenafil is controversial: although several studies have proven the efficacy of both high-dose on-demand and OaD administration, a 2016 randomized study denies any benefit of sildenafil OaD in restoring ED post-RP [44].

Vardenafil 10 mg and tadalafil 20 mg on-demand are both effective on improving the erectile function of patients who underwent NS prostatectomy [42–45]. Tadalafil 5 mg OaD showed the same effectiveness. In addition, if introduced as a therapy immediately after surgery, it helps the recovery of post-operative erectile function and the maintaining of penile length. In contrast, tadalafil on-demand has not showed these features [46]. However, the therapeutic effects are lost once the drug is discontinued, even after 9 months of treatment [47].

4.1.2 Vacuum Erection Devices

Vacuum device is a manual or electric pump used to obtain mechanical erection in a vacuum chamber. The dispositive consists in a plastic tube where the penis is allocated. When the patient starts the device, the chamber reaches vacuum and the penis is engorged with venous blood. A constriction ring can be placed at the base of the penis in order to keep the erection during a sexual intercourse. Differently from a physiological or pharmacologically induced erection, the portion of the penis next to the ring is not rigid. It may lead to a penile bend effect, moreover the penis skin can result cold and dusky. The ejaculation can be difficult due to the uncomfortable and painful ring positioning. As described by *Montague* et al., an extreme negative pressure can lead to penile injury. Thus patients with bleeding disorders or on anticoagulant therapy should avoid vacuum therapy [48].

In the literature, minor complications such as inability to ejaculate, bruising, petechiae, numbness, and pain are described. Skin necrosis as a major complication can usually be avoided by removing the ring within 30 min [49].

Vacuum device therapy has a satisfaction rates range between 27% and 94% despite the cause of ED [49, 50]. However, a percentage from 50% to 64% patients stop the treatment after 2 years [51].

Patients with infrequent sexual intercourse and comorbidities may benefit from the treatment described below, as it is drug-free and non-invasive [49, 50, 52].

4.1.3 Alprostadil

Prostaglandine E-1 and its synthetic formulation known as alprostadil is the only intracavernous and transurethral therapy, approved by FDA, to treat ED. The drug is absorbed by the urethra to the corpus spongiosum and then to the corpus cavernosum.

Alprostadil operates stimulating adenyl cyclase. The latter increases the cAMP level and decreases the intracellular calcium involving the subsequent relaxation of arterial and trabecular smooth muscle [53].

4.1.3.1 Topical Route

The topical route (200 and 300 μg VITAROS) is less invasive than the other formulations. It is a cream with a permeation enhancer that facilitates the urethral absorption. Patients suffering from mild-to-severe erectile dysfunction can benefit from this treatment. Although the literature is not rich in data, significant improvement in IIEF-Erectile Function domain score are reported vs placebo [54]. Systemic side effects are infrequent while local effects such as penile erythema, penile burning, and pain are usually self-limiting within 2 h [55, 56].

4.1.3.2 Intraurethral Route

The intraurethral route (125–1000 μg MUSE, medicated urethral system for erection) consists of small semisolid pellets managed into the distal urethra using an adequate device.

If penile rigidity is not reached, a ring at the root of the penis can be useful to keep erection enhancing the veno-occlusive mechanism.

Patients reported a successful rate about 50% [57]. One-third of patients reported penile and/or scrotal pain or discomfort. About 10% of patient's partners using intraurethral alprostadil reported vaginal discomfort after ejaculation. Hypotension and syncope have also been described in 1–5.8%. Local pain is the most common side effect reported (29–41%), while hypotension occurs in about 1.9% and 14% of cases. Urethral bleeding and urinary tract infection (UTI) are reported in 5% and 0.2% of cases respectively and are strictly related to the mode of administration. Priapism is extremely rare, reported in less than 1% of cases [58–60].

4.1.3.3 Intracavernous Injection

Intracavernous injection (ICI) allows the chemical erection of the corpora cavernosa.

It is considered the most effective non-surgical treatment for PDE5-I non-responders (approximately 25% of patients [61]) or those that cannot tolerate side effects of oral agents [62, 63].

ICI treatment does not present systemic side effects (since no change in peripheral blood vessels are observed) or drug interactions. The onset is rapid and independent from sexual stimulations [61].

Alprostadil is the only drug approved by FDA for intracavernous injections with a success rate of 70–75% with a median dose of 12–15 mg [53]. Once injected in the corpora cavernosa the drug allows relaxation of smooth muscle fibres and the consequential vasodilatation that lead to the erectile mechanism. Alprostadil is metabolized within 60 min by the 15-hydroxy dehydrogenase, which is very active in human corpora cavernosa [53].

The most common side effects reported are pain or burning sensation usually at the injection site or during the erection (11–15%). Fibrosis and small hematomas are reported too. Priapism is considered the most severe side effect, but it is reported in only 1–3% of patients [64].

Fibrosis (1–3%) can lead to nodule, diffuse scarring, plaque, or curvature. A 5 min compression above the injection site could prevent scar tissue formation [65].

4.1.4 Extracorporeal Shockwave Therapy

4.1.4.1 Introduction

The shockwaves (SW) are acoustic waves that deliver energy when focused on an anatomical target. The focused SW simulate a microtrauma in the tissues that eventually stimulate the release of endothelial nitric oxide synthase (eNOS), vascular endothelial growth factor (VEGF) and proliferating nuclear cell antigen (PCNA) [66]. Thus neo-angiogenesis and subsequent improvement of bloodstream are facilitated [67, 68].

4.1.4.2 ESWT and Vascularization

The effect of SW has been under investigation for a long time. Both in vitro and in vivo studies are present in the literature investigating whether the shockwaves improve the vascularization. The cavitation and shear-stress are the main physical mechanisms involved. The cavitation is provoked by the compression of the positive phase of the SW, followed by the rapid expansion of the tissue. As the cavitation is highly focused, the SW stress the cellular wall of the endotheliocytes [69, 70].

Several studies demonstrated the biochemical effects of the SW, such as the hyperpolarization of the cellular membrane and the activation of RAS and eNOS [71–73].

The rationale of applying the SW to treat the ED comes from several studies on animals: the hypothesis is to improve the endothelial function and angiogenesis in the corpora cavernosa.

4.1.4.3 ESWT and Stem Cells

The SW stimulate the recruitment of the circulating epithelial progenitor cells (EPC) through the expression of chemotactic factors (SDF-1, VEGF) [74]. Evidence suggests the role of the SW in the differentiation of mesenchymal stem cell in bone-forming cell in the bone tissue. This process might be mediated by TGF-beta and VEGF-A [75].

Nurzynska et al. [76] observed that SW promote the proliferation and differentiation of cardiomyocytes, smooth-muscle cells, and endotheliocytes.

4.1.4.4 ESWT and Erectile Dysfunction

Some studies on animal models of ED dysfunction induced by diabetes demonstrated that SW induce regeneration of nerves, endothelium, and smooth muscle [67, 77].

A recent metanalysis of seven randomized controlled trials on 602 men showed a significant improvement of the IIEF-Erectile Function domain score after SW therapy. The mean improvement of the score was 4.17. This improvement was clinically significant [78].

However, the patient must be selected to maximize the effect of SW: age, comorbidities, longtime ED, low IIEF-EF domain score, and poor response to PDE5-i might negatively affect the outcome of SW therapy [79, 80].

In 2015, an analysis of eight studies by *Feldman* et al. [81] on 604 patients showed that SW are safe and effective in both responders and non-responders to PDE-5I.

4.1.4.5 ESWT Protocol

For the treatment of ED, the delivery of 14,400 shockwaves in 4 weeks is suggested. In each session, 3600 hits are delivered with an energy flux density of 0.09 mJ/mm, 1800 are delivered on the shaft (900 for each corpus cavernosum), and 1800 are delivered to the perineum (900 for each crus penis). Each session lasts about 20 min and is performed in office without anaesthesia [79].

4.1.4.6 ESWT Adverse Effects

The shockwaves therapy has virtually no adverse effects. On animal models of cardiac ischemia, no adverse effects were observed [82].

In a recent metanalysis, *Feldman* et al. [81] involving 604 patient only observed mild adverse effects, self-limiting, and self-resolving.

References

1. Frühauf S, Gerger H, Schmidt HM, Munder T, Barth J. Efficacy of psychological interventions for sexual dysfunction: a systematic review and meta-analysis. Arch Sex Behav. 2013;42(6):915–33. https://doi.org/10.1007/S10508-012-0062-0.
2. Hatzimouratidis K, et al. Pharmacotherapy for erectile dysfunction: recommendations from the fourth International Consultation for Sexual Medicine (ICSM 2015). J Sex Med. 2016;13(4):465–88. https://doi.org/10.1016/J.JSXM.2016.01.016.
3. Carson CC. Phosphodiesterase type 5 inhibitors: state of the therapeutic class. Urol Clin North Am. 2007;34(4):507–15. https://doi.org/10.1016/J.UCL.2007.08.013.
4. Dunn ME, Althof SE, Perelman MA. Phosphodiesterase type 5 inhibitors' extended duration of response as a variable in the treatment of erectile dysfunction. Int J Impot Res. Mar. 2007;19(2):119–23. https://doi.org/10.1038/SJ.IJIR.3901490.
5. Alan LRK, Wein J, Partin AW, Peters CA. Campbell-Walsh urology. Elsevier; 2015.
6. Goldstein I, Lue TF, Padma-Nathan H, Rosen RC, Steers WD, Wicker PA. Oral sildenafil in the treatment of erectile dysfunction. Sildenafil Study Group. N Engl J Med. 1998;338(20):1397–404. https://doi.org/10.1056/NEJM199805143382001.
7. Giuliano F, Jackson G, Montorsi F, Martin-Morales A, Raillard P. Safety of sildenafil citrate: review of 67 double-blind placebo-controlled trials and the postmarketing safety database. Int J Clin Pract. 2010;64(2):240–55. https://doi.org/10.1111/J.1742-1241.2009.02254.X.

8. Goldstein I, Tseng LJ, Creanga D, Stecher V, Kaminetsky JC. Efficacy and safety of sildenafil by age in men with erectile dysfunction. J Sex Med. 2016;13(5):852–9. https://doi.org/10.1016/J.JSXM.2016.02.166.

9. Gupta M, Kovar A, Meibohm B. The clinical pharmacokinetics of phosphodiesterase-5 inhibitors for erectile dysfunction. J Clin Pharmacol. 2005;45(9):987–1003. https://doi.org/10.1177/0091270005276847.

10. Goldstein I, Lue TF, Padma-Nathan H, Rosen RC, Steers WD, Wicker PA. Oral sildenafil in the treatment of erectile dysfunction. 1998. J Urol. 2002;167(2 Pt 2) https://doi.org/10.1016/S0022-5347(02)80386-X.

11. Capogrosso P, et al. Time of onset of vardenafil orodispersible tablet in a real-life setting—looking beyond randomized clinical trials. Expert Rev Clin Pharmacol. 2017;10(3):339–44. https://doi.org/10.1080/17512433.2017.1288567.

12. Chung E, Brock GB. A state of art review on vardenafil in men with erectile dysfunction and associated underlying diseases. Expert Opin Pharmacother. 2011;12(8):1341–8. https://doi.org/10.1517/14656566.2011.584064.

13. Sperling H, Debruyne F, Boermans A, Beneke M, Ulbrich E, Ewald S. The POTENT I randomized trial: efficacy and safety of an orodispersible vardenafil formulation for the treatment of erectile dysfunction. J Sex Med. 2010;7(4 Pt 1):1497–507. https://doi.org/10.1111/J.1743-6109.2010.01806.X.

14. Debruyne FMJ, Gittelman M, Sperling H, Börner M, Beneke M. Time to onset of action of vardenafil: a retrospective analysis of the pivotal trials for the orodispersible and film-coated tablet formulations. J Sex Med. 2011;8(10):2912–23. https://doi.org/10.1111/J.1743-6109.2011.02462.X.

15. Daugan A, et al. The discovery of tadalafil: a novel and highly selective PDE5 inhibitor. 2: 2,3,6,7,12,12a-Hexahydropyrazino[1′,2′ :1,6]pyrido[3,4-b]indole-1,4-dione analogues. J Med Chem. 2003;46(21):4533–42. https://doi.org/10.1021/JM0300577/SUPPL_FILE/JM0300577_S.PDF.

16. Coward RM, Carson CC. Tadalafil in the treatment of erectile dysfunction. Ther Clin Risk Manag. 2008;4(6):1315–29. https://doi.org/10.2147/TCRM.S3336.

17. Wang R, et al. Selectivity of avanafil, a PDE5 inhibitor for the treatment of erectile dysfunction: implications for clinical safety and improved tolerability. J Sex Med. 2012;9(8):2122–9. https://doi.org/10.1111/J.1743-6109.2012.02822.X.

18. Kyle JA, Brown DA, Hill JK. Avanafil for erectile dysfunction. Ann Pharmacother. 2013;47(10):1312–20. https://doi.org/10.1177/1060028013501989.

19. Rajfer J, Aliotta PJ, Steidle CP, Fitch WP, Zhao Y, Yu A. Tadalafil dosed once a day in men with erectile dysfunction: a randomized, double-blind, placebo-controlled study in the US. Int J Impot Res. 2007;19(1):95–103. https://doi.org/10.1038/SJ.IJIR.3901496.

20. Porst H, Padma-Nathan H, Giuliano F, Anglin G, Varanese L, Rosen R. Efficacy of tadalafil for the treatment of erectile dysfunction at 24 and 36 hours after dosing: a randomized controlled trial. Urology. Jul. 2003;62(1):121–5. https://doi.org/10.1016/S0090-4295(03)00359-5.

21. Taylor J, Baldo OB, Storey A, Cartledge J, Eardley I. Differences in side-effect duration and related bother levels between phosphodiesterase type 5 inhibitors. BJU Int. 2009;103(10):1392–5. https://doi.org/10.1111/J.1464-410X.2008.08328.X.

22. Kedia GT, Ückert S, Assadi-Pour F, Kuczyk MA, Albrecht K. Avanafil for the treatment of erectile dysfunction: initial data and clinical key properties. Ther Adv Urol. 2013;5(1):35–41. https://doi.org/10.1177/1756287212466282.

23. Hellstrom WJG, et al. Efficacy of avanafil 15 minutes after dosing in men with erectile dysfunction: a randomized, double-blind, placebo controlled study. J Urol. 2015;194(2):485–92. https://doi.org/10.1016/J.JURO.2014.12.101.

24. Wang H, Yuan J, Hu X, Tao K, Liu J, Hu D. The effectiveness and safety of avanafil for erectile dysfunction: a systematic review and meta-analysis. Curr Med Res Opin. 2014;30(8):1565–71. https://doi.org/10.1185/03007995.2014.909391.

25. Chen L, et al. Phosphodiesterase 5 inhibitors for the treatment of erectile dysfunction: a trade-off network meta-analysis. Eur Urol. 2015;68(4):674–80. https://doi.org/10.1016/J.EURURO.2015.03.031.

26. Swearingen D, Nehra A, Morelos S, Peterson CA. Hemodynamic effect of avanafil and glyceryl trinitrate coadministration. Drugs Context. 2013;2013:212248. https://doi.org/10.7573/DIC.212248.

27. Yuan J, et al. Comparative effectiveness and safety of oral phosphodiesterase type 5 inhibitors for erectile dysfunction: a systematic review and network meta-analysis. Eur Urol. 2013;63(5):902–12. https://doi.org/10.1016/J.EURURO.2013.01.012.

28. Kloner RA, Goldstein I, Kirby MG, Parker JD, Sadovsky R. Cardiovascular safety of phosphodiesterase type 5 inhibitors after nearly 2 decades on the market. Sex Med Rev. 2018;6(4):583–94. https://doi.org/10.1016/J.SXMR.2018.03.008.

29. McCullough AR, Barada JH, Fawzy A, Guay AT, Hatzichristou D. Achieving treatment optimization with sildenafil citrate (Viagra) in patients with erectile dysfunction. Urology. 2002;60(2 Suppl 2):28–38. https://doi.org/10.1016/S0090-4295(02)01688-6.

30. Rosen RC, Padma-Nathan H, Shabsigh R, Saikali K, Watkins V, Pullman W. Determining the earliest time within 30 minutes to erectogenic effect after tadalafil 10 and 20 mg: a multicenter, randomized, double-blind, placebo-controlled, at-home study. J Sex Med. 2004;1(2):193–200. https://doi.org/10.1111/J.1743-6109.2004.04028.X.

31. Padma-Nathan H, Stecher VJ, Sweeney M, Orazem J, Tseng LJ, DeRiesthal H. Minimal time to successful intercourse after sildenafil citrate: results of a

randomized, double-blind, placebo-controlled trial. Urology. 2003;62(3):400–3. https://doi.org/10.1016/S0090-4295(03)00567-3.

32. Marchal-Escalona C, et al. PDE5A polymorphisms influence on sildenafil treatment success. J Sex Med. 2016;13(7):1104–10. https://doi.org/10.1016/J.JSXM.2016.04.075.

33. Costa P, Grivel T, Gehchan N. Tadalafil once daily in the management of erectile dysfunction: patient and partner perspectives. Patient Prefer Adherence. 2009;3:105–11. https://doi.org/10.2147/PPA.S3937.

34. Dean J, et al. Psychosocial outcomes and drug attributes affecting treatment choice in men receiving sildenafil citrate and tadalafil for the treatment of erectile dysfunction: results of a multicenter, randomized, open-label, crossover study. J Sex Med. 2006;3(4):650–61. https://doi.org/10.1111/J.1743-6109.2006.00261.X.

35. Hatzimouratidis K, et al. Psychosocial outcomes after initial treatment of erectile dysfunction with tadalafil once daily, tadalafil on demand or sildenafil citrate on demand: results from a randomized, open-label study. Int J Impot Res. 2014;26(6):223–9. https://doi.org/10.1038/IJIR.2014.15.

36. Lin G, et al. Up and down-regulation of phosphodiesterase-5 as related to tachyphylaxis and priapism. J Urol. 2003;170(2 Pt 2):S15–8. https://doi.org/10.1097/01.JU.0000075500.11519.E8.

37. Vernet D, Magee T, Qian A, Nolazco G, Rajfer J, Gonzalez-Cadavid N. Phosphodiesterase type 5 is not upregulated by tadalafil in cultures of human penile cells. J Sex Med. 2006;3(1):84–95. https://doi.org/10.1111/J.1743-6109.2005.00197.X.

38. Washington SL, Shindel AW. A once-daily dose of tadalafil for erectile dysfunction: compliance and efficacy. Drug Des Devel Ther. 2010;4:159–71. https://doi.org/10.2147/DDDT.S9067.

39. Mirone V, et al. An evaluation of an alternative dosing regimen with tadalafil, 3 times/week, for men with erectile dysfunction: SURE study in 14 European countries. Eur Urol. 2005;47(6):846–54. https://doi.org/10.1016/J.EURURO.2005.02.019.

40. Conaglen HM, Conaglen JV. Investigating women's preference for sildenafil or tadalafil use by their partners with erectile dysfunction: the partners' preference study. J Sex Med. 2008;5(5):1198–207. https://doi.org/10.1111/J.1743-6109.2008.00774.X.

41. Salonia A, et al. Prevention and management of postprostatectomy sexual dysfunctions. Part 1: choosing the right patient at the right time for the right surgery. Eur Urol. Aug. 2012;62(2):261–72. https://doi.org/10.1016/J.EURURO.2012.04.046.

42. Montorsi F, et al. Tadalafil in the treatment of erectile dysfunction following bilateral nerve sparing radical retropubic prostatectomy: a randomized, double-blind, placebo controlled trial. J Urol. 2004;172(3):1036–41. https://doi.org/10.1097/01.JU.0000136448.71773.2B.

43. Salonia A, et al. Sexual and reproductive health EAU guidelines. 2021. p. 282. https://uroweb.org/guideline/sexual-and-reproductive-health/#10.

44. Kim DJ, et al. A prospective, randomized, placebo-controlled trial of on-Demand vs. nightly sildenafil citrate as assessed by Rigiscan and the international index of erectile function. Andrology. 2016;4(1):27–32. https://doi.org/10.1111/ANDR.12118.

45. Nehra A, Grantmyre J, Nadel A, Thibonnier M, Brock G. Vardenafil improved patient satisfaction with erectile hardness, orgasmic function and sexual experience in men with erectile dysfunction following nerve sparing radical prostatectomy. J Urol. 2005;173(6):2067–71. https://doi.org/10.1097/01.JU.0000158456.41788.93.

46. Moncada I, et al. Effects of tadalafil once daily or on demand versus placebo on time to recovery of erectile function in patients after bilateral nerve-sparing radical prostatectomy. World J Urol. 2015;33(7):1031–8. https://doi.org/10.1007/S00345-014-1377-3.

47. Montorsi F, et al. Effects of tadalafil treatment on erectile function recovery following bilateral nerve-sparing radical prostatectomy: a randomised placebo-controlled study (REACTT). Eur Urol. 2014;65(3):587–96. https://doi.org/10.1016/J.EURURO.2013.09.051.

48. Montague DK, et al. Clinical guidelines panel on erectile dysfunction: summary report on the treatment of organic erectile dysfunction. The American Urological Association. J Urol. 1996;156(6):2007–11. https://doi.org/10.1016/S0022-5347(01)65419-3.

49. Yuan J, Hoang AN, Romero CA, Lin H, Dai Y, Wang R. Vacuum therapy in erectile dysfunction—science and clinical evidence. Int J Impot Res. 2010;22(4):211–9. https://doi.org/10.1038/IJIR.2010.4.

50. Levine LA, Dimitriou RJ. Vacuum constriction and external erection devices in erectile dysfunction. Urol Clin North Am. 2001;28(2):335–42. https://doi.org/10.1016/S0094-0143(05)70142-7.

51. Cookson MS, Nadig PW, Moul J. Long-term results with vacuum constriction device. J Urol. 1993;149(2):290–4. https://doi.org/10.1016/S0022-5347(17)36059-7.

52. Pajovic B, Dimitrovski A, Fatic N, Malidzan M, Vukovic M. Vacuum erection device in treatment of organic erectile dysfunction and penile vascular differences between patients with DM type I and DM type II. Aging Male. 2017;20(1):49–53. https://doi.org/10.1080/13685538.2016.1230601.

53. Hanchanale V, Eardley I. Alprostadil for the treatment of impotence. Expert Opin Pharmacother. 2014;15(3):421–8. https://doi.org/10.1517/14656566.2014.873789.

54. Cai T, et al. The intra-meatal application of alprostadil cream (Vitaros®) improves drug efficacy and patient's satisfaction: results from a randomized, two-administration route, cross-over clinical trial.

Int J Impot Res. 2019;31(2):119–25. https://doi.org/10.1038/s41443-018-0087-6.

55. Anaissie J, Hellstrom WJG. Clinical use of alprostadil topical cream in patients with erectile dysfunction: a review. Res Rep Urol. 2016;8:123–31. https://doi.org/10.2147/RRU.S68560.

56. Rooney M, Pfister W, Mahoney M, Nelson M, Yeager J, Steidle C. Long-term, multicenter study of the safety and efficacy of topical alprostadil cream in male patients with erectile dysfunction. J Sex Med. 2009;6(2):520–34. https://doi.org/10.1111/J.1743-6109.2008.01118.X.

57. Mulhall JP, Jahoda AE, Ahmed A, Parker M. Analysis of the consistency of intraurethral prostaglandin E(1) (MUSE) during at-home use. Urology. 2001;58(2):262–6. https://doi.org/10.1016/S0090-4295(01)01164-5.

58. Garrido Abad P, Sinués Ojas B, Martínez Blázquez L, Conde Caturla P, Fernández Arjona M. Safety and efficacy of intraurethral alprostadil in patients with erectile dysfunction refractory to treatment using phosphodiesterase-5 inhibitors. Actas Urol Esp. 2015;39(10):635–40. https://doi.org/10.1016/J.ACURO.2015.04.007.

59. Costa P, Potempa AJ. Intraurethral alprostadil for erectile dysfunction: a review of the literature. Drugs. 2012;72(17):2243–54. https://doi.org/10.2165/11641380-000000000-00000.

60. Kongkanand A, et al. Evaluation of transurethal alprostadil for safety and efficacy in men with erectile dysfunction. J Med Assoc Thai. 2002;85(2):223–8. https://pubmed.ncbi.nlm.nih.gov/12081123/. Accessed 5 Feb 2022.

61. Nagai A, et al. Intracavernous injection of prostaglandin E1 is effective in patients with erectile dysfunction not responding to phosphodiseterase 5 inhibitors. Acta Med Okayama. 2005;59(6):279–80. https://doi.org/10.18926/AMO/31956.

62. Alexandre B, Lemaire A, Desvaux P, Amar E. Intracavernous injections of prostaglandin E1 for erectile dysfunction: patient satisfaction and quality of sex life on long-term treatment. J Sex Med. 2007;4(2):426–31. https://doi.org/10.1111/J.1743-6109.2006.00260.X.

63. Rajpurkar A, Dhabuwala CB. Comparison of satisfaction rates and erectile function in patients treated with sildenafil, intracavernous prostaglandin E1 and penile implant surgery for erectile dysfunction in urology practice. J Urol. 2003;170(1):159–63. https://doi.org/10.1097/01.JU.0000072524.82345.6D.

64. Earle CM, Stuckey BGA, Ching HL, Wisniewski ZS. The incidence and management of priapism in Western Australia: a 16 year audit. Int J Impot Res. 2003;15(4):272–6. https://doi.org/10.1038/SJ.IJIR.3901018.

65. Chew KK, Stuckey BGA, Earle CM, Dhaliwal SS, Keogh EJ, Porst H. Penile fibrosis in intracavernosal prostaglandin E1 injection therapy for erectile dysfunction. Int J Impot Res. 1997;9(4):225–30. https://doi.org/10.1038/SJ.IJIR.3900296.

66. Zhao JC, Zhang BR, Hong L, Shi K, Wu WW, Yu JA. Extracorporeal shock wave therapy with low-energy flux density inhibits hypertrophic scar formation in an animal model. Int J Mol Med. 2018;41(4):1931–8. https://doi.org/10.3892/IJMM.2018.3434.

67. Qiu X, et al. Effects of low-energy shockwave therapy on the erectile function and tissue of a diabetic rat model. J Sex Med. 2013;10(3):738–46. https://doi.org/10.1111/JSM.12024.

68. Lee M-C, El-Sakka AI, Graziottin TM, Ho H-C, Lin C-S, Lue TF. The effect of vascular endothelial growth factor on a rat model of traumatic arteriogenic erectile dysfunction. J Urol. 2002;167(2 Pt 1):761–9. https://doi.org/10.1097/00005392-200202000-00080.

69. Apfel RE. Acoustic cavitation: a possible consequence of biomedical uses of ultrasound. Br J Cancer Suppl. Mar. 1982;5:140–6.

70. Ogden JA, Tóth-Kischkat A, Schultheiss R. Principles of shock wave therapy. Clin Orthop Relat Res. 2001;(387):8–17. https://doi.org/10.1097/00003086-200106000-00003.

71. Gotte G, Amelio E, Russo S, Marlinghaus E, Musci G, Suzuki H. Short-time non-enzymatic nitric oxide synthesis from L-arginine and hydrogen peroxide induced by shock waves treatment. FEBS Lett. 2002;520(1–3):153–5. https://doi.org/10.1016/S0014-5793(02)02807-7.

72. Mariotto S, de Prati A, Cavalieri E, Amelio E, Marlinghaus E, Suzuki H. Extracorporeal shock wave therapy in inflammatory diseases: molecular mechanism that triggers anti-inflammatory action. Curr Med Chem. 2009;16(19):2366–72. https://doi.org/10.2174/092986709788682119.

73. Hatanaka K, et al. Molecular mechanisms of the angiogenic effects of low-energy shock wave therapy: roles of mechanotransduction. Am J Physiol Cell Physiol. 2016;311(3):C378–85. https://doi.org/10.1152/AJPCELL.00152.2016.

74. Aicher A, Heeschen C, Sasaki KI, Urbich C, Zeiher AM, Dimmeler S. Low-energy shock wave for enhancing recruitment of endothelial progenitor cells: a new modality to increase efficacy of cell therapy in chronic hind limb ischemia. Circulation. 2006;114(25):2823–30. https://doi.org/10.1161/CIRCULATIONAHA.106.628623.

75. Chen YJ, et al. Recruitment of mesenchymal stem cells and expression of TGF-beta 1 and VEGF in the early stage of shock wave-promoted bone regeneration of segmental defect in rats. J Orthop Res. 2004;22(3):526–34. https://doi.org/10.1016/J.ORTHRES.2003.10.005.

76. Nurzynska D, et al. Shock waves activate in vitro cultured progenitors and precursors of cardiac cell lineages from the human heart. Ultrasound Med Biol. 2008;34(2):334–42. https://doi.org/10.1016/J.ULTRASMEDBIO.2007.07.017.

77. Jeong HC, et al. Effects of next-generation low-energy extracorporeal shockwave therapy on erectile dysfunction in an animal model of diabetes.

World J Mens Health. 2017;35(3):186. https://doi.org/10.5534/WJMH.17024.

78. Rosen RC, Allen KR, Ni X, Araujo AB. Minimal clinically important differences in the erectile function domain of the International Index of Erectile Function scale. Eur Urol. 2011;60(5):1010–6. https://doi.org/10.1016/J.EURURO.2011.07.053.

79. Reisman Y, Hind A, Varaneckas A, Motil I. Initial experience with linear focused shockwave treatment for erectile dysfunction: a 6-month follow-up pilot study. Int J Impot Res. 2015;27(3):108–12. https://doi.org/10.1038/IJIR.2014.41.

80. Kitrey ND, Gruenwald I, Appel B, Shechter A, Massarwa O, Vardi Y. Penile low intensity shock wave treatment is able to shift PDE5i nonresponders to responders: a double-blind, sham controlled study. J Urol. 2016;195(5):1550–5. https://doi.org/10.1016/J.JURO.2015.12.049.

81. Feldman R, Denes B, Appel B, Vasan SS, Shultz T, Burnett A. PD45-10 the safety and efficacy of LI-ESWT in 604 patients for erectile dysfunction: summary of current and evolving evidence. J Urol. 2015;193(4S):e905–6. https://doi.org/10.1016/J.JURO.2015.02.2582.

82. Nishida T, et al. Extracorporeal cardiac shock wave therapy markedly ameliorates ischemia-induced myocardial dysfunction in pigs in vivo. Circulation. 2004;110(19):3055–61. https://doi.org/10.1161/01.CIR.0000148849.51177.97.

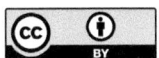

Carlo Bettocchi, Fabio Castiglione,
Omer Onur Cakir, Ugo Falagario,
and Anna Ricapito

5.1 Erectile Dysfunction: Surgical Therapy

5.1.1 Introduction

Erectile dysfunction (ED) is defined as the failure to achieve and/or maintain a penile erection that is satisfactory for sexual intercourse [1]. It is postulated that more than 40% of men between the ages of 40 and 80 could suffer from different grades of ED [2]. The causes of ED are numerous but only in very few cases, ED is truly curable, such as the psychogenic one. In most cases, ED is only treatable [2].

Supplementary Information The online version contains supplementary material available at [https://doi.org/10.1007/978-3-031-11701-5_5].

C. Bettocchi (✉)
Andrology and Male Genitalia Reconstructive Surgery Unit, University of Foggia, Policlinico "Riuniti" Foggia, Foggia, Italy
e-mail: carlo.bettocchi@unifg.it

F. Castiglione · O. O. Cakir
Department of Urology, University College London Hospitals NHS Trust, London, UK

U. Falagario
Department of Urology and Organ Transplantation, University of Foggia, Foggia, Italy

A. Ricapito
Department of Urology and Organ Transplantation, "Policlinico Riuniti", University of Foggia, Foggia, Italy

Regardless of the cause, chronic ED is characterized by anatomical and functional alterations in the erectile cavernous tissue characterized by fibrosis [3]. Historically, the concept of penile fibrosis has been entirely linked to Peyronie's disease and urethral stricture [4]. On the other hand, corpus cavernosum (CC) fibrosis was considered a rare disorder that was only seen after penile fracture or after prolonged erection [5].

However, recently, several studies have demonstrated that CC fibrosis is a common pathological sign underlying most cases of vasculogenic and/or neurogenic ED. The penile erection is regulated by a complex mechanism that involves the synergy of the nitrergic and adrenergic neuronal system, endothelium, and smooth muscle cells of the CC. Pathological disorders affecting one or more of these elements could cause CC fibrosis [6]. An impaired elasticity of the CC due to fibrosis leads to a diminished filling of the sinusoids and inadequate compression of the subtunical venules. This lack of compression will result in blood leaking out of the CC during an erection, which makes the penis incapable to become entirely erected.

The ED treatment has been standard for many years, and it was characterized by a limited range of therapeutic agents. First-level approach consists of lifestyle modification followed by medical therapy with phosphodiesterase-5 (PDE5i) inhibitors. For refractory patients, or those with intolerable side effects, European guidelines [7] suggest second- and third-level treatments such as vacuum devices, self-administered intracavernous injection of erectogenic substances, intraurethral creams, and placement of penile prostheses [8].

5.1.2 History of Penile Prosthesis

The world of penile prosthesis was born more than a hundred years ago, and the actual devices are the ultimate evolution of the earliest systems. The first mechanism similar to a penile prosthesis was created in 1930s by Bogoras, who implanted rib cartilage into an abdominal tube pedicle graft during war [9]. This technique evolved during years, but the material was not considered ideal, due to its firmness and its high risk of extrusion and reabsorption. In 1952, Goodwin implanted the first non-autologous device, made of an acrylic rob outside the corpora cavernosa, then replaced by the first silicone implants by Beheri in 1966, who used polyethylene rob into the corpora cavernosa [9, 10]. The modern era of penile prosthesis started in 1974 at the AUA Meeting, where Carrion proposed the silicone gel-filled penile implant, inspired by silicone gel-filled breast implants, with excellent outcomes: this was the ancestor of the actual semi-rigid prosthesis [9]. In 1970s, Scott, Timm, and Bradley laid the foundations of the first inflatable penile prosthesis, utilizing a fluid-based system to inflate an expandable cylinder in the corpora cavernosa [11]. Many adjustments have been made during the last 40 years, up until the current models, which remain recognizable from the original prototype.

5.1.3 Penile Prosthesis Implant

The implantation of a penile prosthesis may be considered in patients who are not suitable for different pharmacotherapies and do not respond to the first and the second line of treatment, that are pharmacological therapies [7]. An appropriate patient selection and preoperative counselling are required to achieve solid outcomes.

5.1.4 Types of Devices and Differences

Penile prosthesis can be divided in two main types: non-inflatable or malleable and inflatable (Table 5.1).

Non-inflatable or malleable penile prosthesis consists of a pair of rods made of spiral wire or silicone material, wrapped in fabric, like silicone (Fig. 5.1). There have been many features, that improved these kinds of devices: articulated segments, held by a central spring, providing a positional memory, and allowing the rods to remain hidden when not in use; a hydrophilic coating, which allows the choice of any antibiotic as a device preparation [12]. Malleable devices require less manual dexterity by the patient, given

Table 5.1 Different types of penile prostheses

Semi-rigid prostheses	Inflatable prostheses		
	Single-piece	Two-piece	Three-piece
Boston Scientific AMS Tactra	Boston Scientific AMS Hydroflex[a]	Boston Scientific AMS Ambicor[a]	Coloplast Titan (OTR NB, Zero Degree)
Coloplast Genesis	Surgitek Flexi-Flate[a]		Boston Scientific AMS 700 (CX, LGX, CXR)
Rigicon Rigi10™			Rigicon INFLA10®
Zephyr ZSI 100			Zephyr ZSI 475

[a]Not available

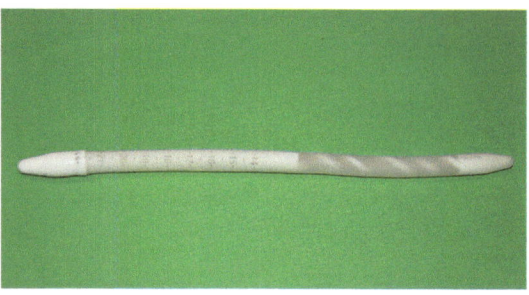

Fig. 5.1 Malleable penile prosthesis

their malleable nature, they are less prone to malfunction; they are permanently firm and have lower overall satisfaction, also having a higher risk of erosion and chronic pain [13].

Inflatable devices consist of a pair of cylinders implanted in the corpora cavernosa and connected to a pump: when the pump is squeezed and released multiple times, the cylinders are filled with normal sterile saline, stimulating the corpora blood filing during erection. They can be distinguished into one-piece, two-piece, and three-piece implants, based on the dimension and the site of the reservoir. The single-piece penile prosthesis has a small reservoir in the end of each cylinder, that allows the transition of a small volume of fluid into a central core [12]. These prostheses have been shown inferior to two- and three-piece inflatable prostheses, due to their poor mechanical reliability and patients' satisfaction rates [14].

The two-piece system consists of corporal cylinders and a pump-reservoir. The pump transfers fluid from the small reservoir in the proximal portion of the cylinders to the inflatable distal portion of them, causing an erection. With the lack of a distinct reservoir, the two-piece devices do not permit complete deflation of the penile cylinders. The main indications for the two-piece device is represented by patients with little dexterity, since its easier mechanism of inflation and deflation; prior abdominal or pelvic surgery, due to obliteration of the Retzius space; pelvic organ transplantation recipients, since the absence of the reservoir; female-to-male transgender patients, due to absence of the reservoir, although its more difficult pump mechanism [12, 15].

The three-piece system (Fig. 5.2), instead, consists of corporal cylinders, a scrotal pump, and a separate reservoir, placed in abdomen, which allows the patient to press the button once, then squeezing the cylinders in one single time, making the deflation easier. Many improvement have been made in many three-piece models: a three-layered fabric was introduced, to reduce the cylinder aneurism formation and mechanical failure; an additional coating to the surface of the silicone to increase the lubricity of silicone itself;

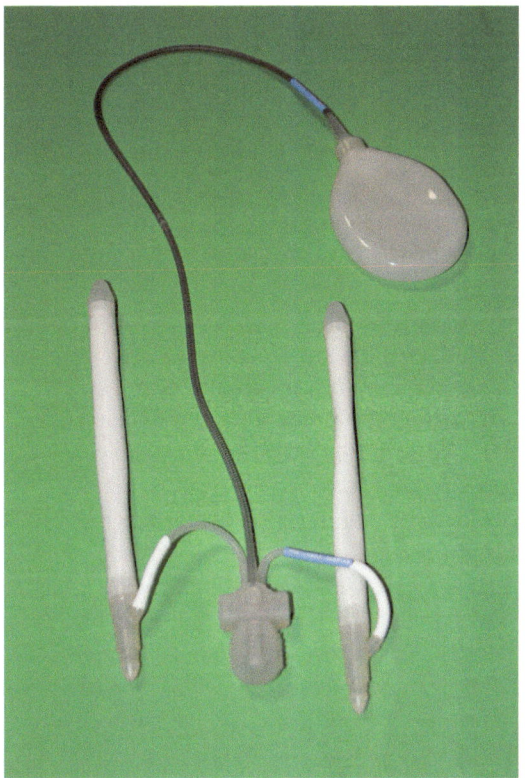

Fig. 5.2 Three components inflatable penile prosthesis

a lock-out valve has been incorporated into the pump to prevent auto-inflation of the cylinders in case of sudden high pressure within the reservoir; permanent antibiotic elution device, that is an antibiotic formulation impregnated onto the external surface of prosthesis; hydrophilic coating, which reduces bacterial attachments and binds strongly the antibiotic with a low rate of infection; the momentary-squeeze pump, which allows the deflation only pressing once the button with a quick squeeze, avoiding the patient to hold continuingly the deflation button. The most common device implanted in penile surgery is the three-piece IPP, since its mechanical reliability and very high satisfaction rates. This represents the best option in case of Peyronie's disease, since its greater rigidity; in patients with severe corporal fibrosis, due to the little elasticity of tissues; in case of long narrow penises, because of decreased axial support [12, 13, 16, 17].

5.1.5 Surgical Approach

There are many different techniques of penile prosthesis, but the most used approaches are mainly three as follows: the **infrapubic approach**, first applied by Scott in 1972, the **penoscrotal approach**, first described by Barry and Scott in 1979, and the **subcoronal approach**, popularized by Egidio in 2016 [18].

All the procedures start with accurate disinfection of the field and bladder drainage inserting a 16 Fr Foley urethral catheter (Video 5.1). The skin incision represents the next step: in the penoscrotal approach, after positioning a Scott ring retractor, a longitudinal skin incision (about 3–4 cm) at the penoscrotal junction is made (Video 5.2), exposing and then incising the dartos, placing six hooks for retraction, until the tunica albuginea appears and the dartos is incised; while in the infrapubic approach, an infrapubic 2 cm skin incision is made about 1 cm above the penopubic junction; in case of the subcoronal technique, a distal sub-coronal "circumcision" incision is made 2 cm proximal to the coronal sulcus of the glans, then degloving the penis to the level of the penoscrotal junction, placing silk sutures on the everted dartos (at 3, 6, 9, and 12 o'clock).

Corporotomy may now start: in the penoscrotal technique, four absorbable Vicryl 2.0 stay sutures are placed in both corpora cavernosa and a 2 cm longitudinal tunical incision is made in each corpus between the stay sutures (Video 5.3); during the infrapubic approach, the Scarpa fascia is opened with the guidance of the finger and, once isolated, the two corpora cavernosa, the bilateral corporotomies (1.5 cm each) are made, after positioning, two stay stitches on each corpus, that must be not too large preventing their bunching up during the tunica closing; in the subcoronal technique stay, sutures are placed proximal to the penoscrotal junction, taking care that the corporotomy will be proximal enough, then a corporotomy is made between the stay suture.

Thereafter, dilatators are then used to create the intracorporeal space and a Furlow insertion tool is used to measure the corpora length to choose the cylinder size (Video 5.4). At this point, irrigation of the site with rifampicin solution is demanded to prevent infections and to check for any urethral injury. Measurements of each corpus are performed both proximal and distal, and a rear-tip extender (RTE) is selected, according to the difference between the proximal and distal measurements.

After cycling and plumping the cylinders with saline solution to remove air bubbles and positioning the chosen RTE on both cylinders, one cylinder at time is placed in the corpora cavernosa with the guide of the insertion instrument laterally in the corpora to avoid urethral injury, placing it proximally and then distally. In case of subcoronal approach, the proximal end of the prosthesis is placed into the corpora, proximal to the penoscrotal junction, and then the distal tips of the prosthesis are pulled through the remaining corpora to the mid glans. The corporotomy closure begins with 2.0 Vycril horizontal sutures.

The next step consists of the pump placement (Video 5.5): in the penoscrotal approach, the pump space is created in the scrotum between both testes with the deflation button anteriorly; during the infrapubic approach, the pump is positioned in a dartos pouch in the scrotum, then brought down; in the subcoronal technique, a scrotal pouch is created posterior to the testes for placement of the pump, then placing the pump easily into the scrotum without a nasal speculum.

The reservoir placement is an essential step during the penile prosthesis implant (Video 5.6). During the penoscrotal approach, the reservoir usually is positioned into the Retzius space with the index finger as a guidance and, once pierced the transversalis fascia, a space near the bladder is made. The reservoir space during the subcoronal approach is created in the same way. In case of previous pelvic surgery, such as radical prostatectomy, the scarring of the prevesical space and effective "peritonealization" of the bladder, traditional three-piece IPP reservoir placement blindly into the space of Retzius via the external inguinal ring can take to severe complications given the close proximity of bowel, bladder, and major vascular structures. The reservoir can so be positioned ectopically, that is, above the transversalis fascia and below the transversus abdominis muscle. Another location of the reservoir is the submuscular or high submuscular (HSM) position, posterior to the rectus muscle but anterior to the transversalis fascia which can be achieved through a penoscrotal incision via the external inguinal ring, eliminating the risk of intraperitoneal placement and associated bowel, bladder, or vascular complications. The HSM technique is characterized by the so-called five steps: the first one consists of the access to the external inguinal ring with the index through the penoscrotal incision and the transversalis fascia is earned; then the 2/3 of the HSM tunnel is created by manual dissection, while in the next step, the remaining portion of the tunnel is obtained with a curved sponge stick, lifting the fibres of the rectus muscle from the transversalis fascia. At this point, the deflated reservoir is delivered into the newly created pocket and then filled with 120 cc, to flatten the reservoir and ensure the space; so the excess of saline is removed and then connected to the other components. In case of an infrapubic approach, the reservoir is positioned in a paravesical space, obtained with a nasal speculum, which passes through the external inguinal ring and then across the fascia transversalis, after blunting dissecting the fat off the pubic rami. In patients with compromised pelvis, the speculum is advanced less distance into the ring and thrust upward into the space anterior to transversalis fascia.

The cylinders, pump, and reservoir are all interconnected with kink-resistant tubes, and inflation and deflation of the device is done multiple times for testing the correct functioning and positioning (Video 5.7). A closed suction drain is placed in the scrotum, in case of the penoscrotal approach. The wounds are closed in two layers, that is, dartos fascia and the skin in the PS and IF approach; in the subcoronal technique, the dartos is reapproximated at the level of the glans and the sub-coronal skin incision is closed [13, 19–21].

5.1.6 Comparison Between the Three Techniques

The three main penile prosthesis implant techniques have all important advantages, but also considerable critical issues. The penoscrotal approach presents a minimal risk of dorsal nerve injury, compared to the infrapubic approach, even if this one allows a shorter operative time, which leads to a reduced risk of infections. This could be explained by the fact that, compared to the PS surgery, several steps are omitted in the IP approach, such as in the IP technique, the dilatation and measurement of the corpora is performed in a single step. The pump placement in the scrotum is quite easier in the penoscrotal technique, since in the infrapubic procedure, a pouch must be created ex novo and great attention is needed during the positioning and the orientation of the activator of the pump itself: the patient, in fact, can find more difficult to manage the pump compared to the penoscrotal system. In particular in obese patients, this last technique allows a better corporal exposure, in order to obtain a correct corporotomy and an appropriate measurement of the length of each corpus, allowing a more precise cylinder choice and positioning, while patients with previous abdominal surgical procedures, for whom reservoir placement can be difficult, may better benefit with the IP approach. As previously described, the reservoir placement both in the infrapubic and in the subcoronal approach is characterized by a direct visualization, avoiding pelvic organs and vessels injury, compared to the penoscrotal approach, where this procedure is completely blind and requires high precision and dexterity by the surgeon. The infrapubic technique includes a skin incision that inevitably creates a less acceptable cosmetic result, since the penoscrotal incision remains quite hidden on the scrotum. Urethral injury represents an issue, in particular during the penoscrotal technique, during the dissection of the corpora cavernosa at the level of the penoscrotal junction anteriorly. The penoscrotal approach seems to be more indicated in case of corporal fibrosis, mainly secondary to prior implant removal due to infection, as it allows more complete access to the corpora proximally and distally. About subcoronal approach, excellent visibility of corpora cavernosa and urethra are guaranteed and additional surgical reconstructive procedure, such as Peyronie's disease, can be easily performed; however, it requires more operative time, compared to the two other techniques, and the degloving of the penis may cause sensorial alteration or skin loss; it is also limited by the number of studies about the surgical approach and the follow [13, 18].

5.1.7 Complications

Penile prosthesis implant complications can be distinguished into intraoperative and postoperative.

5.1.7.1 Intraoperative Complications

About intraoperative complications, we may include first a hematoma formation, typically in the scrotum, which can be prevented using a compressive dressing and placing a drainage; floppy glans represents an issue, due to inadequate prosthetic cylinder sizing or positioning, causing insufficient venous compression between Buck's fascia and the corpora cavernosa; it is usually adjusted with the normal healing and so it is quite easily resolved. A relevant complication is corporal fibrosis, defined as the replacement of smooth muscle cells with fibrotic tissue within the corporal bodies: it is common in diabetic patients and in ones with a history of ischemic priapism and usually requires increased effort during corporal dilatation, increasing though the likelihood of perforation and so requiring high levels of accuracy. Corporal crossover may occur mostly during corporal dilatation or cylinder placement: the contralateral cylinder perforation may be caused by the needle used in the ipsilateral cylinder placing; to prevent this, both the needles should be placed correctly before placing the cylinders and it is safer to start the corpora dilatation laterally and gradually. Another issue is represented by perforation of the corpora cavernosa: proximal perforation of the corpora can be detected as a sudden loss of resistance during dilatation, and it can be treated by inserting corporotomy sutures, preventing the proximal migration of the prosthesis; distal perforation represents a more serious issue due to the risk of

urethral injury and it is safe to interrupt the procedure. The rate of urethral injury is very low (0.1–0.4%) and it may be avoided staying as lateral as possible during the dilatation of the corpora; it should be repaired with a catheter and the procedure rescheduled after 6 weeks at least.

Bladder, vascular, and bowel injury are the most dangerous events: bladder injury, evident because of blood in the catheter, should be prevented by fully emptying the bladder itself before reservoir placing; while in case of both vascular and bowel damage, the procedure must be stopped to consult the specialists (general surgeons) [13, 22].

5.1.7.2 Postoperative Complications

Infection represents a serious issue: its rate reaches 4% and the most common organism involved is Staphylococcus epidermidis, due to the contamination of the skin flora during the procedure; risk factors are long operative time, immunosuppressed or transplanted patients and diabetic population. The main tips to prevent infections are intraoperatively the genital region bathing with an antiseptic soap and the use of a chlorhexidine-alcohol skin preparation, while perioperatively the administration of intravenous antibiotics (vancomycin) starting an hour prior the operation and continuing up to 24 h, constant irrigation of the field with antibiotic solution and the no-skin touch technique during surgery. In case of infection, resistant to antibiotic therapy, the removal of the prosthesis must be considered. Impending erosion, instead, can start from distal lateral corpora, urethra and glans and its rate increases in case of intraoperative urethral damage and in patients with spinal cord injuries, because of the absolute need of the catheter, which can easy the erosion mechanism. Then, glandular ischemia can be considered a very rare complication, more likely in patients with CVD, diabetes, and history of smoking; it can lead to penile gangrene and it is induced in case of an interruption of the blood supply to the glans through the dorsal penile arteries [13, 22].

5.2 Regenerative Therapies for Erectile Dysfunction

5.2.1 Introduction

Over the last decades, there has been an increasing interest in the hypothesis of "regenerative" cures for ED aimed at decreasing fibrosis of the CC and rebuilding their normal biological architecture. These new regenerative treatments include stem cell injections, platelet-rich plasma, and low-intensity shock wave therapy (Li-SWT). There are numerous data obtained on animal models of ED that indicate that these methods can result in angiogenesis and reducing fibrosis, thus "restoring" dysfunctional CC tissue [23].

To date, there are limited clinical data to support regenerative therapies as a first-line treatment for ED. However, evidence is growing every year, and these regenerative therapies are becoming a realty in the ED treatment clinical scenario.

5.2.2 Li-SWT for Erectile Dysfunction

In the last 10 years, the use of LI-SWT has been increasingly offered as an alternative treatment for vasculogenic ED, being the only currently approved therapy that might provide a "cure," which is the most wanted result for men affected by ED. LI-SWT has gotten recognition in the treatment of ED, based on the assumption that LI-SWT application may result in neoangiogenesis and thus increased blood flow to the corpora cavernosa. The usage of LI-SWT was for long time against the EAU guidelines; however, the last 2020 EAU guideline on sexual health [7] promoted LI-SWT as treatment for ED. EAU Guideline suggested to use LI-SWT in patients with mild vasculogenic ED or as an alternative first-line therapy in well-informed patients who do not wish or are not suitable for oral vasoactive therapy or desire a curable option. More importantly, a recent study has shown that an increased proportion of urologist had suggested a wider use of LISWT, and some even encouraged its application in neovasculogenic ED [7].

5.2.2.1 Mechanism of Action

A shockwave is defined as a high-pressure acoustic wave with the capacity to conduct energy and spread through a medium [24]. The waveform itself is characterized by a high peak pressure inducing a focal tissue compression followed by extension. This causes tissue injury which is postulated to induce a wound healing process activation characterized by neovascularization and activation of local stem cells. Another theory is the shockwaves can activate the neovascularization using a process called "mechanotransduction" [25], which is defined as a biochemical response to mechanical stimuli [26].

Several basic *science reports showed* LI-SWT improved levels of VEGF and endothelial nitric oxide synthase (eNOS), and that caveolin-1 and ß$_1$-integrin, constitutive proteins of caveolae, which are invaginated organelles found in the plasma membrane and accountable for cell homing, are integral for LI-SWT-induced angiogenesis [25].

LI-SWT can promote neurogenesis through local mechanisms [27]. In a rat model of pelvic neurovascular injuries, a recent report proved that LI-SWT amended erectile function by penile nerve regeneration [28].

In conclusion, the mechanism of action at the base of LI-SWT regenerative effects on CC tissue is not totally comprehended but likely include angiogenesis and neurogenesis. Local activation and recruitment of stem cells may also play a role. Thus, from a theoretical point of view, LI-SWT has the potential to cure ED conversely to the other standard treatment.

5.2.2.2 Type of Li-SWT Machine

These waves are generated by machines called lithotripters. There are mainly three types of lithotripters in common use: electrohydraulic, electromagnetic, and piezoelectric (Table 5.2).

Table 5.2 Type of lithotripters

Type of lithotripters	Mechanism of action
Electrohydraulic	Electrohydraulic waves are generated by applying high voltage to electrodes to generate a spark
Electromagnetic	Electromagnetic waves are generated by separating a metal membrane away from an electromagnetic coil using a high voltage electric pulse. The fast forward movement of the membrane produces a planar acoustic pulse, and the shockwave is focused by an acoustic reflector
Piezoelectric	This machine uses piezoelectric crystals that enlarge quickly and at the same time, when a high-voltage electric pulse is applied to them, generating a pressure wave. These crystals are allocated in a spherical way to focus the energy not needing a reflector

Table 5.3 Characteristic of lithotripters available in the market for ED

Machine	PiezoWave 2 (Richard Wolf GmbH, Knittlingen, Germany)	Renova (Direx System GmbH, Wiesbaden, Germany)	Aries 2 (Dornier MedTech GmbH, Wessling, Germany)	Duolith SD1 (Storz Medical AG, Tägerwilen, Switzerland)	Omnispec ED 1000 (Medispec, MD, USA)
Type of lithotripters	Piezoelectric	Electromagnetic	Electromagnetic	Electromagnetic	Electrohydraulic
Focus penetration depth (mm)	0–80	0–125	0–50	0–40	0–40
Frequency (Hz)	1–3	1–8	1–5	1–5	1–8
Maximal energy density (mJ/mm^2)	0.23	1.24	0.31	0.9	1.05

Contemporary lithotripter machines differ from each other regarding specific settings, namely energy flux density (EFD), penetration depth, and frequency (Table 5.3).

Also, each company has its own suggested protocol, including number and frequency of sessions and number of shocks per each session. Disparities amongst machine protocols or type of lithotripters and the lack of head-to-head reports make it puzzling to define the advantage of one machine and/or protocol over another [29].

5.2.2.3 Efficacy

Numerous single-arm studies have reported encouraging effects of LI-SWT on ED patients. However, results from randomised prospective are contradictory, and many issues wait to be solved specifically because of the several types of lithotripters used; type of energy or frequency parameters and treatment protocols [30]. The large part of the studies has reported that LI-SWT can significantly increase the IIEF in patients with vasculogenic ED [7]. More impor-

tantly, few studies have demonstrated an enhancement in penile haemodynamic at penile doppler after LI-SWT. Likewise, several reports suggest that LI-SWT could improve erectile function even in severe ED men who are PDE5Is non-responders, thus dropping the urgent need for second-line treatments like injection or penile implant insertion [31].

On the other hand, high-quality prospective randomize trials with long follow-up are needed to provide urologists and sexual medicine clinicians with more assurance concerning the efficacy of LI-SWT. Further clarity is also needed in defining treatment protocols that can result in greater clinical benefits [31].

5.3 Platelet-Rich Plasma for Erectile Dysfunction

Platelet-rich plasma (PRP) is defined as autologous blood plasma with supraphysiologic concentrations of activated platelets. Its regenerative capacities were first reported in the 1987 within the field of reconstructive surgery. In the last four decades, PRP has been utilized in a myriad of fields such as plastic surgery, cardio surgery, dermatology, and more recently in andrology [32].

5.3.1 Mechanism of Action

Notwithstanding PRP's extensive usage, its biological characteristics and outcomes continue to be inadequately comprehended and debateable.

The preparation of PRP is very simple, and it can be done in outpatient setting. Autologous blood is drawn and centrifuged to obtain a platelet-rich plasma fluid with a concentration reaching up to seven times physiological levels (Fig. 5.3) [33]. Preclinical results show that PRP can release in the system a wide range of growth factors (Fig. 5.4) and activated platelets which act synergistically to assist mitogenesis and neoangiogenesis, thus reconstructing injured tissues. Other constituents inside PRP have also been reported to work as a scaffold for healing process [34].

PROCESS OF PRP THERAPY

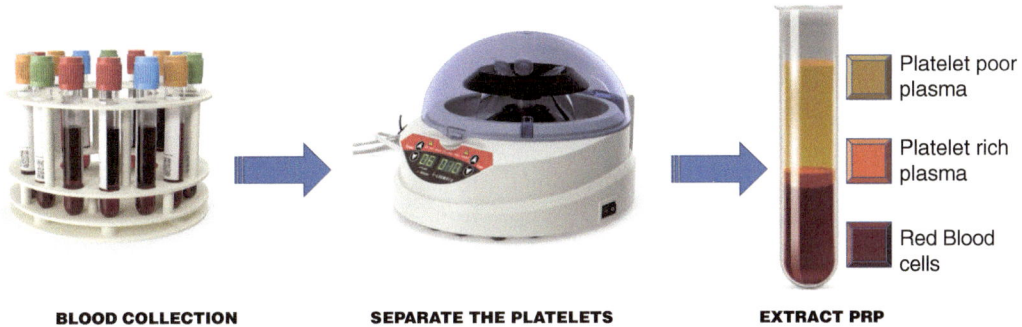

Fig. 5.3 Process of platelet-rich plasma therapy

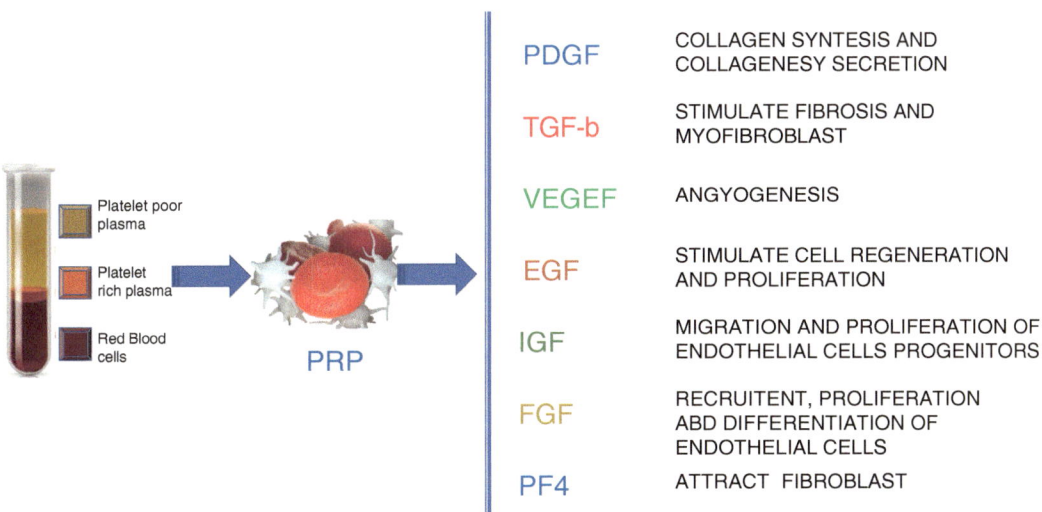

Fig. 5.4 Overview of PRP content. *PRP* platelet-rich plasma, *PDGF* platelet-derived growth factor, *TGF-b* transforming growth factor beta, *VEGF* vascular endothelial growth factor, *EGF* epidermal growth factor, *IGF* insulin-like growth factor, *FGF* fibroblast growth factor, *PF-4* platelet-factor 4, *VSM* vascular smooth muscle

5.3.2 Effectiveness

Up to the present time, few basic science studies have assessed PRP efficacy in ED animal model. Based on their results, PRP was able to (1) increase erectile function, (2) boost neural regeneration, and (3) decrease expression of pro-fibrotic molecules within the corporal cavernosa tissue. Nevertheless, these reports are characterized by several limitations that can jeopardize the value of the results like (1) reduced sample sizes, (2) dissimilar methods of PRP extraction, and (3) poor regulation of PRP concentrations [33–39]. In humans, conversely, PRP proved promising results on ED. In fact, few small reports and phase 1–2 trials showed that PRP injections significantly improved EF based on intracavernosal peak systolic velocity (PSV), IIEF-5, and sexual encounter profile scores independently of whether PRP was activated by calcium or used in conjunction to another treatment. It appears that the concurrent use of PRP could prolong Li-ESWT notable improvements for up to 6 months [32].

Notwithstanding early excitement for PRP as a regenerative cure for ED, the existing data to support its value in the ED therapy is deficient. Solid records on its safety and efficacy are still missing with only two clinical trials completed until now. The largest clinical trial assessing the efficacy of PRP involved in only 75 men with heterogeneous of ED severities [40].

Presently, no randomized controlled blinded clinical trials have delivered enough proof to sustain the extensive use of PRP for ED therapy. More importantly, approximately half of the clinical reports are abstracts and needed important details. Also, protocols required homogeneity; it is crucial to offer longer follow-up to allow beneficial outcomes to establish. Furthermore, PRP extraction varied noticeably. While, reports described a supplement of hyaluronic acids to the PRP, one reported on the efficacy of Li-ESWT combined with $CaCl_2$-activated PRP [32].

5.4 Stem Cells for Erectile Dysfunction

5.4.1 Introduction

In the context of ED, the effects of stem cells from a broad range of sources have been reported, including adipose-derived stem cells (ADSCs), bone marrow stem cells (BMSCs), embryonic stem cells (ESCs), endothelial progenitor cells (EPCEPCs), urine-derived stem cells (USCs), skeletal muscle-derived stem cells (SkMSCs), and stromal vascular fraction (SVF) (Table 5.4). In the past decade, several studies

Table 5.4 Subtypes of stem cells

Type of cells	Definition
Totipotent stem cells	These stem cells have the capacity to divide and develop into cells from all three germ cell layers and into extraembryonic tissues (for example, placenta). The zygote is an example of such a cell
Pluripotent stem cells	These stem cells have the capacity to divide and develop into cells from all three germ cell layers, but not into extraembryonic tissues (for example, placenta). Embryonic stem cells are examples of such cells
Multipotent stem cells	These stem cells have the capacity to divide and develop into cells from a specific tissue or organ. Most adult stem cells are examples of such cells
Mesenchymal stem cells	Multipotent stromal cells (MSCs) with the ability to differentiate into several cell types within their germ layer: Osteoblasts, chondrocytes, myocytes, and adipocytes
Stromal vascular fraction	Stromal vascular fraction (SVF) is a component of the lipoaspirate obtained from liposuction of excess adipose tissue, which contains a large population of adipose derived stem cells (ADSCs)
Embryonic stem cells	Embryonic stem cells (ESCs) are pluripotent and can produce all germinal layers

have evaluated the effect of stem cell therapy on the recovery of erectile function in several animal models of ageing, diabetes mellitus, and cavernous nerve injury [41]. More important several phase 1 and phase 2 studies have evaluated the safety and the efficacy of stem cell-based therapy in man suffering ED [42–47].

5.4.2 Mechanism of Action

The mechanism of action of stem cells in the treatment of ED has generated, in the last 15 years, considerable attention in molecular biology, genetics, and bioengineer. Stem cells are well known for capacity of self-renewal and their potential for differentiation into mature cell types or tissue. Depending on their potential for differentiation, stem cells are classified as totipotent stem cells, pluripotent stem cells, or multipotent stem cells. ESCs are an example of pluripotent whereas Mesenchymal stem cells are multipotent stem cells. MSC can be isolated from organs and can differentiate into any cell type within their germ tissue. ESCs have two main advantages over MSCs and SVF, the first of which is their ability to proliferate for longer periods of time, and the second is their capacity to differentiate into a broader range of cell types [3]. However, owing to the ethical conflict that surrounds ESCs, their use in research has been limited and, as such, MSCs and SVF are a more feasible option for research and therapeutic applications.

Although the mechanism of action of stem cells on ED is not yet very well understood, it is one of the most popular targets of both preclinical studies and clinical trials in the current decade. Despite their potential for differentiation into mature cell types or tissue, there is another capacity of the stem cells that makes them appealing for therapeutic purpose. The latest theory identified stem cells as a sort of drug store able to secrete several different molecules acting via paracrine way di complex mechanisms including, modulation of the innate and adaptive immune system, stimulation of neoangiogenesis and neurogenesis, reducing apoptosis, fibrosis, and myofibroblast activation [3, 48] (Fig. 5.5).

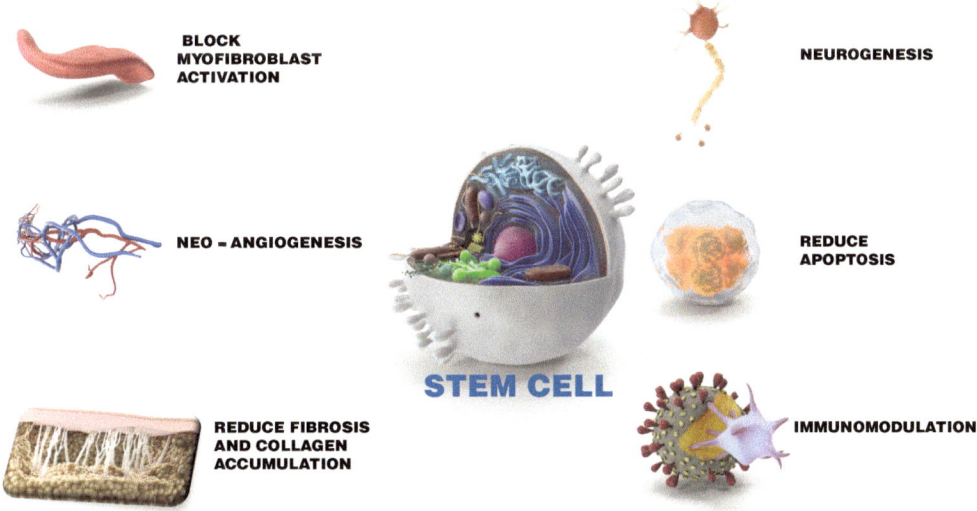

Fig. 5.5 Stem cells paracrine effects

5.4.3 Efficacy

While basic science results for stem cells and SVF are encouraging and have generated significant findings about the mechanisms of penile tissue regeneration, clinical results are limited and not robust. There are quite a few of small trial sharing similar protocols and involving few patients. Two studies looked at ESC. One involving seven diabetic patients who had regained morning erections and two who achieved erections hard enough for sexual penetrative intercourse [47]. The other recruited eight patients with organic ED for at least 6 months and those with baseline IIEF scores of 21 or higher were treated with placental matrix derived stem cells injected into the corpora cavernosal [49]. This trial showed a significantly improved systolic velocity (PSV) at penile Doppler ultrasonography [49].

INtra-cavernous STem-cell INjection (INSTIN) clinical trial [45] focused on men suffering from post-radical prostatectomy (RP) iatrogenic ED. This was a phase 1 trial that used bone marrow-derived stem cells. The authors reported no adverse events. At 180 days, they reported significant progresses in the sexual satisfaction and erectile function domains of the IIEF-15 and EHS. It should be noted that these trials were phase 1, powered only for safety, and adverse events were no reported. Notably, the group reported a decline in the improved erectile function over time, advocating a role for multiple SC treatments. Similarly, at 2 years post RP, no PSA recurrence was reported. Consequently, this trial indicates a relative safety of stem cell treatment in prostate cancer patients.

Two clinical studies published looking at SVF [43, 44]. One study investigated SVF treatment in 21 men suffering from ED post RP, and another trial in 30 patients [43]. No serious adverse events were observed. The most common being bruising or pain at the site of SVF injection or liposuction within the first 48 h. In both studies, IIEF-5 scores demonstrated an improvement.

Notwithstanding the encouraging outcomes of these phase 1–2 trials, it is imperative to acknowledge that these studies include small number of patients, are open label, and asses the safety rather than the efficacy of stem cells. All together, these trials involve around 70 ED patients treated with different protocols and type of stem cells. Most studies evaluated the safety as the primary end point and no trial reported any significant adverse event. Consequently, to overcome the substantial bias that characterized this research, the next studies need to be larger, placebo-controlled, double-blinded, and randomized trials.

References

1. Castiglione F, Montorsi F, Briganti A. Tadalafil for erectile dysfunction prevention after radiotherapy for prostate cancer. JAMA. 2014;312:748. https://doi.org/10.1001/jama.2014.7920.
2. Goldstein I, Goren A, Li VW, Tang WY, Hassan TA. Epidemiology update of erectile dysfunction in eight countries with high burden. Sex Med Rev. 2020;8:48–58. https://doi.org/10.1016/J.SXMR.2019.06.008.
3. Milenkovic U, Albersen M, Castiglione F. The mechanisms and potential of stem cell therapy for penile fibrosis. Nat Rev Urol. 2019;16:79–97. https://doi.org/10.1038/s41585-018-0109-7.
4. Pozzi E, Muneer A, Sangster P, Alnajjar HM, Salonia A, Bettocchi C, et al. Stem-cell regenerative medicine as applied to the penis. Curr Opin Urol. 2019;29:443–9. https://doi.org/10.1097/MOU.0000000000000636.
5. Capece M, la Rocca R, Mirone V, Bivalacqua TJ, Castiglione F, Albersen M, et al. A systematic review on ischemic priapism and immediate implantation: do we need more data? Sex Med Rev. 2019;7:530–4. https://doi.org/10.1016/j.sxmr.2018.10.007.
6. Milenkovic U, Albersen M, Castiglione F. The mechanisms and potential of stem cell therapy for penile fibrosis. Nat Rev Urol. 2018;16:79–97. https://doi.org/10.1038/s41585-018-0109-7.
7. Compilations of all guidelines | Uroweb n.d.. https://uroweb.org/guidelines/compilations-of-all-guidelines/. Accessed 4 Nov 2021.
8. Hazir B, Haberal HB, Asci A, Muneer A, Gudeloglu A. Erectile dysfunction management: a critical appraisal of clinical practice guidelines with the AGREE II instrument. Int J Impot Res. 2021;34(5):471–9. https://doi.org/10.1038/S41443-021-00442-7.
9. Carrion H, Martinez D, Parker J, Hakky T, Bickell M, Boyle A, et al. A history of the penile implant to 1974. Sex Med Rev. 2016;4:285–93. https://doi.org/10.1016/J.SXMR.2016.05.003.
10. Beheri GE. Surgical treatment of impotence. Plast Reconstr Surg. 1966;38:92–7. https://doi.org/10.1097/00006534-196608000-00002.

11. Brantley Scott F, Bradley WE, Timm GW. Management of erectile impotence. Use of implantable inflatable prosthesis. Urology. 1973;2:80–2. https://doi.org/10.1016/0090-4295(73)90224-0.

12. Chung E. Penile prosthesis implant: scientific advances and technological innovations over the last four decades. Transl Androl Urol. 2017;6:37–45. https://doi.org/10.21037/TAU.2016.12.06.

13. Ignacio MI, Pramod K. Textbook of urogenital prosthetic surgery: erectile restoration & urinary incontinence 2021.

14. Wilson SK, Cleves M, Delk JR II. Long-term results with Hydroflex and Dynaflex penile prostheses: device survival comparison to multicomponent inflatables. J Urol. 1996;155(5):1621–3. https://pubmed.ncbi.nlm.nih.gov/8627837/. Accessed 19 Dec 2021.

15. Kocjancic E, Jaunarena JH, Schechter L, Acar Ö. Inflatable penile prosthesis implantation after gender affirming phalloplasty with radial forearm free flap. Int J Impot Res. 2020;32:99–106. https://doi.org/10.1038/S41443-019-0153-8.

16. Abdelsayed GA, Levine LA. Ambicor 2-piece inflatable penile prosthesis: who and how? J Sex Med. 2018;15:410–5. https://doi.org/10.1016/J.JSXM.2017.12.010.

17. Levine LA, Becher EF, Bella AJ, Brant WO, Kohler TS, Martinez-Salamanca JI, et al. Penile prosthesis surgery: current recommendations from the international consultation on sexual medicine. J Sex Med. 2016;13:489–518. https://doi.org/10.1016/j.jsxm.2016.01.017.

18. Otero JR, Manfredi C, Wilson SK. The good, the bad, and the ugly about surgical approaches for inflatable penile prosthesis implantation. Int J Impot Res. 2020;34:128–37. https://doi.org/10.1038/S41443-020-0319-4.

19. Weinberg AC, Pagano MJ, Deibert CM, Valenzuela RJ. Sub-coronal inflatable penile prosthesis placement with modified no-touch technique: a step-by-step approach with outcomes. J Sex Med. 2016;13:270–6. https://doi.org/10.1016/J.JSXM.2015.12.016.

20. Baumgarten AS, Kavoussi M, VanDyke ME, Ortiz NM, Khouri RK, Ward EE, et al. Avoiding deep pelvic complications using a "Five-Step" technique for high submuscular placement of inflatable penile prosthesis reservoirs. BJU Int. 2020;126:457–63. https://doi.org/10.1111/BJU.15106.

21. Vollstedt A, Gross MS, Antonini G, Perito PE. The infrapubic surgical approach for inflatable penile prosthesis placement. Transl Androl Urol. 2017;6:620–7. https://doi.org/10.21037/TAU.2017.07.14.

22. Scherzer ND, Dick B, Gabrielson AT, Alzweri LM, Hellstrom WJG. Penile prosthesis complications: planning, prevention, and decision making. Sex Med Rev. 2019;7:349–59. https://doi.org/10.1016/J.SXMR.2018.04.002.

23. Towe M, Peta A, Saltzman RG, Balaji N, Chu K, Ramasamy R. The use of combination regenerative therapies for erectile dysfunction: rationale and current status. Int J Impot Res. 2021; https://doi.org/10.1038/S41443-021-00456-1.

24. Katz JE, Clavijo RI, Rizk P, Ramasamy R. The basic physics of waves, soundwaves, and shockwaves for erectile dysfunction. Sex Med Rev. 2020;8:100–5. https://doi.org/10.1016/J.SXMR.2019.09.004.

25. Hatanaka K, Ito K, Shindo T, Kagaya Y, Ogata T, Eguchi K, Kurosawa R, Shimokawa H. Molecular mechanisms of the angiogenic effects of low-energy shock wave therapy: roles of mechanotransduction. Am J Physiol Cell Physiol. 2016;311:C378–85. https://doi.org/10.1152/AJPCELL.00152.2016.

26. Young Academic Urologists Men's Health Group, Fode M, Hatzichristodoulou G, Serefoglu EC, Verze P, Albersen M. Low-intensity shockwave therapy for erectile dysfunction: is the evidence strong enough? Nat Rev Urol. 2017;14:593–606. https://doi.org/10.1038/NRUROL.2017.119.

27. Murata R, Ohtori S, Ochiai N, Takahashi N, Saisu T, Moriya H, Takahashi K, Wada Y. Extracorporeal shockwaves induce the expression of ATF3 and GAP-43 in rat dorsal root ganglion neurons. Auton Neurosci. 2006;128:96–100. https://doi.org/10.1016/J.AUTNEU.2006.04.003.

28. Li H, Matheu MP, Sun F, Wang L, Sanford MT, Ning H, Banie L, Lee Y-C, Xin Z, Guo Y, Lin G, Lue TF. Low-energy shock wave therapy ameliorates erectile dysfunction in a pelvic neurovascular injuries rat model. J Sex Med. 2016;13:22–32. https://doi.org/10.1016/J.JSXM.2015.11.008.

29. Porst H. Review of the current status of low intensity extracorporeal shockwave therapy (Li-ESWT) in erectile dysfunction (ED), Peyronie's disease (PD), and sexual rehabilitation after radical prostatectomy with special focus on technical aspects of the different marketed ESWT devices including personal experiences in 350 patients. Sex Med Rev. 2021;9:93–122. https://doi.org/10.1016/J.SXMR.2020.01.006.

30. Capogrosso P, Frey A, Jensen CFS, Rastrelli G, Russo GI, Torremade J, Albersen M, Gruenwald I, Reisman Y, Corona G. Low-intensity shock wave therapy in sexual medicine-clinical recommendations from the European Society of Sexual Medicine (ESSM). J Sex Med. 2019;16:1490–505. https://doi.org/10.1016/J.JSXM.2019.07.016.

31. Liu JL, Chu KY, Gabrielson AT, Wang R, Trost L, Broderick G, Davies K, Brock G, Mulhall J, Ramasamy R, Bivalacqua TJ. Restorative therapies for erectile dysfunction: position statement from the Sexual Medicine Society of North America (SMSNA). Sex Med. 2021;9:100343. https://doi.org/10.1016/J.ESXM.2021.100343.

32. Scott S, Roberts M, Chung E. Platelet-rich plasma and treatment of erectile dysfunction: critical review of literature and global trends in platelet-rich plasma clinics. Sex Med Rev. 2019;7:306–12. https://doi.org/10.1016/J.SXMR.2018.12.006.

33. Epifanova MV, Gvasalia BR, Durashov MA, Artemenko SA. Platelet-rich plasma therapy for male sexual dysfunction: myth or reality? Sex Med Rev. 2020;8:106–13. https://doi.org/10.1016/J.SXMR.2019.02.002.

34. Alkandari MH, Touma N, Carrier S. Platelet-rich plasma injections for erectile dysfunction and Peyronie's disease: a systematic review of evidence. Sex Med Rev. 2021;10:341–52. https://doi.org/10.1016/J.SXMR.2020.12.004.

35. Jung G, Kwak J, Yoon S, Yoon J, Lue T. IGF-I and TGF-β2 have a key role on regeneration of nitric oxide synthase (NOS)-containing nerves after cavernous neurotomy in rats. Int J Impot Res. 1999;11:247–59. https://doi.org/10.1038/sj.ijir.3900402.

36. Ding XG, Li SW, Zheng XM, Hu LQ, Hu WL, Luo Y. The effect of platelet-rich plasma on cavernous nerve regeneration in a rat model. Asian J Androl. 2009;11:215–21. https://doi.org/10.1038/AJA.2008.37.

37. Lee H-W, Reddy MS, Geurs N, Palcanis KG, Lemons JE, Rahemtulla FG, et al. Efficacy of platelet-rich plasma on wound healing in rabbits. J Periodontol. 2008;79:691–6. https://doi.org/10.1902/JOP.2008.070449.

38. Wu CC, Wu YN, Ho HO, Chen KC, Sheu MT, Chiang HS. The neuroprotective effect of platelet-rich plasma on erectile function in bilateral cavernous nerve injury rat model. J Sex Med. 2012;9:2838–48. https://doi.org/10.1111/J.1743-6109.2012.02881.X.

39. Hu Z, Qu S, Zhang J, Cao X, Wang P, Huang S, et al. Efficacy and safety of platelet-rich plasma for patients with diabetic ulcers: a systematic review and meta-analysis. Adv Wound Care (New Rochelle). 2019;8:298–308. https://doi.org/10.1089/WOUND.2018.0842.

40. Epifanova MV, Chalyi ME, Krasnov AO. [Investigation of mechanisms of action of growth factors of autologous platelet-rich plasma used to treat erectile dysfunction]. Urologiia. 2017;(4):46–8. https://pubmed.ncbi.nlm.nih.gov/28952692/. Accessed 4 Nov 2021.

41. Soebadi MA, Moris L, Castiglione F, Weyne E, Albersen M. Advances in stem cell research for the treatment of male sexual dysfunctions. Curr Opin Urol. 2016;26:129–39. https://doi.org/10.1097/MOU.0000000000000255.

42. Castiglione F, Albersen M, Hedlund P, Gratzke C, Salonia A, Giuliano F. Current pharmacological management of premature ejaculation: a systematic review and meta-analysis. Eur Urol. 2016;69:904–16. https://doi.org/10.1016/j.eururo.2015.12.028.

43. Haahr MK, Jensen CH, Toyserkani NM, Andersen DC, Damkier P, Sørensen JA, Sheikh SP, Lund L. A 12-month follow-up after a single intracavernous injection of autologous adipose-derived regenerative cells in patients with erectile dysfunction following radical prostatectomy: an open-label phase I clinical trial. Urology. 2018;121:203.e6–13. https://doi.org/10.1016/J.UROLOGY.2018.06.018.

44. Haahr MK, Jensen CH, Toyserkani NM, Andersen DC, Damkier P, Sørensen JA, Lund L, Sheikh SP. Safety and potential effect of a single intracavernous injection of autologous adipose-derived regenerative cells in patients with erectile dysfunction following radical prostatectomy: an open-label phase I clinical trial. EBioMedicine. 2016;5:204–10. https://doi.org/10.1016/J.EBIOM.2016.01.024.

45. Yiou R, Hamidou L, Birebent B, Bitari D, Le Corvoisier P, Contremoulins I, Rodriguez A, Augustin D, Roudot-Thoraval F, De la Taille A, Rouard H. Intracavernous injections of bone marrow mononucleated cells for postradical prostatectomy erectile dysfunction: final results of the INSTIN clinical trial. Eur Urol Focus. 2017;3:643–5. https://doi.org/10.1016/J.EUF.2017.06.009.

46. Yiou R, Hamidou L, Birebent B, Bitari D, Lecorvoisier P, Contremoulins I, Khodari M, Rodriguez A-M, Augustin D, Roudot-Thoraval F, de la Taille A, Rouard H. Safety of intracavernous bone marrow-mononuclear cells for postradical prostatectomy erectile dysfunction: an open dose-escalation pilot study. Eur Urol. 2016;69:988–91. https://doi.org/10.1016/J.EURURO.2015.09.026.

47. Al Demour S, Jafar H, Adwan S, AlSharif A, Alhawari H, Alrabadi A, Zayed A, Jaradat A, Awidi A. Safety and potential therapeutic effect of two intracavernous autologous bone marrow derived mesenchymal stem cells injections in diabetic patients with erectile dysfunction: an open label phase I clinical trial. Urol Int. 2018;101:358–65. https://doi.org/10.1159/000492120.

48. Soebadi MA, Milenkovic U, Weyne E, Castiglione F, Albersen M. Stem cells in male sexual dysfunction: are we getting somewhere? Sex Med Rev. 2017;5:222–35. https://doi.org/10.1016/j.sxmr.2016.11.002.

49. Levy JA, Marchand M, Iorio L, Cassini W, Zahalsky MP. Determining the feasibility of managing erectile dysfunction in humans with placental-derived stem cells. J Am Osteopath Assoc. 2016;116:e1–5. https://doi.org/10.7556/JAOA.2016.007.

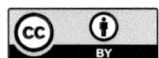

Fabrizio Palumbo, Francesco Sebastiani,
Alessandro Procacci, Nicola D'Altilia,
Anna Ricapito, and Luigi Cormio

6.1 Introduction

Peyronie's disease (PD), also known as *induration penis plastica* (IPP), is a clinical condition characterized by the formation of fibrotic plaques onto the tunica albuginea of the penis, which may result into abnormal penile curvature and deformity, erectile dysfunction (ED), and loss of penile length. The combination of these events may result in the impossibility of performing penetrative intercourse [1].

PD is thought to be a form of connective tissue disease deriving from excessive scarring of the tunica albuginea or of the septum of the corpora cavernosa as a reaction to penile trauma; nevertheless, not all patients recall such episodes when reporting their clinical history [2]. Patients suffering from PD most commonly present diabetes, hypertension, hyperlipidemia as comorbidities and smoking, sexually transmitted diseases, and genital tract surgery as risk factors [3].

PD is not rare even though its occurrence is probably underreported. Indeed, its prevalence has been reported ranging between 0.4% and 7% [4] and up to 16% in the subset of patients undergone radical prostatectomy [5]. PD may be an incidental finding in asymptomatic patients or diagnosed in patients with acquired penile curvature or/and ED, taking a complete medical and andrological history and a focused physical examination of the penile shaft. The correct assessment of the entity of the penile curvature and deformity, as well as of erectile function, especially prior to a planned surgical treatment, requires the evaluation of the penis during erection. So, intracavernous injection and penile Doppler ultrasonography (PDUS) [6] represent the gold-standard diagnostic evaluation.

F. Palumbo · F. Sebastiani · A. Procacci
Department of Urology, Di Venere Hospital,
Bari, Italy

N. D'Altilia
Department of Urology and Renal Transplantation,
Policlinico Riuniti di Foggia, University of Foggia,
Foggia, Italy

A. Ricapito
Department of Urology and Organ Transplantation,
"Policlinico Riuniti", University of Foggia, Foggia,
Italy

L. Cormio (✉)
Department of Urology and Andrology, University of
Foggia, "L. Bonomo" Teaching Hospital Andria,
Andria, Italy

6.2 Pathophysiology

Although PD was first described by the French surgeon Francois Gigot de la Peyronie in 1743 [7], its pathophysiology remains under investigation. The progression of the disease seems to reflect an alteration of the physiological balance between fibrosis and fibrinolysis in tissue repair processes, resulting in the formation of fibrotic

© The Author(s) 2023
C. Bettocchi et al. (eds.), *Practical Clinical Andrology*,
https://doi.org/10.1007/978-3-031-11701-5_6

plaques [8]. The underlying mechanisms are thought not to be exclusive to PD, given a significant overlap in pathology, occurrence, and epidemiology between PD and other localized fibrosing afflictions such as Dupuytren and Ledderhose disease [9].

PD evolution includes two distinct phases: the acute phase is defined by the presence of inflammation and pain, while the chronic phase mainly leads to fibrosis and calcification, with resolution of pain and stabilization of penile deformity [10].

The acute phase is believed to be triggered by microtrauma delivered to the penile tunica albuginea, most commonly during sexual activity. The structure of the tunica albuginea is damaged through delamination of fascial layers. This results in a release of pro-inflammatory mediators (TGF-β, IL-1, FGF, PDGF, PAI-1 as well as reactive oxygen species) involved in wound healing which generate platelet aggregation, clot formation, and local recruitment of inflammatory cells [11]. Alterations in the levels of growth factors and cytokines released in these instances are responsible for the imbalance between extracellular matrix (ECM) deposition, myofibroblast proliferation, and myofibroblast apoptosis which is at the core of this phase [12].

The altered repair processes of the first phase result in the formation of dense fibrotic plaques which may also progress to calcification, stabilizing, or worsening the penile curvature [13]. The bone-like nature of the calcified tissue is thought to be due to the recruitment of osteoblast-like cells from the vascular lumen or to the up-regulation of the osteoblast-specific factor 1 gene [14, 15]. Cavernosal hypoxia is also considered as a possible explanation for the aberrations in local collagen deposition, such as those found in patients who underwent radical prostatectomy and developed PD afterwards [16].

Current knowledge on the matter of molecular pathways of inflammation and fibrosis still seems not enough clear. Indeed, penile trauma does not always result in PD [17], and PD patients do not always have a history of penile trauma. This fact, along with an uneven prevalence across ethnicities and the noted correlations with other fibroproliferative diseases, has prompted research in genetics, mainly in the fields of HLA group antigens, autoimmunity, single nucleotide polymorphisms and karyotype aberrations. Nevertheless, results in this field have been inconclusive [18].

6.3 Epidemiology

PD shows variable rates of occurrence depending on country of origin and age group. Its reported prevalence in general male population ranges between 0.4% and 7%, but is likely to be underestimated due to underreporting [4]. As for ethnic differences, the reported prevalence is 0.4–3.2% of men in the United States [19], as opposed to 0.6% of Japanese men [20]. Indeed, it seems to be more frequent in Caucasians [21].

PD distribution also changes with age. A large study performed in Germany on over 8000 patients by administration of a questionnaire showed that PD prevalence was 1.5% in 30–39 year-old males, 3.0% in 40–59 year-old males, 4.0% in 60–69 year-old males, and 6.5% in men older than 70 years [19]. It is worth mentioning that PD can also occur in teenagers (15–19 years old), often causing high emotional distress levels and more commonly appearing with an increased number of plaques at presentation [22].

Comorbidities associated with PD include diabetes [23], smoking [24], and Dupuytren's disease [25]. Patients suffering from diabetes seem more prone to experience severe PD [23]. Hypertension and hyperlipidemia have been inconstantly associated with PD [24] while there seems to be a strong link between obesity and PD [26]. Penile trauma, both deriving from sexual activity or iatrogenic in nature (catheterization, cystoscopy, and TURP) is the most reported risk factor for PD [24, 27] reaching a 16% incidence in men having undergone radical prostatectomy for prostate cancer (16%) [5].

6.4 Clinical Presentation and Medical Evaluation

PD patients usually seek medical evaluation because of penile pain during the erection, penile bending or complex deformity, loss of penile length, and presence of palpable areas of induration on the penile shaft [28]. Patients may come to the attention of the specialist during the acute phase, in which penile pain and progressive deformity are the main complaints, or during the chronic phase, in which pain is mostly absent and complaints include penile deformities and the impossibility of having regular penetrative intercourse due to excessive bending or penile structural instability [2]. Erectile dysfunction is also present in up to half of men with PD, though it is still object of debate whether PD is a cause of ED or the other way around [29].

PD may generate a significant psychological distress in the affected patient leading to depression, anxiety, avoidance, and lowered self-esteem in intimate situations, partner and relationship problems, and dissatisfaction with sexual activity [30].

History and physical examination are needed to a correct diagnosis and evaluation of PD [31]. History taking should include past medical occurrences and identification of known PD risk factors such as penile trauma, palmar or plantar fibrosis, diabetes, hypertension, and smoking habit. The patient should be asked about the presence or absence of penile pain, and time of deformity onset or eventual stability in order to initially define whether the disease is in an acute or chronic phase. There are specific questionnaires which may aid the specialist in keeping track of all valuable information, such as the Peyronie's disease questionnaire (PDQ) [32]. Other ancillary questionnaires such as the International Index of Erectile Function (IIEF) or Erection Hardness Score (EHS) may prove useful in objectively assessing the sexual function of the patient [2].

Laboratory testing may turn useful in identifying underlying diseases related to PD and ED; they include a complete blood count, a glucose and lipid profile, and total testosterone [33]. Given the usual patients' age, it is worth assessing also serum Prostate-specific Antigen (PSA).

When performing a physical examination in a patient with suspected PD, the focus should be on the penile shaft with palpatory assessment of deformities and areas of abnormal consistency or plaques. The examination should be carried out along the entire length of the shaft, from the pubis to the glans, and may include a Stretched Penile Length (SPL) measurement in the usual fashion—from the pubis to the coronal sulcus—for future reference [2].

The objective evaluation of the degree and entity of the penile curvature or deformity necessitates measurements to be taken when the penis is erect. Patient-provided self-photographs are a viable solution but the quality of the images may be insufficient, leading to incorrect assessments [34]. This may be of utmost importance in patients seeking active curative interventions, in which accurate evaluation of penile deformity is required to choose the correct therapeutic strategy. In-office intracavernous administration (ICI) of an erectogenic agent allows a specialist to perform objective assessment not only of erectile function but also of penile curvature, for example, with the aid of a goniometer, establishing the point of maximum curvature, the degree of penile torsion, and the presence of indentation, hourglass deformity, or "hinge" effect in the case of a planned surgical intervention [31].

As for imaging in PD evaluation, PDUS may aid in the detection and measurement of plaques and their size, although it is often inaccurate and operator-dependent [35]. Most importantly, it can be useful prior to treatment in order to assess penile hemodynamics, especially in the presence of ED. Information obtained through PDUS can be useful for the specialist when selecting the best therapeutic approach while correctly managing the patient's expectations [36].

The other available imaging techniques are not suitable for everyday clinical practice and anyway are all considered inferior to in-office US. Computed Tomography (CT) allows for good visualization of calcified penile plaques, but it is less useful in non-calcified plaques and in the evaluation of soft tissue and degree of inflammation. It is also expensive in terms of time and resources. Magnetic Resonance Imaging (MRI) is the best instrument when needing to visualize soft tissue, areas of inflammations, and non-calcified plaques but its high cost of money, time, and resources far outweighs its benefits [37].

6.5   Non-surgical Treatment for Peyronie's Disease

The main objective of conservative treatment is to prevent disease progression and relieve pain in patients in early stage or in patients who decline other treatments during the active phase.

Non-surgical treatments are as follows: oral medications, topical medications, traction therapy, extracorporeal shock wave therapy, electromotive drugs, intralesional injections, and vacuum erection device. There are several studies on conservative treatments and often their results are contradictory, not allowing to provide recommendations in real life.

6.5.1   Oral Medications

6.5.1.1 Phosphodiesterase Type 5 Inhibitors (PDE5is)

PDE5is are thought to reduce collagen deposition and increase apoptotic index through the inhibition of TFG-b1 [38, 39].

In a retrospective study, PDE5is were administered to 65 patients with penile septal scars; the results showed that those who received therapy had improvement in erectile function, in the reduction of the curvature and resolution of scars (69%) [40]. Unfortunately, there is no prospective RCT that compares PDE5is with placebo.

6.5.1.2 Nonsteroidal Anti-inflammatory Drugs (NSAIDs)

NSAIDs should be offered in active phase of PD to manage penile pain.

6.5.1.3 Coenzime Q10

Coenzime Q10 is hypothesized to prevent the accumulation of free radicals and scar formation in acute PD. One RCT compared Q10 with placebo and found a statistically significant improvement in erectile function and reduction in mean plaque size (40%) in patients to whom was administered Q10. The EAU does not support this treatment.

6.5.1.4 Vitamin E

Vitamin E has antioxidant activity and is hypothesized to have antifibrotic effect reducing circulating free radicals. Vitamin E lacks sufficient evidence. One clinical trial compared Vitamin E with placebo: the results indicated that there was no statistically significant reduction in angulation, pain, or plaque size [41]. The EAU Panel does not support it because of its lack of efficacy.

6.5.1.5 Colchicine

Colchicine is thought to have antifibrotic effects by activating collagenase production and preventing collagen synthesis [42]. Unfortunately, the only RCT available that compares colchicine with placebo does not show significant reductions in angulation, pain, or plaque size [43]. The EAU panel does not support it because of its lack of efficacy.

6.5.1.6 Para-aminobenzoacidic Potassium (POTABA)

POTABA has anti-inflammatory and antifibrotic effects [44]. It is suggested that POTABA can reduce collagen formation. There is only one RCT which concluded that POTABA may reduce plaque size compared to placebo, with no improvement in penile curvature [45]. POTABA has a large amount of side effects; the most common is gastrointestinal distress. The evidence of this treatment is weak, in fact the EAU Panel does not support it.

6.5.1.7 Carnitine

Carnitine has an anti-inflammatory and antifibrotic effect. One RCT compared Carnitine with placebo and found no statistical differences in penile angulation, pain, or plaque size. The EAU Panel does not support this oral medication because of its lack of evidence.

6.5.1.8 Tamoxifen

Tamoxifen is thought to reduce fibrogenesis by increasing the TGF-Beta concentration. The only one RCT that compared tamoxifen with placebo found no statistical difference in penile angulation and pain [46]. Because of its lack of efficacy, the EAU Panel does not recommend tamoxifen for PD.

6.5.2 Topical Medications

There isn't enough scientific evidence that topical treatments (Verapamil, H-100 Gel) applied to the penile shaft with or without iontophoresis can be absorbed by the tunica albuginea and change the course of PD. The EAU Panel in fact does not support this type of treatment for PD.

6.5.3 Extracorporeal Shock Wave Therapy (ESWT)

The exact mechanism of action of Li-ESWT is not known: it is assumed that shock waves may generate nitric oxide and increase vascular endothelial growth factor (VEGF) [47]. Four RCT and one meta-analysis assessed the efficacy of ESWT for PD: from these studies, the only consistent outcome is improvement in pain [48–51].

6.5.4 Mechanical Devices

6.5.4.1 Penile Traction Therapy

Penile traction therapy (PTT) is based on mechanotransduction, according to which stretching forces cause collagen remodeling through decreasing myofibroblast activity and upregulating matrix metalloproteinase [52, 53]. There are two prospective randomized trials on PTT [54, 55] that found improvements in curvature and in stretched penile length. The treatment can result in discomfort due to use of the device for 2–8 h daily. Side effects are generally mild, including local discomfort or glans numbness. PTT seems to be effective and safe, but it is not possible to give any definitive recommendation because of the heterogeneity of the study designs and non-standardized inclusion and exclusion criteria that not allow to draw any definitive conclusions.

6.5.4.2 Vacuum Erection Device

Vacuum erection device seems to affect intracorporeal molecular markers like TGF-b1, collagenase, hypoxia-inducible factor-1a, eNOS. There are no randomized controlled trials using VED to treat PD. The limited data available appear to support improvement in penile curvature and stretched penile length, but further investigation is needed [56].

6.5.5 Intraplaque Injection

6.5.5.1 Collagenase Clostridium Histolyticum (CCH)

CCH is a purified bacterial enzyme that degrades collagen that is the primary component of the PD plaque. In 2014, the EMA approved CCH for the nonsurgical treatment of stable phase PD in men with dorsal palpable penile plaque of 30–90°. Two trials, IMPRESS I and IMPRESS II, found improvement in curvature and PDQ scale (used to assess QoL in PD), with no change in pain or erectile function [57]. During these studies, patients underwent two injections 24–72 h apart, repeated in four treatment cycles with penile modeling. The greatest chance of curvature improvement is for curvatures between 30° and 60°, no calcification, IIEF > 17, longer duration of disease [58]. Regarding side effects, the studies have found several common mild or moderate adverse reactions localized to the penis (penile hematoma, penile pain, and penile swelling). Serious adverse events (0.9%) include penile hematoma and corporeal rupture that require surgical treatment; to avoid these adverse events, the patient should be advised to avoid sexual intercourse in the 4 weeks following injection. Recently, the company has withdrawn the product form the European market.

6.5.5.2 Interferon Alpha

IFN-alpha 2b is hypothesized to treat PD through a fibroblast proliferation decreasing. Furthermore, it seems to reduce extracellular matrix and collagen production, increasing collagenase synthesis by fibroblast [59].

One study found greater improvement in curvature and plaque size among men treated with INF-alpha 2 vs placebo [60]. Intraplaque injection with INF-alpha 2b provides a >20% reduction in curvature, regardless of plaque location. The EAU panel recommends this treatment for stable phase PD.

6.5.5.3 Calcium Channel Blockers (Verapamil, Nicardipine)

CCBs is hypothesized to inhibit calcium dependent extracellular collagen transport and to upgrade the collagenase activity [61]. FDA has not approved verapamil in the treatment of PD. One trial exists for nicardipine with promising results.

6.6 Surgical Treatment for Peyronie's Disease

Surgery represents the most effective treatment for severe penile curvature caused by Peyronie's disease. Its aim is to obtain a penis straight enough for a satisfactory intercourse while preserving sufficient rigidity.

Surgery is recommended when penile deformity and/or reduced erectile function make intercourse difficult or impossible or painful for the partner (dyspareunia). Surgery should be carried out when the disease is "stable" meaning there has been no change in the curvature over the last 6 months, otherwise the "wait and see" attitude is preferred [62, 63].

As mentioned above, dynamic penile color-Doppler sonography allows proper assessment of the integrity of arterial inflow and veno-occlusive mechanism, site and degree of curvature, penile length, and overall deformity such as hinge or hourglass. All such data are useful in choosing the ideal surgical procedure [36, 64].

Accurate patient counselling is essential to explain potential sequelae such as penile shortening, erectile dysfunction, recurrence of curvature, and palpation of stitches underneath the skin. The patient should also understand that surgery is not meant to fully restore the penis to its original shape and dimension, but rather to allow a return to satisfactory sexual intercourse [65, 66].

Based on clinical data and patient's counselling, surgery may consist in:

- Shortening procedures
- Lengthening procedures with grafting
- Penile prosthesis implant potentially associated to further manoeuvres [67]

The choice between techniques is based on curvature shape and severity as well as erectile function.

6.6.1 Tunical Shortening Procedure

Shortening procedures are offered to patients with a <60° curvature, no hinge or hourglass deformity, no erectile dysfunction, and a penis long enough not to suffer from the expected shortening [67].

Shortening procedures aim at giving the long (convex) side of the penis the same length of its short (concave) side [68].

In 1965, Nesbit described a procedure for the correction of congenital penile curvature based on an elliptical excision of the tunica albuginea of the long side of the penis at the site of the angle of greatest curvature. The tunical defect was closed with permanent sutures and additional absorbable sutures if needed [69].

Yachia proposed a modification whereby Nesbit's elliptical excision was replaced by a full-thickness longitudinal incision of the albuginea, which was then closed horizontally according to the Heineke-Mikulicz procedure. Depending on the degree of curvature, one or more incisions are needed; in any case, the incisions should be shorter than 1 cm to avoid creating a "dog ears" effect [70].

Non-incisional procedures in which tunical shortening is obtained by plication without incision have been developed to avoid any potential damage to the underlying erectile tissue. Essed and Schroder proposed tunical plication by placing non-resorbable figure-of-eight sutures that should reduce the perception of the knots at penile palpation [71]. In 2002, Gholami and Lue introduced the 16-stitch (two pairs) or 24-stitch (three pairs) procedure, depending on the length of the side of the penis and the degree of angulation of the curvature, as a different mean of plicating tunica albuginea. The rationale of this procedure was distributing tension to a greater surface area of tunica albuginea contralateral to the fibrotic plaque. They reported a 96% satisfaction rate and a 93%

straightening rate in 116 patients. In this series, the shortening rate was 41% and the estimated recurrence rate 15% [72].

In 1985, Ebbehoj and Metz proposed a plication technique in which an "introflecting" double cross-over stitch of 2/0 Prolene grasping deep into the tunica in four positions was used. The employment of an introflecting knot greatly reduced the perception of penile shaft knots by the patients: in fact, this principle has been widely adopted in following adaptations of tunical plication techniques [66].

For all procedures, the first step should be exposure of Buck's fascia. Circumcision and degloving are usually preferred but, occasionally, longitudinal penile shaft incisions may be used in patients with minor curvatures who would like to avoid circumcision. For dorsal and ventral curvatures, mobilization of urethra or neurovascular bundle, respectively, are recommended to properly expose the curvature to be treated. Artificial erection is needed throughout the procedure and is usually obtained by injection of saline into the corpora while manually compressing the crura; avoiding the use of a tourniquet at the base of the penis provides a more reliable profile of the erect penis [73].

Compared to lengthening procedures, shortening procedures require less surgical time. Shortening procedures provide good aesthetic results, reduce risk of postoperative stiffness loss, and constitute a simple and safe solution with effective straightening. The overall short- and long-term results of shortening techniques are satisfactory with surgical straightening achieved in 79–100% of patients.

Reduction of the final penile length and difficulty in correcting complex curves such as hourglass or hinge curves are considered the main disadvantages. Especially the former can sometimes lead to patients' dissatisfaction, because of subjective comparisons with the size and the shape of their penis as remembered before the development of the Peyronie's disease. Other less common complications include hematoma in up to 9%, decreased sensitivity from 4% to 21%, urethral injury in less than 2%, and phimosis in up to 5% of patients.

Additional penile shrinkage up to 17% has been reported and recurrence of significant penile curvature deformity has been reported up to 12%. In addition, eventual suture granuloma can generate pain at the affected site. The reported risk of new EDs ranges from 0% to 38% and often depends on baseline functional data.

ED can be explained by the fact that the scarring of a healthy tissue may result in anatomical and functional damage to the corpus cavernosum [74–76].

To this day, no technique has been proven clearly superior. The International Consultation on Sexual Medicine (ICSM) of 2010 states, in regard to penile shortening procedures, that there is no evidence that one surgical approach provides better results than another, but curvature correction with less risk of new EDs can be expected compared to grafting procedures [66].

6.6.2 Tunical Lengthening Procedure

Tunical lengthening procedures are suggested in case of severe curvature (>60°) without erectile dysfunction. Their goal is to incise the plaque, lengthen the short or concave side of the penis, and create a defect in the tunica which will be covered by a graft [67].

Tunical lengthening procedures include both plaque incision and graft (PIG) and plaque excision and graft (PEG). Originally, it was thought that plaques could fuel the evolution of disease, so excision was necessary for healing [36, 77]. However, important evidence emerged: the removal of the plaque enhanced the process of fibrosis of the corpora cavernosa and further damaged the delicate mechanism of the veno-occlusive system. Over time, it was realized that these were the two most important factors contributing to postoperative erectile deficit. For this reason, excision and grafting procedures were replaced by new techniques [78].

Plaque excision may be considered in those patients in whom the area of maximum deformity is excised, particularly if it is associated with severe indentation [79].

The area created by the geometric incision of the tunica albuginea should be covered with a graft. The ideal characteristics of the graft should be as similar as possible to the tissue being replaced. Although elasticity and strength summarize the two major capabilities of albuginous tissue, the ideal graft should also be readily available and not very expensive. It should be biocompatible with the target tissue to avoid excessive fibrotic reactions with low risk of infection, antigenicity, and minimal tissue reaction.

It must also be easy to suture, pliable, and compliant, resistant to intracavernous pressures exerted during erections. It should also not be too thick or too thin to avoid bulging or gap formation along the surface of the albuginea with the appearance of new shapes and/or curves after surgery [80, 81].

Several types of grafts have been proposed:

- Heterologous: of human origin but from a deceased donor, including the pericardium, fascia lata, and dura mater
- Biological xenografts: processed bovine pericardium, porcine intestinal submucosa, and porcine dermis and Tachosil® (matrix of equine collagen) [53–58]
- Autologous: taken from the individual himself, they include the dermis, vein, temporalis fascia, fascia lata, tunica vaginalis, tunica albuginea, and buccal mucosa
- Synthetic: Dacron® and Gore-Tex® [67]

Pericardial grafts have adequate thickness, resistance to traction and low risk of contracture, with lower rates of infection and rejection reactions. Many studies evidenced persistent ability to have satisfactory sexual intercourse and poor evidence of insufficient penile straightening [82].

When it comes to biological xenografts, the small intestinal submucosa graft showed similar advantages to the pericardium in terms of sexual satisfaction. This matrix contains angiogenic growth factors that are thought to promote rapid infiltration of host cells and early revascularization, serving as a scaffold for differentiation. In case of large tunica defects, though, decreased stiffness is more common, together with curve

recurrence and postoperative complications such as hematomas and infections [67, 83].

Their main disadvantages are due to cost, biocompatibility, possible infection, and immunologic responses. In addition, they may develop excessive scarring retraction with recurvatum or penile shortening and erectile deficiency on a veno-occlusive basis [84, 85].

Among biological xenografts, the novel collagen fleece synthetic graft (Tachosil®) is currently raising scientific interest. The main feature is the ease of use: application is advertised to be suture-less as the graft has self-adhesive properties. This leads to shorter operating time and reduction of the eventual risk of damaging a penile prosthesis in the case of simultaneous implantation. Retraction and scarring also have been reported to be fairly rare occurrences, but randomized comparison trials with other materials are still needed for a conclusive evaluation [67].

Autologous grafts require preparation of a second surgical site intraoperatively for graft harvest and this potentially lengthens operating room time. In addition, harvesting in the same patient is not free from possible side effects in terms of healing, aesthetic results, and lymphedema. In other cases, the extent of the harvest may be limited by the anatomical site, thus reducing the possibility of obtaining enough tissue to cover large defects [67].

Several series have reported excellent results with the use of autologous vein grafting in the short term (1 year) with a 90% satisfaction rate and a curvature correction rate of 59–96%. On the other hand, these results were not confirmed in the long term with a significant decrease in patient satisfaction after 5 years due to erectile dysfunction (22.5%) or penile shortening (35%) [86].

Buccal mucosa as an autologous graft presented extraordinary characteristics, namely, increased elasticity, best enlargement, and elongation coefficient. At an average follow-up of about 3 years, 24 out of 26 patients (92.3%) achieved complete straightening of the penis with a rate of postoperative recurvature and erectile dysfunction as low as 7.7% with a loss of penile length in 15.4% of cases [87] but plaque excision was carried out. A subsequent study pointed out plaque incision and buccal mucosa grafting was associated with 100% penile straightening, no curvature recurrence or de novo erectile dysfunction, and patient and partner satisfaction of 93.3% and 100%, respectively [88]. A subsequent study from the same authors [90] pointed out that, at mean follow-up of 62.01 ± 34.3 months (range 12-135), all of the 72 patients were able to obtain an erection (SEP-1), 97.1% to penetrate (SEP-2), and 89.7% to successfully complete intercourse (SEP-3); 80.9% of them were satisfied with erection hardness (SEP-4) and 86.8% were overall satisfied (SEP-5), with the main reason for dissatisfaction being expectation of better length and rigidity. Available evidence suggest that buccal mucosa grafting provides excellent long-term results probably due to the typical graft characteristics such as the peculiar blood support that reduces the hypoxia time of the patch. Moreover, the limited loss of elasticity reduces of the risk of fibrosis [89].

Synthetic grafts made of polyethylene terephthalate (PETE, Dacron) and polytetrafluoroethylene (PTFE, Teflon) have been used in the past showing a significant risk of inflammation and subsequent adjacent fibrosis have limited success. The hypoxic environment created inside and around synthetic grafts increases the risk of infection and possible allergic reactions [67, 90].

6.6.3 Penile Prosthesis Implant

Penile prosthesis implantation is typically reserved for the treatment of Peyronie's disease in patients with erectile dysfunction, especially when they do not respond to medical therapy [67].

Although all types of penile prostheses can be used, inflatable penile prosthesis implantation appears to be more clinically feasible in these patients. The pressure within the cylinders allows for superior curvature correction with manual shaping, as well as increased circumference [91].

According to the severity of the curvature, different procedures may take place.

In case of mild to moderate curvature (up to 30°), it may be sufficient to insert two cylinders for an excellent result, without further maneuvers [67].

In cases of severe deformity (>30°), "intraoperative shaping" of the corpora cavernosa on the inflated cylinders has been introduced as an effective treatment and if residual curvature remains, no further treatment is recommended, as the prosthesis will act as an expander leading to progressive straightening in a few months. This approach consists of achieving an erection through the prosthesis to maximum rigidity, evaluating the curvature. The system is then sealed with protected hemostats between pump and cylinders, to protect the pump from the high pressures that can occur during manual modeling. The penis is then bent in the contralateral direction to the curvature for approximately 60–90 s.

After modeling, additional liquid can be introduced into the system to evaluate the aesthetic result. Then, the procedure can be repeated until a satisfactory correction of the deformity is achieved. a gradual and progressive moderation is preferable rather than rapid and violent, to avoid lesions of the tunic and excessive traction of the neuro-vascular bundle. This is considered a first-line therapy for curvature correction after prosthetic implantation [67, 92].

The main risk is represented by urethral injuries. To reduce the likelihood of injury, the distal end of the penile shaft must be protected by the flexing hand, leaving the glans free. In this way, the apexes of the corpora cavernosa will be protected from excessive traction by the tips of the cylinders. The other hand will grasp the base of the penis to provide support to this area, reducing the likelihood of breaking the suture line.

Published reports on the use of modeling indicated that 86–100% successful straightening can be expected without a higher incidence of device revision; sensory traction deficit of the nerve bundle after manual modeling may occur but remains a potential complication that should be discussed with the patient prior to surgery [92, 93].

An alternative to manual remodeling would be plication of the contralateral tunic to correct curvature prior to prosthesis placement [94].

The tunical incision is performed with the cylinders deflated, using the low power cautery, to free the tunic with the intent of preserving the cavernous tissue over the implant. Once the incision is made, the cylinders are inflated to evaluate the correction. The modeling procedure can be repeated until the desired result is achieved.

While there is no clearly accepted approach, grafting is recommended if the incisions result in a tunical defect that measures more than 2 cm in any size to reduce scar contracture and cylinder herniation [95].

Synthetic grafts were used in the past, but porcine SIS or pericardium biological grafts are now frequently used, while the use of locally harvested dermal grafts is not recommended, because there is a risk of transferring bacteria to the prosthesis. The frequently encountered post-operative complaint is loss of length. This is particularly disabling in the Peyronie's disease population, who often already have a loss of penis length. To overcome this complication, prolonged post-operative inflation of the cylinder has been recommended to preserve the length of the penis. Furthermore, the inflated prosthesis expands the corpora cavernosa in width and favors the correction of any residual curvatures [67].

Another approach to Peyronie's disease when implanting a penile prosthesis has been proposed by Rolle and is known as "sliding technique." After degloving of dartos and isolation of neurovascular bundle, two longitudinal incisions of the tunica albuginea are carried out on the sides of the two corpora cavernosa: the first incision at 3 o'clock on the left and the second incision at 9 o'clock on the right. A dorsal semicircular incision is made to connect the upper ends of the lateral incisions, and a second semicircular ventral incision is made to connect points of the second incision. After incision and dissection of the tunica albuginea from the cavernous tissue and from the septum, traction is exerted on the glans, thus obtaining a sliding of the distal part of the penis from the proximal one. Two rectangular and bow-shaped defects of tunica albuginea remain: the first, dorsal and proximal and the second, distal and ventral. Then, two cylinders of the prosthesis can be inserted in the two corpora cavernosa and the two losses of substance are covered with two rectangular grafts of porcine small intestinal submucosa [96].

Egydio modified this technique, closing the tunical defects using Buck's fascia rather than a graft and making additional longitudinal tunical incisions to restore penile girth. This has been proven to reduce operative time and improve girth and length, but at the cost of a higher rate of hematoma formation and possible auto-inflation of inflatable prosthesis [97].

An evolution of these approaches has been developed by Egydio himself with the MUST (Multiple-Slit Technique). It consists of performing two longitudinal incisions at 3 and 9 o'clock positions on the tunica albuginea, whose ends are connected with semicircular incisions on the ventral and dorsal part of the penis. Additional semicircular incisions must be placed on the concave penile side, creating multiple small tunica defects. The innovation lies in the fact that the use of grafts to cover large tunical defects is avoided, since the size of the tunical defect is actually distributed among multiple small tunical defects. This seems to help in avoiding potential bulging and gap sensations in the affected areas. Glans necrosis, glans ischemia, and partial loss of sensitivity of glans represent the main complications [98].

References

1. Babu A, Kayes O. Recent advances in managing Peyronie's disease. F1000Res. 2020;9:F1000 Faculty Rev-381. https://doi.org/10.12688/f1000research.20557.1. PMID: 32518629; PMCID: PMC7255896.
2. Ziegelmann MJ, Bajic P, Levine LA. Peyronie's disease: contemporary evaluation and management. Int J Urol. 2020;27(6):504–16. https://doi.org/10.1111/iju.14230. Epub 2020 Apr 6. PMID: 32253786.
3. Al-Thakafi S, Al-Hathal N. Peyronie's disease: a literature review on epidemiology, genetics, pathophysiology, diagnosis and work-up. Transl Androl Urol. 2016;5(3):280–9. https://doi.org/10.21037/tau.2016.04.05. PMID: 27298774; PMCID: PMC4893516.
4. Ostrowski KA, Gannon JR, Walsh TJ. A review of the epidemiology and treatment of Peyronie's disease. Res Rep Urol. 2016;8:61–70. https://doi.org/10.2147/RRU.S65620. PMID: 27200305; PMCID: PMC4857830.
5. Dibenedetti DB, Nguyen D, Zografos L, et al. A population-based study of Peyronie's disease: prevalence and treatment patterns in the United States. Adv Urol. 2011;2011:282503.

6. Chen JY, Hockenberry MS, Lipshultz LI. Objective assessments of Peyronie's disease. Sex Med Rev. 2018;6(3):438–45. https://doi.org/10.1016/j.sxmr.2017.12.006. Epub 2018 Feb 21. PMID: 29477573.

7. Musitelli S, Bossi M, Jallous H. A brief historical survey of "Peyronie's disease". J Sex Med. 2008;5:1737–46.

8. Gonzalez-Cadavid NF, Rajfer J. Mechanisms of disease: new insights into the cellular and molecular pathology of Peyronie's disease. Nat Clin Pract Urol. 2005;2(6):291–7. https://doi.org/10.1038/ncpuro0201.

9. Patel DP, Christensen MB, Hotaling JM, Pastuszak AW. A review of inflammation and fibrosis: implications for the pathogenesis of Peyronie's disease. World J Urol. 2020;38(2):253–61. https://doi.org/10.1007/s00345-019-02815-6. Epub 2019 Jun 12. PMID: 31190155; PMCID: PMC7333524.

10. Di Maida F, Cito G, Lambertini L, Valastro F, Morelli G, Mari A, Carini M, Minervini A, Cocci A. The natural history of Peyronie's disease. World J Mens Health. 2020;39:399. https://doi.org/10.5534/wjmh.200065. PMID: 32648381.

11. Lue TF. Peyronie's disease: an anatomically-based hypothesis and beyond. Int J Impot Res. 2002;14(5):411–3. https://doi.org/10.1038/sj.ijir.3900876.

12. Wynn TA. Cellular and molecular mechanisms of fibrosis. J Pathol. 2008;214(2):199–210. https://doi.org/10.1002/path.2277.

13. Levine L, Rybak J, Corder C, Farrel MR. Peyronie's disease plaque calcification–prevalence, time to identification, and development of a new grading classification. J Sex Med. 2013;10:3121–8.

14. Devine CJ Jr. International conference on Peyronie's disease advances in basic and clinical research. March 17–19, 1993. Introduction. J Urol. 1997;157:272–5.

15. Gonzalez-Cadavid NF, Magee TR, Ferrini M, Qian A, Vernet D, Rajfer J. Gene expression in Peyronie's disease. Int J Impot Res. 2002;14:361–74.

16. Tal R, Heck M, Teloken P, Siegrist T, Nelson CJ, Mulhall JP. Peyronie's disease following radical prostatectomy: incidence and predictors. J Sex Med. 2010;7:1254–61.

17. Zargooshi J. Trauma as the cause of Peyronie's disease: penile fracture as a model of trauma. J Urol. 2004;172:186–8. https://doi.org/10.1097/01.ju.0000132144.71458.86.

18. Gabrielsen JS. Peyronie's disease: is it genetic or not? Transl Androl Urol. 2020;9(Suppl 2):S262–8. https://doi.org/10.21037/tau.2019.10.21. PMID: 32257867; PMCID: PMC7108984.

19. Schwarzer U, Sommer F, Klotz T, Braun M, Reifenrath B, Engelmann U. The prevalence of Peyronie's disease: results of a large survey. BJU Int. 2001;88(7):727–30. https://doi.org/10.1046/j.1464-4096.2001.02436.x. PMID: 11890244.

20. Shiraishi K, Shimabukuro T, Matsuyama H. The prevalence of Peyronie's disease in Japan: a study in men undergoing maintenance hemodialysis and routine health checks. J Sex Med. 2012;9:2716–23.

21. Rhoden EL, Riedner CE, Fuchs SC, Fuchs S, Ribeiro EP, Halmenschlager G. A cross-sectional study for the analysis of clinical, sexual and laboratory conditions associated to Peyronie's disease. J Sex Med. 2010;7(4 pt 1):1529–37.

22. Tal R, Hall MS, Alex B, Choi J, Mulhall JP. Peyronie's disease in teenagers. J Sex Med. 2012;9(1):302–8. https://doi.org/10.1111/j.1743-6109.2011.02502.x. Epub 2011 Oct 7. PMID: 21981606.

23. Kendirci M, Trost L, Sikka SC, Hellstrom WJG. Diabetes mellitus is associated with severe Peyronie's disease. BJU Int. 2007;99:383–6.

24. Bjekic MD, Vlajinac HD, Sipetic SB, Marinkovic JM. Risk factors for Peyronie's disease: a case-control study. BJU Int. 2006;97:570–4.

25. Nugteren HM, Nijman JM, de Jong IJ, van Driel MF. The association between Peyronie's and Dupuytren's disease. Int J Impot Res. 2011;23(4):142–5.

26. Segundo A, Glina S. Prevalence, risk factors, and erectile dysfunction associated with Peyronie's disease among men seeking urological care. Sex Med. 2020;8(2):230–6. https://doi.org/10.1016/j.esxm.2019.11.002. Epub 2020 Jan 30. PMID: 32007472; PMCID: PMC7261680.

27. Chung E, Ralph D, Kagioglu A. Evidence-based management guidelines on Peyronie's disease. J Sex Med. 2016;13:905–23.

28. Chung PH, Han TM, Rudnik B, Das AK. Peyronie's disease: what do we know and how do we treat it? Can J Urol. 2020;27(S3):11–9. PMID: 32875997.

29. Burri A, Porst H. The relationship between penile deformity, age, psychological bother, and erectile dysfunction in a sample of men with Peyronie's disease (PD). Int J Impot Res. 2018;30(4):171–8. https://doi.org/10.1038/s41443-018-0029-3. Epub 2018 May 25. PMID: 29795530.

30. Goldstein I, Hartzell R, Shabsigh R. The impact of Peyronie's disease on the patient: gaps in our current understanding. J Sex Marital Ther. 2016;42(2):178–90. https://doi.org/10.1080/0092623X.2014.985351. Epub 2015 Jan 9. PMID: 25405853.

31. EAU Guidelines. Edn. presented at the EAU Annual Congress Milan 2021. ISBN 978-94-92671-13-4.

32. Serefoglu EC, Smith TM, Kaufman GJ, Liu G, Yafi FA, Hellstrom WJG. Factors associated with erectile dysfunction and the Peyronie's disease questionnaire in patients with Peyronie disease. Urology. 2017;107:155–60. https://doi.org/10.1016/j.urology.2017.05.029. Epub 2017 May 26. PMID: 28554517.

33. Allen MS, Walter EE. Erectile dysfunction: an umbrella review of meta-analyses of risk-factors, treatment, and prevalence outcomes. J Sex Med. 2019;16(4):531–41. https://doi.org/10.1016/j.jsxm.2019.01.314. Epub 2019 Mar 2. PMID: 30833150.

34. Nascimento B, Cerqueira I, Miranda EP, Bessa J Jr, Ivanovic RF, Guglielmetti G, Nahas WC, Srougi M, Chiesa GAE, Cury J. Impact of camera deviation on penile curvature assessment using 2D pictures. J Sex

Med. 2018;15(11):1638–44. https://doi.org/10.1016/j.jsxm.2018.08.017. PMID: 30415815.

35. McCauley JF, et al. Diagnostic utility of penile ultrasound in Peyronie's disease. World J Urol. 2020;38:263.

36. Kadioglu A, et al. Color Doppler ultrasound assessment of penile vascular system in men with Peyronie's disease. Int J Impot Res. 2000;12(5):263–7.

37. Parmar M, Masterson JM, Masterson TA 3rd. The role of imaging in the diagnosis and management of Peyronie's disease. Curr Opin Urol. 2020;30(3):283–9. https://doi.org/10.1097/MOU.0000000000000754. PMID: 32205808.

38. Ferrini MG, et al. Effects of long-term vardenafil treatment on the development of fibrotic plaques in a rat model of Peyronie's disease. BJU Int. 2006;97:625.

39. Ilg MM, et al. Phosphodiesterase type 5 inhibitors and selective estrogen receptor modulators can prevent but not reverse myofibroblast transformation in Peyronie's disease. J Sex Med. 2020;17:1848.

40. Chung E, Deyoung L, Brock GB. The role of PDE5 inhibitors in penile septal scar remodeling: assessment of clinical and radiological outcomes. J Sex Med. 2011;8:1472–7.

41. Safarinejad MR, Hosseini SY, Kolahi AA. Comparison of vitamin E and propionyl-L-carnitine, separately or in combination, in patients with early chronic Peyronie's disease: a double-blind, placebo controlled, randomized study. J Urol. 2007;178:1398–403.

42. Akkus E, Carrier S, Rehman J, et al. Is colchicine effective in Peyronie's disease? A pilot study. Urology. 1994;44:291–5.

43. Safarinejad MR. Therapeutic effects of colchicine in the management of Peyronie's disease: a randomized double-blind, placebo-controlled study. Int J Impot Res. 2004;16:238–43.

44. Zarafonetis CJ, Horrax TM. Treatment of Peyronie's disease with potassium para-aminobenzoate (potaba). J Urol. 1959;81:770–2.

45. Weidner W, Hauck EW, Schnitker J. Potassium Para-aminobenzoate (POTABATM) in the treatment of Peyronie's disease: a prospective, placebo-controlled, randomized study. Eur Urol. 2005;47:530–53.

46. Teloken C, Rhoden EL, Grazziotin TM, et al. Tamoxifen versus placebo in the treatment of Peyronie's disease. J Urol. 1999;162:2003–5.

47. Frairia R, Berta L. Biological effects of extracorporeal shock waves on fibroblasts. A review. Muscles Ligaments Tendons J. 2011;1:138–47.

48. Palmieri A, et al. A first prospective, randomized, double-blind, placebo-controlled clinical trial evaluating extracorporeal shock wave therapy for the treatment of Peyronie's disease. Eur Urol. 2009;56:363.

49. Chitale S, et al. Limited shock wave therapy vs sham treatment in men with Peyronie's disease: results of a prospective randomized controlled double-blind trial. BJU Int. 2010;106:1352.

50. Hatzichristodoulou G, et al. Extracorporeal shock wave therapy in Peyronie's disease: results of a placebo-controlled, prospective, randomized, single-blind study. J Sex Med. 2013;10:2815.

51. Gao L, et al. A meta-analysis of extracorporeal shock wave therapy for Peyronie's disease. Int J Impot Res. 2016;28:161.

52. Gelbard M. Myofibroblasts and mechanotransduction: do forces in the tunica albuginea contribute to Peyronie's disease? J Sex Med. 2008;5:2974.

53. Chung E, et al. Peyronie's disease and mechanotransduction: an in vitro analysis of the cellular changes to Peyronie's disease in a cell-culture strain system. J Sex Med. 2013;10:1259.

54. Moncada I, Krishnappa P, Romero J, et al. Penile traction therapy with the new device "Penimaster PRO" is effective and safe in the stable phase of Peyronie's disease: a controlled multicentre study. BJU Int. 2019;123:694–702.

55. Ziegelmann M, Savage J, Toussi A, et al. Outcomes of a novel penile traction device in men with Peyronie's disease: a randomized, single-blind, controlled trial. J Urol. 2019;202:599–610.

56. Raheem AA, et al. The role of vacuum pump therapy to mechanically straighten the penis in Peyronie's disease. BJU Int. 2010;106:1178.

57. Gelbard M, Goldstein I, Hellstrom WJG, et al. Clinical efficacy, safety and tolerability of collagenase clostridium histolyticum for the treatment of peyronie disease in 2 large double-blind, randomized, placebo controlled phase 3 studies. J Urol. 2013;190:199–207.

58. Masterson TA, et al. Characteristics predictive of response to collagenase clostridium histolyticum for Peyronie's disease: a review of the literature. World J Urol. 2020;38(2):279–85.

59. Duncan MR, Berman B, Nseyo UO. Regulation of the proliferation and biosynthetic activities of cultured human Peyronie's disease fibroblasts by interferons-alpha, -beta and -gamma. Scand J Urol Nephrol. 1991;25:89–94.

60. Hellstrom WJG, Kendirci M, Matern R, et al. Single-blind, multicenter, placebo controlled, parallel study to assess the safety and efficacy of intralesional interferon alpha-2B for minimally invasive treatment for Peyronie's disease. J Urol. 2006;176:394–8.

61. Levine LA, Merrick PF, Lee RC. Intralesional verapamil injection for the treatment of Peyronie's disease. J Urol. 1994;151:1522–4.

62. Htzimouratidis K. EAU guidelines on penile curvature. Eur Urol. 2012;62(3):543–52.

63. Levine LA. Surgery for Peyronie's disease. Asian J Androl. 2013;15(1):27–34.

64. Porst H. Standards for clinical trials in male sexual dysfunctions. J Sex Med. 2010;7(1):414–44.

65. Wein AJ, Kavoussi LR, Partin AW, Peters CA. "Campbell-Walsh Urology: 4-Volume Set (11th Ed.)". Faculty Bookshelf. 2016:69. https://doi.org/9781455775675.

66. Ralph D, Gonzalez-Cadavid N, Mirone V, Perovic S, Sohn M, Usta M, Levine L. The management of Peyronie's disease: evidence-based 2010 guidelines. J Sex Med. 2010;7(7):2359-74. https://doi.org/10.1111/

j.1743-6109.2010.01850.x. Epub 2010 May 19. PMID:20497306.

67. EAU guidelines. 2021.

68. Syed AH. Nesbit procedure for disabling Peyronie's curvature: a median follow-up of 84 months. Urology. 2003;61:999–1003.

69. Nesbit RM. Congenital curvature of the phallus: report of three cases with description of corrective operation. J Urol. 1965;93:230–2.

70. Yachia D. Modified corporoplasty for the treatment of penile curvature. J Urol. 1990;1443(1):80–2.

71. Essed E. New surgical treatment for Peyronie's disease. Urology. 1985;25(6):582–7.

72. Ghoami SS. Correction of penile curvature using the 16-dot plication technique: a review of 132 patients. J Urol. 2002;167:2066–9.

73. Yosef B. Midline forsal plication technique for penile curvature repair. J Urol. 2004;172:1368–9.

74. Van Der Horst C. Treatment of penile curvature with Essed-Schroder tunical plication: aspects of quality of life from patients' perspective. BJU. 2004;93:105–9.

75. Larsen AM. Surgery for Peyronie's disease. Asian J Androl. 2013;15:27–34.

76. Ding S. A novel modification for tunical plication by plaque thinning: long-term results in treating penile curvature of Peyronie's disease. Int Urol Nephrol. 2010;42:597–602.

77. Kndirci M. Critical analysis of surgery for Peyronie's disease. Curr Opin Urol. 2004;14:381–8.

78. Dalton B. Venoenic impotence followin dermal graft repair for Peyronie's disease. J Urol. 1991;146:849–51.

79. Levine LA. Partial plaque excision and grafting (PEG) for Peyronie's disease. J Sex Med. 2011;8:1842–5.

80. Carson C. Outcomes of surgical treatment of Peyronie's disease. BJU Int. 2014;113(5):704–13.

81. Kadioglu A. Graft materials in Peyronie's disease surgery: a comprehensive review. J Sex Rev. 2007;4:581–95.

82. Chun J. A comparsion of dermal and cadaveric pericardial grafts in the modified Horton-Devine procedure for Peyronie's disease. J Urol. 2001;166(1):185–8.

83. Voytik-Harbin S. Identification of extractable growth factors from small intestinal submucosa. J Cell Biochem. 1997;67:478–91.

84. Nagele U. In vitro investigations of tissue-engineered multilayered urothelium established from bladder washings. Eur Urol. 2008;54(6):1414–22.

85. Breyer BN. Complications of porcine small intestine submucosa graft for Peyronie's disease. J Urol. 2007;177(2):589–91.

86. El-Sakka AL. Effect of incision and saphenous vein grafting for Peyronie's disease on penile length and sexual satisfaction. J Urol. 2001;166:1769–73.

87. Kakonashivili A. Substitution of tunica albuginea penis by different autotransplant: an experimental study. Georgian Med News. 2003;10:38–42.

88. Combined Plaque Incision, Buccal Mucosa Grafting, and Additional Tunica Albuginea Plication for Peyronie's Disease, Cormio et al., Sex Med, 2019 - https://doi.org/10.1016/j.esxm.2018.11.002.

89. Cormio L. Combined plaque incision, buccal mucosa grafting and additional tunica albuginea plication for Peyronie's disease*ex*. Sex Med Rev. 2019;7(1):48–53.

90. Bokarica P. Surgical treatment of Peyronie's disease based on penile length and degree of curvature. Int J Impot. 2005;17:170–4.

91. Montorsi F. AMS CX 700 inflatable penile implants for Peyronie's disease: functional results, morbidity and patient-partner satisfaction. Int J Impot Res. 1996;8(2):81–5.

92. Wilson S. Long-term follow-up of treatment for Peyronie's disease: modeling the penis over an inflatable penile prosthesis. J Urol. 2001;165(3):825–9.

93. Montague D. AMS 3-piece inflatable penile prosthesis implantation in men with Peyronie's disease: comparison of CX and Ultrex cylinders. J Urol. 1996;156:1633–5.

94. Rahman N. Combined penile plication surgery and insertion of penile prosthesis for severe penile curvature and erectile dysfunction. J Urol. 2004;171:2346–8.

95. Levine LA. Inflatable penile prosthesis placement in men with Peyronie's disease and drug-resistant erectile dysfunction: a single-centre study. J Sex Med. 2010;7:3775–83.

96. Rolle L. A new, innovative, lengthening surgical procedure for Peyronie disease by penile prosthesis implantation with double dorsal-ventral patch graft: the "sliding technique". J Sex Med. 2012;9:2389–95.

97. Hegydio P. Penile lengthening and widening without grafting according to a modified "sliding" technique. BJUI. 2015;116:965–72.

98. Egydio P. The multiple-slit technique (MUST) for penile length and girth restoration. J Sex Med. 2017;15:261–9.

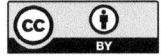

Federico Belladelli, Edoardo Pozzi,
Giuseppe Fallara, Paolo Capogrosso,
and Andrea Salonia

7.1 Anatomy and Physiology of Orgasm and Ejaculation

There is no standard definition of orgasm, although it has been defined as an intense transient peak sensation of pleasure alternating the state of consciousness and associated with reported physical changes. It is commonly combined with ejaculation [1] although the experience of orgasm is a distinct cortical event, associated with the perception of striated muscle contractions and resulting in semen expelled during ejaculation, mediated through sensory neurons in the pelvic region. During orgasm, hyperventilation up to 40 breaths/min, tachycardia, and high blood pressure could occur [1]. Both ejaculation and orgasm are based on a complex interplay between the central nervous system and the peripheral nervous system, with the involvement of several neurotransmitters, thus including dopamine, norepinephrine, serotonin, acetylcholine, gamma-aminobutyric acid (GABA), and nitric oxide (NO) [2]; moreover,

hormonal pathways may influence the process of ejaculation with an active role played by oxytocin, prolactin, thyroid hormones, glucocorticoids, and sexual steroid hormones [2]. Different studies using positron emission tomography (PET) have identified areas of activation in the brain during orgasm. Primary intense activation areas are noted to be in the mesodiencephalic transition zones, which include the midline, the zona incerta, ventroposterior and intralaminar thalamic nuclei, the lateral segmental central field, the suprafascicular nucleus, and the ventral tegmental area. Strong increases were seen in the cerebellum. Decreases were noted at the entorhinal cortex and the amygdala [3]. In men, a period of inhibition normally follows orgasm, called the refractory period. This is a poorly understood phenomenon, with some investigators suggesting a central rather than spinal mechanism to be involved [4].

Ejaculation is a different physiological process mainly under the regulation of the autonomic nervous system. It consists of two main phases: emission and expulsion. The first step in the emission phase is the closure of bladder neck to prevent retrograde spillage of the seminal fluid into the bladder. This is followed by the ejection of prostatic secretions, mixed with spermatozoa from the vas deferens into the prostatic urethra [5]. The organs involved in the ejaculation process receive dense autonomic nerve supply, both sympathetic and parasympathetic, from the pelvic plexus. The sympathetic neurons play the pre-

---

F. Belladelli · E. Pozzi · G. Fallara · A. Salonia (✉)
Division of Experimental Oncology/Unit of Urology,
URI-Urological Research Institute, IRCCS Ospedale
San Raffaele, Milan, Italy

University Vita-Salute San Raffaele, Milan, Italy
e-mail: salonia.andrea@hsr.it

P. Capogrosso
Department of Urology and Andrology, Ospedale di
Circolo and Macchi Foundation, Varese, Italy

© The Author(s) 2023
C. Bettocchi et al. (eds.), *Practical Clinical Andrology*,
https://doi.org/10.1007/978-3-031-11701-5_7

dominant role in the ejaculation process. Input from genital stimulation is integrated at the neural sacral spinal level to produce emission [6]. The emission phase of ejaculation is also under a considerable cerebral control, and can be induced through physical or visual erotic stimulation [7]. Expulsion follows emission and refers to the ejection of semen through the urethral meatus. The semen is propelled through a number of rhythmic contractions of the pelvic striated muscles in addition to the bulbospongiosus and ischiocavernosus muscles [1]. To achieve antegrade semen expulsion, the bladder neck remains closed, whereas the external urethral sphincter is open.

7.2 Premature Ejaculation (PE)

7.2.1 Aetiology

The International Society for Sexual Medicine (ISSM) elaborated the most comprehensive and widely considered definition of PE, which indeed is defined as a male sexual dysfunction where ejaculation always or almost always occurs prior to or within about 1 min of penetration. It is a condition characterized by the inability to delay ejaculation during sexual activity all (or nearly all) of the time, that causes personal distress and may even lead to the avoidance of sexual intimacy [8]. Overall, the most widely used classification for PE is as follows:

1. Lifelong PE (LPE): occurring since an individual's first sexual encounter.
2. Acquired PE (APE): it begins occurring at some point later in a person's life.

According to this definition, PE prevalence could affect about 4% of the male population [9–13]. Few of these men typically seek treatment for their condition. Up to approximately 30% of men with PE suffer from concurrent erectile dysfunction (ED), which typically may result in early ejaculation without full erection [11, 14, 15]. A wide range of severity is seen, with patients ejaculating on or prior to penetration in the most severe cases. Although this holds true, PE pathophysiology remains an undoubtedly complex topic even though compelling evidence has accumulated over the years, both on animal and human models.

7.2.1.1 Hereditary PE

Hereditary and genetic factors have been supported and correlated with PE onset, thanks to results of familial studies, whereby the risk of PE between family members was higher than the risk expected solely based on prevalence rates in the population [16]. Furthermore, other studies investigating twins, demonstrated a substantial genetic effect on LPE, representing 22% [17] to 28% [17–19] of the variance, as well as on undifferentiated PE observed in young adults (mean age 29.9 years), representing 28–31.5% of the variance [17, 18].

7.2.1.2 Neurobiology of PE

Serotonin (5-HT) is the neurotransmitter of greatest interest in the control of ejaculation. Robust data on animal and human models have been published over the years. As such, it has been hypothesized and subsequently demonstrated that LPE in humans may be explained by a hyposensitivity of the 5-HT2C and/or hypersensitivity of the 5-HT1A receptors. In this context, serotonin per se is known to delay ejaculation; in fact, men with low circulating levels of 5-HT or with 5-HT2C receptor hyposensitivity are known to have lower ejaculatory thresholds. Indeed, it has been demonstrated the presence of a neural network at the peripheral level (within the spinal cord) responsible for the ejaculatory reflex whereby serotonin plays a major role in controlling ejaculation [20]. From this, many therapeutic approaches have been tried and validated. Additionally, both dopamine and oxytocin also appear to play important roles in ejaculation; the biology of these neurotransmitters in relation to ejaculation is less well studied, but in animal models, both appear to have a stimulatory effect on ejaculation [21]. To conclude, the well-documented efficacy of selective serotonin reuptake inhibitors (SSRIs)—such as paroxetine and the on-demand on label molecule dapoxetine—in increasing intravaginal ejaculatory latency time (IELT) in men with PE supports the role of an impairment over the serotonergic inhibitory control of the ejaculatory process, at least in some men with PE [21].

7.2.1.3 Hormones and PE

Animal studies show the biological interactions between 5-HT, dopamine, and the hypothalamic-pituitary axis. Specifically, the hypothalamic-pituitary-thyroid axis is involved [22–24]. Corona et al. and Carani et al. reported a significant correlation between APE and suppressed thyroid-stimulating hormone (TSH) and high thyroid hormone values [25–28]. After normalizing thyroid function in hyperthyroid men, the prevalence of APE fells from 50% to 15% [26]. Interestingly, no case of hyperthyroidism was found in 620 men with LPE, demonstrating that the association of PE with hyperthyroidism is obviously restricted to men with APE [29]. Furthermore, more recently published studies indicate that prolactin (PRL) hormone is somehow connected with ejaculatory control. Particularly, by analysing data of 25,321 patients seeking first medical help for sexual dysfunctions, lowest interquartile levels of PRL were registered with APE and anxiety symptoms [30]. Lastly, testosterone levels have also been correlated with PE onset. More in details, lower levels of testosterone have been linked with delayed ejaculation [31]. Even though the aforementioned statements are true, hyperprolactinemia and high testosterone levels cannot be considered causative factors for APE onset.

7.2.1.4 Chronic Prostatitis and Chronic Pelvic Pain Syndrome (CPPS)

It has been shown how men with chronic prostatitis or CPPS have a higher probability of reporting PE [32, 33]. Studies investigating prevalence of PE among patients with lower urinary tract symptoms (LUTS) associated with CPPS, showed a prevalence of PE in LUTS ranging from 12% to 77% [34]. In this context, the patho-physiological mechanism remains unclear with many hypotheses postulated. Although this holds true, considering the role of the prostate in the ejaculatory mechanism, a direct influence of the local inflammation in the pathogenesis of a few cases of APE seems possible [33, 35–38].

7.2.1.5 Psychological Factors

Psychological and interpersonal factors may cause or exacerbate symptoms of APE and LPE [39]. In this context, robust data exist regarding the true association of a specific psychological distress and PE onset. As such, the well-known bidirectional influence of PE and psychological distress makes it extremely difficult to detect the true causative agent. Although this holds true, sexual abuse, attitudes toward sex internalized during childhood, individual psychological factors (e.g., body image, depression, performance anxiety, alexithymia), and/or relationship factors (e.g., decreased intimacy, partner conflict) have all been related to PE [40–42].

7.2.1.6 Pharmacology and PE

Possible interactions between opioid withdrawal and APE onset have been postulated [43]. As such, endogenous opioids have been demonstrated to influence (in rats) the inhibition of the ejaculatory reflex at the spinal level. Furthermore, in several placebo-controlled trials, tramadol per se, significantly improved the IELT of men with LPE. Lastly, it has been reported that APE could occur when SSRIs or norepinephrine re-uptake inhibitors are interrupted without a proper decalage.

7.2.2 Diagnosis

7.2.2.1 History and Questionnaires

The diagnosis of PE should start with a comprehensive and detailed medical and sexual history. Moreover, classification of APE, LPE situational, and consistent PE should be made at first clinical assessment. Specific focus should be put on the duration of ejaculation, the impact on patient's quality of life (QoL), and any concomitant use of specific drugs or the abuse of recreational substances. As a whole, IELT alone is not sufficient for the diagnosis of PE. In fact, it has been reported that there is a significant overlap between men with PE and without PE by using the IELT [44]. In this context, the correct evaluation of QoL is mandatory for the diagnosis. As such, notwithstanding not indicated for diagnosis in clinical practice, a number of questionnaires have been developed over the years. Of those, two validated questionnaires are suggested by the clinical guidelines, such as:

1. Premature Ejaculation Diagnostic Tool (PEDT) [45]: a five-item questionnaire based upon interviews made in USA, Germany, and Spain. A score of >11 is suggestive of PE. A score of 9 or 10 shows a probable PE, whereas a score <8 is indicative of non-PE.
2. Arabic Index of Premature Ejaculation (AIPE) [46]: a seven-item questionnaire developed in Saudi Arabia. A cut-off of 30 shows PE. Severity of PE can also be assessed using the AIPE.

7.2.2.2 Physical Examination

Physical examination should be part of the initial assessment of a patient complaining of PE. As such, penile and genital abnormalities should be carefully assessed, along with other urological, endocrinological, and neurological conditions [44]. Other urological disorders such as ED, Peyronie's disease (PD), urethritis, and prostatitis should be carefully assessed. Lastly, there is no need to ask for laboratory exams unless an underlying aetiology that should be confirmed or excluded is present (e.g., dysthyroidism). During assessment, checking for specific triggers of APE is recommended (e.g., anxiety, guilt, and fear of being caught). As such, the involvement of the partner is often strongly suggested [44].

7.2.3 Treatments

Management depends upon the aetiology, but the most useful available drugs include:

1. *Selective Serotonin Reuptake Inhibitors (SSRIs)* [39]. SSRIs include Paroxetine (10–40 mg/day), Sertraline (50–200 mg/day), Fluoxetine (20–40 mg/day), Citalopram (20–40 mg/day), and Escitalopram (10–20 mg/day) [47]. SSRIs should be started at the lowest dose and up-titrated as needed at 3- to 4-week intervals. Among those, in a meta-analysis, paroxetine has been found to be the most effective in delaying ejaculation when considered as a continuous daily treatment [48]. Additionally, dapoxetine was the first drug patented for the specific treatment of PE; evidence has accumulated upon five trials (including over 6000 men) who were randomly assigned to placebo vs. dapoxetine (30 mg or 60 mg/prn) [49]. Unlike other SSRIs, which are most effective when taken daily, dapoxetine is taken on-demand, ideally 2–3 h before intercourse in the everyday scenario. Specific attention should be maintained regarding the full therapeutic effect of SSRIs. It is typically not seen if not after 2–3 weeks of continuous therapy, and symptoms return if treatment is stopped (although is strictly recommended not to abruptly discontinue any SSRI). Lastly, if SSRIs are not well tolerated or they are ineffective, serotoninergic tricyclic antidepressants (TCA) (e.g., tricyclic clomipramine (12.5–50 mg/day)) could be tried as a second-line alternative [50].
2. *Topical Anaesthetics* [51]. Among this class of available PE treatments, lidocaine-prilocaine spray is the predominant topical treatment given to PE patients in routine clinical-practice [52]. In this context, multicentric trials have shown its superior efficacy at improving ejaculatory control, ejaculatory latency, and eventually overall patients' satisfaction [52].
3. *Psychotherapy*, when psychogenic and/or relationship factors are predominant or co-existing [53]. In this context, behavioural and psychological therapies are effective in some men. These interventions are designed to achieve several goals: improve self-confidence and communication in the relationship and, ultimately, increase the ejaculation latency. Of note, combination therapy (e.g., topical therapy + behavioural therapy) has been shown to be more effective when psychological distress is particularly predominant.

Other available treatments are as follows:

1. *Phosphodiesterase type 5 inhibitors (PDE5i)* [54]. This class of drugs is particularly relevant whenever PE is coexisting with ED. In this context, two meta-analyses have shown the efficacy of PDE5i for PE [55, 56]. The main findings were: (a) both SSRIs and PDE5i are more effective than placebo; (b) PDE5i are either as effective as SSRIs or slightly more effective; and (c) combined therapy is more effective than either therapy alone.

2. *Topical Alprostadil cream (200/300 μg)* [57]. In this context, one available study (multicentre, open-label, long-term study) analysing 1161 patients has shown beneficial effects in terms of delaying ejaculation.

3. *Tramadol* [58, 59]. Tramadol exerts its effect on the opioid receptors along with weak inhibition of serotonin and norepinephrine reuptake. Tramadol can be used as an alternative to SSRIs and TCA anti-depressants. In this context, tramadol's effects on PE have previously been evaluated by three systematic reviews [60–62], two of which have pooled data in a meta-analysis [61, 62]. Of the two meta-analyses, one [60] pooled data across different study types (observational studies and RCTs) [60]. The other one reviewed pooled IELT effect estimates across studies using a standardized mean difference [61]. In conclusion, tramadol appeared to be more effective than placebo or behavioural therapy in the treatment of PE. However, these findings should be interpreted with caution given the observed levels of between-study heterogeneity and the methodological quality of the available evidence. Overall, meticulous attention should be used when prescribing this drug in the everyday clinical setting.

4. *Alpha Blockers* [63]. Patients with LUTS are often diagnosed with sexual dysfunctions (thus including PE) [36]. As such, treatment of LUTS with Alfuzosin has been shown to reduce ejaculatory dysfunctions.

7.3 Delayed Ejaculation (DE)

7.3.1 Aetiology

The American Psychiatric Association defines delayed ejaculation (DE) as requiring one of two symptoms as follows: marked delay, infrequency, or absence of ejaculation on 75–100% of occasions, that persists for at least 6 months, and which causes personal distress [64]. Although this holds true, the definition of DE remains of clinical debate; in this context, compelling evidence has accumulated regarding the true prevalence of DE, thus revealing a 3% prevalence among sexually active men [65, 66]. According to the National Health and Social Life Survey (NHSLS), involving a national probability sample of 1749 women and 1410 men aged 18–59 years, and assessing the prevalence and risk of experiencing sexual dysfunction across various social groups, the prevalence of men having the inability to achieve orgasm climax and ejaculation is around 7.78% [66]. Likewise, another national probability sample study reporting sexual function problems among 11,161 men and women aged 16–44 years in Britain found that 0.7% of men reported inability of achieving an orgasm [67]. Additionally, in an international survey of sexual problems among 13,618 men aged 40–80 years from 29 countries, 1.1–2.8% of men reported that they frequently experience inability to reach orgasm [68]. Although the evidence is limited, the prevalence of lifelong and acquired DE is estimated around 1% and 4%, respectively [69]. Regarding the pathophysiology of DE, experimental evidence shows how 5-HT, throughout brain interconnection pathways (descending), exerts an inhibitory role on ejaculation. Up to date, three main serotonin receptor subtypes (5-HT1A, 5-HT1B, and 5-HT2C) have been postulated to control the ejaculatory reflex. It has been suggested that the presynaptic 5-HT1A somatodendritic auto-receptors, located in the mesencephalic and medullary raphe nuclei and responsible for decreasing 5-HT release into the synapse, decrease ejaculatory latency. In contrast, the postsynaptic 5-HT1B and 5-HT2C receptors have been shown to prolong ejaculatory latency [70, 71]. In this context, the true pathophysiological mechanisms behind DE remain unclear. There are mainly three aetiological factors which are well-recognized in the context of DE [44].

1. Aging: degeneration of penile afferent nerves inhibits ejaculation.
2. Congenital: Mullerian duct cyst, Wolffian duct abnormalities, Prune Belly Syndrome, imperforate anus, and genetic abnormalities.
3. Anatomic causes: transurethral resection of prostate, bladder neck incision, circumcision, and ejaculatory duct obstruction (can be congenital or acquired).
4. Neurogenic causes: diabetic autonomic neuropathy, multiple sclerosis, spinal cord injury, radical prostatectomy, proctocolectomy, bilateral sympathectomy, abdominal aortic aneurysmectomy, and para-aortic lymphadenectomy.
5. Infective/inflammatory causes: urethritis, genitourinary tuberculosis, schistosomiasis, prostatitis, and orchitis.
6. Endocrine causes: hypogonadism, hypothyroidism, and prolactin disorders.
7. Medications: antihypertensives, thiazide diuretics, alpha-adrenergic blockers, antipsychotics, antidepressants, alcohol, antiandrogens, ganglion blockers, and SSRIs.
8. Psychological: acute psychological distress, relationship distress, psychosexual skill deficit, disconnect between arousal and sexual situations masturbation style.

7.3.2 Diagnosis of DE

Patients should be assessed with a full medical and sexual history. Comprehensive physical examination should exclude anatomical and congenital abnormalities of male genitalia. Understanding the details of patients' ejaculation, as well as sexual habits, might be useful during the patients work-up. In this context, the impact of the disease is also useful to better tailor the therapeutic approach. Psychological evaluation might be useful if psychological distress appears to be relevant [44].

7.3.3 Treatment

1. *Psychological support:* patients with DE should be counselled by a psychology expert dealing with sexual issues. A basic understanding of the sexual cycle for their respective partners can assist men and women in managing expectations and evaluating their own sexual practices [72].
2. *Pharmacotherapy:* many therapeutic options exist in the context of DE. As such, even though neither the European Medicine Agency (EMA) nor the Food and Drug Administration (FDA) approval exist, agents like cabergoline, bupropion, alpha-1-adrenergic agonists, buspirone, oxytocin, testosterone, bethanechol, yohimbine, amantadine, cyproheptadine, and apomorphine have been used to treat DE, with varied success rates [73].
3. *Penile vibratory stimulation:* this should be used in selected cases (e.g., men with spinal cord-injuries) in conjunction with pharmacological therapy [74]. In this context, penile vibrators fall into two categories; (a) high-amplitude vibrators (tend to be more effective because they cover more surface area) and (b) low-amplitude vibrators. In this context, the Miami Project to Cure Paralysis estimated that 30–40% of men with spinal cord injury can ejaculate using a low-amplitude vibrator [75]. For men using a high-amplitude vibrator, the estimate is 55–85%. Penile vibratory stimulation may take place in a doctor's office or at home.

7.4 Retrograde Ejaculation

7.4.1 Aetiology

Retrograde ejaculation is a condition in which patients are unable to release semen since in the posterior urethra, it flows back into the bladder, as diagnosed by five or more spermatozoa/HPF in the urine sediment immediately after masturbation. Among the different causes of RE is possible to find spinal cord injuries, diabetic neuropathies, colorectal surgeries, aortic aneurysm surgeries, thoracolumbar sympathectomies, retroperitoneal lymph node dissection surgeries, transurethral prostatectomies, and transurethral bladder neck incisions. Transurethral prostatectomies (e.g., TURP, THULEP, or HOLEP) are probably the most common surgical causes of RE. It affects more than 80% of patients undergoing these procedures [76]. Also, bladder neck surgery may cause RE, especially if performed in childhood [77]. Pharmacological aetiology is mainly related to antihypertensives, thiazide diuretics, α-1-adrenoceptor antagonists, antipsychotics, and antidepressants [73].

7.4.2 Diagnosis of RE

Men with RE present with reduced ejaculation or dry orgasm, cloudy urine post orgasm, due to the mixing of semen in the bladder with urine. A thorough history is essential in order to identify the underlying cause. The lower reference limit for semen volume is 1.5 mL (fifth centile, 95% confidence interval (CI) 1.4–1.7) as defined by the World Health Organization (WHO) [78]. Hypospermia or aspermia should highlight to the clinician the possibility of RE. Vroege et al. suggested that the analysis and confirmation of sperm in a post orgasmic urine sample could help differentiate between a failure of semen emission and RE [79]. Presence in the post-orgasmic urine of 10–15 sperm per high-power field would confirm the diagnosis of RE [80].

7.4.3 Treatment

Several medical approaches have been investigated in order to achieve antegrade ejaculation for natural reproduction in patients with RE. The tested substances include imipramine (tri-cyclic antidepressant), amoxapine (tri-cyclic antidepressant), B12 vitamin, pseudoephedrine (stimulation of α and β receptors in the urinary tract) as well as injection of collagen within the bladder neck [81–85]. One cross-over RCT treated 26 patients with amoxapine (50 mg daily) and B12

vitamin (500 μg three times per day), separately for a period of 4 weeks with each drug [82]. Amoxapine, which acts as a noradrenaline reuptake inhibitor, was effective in 80% of patients compared to only 16% success obtained in the vitamin B12 group. In another study, comparing the effects of imipramine 25 mg twice per day and pseudoephedrine 120 mg twice per day on RE in diabetic men, Arafa et al. [84] found a more moderate success rate of 38.5% with imipramine. However, the use of pseudoephedrine resulted in almost half of the patients having antegrade ejaculation and this increased to 61.5% when combining the two drugs. Of note, the side effects of sympathomimetics include dryness of mucous membranes and hypertension. Exploring a different approach to the problem, Kurbatov et al. injected collagen into the bladder neck to increase the constriction of the internal sphincter [83]. A total of 24 diabetic men were randomized to either a collagen or a saline injection, showing a small increase in antegrade ejaculate with a mean difference of 0.71 mL in favour of patients receiving collagen ($p < 0.05$).

Beyond the use of drugs, other methods have been proposed in order to manage infertility in RE. Standard sperm-retrieval techniques, such as testicular sperm extraction (TESE), and two different methods of sperm acquisition have been proposed [44]. Those include the following:

1. Centrifugation and resuspension of post-ejaculatory urine specimens: post-orgasmic urine sample is collected by introducing a catheter or spontaneous voiding. This sample is then centrifuged and suspended in a medium. The resultant modified sperm mixture can then be used in assisted reproductive techniques. A systematic review of studies is done in couples in which male partner had RE found a 15% pregnancy rate per cycle (0–100%) [86].
2. The Hotchkiss (or modified Hotchkiss) technique, which involves emptying the bladder prior to ejaculation, using a catheter, and then washing out and instilling a small quantity of Lactated Ringers to improve the ambient condition of the bladder. The patient then

ejaculates, and semen is retrieved by catheterization or voiding [87]. Modified Hotchkiss methods involve variance in the instillation medium. Pregnancy rates were 24% per cycle (0–100%) [86].

7.5 Anejaculation and Anorgasmia

7.5.1 Aetiology

The Diagnostic Manual of Mental Disorders defines inhibited ejaculation as the persistent or recurrent absence of attaining orgasm following sufficient sexual stimulation, which causes personal distress [64]. On the other hand, anejaculation can be classified as either a lifelong or acquired, or as global or situational. Any single or combination of psychological or medical disease, surgical procedure or drug which interferes with either central control of ejaculation, the afferent or efferent nerve supply to the vas, bladder neck, pelvic floor, or the penis, can result in inhibited ejaculation, anejaculation, and anorgasmia. Among the different aetiologies, a prominent role is occupied by multiple sclerosis, a demyelinating disease affecting the central nervous system—both the brain and the spinal cord [88]. Its effect on sexual function depends on the location of plaques in the central nervous system with ejaculatory dysfunction appearing in almost 50% of men with this condition [89].

7.5.2 Diagnosis

Medical/psychosexual history, social/religious history, medication list, and physical exam are the main part of the diagnosis. Penile sensitivity must be addressed, especially in men at risk for penile sensation loss such as those with diabetes mellitus. Symptoms and signs of endocrinopathies, such as testosterone deficiency, hypothyroidism, and hyperprolactinemia, should be sought. Masturbatory style is another useful line of inquiry as frequent masturbation or idiosyncratic masturbatory styles may play a role.

Furthermore, identifying the onset is critical, whether lifelong or acquired. Next, understanding whether the condition is generalized or situational is also critical to understand the pathophysiology [90]. The role of laboratory testing, such a testosterone and TSH levels, is optional and is applied depending on patient symptoms. In patients complaining of loss of penile sensitivity, bio-thesiometry and/or pudendal somatosensory evoked potentials (SSEP) might be warranted [91].

7.5.3 Treatment

Although multiple psychodynamic and behavioural treatments for anorgasmia and anejaculation have been suggested, empirical evidence to support treatment efficacy is lacking [92]. Most reports are uncontrolled case reports with treatment ranging from a few brief sessions of sex education to the nearly 2 years of multiple-modality treatment in more complex multiple aetiologic cases. There has been limited success with pharmacologic therapies for the treatment of anejaculation. Cabergoline and bupropion are the two most trialled medications, though neither has been officially approved. Cabergoline is a potent dopamine receptor agonist. By increasing dopamine neurotransmission, it is thought to promote ejaculation. One study found that cabergoline in the treatment of 72 anorgasmic men showed improvement in 69% of men [93]. On the other hand, Bupropion blocks the reuptake of both norepinephrine and dopamine, is commonly used in depressed men when SSRIs cause delayed or anejaculation [94].

Another proposed therapeutic approach is the vibratory stimulation of the dorsal penile nerve. Three studies have investigated success rates and achieved successful retrieval in 32–96% of the patients [95–97]. Success was primarily dependent on amplitude of the stimulation. In a cohort of 66 men with spinal cord injury and anejaculation, Sønksen et al. [97] found better success rates with a 100 Hz frequency and an increasing amplitude of the stimulation plate spanning from 32% with an amplitude of 1 mm, to 96% with an amplitude of 2.5 mm. In a similar setting with 211 spinal cord injury men, Brackett et al. [96] managed good results using an amplitude of 2.5 mm, resulting in sperm retrieval in 54.4% of the cases. Interestingly, there seem to be a better sperm quality with PVS as compared to EEJ [98].

References

1. Gerstenberg TC, Levin RJ, Wagner G. Erection and ejaculation in man. Assessment of the electromyographic activity of the bulbocavernosus and ischiocavernosus muscles. Br J Urol. 1990;65:395–402. https://doi.org/10.1111/j.1464-410x.1990.tb14764.x.
2. Alwaal A, Breyer BN, Lue TF. Normal male sexual function: emphasis on orgasm and ejaculation. Fertil Steril. 2015;104:1051–60. https://doi.org/10.1016/j.fertnstert.2015.08.033.
3. Holstege G, Georgiadis JR, Paans AMJ, Meiners LC, van der Graaf FHCE, Reinders AATS. Brain activation during human male ejaculation. J Neurosci. 2003;23:9185–93.
4. Levin RJ. Revisiting post-ejaculation refractory time-what we know and what we do not know in males and in females. J Sex Med. 2009;6:2376–89. https://doi.org/10.1111/j.1743-6109.2009.01350.x.
5. Master VA, Turek PJ. Ejaculatory physiology and dysfunction. Urol Clin North Am. 2001;28(363–75):x. https://doi.org/10.1016/s0094-0143(05)70145-2.
6. Ver Voort SM. Ejaculatory stimulation in spinal-cord injured men. Urology. 1987;29:282–9. https://doi.org/10.1016/0090-4295(87)90072-0.
7. Comarr AE. Sexual function among patients with spinal cord injury. Urol Int. 1970;25(2):134–68. https://pubmed.ncbi.nlm.nih.gov/5422714/. Accessed 2 Mar 2022.
8. Serefoglu EC, McMahon CG, Waldinger MD, Althof SE, Shindel A, Adaikan G, et al. An evidence-based unified definition of lifelong and acquired premature ejaculation: report of the Second International Society for Sexual Medicine Ad Hoc Committee for the definition of premature ejaculation. J Sex Med. 2014;11:1423–41. https://doi.org/10.1111/jsm.12524.
9. Rosen RC, Heiman JR, Long JS, Fisher WA, Sand MS. Men with sexual problems and their partners: findings from the international survey of relationships. Arch Sex Behav. 2016;45:159–73. https://doi.org/10.1007/s10508-015-0568-3.
10. Patrick DL, Althof SE, Pryor JL, Rosen R, Rowland DL, Ho KF, et al. Premature ejaculation: an observational study of men and their partners. J Sex Med. 2005;2:358–67. https://doi.org/10.1111/j.1743-6109.2005.20353.x.
11. Rosen RC, McMahon CG, Niederberger C, Broderick GA, Jamieson C, Gagnon DD. Correlates to the clinical diagnosis of premature ejaculation: results from a large observational study of men and their partners. J Urol. 2007;177:1059–64; discussion 1064. https://doi.org/10.1016/j.juro.2006.10.044.
12. Côté-Léger P, Rowland DL. Estimations of typical, ideal, premature ejaculation, and actual latencies by men and female sexual partners of men during partnered sex. J Sex Med. 2020;17:1448–56. https://doi.org/10.1016/j.jsxm.2020.04.317.
13. Coskuner ER, Ozkan B. Premature ejaculation and endocrine disorders: a literature review. World J Mens Health. 2022;40:38–51. https://doi.org/10.5534/wjmh.200184.
14. Patrick DL, Chiang YP. Measurement of health outcomes in treatment effectiveness evaluations: conceptual and methodological challenges. Med Care. 2000;38:II14–25. https://doi.org/10.1097/00005650-200009002-00005.
15. Corona G, Rastrelli G, Limoncin E, Sforza A, Jannini EA, Maggi M. Interplay between premature ejaculation and erectile dysfunction: a systematic review and meta-analysis. J Sex Med. 2015;12:2291–300. https://doi.org/10.1111/jsm.13041.
16. Santtila P, Jern P, Westberg L, Walum H, Pedersen CT, Eriksson E, et al. The dopamine transporter gene (DAT1) polymorphism is associated with premature ejaculation. J Sex Med. 2010;7:1538–46. https://doi.org/10.1111/j.1743-6109.2009.01696.x.
17. Santtila P, Sandnabba NK, Jern P. Prevalence and determinants of male sexual dysfunctions during first intercourse. J Sex Marital Ther. 2009;35:86–105. https://doi.org/10.1080/00926230802712293.
18. Jern P, Santtila P, Witting K, Alanko K, Harlaar N, Johansson A, et al. Premature and delayed ejaculation: genetic and environmental effects in a population-based sample of Finnish twins. J Sex Med. 2007;4:1739–49. https://doi.org/10.1111/j.1743-6109.2007.00599.x.
19. Jern P, Santtila P, Johansson A, Varjonen M, Witting K, von der Pahlen B, et al. Evidence for a genetic etiology to ejaculatory dysfunction. Int J Impot Res. 2009;21:62–7. https://doi.org/10.1038/ijir.2008.61.
20. Salonia A, Saccà A, Briganti A, Del Carro U, Dehò F, Zanni G, et al. Quantitative sensory testing of peripheral thresholds in patients with lifelong premature ejaculation: a case-controlled study. J Sex Med. 2009;6:1755–62. https://doi.org/10.1111/j.1743-6109.2009.01276.x.
21. Rowland DL. Psychophysiology of ejaculatory function and dysfunction. World J Urol. 2005;23:82–8. https://doi.org/10.1007/s00345-004-0488-7.
22. Tannenbaum J, Youssef M, Attia AS, Hsieh T-C, Raheem O. Hyperthyroidism as an underlying cause of premature ejaculation. Sex Med Rev. 2022;10:108–12. https://doi.org/10.1016/j.sxmr.2021.03.005.
23. Chen T, Wu F, Wang X, Ma G, Xuan X, Tang R, et al. Different levels of estradiol are correlated with sexual dysfunction in adult men. Sci Rep. 2020;10:12660. https://doi.org/10.1038/s41598-020-69712-6.

24. Fiala L, Lenz J. Psychosocial stress, somatoform dissociative symptoms and free testosterone in premature ejaculation. Andrologia. 2020;52:e13828. https://doi.org/10.1111/and.13828.

25. Corona G, Jannini EA, Lotti F, Boddi V, De Vita G, Forti G, et al. Premature and delayed ejaculation: two ends of a single continuum influenced by hormonal milieu. Int J Androl. 2011;34:41–8. https://doi.org/10.1111/j.1365-2605.2010.01059.x.

26. Carani C, Isidori AM, Granata A, Carosa E, Maggi M, Lenzi A, et al. Multicenter study on the prevalence of sexual symptoms in male hypo- and hyperthyroid patients. J Clin Endocrinol Metab. 2005;90:6472–9. https://doi.org/10.1210/jc.2005-1135.

27. Hirshfield S, Chiasson MA, Wagmiller RL, Remien RH, Humberstone M, Scheinmann R, et al. Sexual dysfunction in an internet sample of U.S. men who have sex with men. J Sex Med. 2010;7:3104–14. https://doi.org/10.1111/j.1743-6109.2009.01636.x.

28. Christensen BS, Grønbaek M, Osler M, Pedersen BV, Graugaard C, Frisch M. Sexual dysfunctions and difficulties in Denmark: prevalence and associated sociodemographic factors. Arch Sex Behav. 2011;40:121–32. https://doi.org/10.1007/s10508-010-9599-y.

29. Serefoglu EC, Direk N, Hellstrom WJG. Premature ejaculation and erectile dysfunction prevalence and attitudes in the Asia-Pacific region—a comment. J Sex Med. 2012;9:1488–9. https://doi.org/10.1111/j.1743-6109.2012.02685.x.

30. Corona G, Mannucci E, Jannini EA, Lotti F, Ricca V, Monami M, et al. Original research–endocrinology: Hypoprolactinemia: a new clinical syndrome in patients with sexual dysfunction. J Sex Med. 2009;6:1457–66. https://doi.org/10.1111/j.1743-6109.2008.01206.x.

31. Corona G, Jannini EA, Mannucci E, Fisher AD, Lotti F, Petrone L, et al. Different testosterone levels are associated with ejaculatory dysfunction. J Sex Med. 2008;5:1991–8. https://doi.org/10.1111/j.1743-6109.2008.00803.x.

32. Trinchieri A, Magri V, Cariani L, Bonamore R, Restelli A, Garlaschi MC, et al. Prevalence of sexual dysfunction in men with chronic prostatitis/chronic pelvic pain syndrome. Arch Ital Urol Androl. 2007;79:67–70.

33. Shamloul R, el-Nashaar A. Chronic prostatitis in premature ejaculation: a cohort study in 153 men. J Sex Med. 2006;3:150–4. https://doi.org/10.1111/j.1743-6109.2005.00107.x.

34. Sihotang RC, Alvonico T, Taher A, Birowo P, Rasyid N, Atmoko W. Premature ejaculation in patients with lower urinary tract symptoms: a systematic review. Int J Impot Res. 2021;33:516–24. https://doi.org/10.1038/s41443-020-0298-5.

35. Lotti F, Corona G, Mancini M, Biagini C, Colpi GM, Innocenti SD, et al. The association between varicocele, premature ejaculation and prostatitis symptoms: possible mechanisms. J Sex Med. 2009;6:2878–87. https://doi.org/10.1111/j.1743-6109.2009.01417.x.

36. Chierigo F, Capogrosso P, Boeri L, Ventimiglia E, Frego N, Pozzi E, et al. Lower urinary tract symptoms and depressive symptoms among patients presenting for distressing early ejaculation. Int J Impot Res. 2020;32:207–12. https://doi.org/10.1038/s41443-019-0147-6.

37. Screponi E, Carosa E, Di Stasi SM, Pepe M, Carruba G, Jannini EA. Prevalence of chronic prostatitis in men with premature ejaculation. Urology. 2001;58:198–202. https://doi.org/10.1016/s0090-4295(01)01151-7.

38. McMahon CG, Jannini EA, Serefoglu EC, Hellstrom WJG. The pathophysiology of acquired premature ejaculation. Transl Androl Urol. 2016;5:43449.

39. Shaeer O, Shaeer K. The Global Online Sexuality Survey (GOSS): the United States of America in 2011. Chapter I: erectile dysfunction among English-speakers. J Sex Med. 2012;9:3018–27. https://doi.org/10.1111/j.1743-6109.2012.02976.x.

40. Althof SE, McMahon CG, Waldinger MD, Serefoglu EC, Shindel AW, Adaikan PG, et al. An update of the International Society of Sexual Medicine's guidelines for the diagnosis and treatment of premature ejaculation (PE). J Sex Med. 2014;11:1392–422. https://doi.org/10.1111/jsm.12504.

41. McCabe M, Althof SE, Assalian P, Chevret-Measson M, Leiblum SR, Simonelli C, et al. Psychological and interpersonal dimensions of sexual function and dysfunction. J Sex Med. 2010;7:327–36. https://doi.org/10.1111/j.1743-6109.2009.01618.x.

42. Michetti PM, Rossi R, Bonanno D, De Dominicis C, Iori F, Simonelli C. Dysregulation of emotions and premature ejaculation (PE): alexithymia in 100 outpatients. J Sex Med. 2007;4:1462–7. https://doi.org/10.1111/j.1743-6109.2007.00564.x.

43. Abdollahian E, Javanbakht A, Javidi K, Samari AA, Shakiba M, Sargolzaee MR. Study of the efficacy of fluoxetine and clomipramine in the treatment of premature ejaculation after opioid detoxification. Am J Addict. 2006;15:100–4. https://doi.org/10.1080/10550490500419151.

44. Salonia A, Bettocchi C, Boeri L, Capogrosso P, Carvalho J, Cilesiz NC, et al. European Association of Urology guidelines on sexual and reproductive health—2021 update: male sexual dysfunction. Eur Urol. 2021;80(3):333–57. https://doi.org/10.1016/j.eururo.2021.06.007.

45. Huang Y-P, Chen B, Ping P, Wang H-X, Hu K, Zhang T, et al. The premature ejaculation diagnostic tool (PEDT): linguistic validity of the Chinese version. J Sex Med. 2014;11:2232–8. https://doi.org/10.1111/jsm.12612.

46. Arafa M, Shamloul R. Development and evaluation of the Arabic Index of Premature Ejaculation (AIPE). J Sex Med. 2007;4:1750–6. https://doi.org/10.1111/j.1743-6109.2006.00213.x.

47. Farnia V, Raisi F, Mohseni MG, Atharikia D, Ghafuri Z. On-demand treatment of premature ejaculation with citalopram: a randomized double-blind study. Acta Med Iran. 2009;47(5):353–7.

48. Rowland D, McMahon CG, Abdo C, Chen J, Jannini E, Waldinger MD, et al. Disorders of orgasm and ejaculation in men. J Sex Med. 2010;7:1668–86. https://doi.org/10.1111/j.1743-6109.2010.01782.x.

49. Buvat J, Tesfaye F, Rothman M, Rivas DA, Giuliano F. Dapoxetine for the treatment of premature ejaculation: results from a randomized, double-blind, placebo-controlled phase 3 trial in 22 countries. Eur Urol. 2009;55:957–67. https://doi.org/10.1016/j.eururo.2009.01.025.

50. Waldinger MD, Zwinderman AH, Olivier B. On-demand treatment of premature ejaculation with clomipramine and paroxetine: a randomized, double-blind fixed-dose study with stopwatch assessment. Eur Urol. 2004;46:510–5; discussion 516. https://doi.org/10.1016/j.eururo.2004.05.005.

51. Berkovitch M, Keresteci AG, Koren G. Efficacy of prilocaine-lidocaine cream in the treatment of premature ejaculation. J Urol. 1995;154:1360–1.

52. Boeri L, Pozzi E, Fallara G, Montorsi F, Salonia A. Real-life use of the eutectic mixture lidocaine/prilocaine spray in men with premature ejaculation. Int J Impot Res. 2021;34:289–94. https://doi.org/10.1038/s41443-021-00424-9.

53. Althof SE. Psychosexual therapy for premature ejaculation. Transl Androl Urol. 2016;5:475–81. https://doi.org/10.21037/tau.2016.05.15.

54. Aversa A, Pili M, Francomano D, Bruzziches R, Spera E, La Pera G, et al. Effects of vardenafil administration on intravaginal ejaculatory latency time in men with lifelong premature ejaculation. Int J Impot Res. 2009;21:221–7. https://doi.org/10.1038/ijir.2009.21.

55. Asimakopoulos AD, Miano R, Agrò EF, Vespasiani G, Spera E. Does current scientific and clinical evidence support the use of phosphodiesterase type 5 inhibitors for the treatment of premature ejaculation? A systematic review and meta-analysis. J Sex Med. 2012;9:2404–16. https://doi.org/10.1111/j.1743-6109.2011.02628.x.

56. McMahon CG, McMahon CN, Leow LJ, Winestock CG. Efficacy of type-5 phosphodiesterase inhibitors in the drug treatment of premature ejaculation: a systematic review. BJU Int. 2006;98(2):259–72.

57. Morales A, Barada J, Wyllie MG. A review of the current status of topical treatments for premature ejaculation. BJU Int. 2007;100:493–501. https://doi.org/10.1111/j.1464-410X.2007.07051.x.

58. Frink MC, Hennies HH, Englberger W, Haurand M, Wilffert B. Influence of tramadol on neurotransmitter systems of the rat brain. Arzneimittelforschung. 1996;46:1029–36.

59. Szkutnik-Fiedler D, Kus K, Balcerkiewicz M, Grześkowiak E, Nowakowska E, Burda K, et al. Concomitant use of tramadol and venlafaxine—evaluation of antidepressant-like activity and other behavioral effects in rats. Pharmacol Rep PR. 2012;64:1350–8. https://doi.org/10.1016/s1734-1140(12)70932-5.

60. Wong BLK, Malde S. The use of tramadol "on-demand" for premature ejaculation: a system-atic review. Urology. 2013;81:98–103. https://doi.org/10.1016/j.urology.2012.08.037.

61. Yang L, Qian S, Liu H, Liu L, Pu C, Han P, et al. Role of tramadol in premature ejaculation: a systematic review and meta-analysis. Urol Int. 2013;91:197–205. https://doi.org/10.1159/000348826.

62. Wu T, Yue X, Duan X, Luo D, Cheng Y, Tian Y, et al. Efficacy and safety of tramadol for premature ejaculation: a systematic review and meta-analysis. Urology. 2012;80:618–24. https://doi.org/10.1016/j.urology.2012.05.035.

63. Cavallini G. Alpha-1 blockade pharmacotherapy in primitive psychogenic premature ejaculation resistant to psychotherapy. Eur Urol. 1995;28:126–30. https://doi.org/10.1159/000475036.

64. American Psychiatric Association. Cautionary statement for forensic use of DSM-5. In: Diagnostic and statistical manual of mental disorders. 5th ed; 2013. https://doi.org/10.1176/appi.books.9780890425596.CautionaryStatement.

65. Simons JS, Carey MP. Prevalence of sexual dysfunctions: results from a decade of research. Arch Sex Behav. 2001;30:177–219. https://doi.org/10.1023/a:1002729318254.

66. Laumann EO, Paik A, Rosen RC. Sexual dysfunction in the United States: prevalence and predictors. JAMA. 1999;281:537–44. https://doi.org/10.1001/jama.281.6.537.

67. Mercer CH, Fenton KA, Johnson AM, Copas AJ, Macdowall W, Erens B, et al. Who reports sexual function problems? Empirical evidence from Britain's 2000 National Survey of Sexual Attitudes and Lifestyles. Sex Transm Infect. 2005;81:394–9. https://doi.org/10.1136/sti.2005.015149.

68. Laumann EO, Nicolosi A, Glasser DB, Paik A, Gingell C, Moreira E, et al. Sexual problems among women and men aged 40-80 y: prevalence and correlates identified in the Global Study of Sexual Attitudes and Behaviors. Int J Impot Res. 2005;17:39–57. https://doi.org/10.1038/sj.ijir.3901250.

69. Di Sante S, Mollaioli D, Gravina GL, Ciocca G, Limoncin E, Carosa E, Lenzi A, Jannini EA. Epidemiology of delayed ejaculation. Transl Androl Urol. 2016;5(4):541–8. https://doi.org/10.21037/tau.2016.05.10.

70. de Almeida Kiguti LR, Pacheco TL, Antunes E, Kempinas WG. Lorcaserin administration has pro-ejaculatory effects in rats via 5-HT2C receptors activation: a putative pharmacologic strategy to delayed ejaculation? J Sex Med. 2020;17:1060–71. https://doi.org/10.1016/j.jsxm.2020.02.027.

71. Waldinger MD, Berendsen HH, Blok BF, Olivier B, Holstege G. Premature ejaculation and serotonergic antidepressants-induced delayed ejaculation: the involvement of the serotonergic system. Behav Brain Res. 1998;92:111–8. https://doi.org/10.1016/s0166-4328(97)00183-6.

72. Carvalheira A, Santana R. Individual and relationship factors associated with the self-identified inability to experience orgasm in a community sample of heterosexual men from three European countries. J Sex

Marital Ther. 2016;42:257–66. https://doi.org/10.108 0/0092623X.2015.1010677.

73. Martin-Tuite P, Shindel AW. Management options for premature ejaculation and delayed ejaculation in men. Sex Med Rev. 2020;8:473–85. https://doi.org/10.1016/j.sxmr.2019.09.002.

74. Nelson CJ, Ahmed A, Valenzuela R, Parker M, Mulhall JP. Assessment of penile vibratory stimulation as a management strategy in men with secondary retarded orgasm. Urology. 2007;69:552–5; discussion 555–556. https://doi.org/10.1016/j.urology.2006.02.048.

75. Kleitman N. Under one roof: the Miami Project to Cure Paralysis model for spinal cord injury research. Neuroscientist. 2001;7:192–201. https://doi.org/10.1177/107385840100700304.

76. Grise P, Plante M, Palmer J, Martinez-Sagarra J, Hernandez C, Schettini M, et al. Evaluation of the transurethral ethanol ablation of the prostate (TEAP) for symptomatic benign prostatic hyperplasia (BPH): a European multi-center evaluation. Eur Urol. 2004;46:496–501; discussion 501–502. https://doi.org/10.1016/j.eururo.2004.06.001.

77. Huang Z, Berg WT. Iatrogenic effects of radical cancer surgery on male fertility. Fertil Steril. 2021;116:625–9. https://doi.org/10.1016/j.fertnstert.2021.07.1200.

78. Cooper TG, Noonan E, von Eckardstein S, Auger J, Baker HWG, Behre HM, et al. World Health Organization reference values for human semen characteristics. Hum Reprod Update. 2010;16:231–45. https://doi.org/10.1093/humupd/dmp048.

79. Vroege JA, Gijs L, Hengeveld MW. Classification of sexual dysfunctions: towards DSM-V and ICD-11. Compr Psychiatry. 1998;39:333–7. https://doi.org/10.1016/s0010-440x(98)90044-x.

80. Fedder J, Kaspersen MD, Brandslund I, Højgaard A. Retrograde ejaculation and sexual dysfunction in men with diabetes mellitus: a prospective, controlled study. Andrology. 2013;1:602–6. https://doi.org/10.1111/j.2047-2927.2013.00083.x.

81. Shoshany O, Abhyankar N, Elyaguov J, Niederberger C. Efficacy of treatment with pseudoephedrine in men with retrograde ejaculation. Andrology. 2017;5:744–8. https://doi.org/10.1111/andr.12361.

82. Hu J, Nagao K, Tai T, Kobayashi H, Nakajima K. Randomized crossover trial of amoxapine versus vitamin B12 for retrograde ejaculation. Int Braz J Urol. 2017;43:496–504. https://doi.org/10.1590/S1677-5538.IBJU.2016.0468.

83. Kurbatov D, Russo GI, Galstyan GR, Rozhivanov R, Lepetukhin A, Dubsky S, et al. Correction of retrograde ejaculation in patients with diabetes mellitus using endourethral collagen injection: preliminary results. J Sex Med. 2015;12:2126–9. https://doi.org/10.1111/jsm.13024.

84. Arafa M, El Tabie O. Medical treatment of retrograde ejaculation in diabetic patients: a hope for spontaneous pregnancy. J Sex Med. 2008;5:194–8. https://doi.org/10.1111/j.1743-6109.2007.00456.x.

85. Ochsenkühn R, Kamischke A, Nieschlag E. Imipramine for successful treatment of retrograde ejaculation caused by retroperitoneal surgery. Int J Androl. 1999;22:173–7. https://doi.org/10.1046/j.1365-2605.1999.00165.x.

86. Jefferys A, Siassakos D, Wardle P. The management of retrograde ejaculation: a systematic review and update. Fertil Steril. 2012;97:306–12. https://doi.org/10.1016/j.fertnstert.2011.11.019.

87. Hotchkiss RS, Pinto AB, Kleegman S. Artificial insemination with semen recovered from the bladder. Fertil Steril. 1954;6:37–42. https://doi.org/10.1016/s0015-0282(16)31863-5.

88. Olek MJ. Multiple sclerosis—part I. Overview, pathophysiology, diagnostic evaluation, and clinical parameters. J Am Osteopath Assoc. 1999;99:574–88. https://doi.org/10.7556/jaoa.1999.99.11.574.

89. Haensch C-A, Jörg J. Autonomic dysfunction in multiple sclerosis. J Neurol. 2006;253(Suppl 1):I3–9. https://doi.org/10.1007/s00415-006-1102-2.

90. Jenkins LC, Mulhall JP. Delayed orgasm and anorgasmia. Fertil Steril. 2015;104:1082–8. https://doi.org/10.1016/j.fertnstert.2015.09.029.

91. McMahon CG, Jannini E, Waldinger M, Rowland D. Standard operating procedures in the disorders of orgasm and ejaculation. J Sex Med. 2013;10(1):204–29. https://pubmed.ncbi.nlm.nih.gov/22970767/. Accessed 3 Mar 2022

92. Heiman JR, Meston CM. Empirically validated treatment for sexual dysfunction. Annu Rev Sex Res. 1997;8:148–94.

93. Abdel-Hamid IA, Elsaied MA, Mostafa T. The drug treatment of delayed ejaculation. Transl Androl Urol. 2016;5:576–91. https://doi.org/10.21037/tau.2016.05.05.

94. Dording CM, Mischoulon D, Petersen TJ, Kornbluh R, Gordon J, Nierenberg AA, et al. The pharmacologic management of SSRI-induced side effects: a survey of psychiatrists. Ann Clin Psychiatry. 2002;14:143–7. https://doi.org/10.1023/a:1021137118956.

95. Castle SM, Jenkins LC, Ibrahim E, Aballa TC, Lynne CM, Brackett NL. Safety and efficacy of a new device for inducing ejaculation in men with spinal cord injuries. Spinal Cord. 2014;52:S27–9. https://doi.org/10.1038/sc.2014.110.

96. Brackett NL, Ferrell SM, Aballa TC, Amador MJ, Padron OF, Sonksen J, et al. An analysis of 653 trials of penile vibratory stimulation in men with spinal cord injury. J Urol. 1998;159:1931–4.

97. Sønksen J, Biering-Sørensen F, Kristensen JK. Ejaculation induced by penile vibratory stimulation in men with spinal cord injuries. The importance of the vibratory amplitude. Paraplegia. 1994;32:651–60. https://doi.org/10.1038/sc.1994.105.

98. Meng X, Fan L, Liu J, Wang T, Yang J, Wang J, et al. Fresh semen quality in ejaculates produced by nocturnal emission in men with idiopathic anejaculation. Fertil Steril. 2013;100:1248–52. https://doi.org/10.1016/j.fertnstert.2013.07.1979.

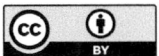

Female Sexual Dysfunctions: A Clinical Perspective on HSDD, FAD, PGAD, and FOD

Alessandra Graziottin, Elisa Maseroli, and Linda Vignozzi

Abbreviations

CBT	Cognitive behavior therapy
cGMP	Cyclic guanosine monophosphate
CNS	Central nervous system
DHEA	Dehydroepiandrosterone
DHT	Dihydrotestosterone
DSDS	Decreased sexual desire screener
DSM	Diagnostic and Statistical Manual (of Mental Disorders)
FCAD	Female cognitive arousal disorder
FGAD	Female genital arousal disorder
fMRI	Functional magnetic resonance imaging
FOD	Female orgasm disorder
FOIS	Female orgasmic illness syndrome
FSD	Female sexual dysfunction
FSFI	Female Sexual Function Index
FSIAD	Female sexual interest/arousal disorder
GPPPD	Genito-pelvic pain/penetration disorder
GSM	Genitourinary syndrome of menopause
HMB	Heavy menstrual bleeding
HPF	Hyperactive pelvic floor
HSDD	Hypoactive sexual desire disorder
IBS	Irritable bowel syndrome
ICD	International Classification of Diseases and Statistics
IDA	Iron deficient anemia
ISSWSH	International Society for Women's Sexual Health
MCR	Melanocortin receptor
MRI	Magnetic resonance imaging
NO	Nitric oxide
PDOD	Pleasure dissociative orgasmic disorder
PF	Pelvic floor
PGAD	Persistent genital arousal disorder
PGAD/GPD	Persistent genital arousal disorder/genito-pelvic dysesthesia

A. Graziottin (✉)
Department of Obstetrics and Gynecology, University of Verona, Verona, Italy

Center of Gynecology and Medical Sexology, H. San Raffaele Resnati, Milan, Italy

Alessandra Graziottin Foundation for the Cure and Care of Pain in Women NPO, Milan, Italy
e-mail: direzione@studiograziottin.it

E. Maseroli
Andrology, Women's Endocrinology and Gender Incongruence Unit, Careggi University Hospital, Florence, Italy

L. Vignozzi
Andrology, Women's Endocrinology and Gender Incongruence Unit, Department of Experimental and Clinical Biomedical Sciences "Mario Serio", University of Florence, Florence, Italy
e-mail: linda.vignozzi@unifi.it

© The Author(s) 2023
C. Bettocchi et al. (eds.), *Practical Clinical Andrology*,
https://doi.org/10.1007/978-3-031-11701-5_8

SFQ	Sexual Function Questionnaire
SHBG	Sex hormone-binding globulin
SNRIs	Serotonin and norepinephrine reuptake inhibitor
SSRIs	Selective serotonin reuptake inhibitors
STP	Sexual tipping point
UTI	Urinary tract infection
VAS	Visual analogue scale
VPA	Vaginal pulse amplitude
VPP	Vaginal photoplethysmography
VVA	Vulvovaginal atrophy
WHO	World Health Organization

8.1 Female Sexual Dysfunctions: A Clinical Perspective

8.1.1 Introduction

Sexual dysfunction encompasses a disturbance in sexual functioning involving one or more phases of the sexual response cycle, including pain associated with sexual activity. Classifications are still evolving; they are a real nosographic "work in progress." Historically, two classification systems have been used for sexual medicine diagnosis: the Diagnostic and Statistical Manual of Mental Disorders (DSM), edited by the American Psychiatric Association, and the International Classification of Diseases and Statistics (ICD), endorsed by the World Health Organization (WHO). In addition, throughout the past decades, sexual medicine experts from various international societies have been constantly working to revise and redefine the nomenclature of female sexual dysfunctions (FSDs), in order to reflect the updated scientific evidence and the ever-changing standards in clinical care for women with sexual problems [1]. Disease classification systems provide a standard and internationally comparable system for use in national and international information and reporting.

However, three major drawbacks persist. First, the aim of perfectly describing the elusive complexity and nuances of female sexual function and dysfunction leads to the usage of complicated definitions that are difficult to use with and be understood by colleagues not specifically trained in sexual medicine. Conversing with patients is even more challenging. Second, it is difficult to translate sophisticated definitions from English to national languages in easy-to-catch words that adhere to the human daily experience. Third, and most importantly, the persisting neglect or scotomization of prominent biological etiologies of FSD. This contributes to maintaining a wide gender bias, overfocusing on the psychodynamic/relational/contextual etiology of FSD.

Commonly accepted diagnostic criteria play a critical role in framing the interpretation of concepts in the medical and epidemiological literature, influencing how healthcare providers organize their thoughts about clinical conditions, how populations are defined in trials, and allowing global information exchange among clinicians, patients, and healthcare systems [1]. The classifications of FSDs followed over the years reflect the evolution of the female sexual response models. In the 1960s, Masters and Johnson published "Human Sexual Response," proposing the first model of the human sexual response cycle in both men and women, consisting of four stages: excitement/arousal, plateau, orgasm, and resolution. In 1979, Kaplan added the concept of desire to be applicable to a non-laboratory setting. Kaplan conceived sexual desire as an "appetitive phase" localized in the brain, initiating a cascade of physiological, genitally-focused events. Both these models are known as "linear," since they postulate that sexual response begins with spontaneous sexual desire and proceeds from one stage to the next; this framework became the basis for the conceptualization, classification, and definitions of FSDs in the DSM-IV [2] and DSM-IV-TR [3]. In the early 2000s, Basson introduced the circular incentive-based model of the female sexual response, suggesting that women may be motivated to engage in sexual activity for many sexual and non-sexual reasons, including wanting to enhance intimacy or bonding, to feel attractive or desired, or to communicate affection for a partner, and therefore may start a sexual experience in a state of "sexual neutrality" [4]. Women can also engage in sexual activity to gain personal and/or economic advantages, starting in a non-aroused state. According to this alternative conceptualization, women may experience desire once sexual stimuli have triggered arousal (concept of "responsive desire"). Arousal and desire often co-occur and reinforce one another. These new concepts, along with several perceived shortcomings of previous models [5], led to suggestions that informed the DSM-V definitions [6].

It should be noted that crucial intra- and inter-individual differences exist in the physiological sexual response and that no single model is universal; however, among women, sexual dysfunction and distress have been reported to be significantly related to the endorsement of the Basson model [7].

8.2 Sexual Interest/Desire Disorders

8.2.1 Pathophysiology of Low Desire

In both sexes, the sexual desire construct underlies cognitive and emotional processes that are ultimately controlled by systems and neurotransmitters in the central nervous system (CNS) that modulate sexual excitation and inhibition. According to the "Sexual Tipping Point" (STP) model®, the continuous interplay between excitation and inhibition generates a dynamic, personal threshold for sexual responsiveness, which is subjected to variations at any given time in the individual [8]. The regions that modulate sexual desire in the CNS are located in the hypothalamus, limbic system, and prefrontal cortex, and include the medial preoptic area, paraventricular nucleus, ventral tegmental area, and nucleus *accumbens* [9]. Neural pathways controlled by dopamine, and secondarily by melanocortin, norepinephrine, and oxytocin, facilitate the processing and response to sexual stimuli [9]. In particular, dopaminergic neurotransmission positively regulates reward-related neural functions, including sexual reward [10]. In contrast, sexual inhibition is modulated by serotonin, opioid, and endocannabinoid systems that are activated dur-

ing the refractory period and can blunt excitatory processes [9]. These conditions (or drugs) that influence neurotransmission in these key regions, resulting in decreased excitation, increased inhibition, or both, may predispose individuals to hypoactive sexual desire disorder (HSDD). Such dynamic alterations can be reinforced by negative sexual experiences, which can potentiate sexual inhibition.

Cumulative evidence from preclinical and clinical studies indicates that sex steroids act as major neurofunctional modulators of sexual desire in women. In mammalian and rodent females, the sexual motivation peak observed during the periovulatory period is probably driven by ovarian hormone actions, triggering central excitatory mechanisms [11]. Estrogenic priming has been reported to be necessary for progesterone-modulating effects on dopaminergic transmission [12]. In female rats, the lordosis reflex is dependent on estrogen, whereas the full expression of appetitive and consummatory behaviors depends on additional activation by progesterone [13].

Evidence that androgens are crucial determinants of women's sexual desire stems mainly from studies on postmenopausal women with HSDD treated with testosterone therapy (see Sect. 8.2.5). Although there is no threshold for any androgen that can be used to diagnose women with FSD, a recent meta-analysis concluded that there appears to be a moderate association between endogenous total testosterone levels and sexual desire [14]. Studies on female rats treated with estradiol, testosterone, and aromatase inhibitors first suggested that aromatization may not be necessary for testosterone to increase the sensitivity of the response to male-related cues [15]. These data were confirmed in subsequent experiments, in which the administration of the non-aromatizable androgen dihydrotestosterone (DHT) in estradiol-primed ovariectomized rats was able to enhance behavioral measures of sexual desire [16]. It is likely that the excitatory role of androgen signalling in the reward system in humans is implicated in such effects on sexual desire. However, sex hormones act among a myriad of other biological and psychological variables to shape sexual motivation.

8.2.2 Nosology and Current Definitions

In the DSM-V, the classical distinct definitions of desire and arousal problems were collapsed into a new entity called "female sexual interest/arousal disorder" (FSIAD) [6]. This revised classification has proven highly controversial among clinicians and experts, mainly because of the little empirical support for new diagnostic categories and the practical consequences on management, with many women with incomplete loss of receptivity likely to be excluded from any diagnosis [17]. Subsequent international panels, the International Consultation in Sexual Medicine [18], and the International Society for Women's Sexual Health (ISSWSH) Nomenclature Committee [19] restored the label of hypoactive sexual desire disorder (HSDD). Specifically, according to the nosology and nomenclature for FSDs recently proposed by ISSWSH, HSDD "manifests as any of the following for at least 6 months: (1) lack of motivation for sexual activity as manifested by decreased or absent spontaneous desire (sexual thoughts or fantasies), decreased or absent responsive desire to erotic cues and stimulation or inability to maintain desire or interest through sexual activity; (2) loss of desire to initiate or participate in sexual activity, including behavioral responses such as avoidance of situations that could lead to sexual activity, that is not secondary to sexual pain disorders and is combined with clinically significant personal distress that includes frustration, grief, incompetence, loss, sadness, sorrow, or worry" (grade B, level of evidence 2–3) [20]. Similarly, in the updated version of the ICD-11, HSDD is characterized by "[...] (1) reduced or absent spontaneous desire (sexual thoughts or fantasies), (2) reduced or absent responsive desire to erotic cues and stimulation, or (3) inability to sustain desire or interest in sexual activity once initiated [...]" [21]. In both definitions, symptoms must be associated with clinically significant distress to constitute dysfunction.

8.2.3 Prevalence and Leading Etiologies of HSDD

HSDD in women is a multifactorial condition that includes biological, psychosexual, and contextual factors. The differences in the design of epidemiological studies assessing the prevalence of HSDD (concerning definitions, settings, and methodologies) have produced estimates ranging from 17% to over 50% [22]. Data from the PRESIDE study, a large population-based survey conducted on more than 50,000 US women, showed that low desire was the most common sexual difficulty, reported in 37.7% of participants, whereas low desire with associated distress (HSDD) was present in 10% of responders [23].

However, the exact biological alterations that determine HSDD have not yet been characterized. Clinically, no neuroimaging or biochemical parameters can identify women with HSDD. Aging is one of the main factors affecting sexual desire; however, the younger the woman, the higher the distress that this loss may cause. Menopause has a further worsening impact, and premature iatrogenic menopause is the most frequent cause of biologically determined generalized loss of desire [24]. This is probably due to the sudden decline in ovarian sex steroids, namely estrogens and androgens [25], since the ovaries contribute more than 50% of androgens during the reproductive life. In a cross-sectional survey of European women aged 20–70 years, surgical menopause was associated with a significantly and clinically relevant higher risk of HSDD than natural menopause and premenopausal status [26].

Several general medical conditions, including neurologic, oncologic, and metabolic disorders, may represent risk factors for HSDD. Indeed, chronic diseases interfere with sexual function through multiple mechanisms, including fatigue and the psychological burden of a lifelong progressive diagnosis [27]. Psychiatric disorders, such as depression, are also major determinants of low sexual desire and display a bidirectional relationship, with depressive symptoms conferring a 50–70% increased risk of HSDD and HSDD being associated with a 130–210% increased risk of depression [22, 28]. Furthermore, a number of medications, i.e., psychotropics (antipsychotics, barbiturates, benzodiazepines, lithium, serotonin reuptake inhibitors, tricyclic antidepressants, and venlafaxine), cardiovascular and antihypertensive drugs, GnRH agonists and analogs, hormonal contraceptives, antiandrogens, tamoxifen, aromatase inhibitors, and chemotherapeutic agents, have been associated with desire disorders [29].

All pathological and physiological conditions that determine lower androgen and free androgen levels, besides iatrogenic menopause, may result in diminished desire [14]. Among these, pregnancy, puerperium, lactation, pathological hyperprolactinemia, hypopituitarism, hypothalamic amenorrhea, adrenal insufficiency, primary ovarian insufficiency, and increased sex hormone-binding globulin (SHBG), which is common in women using hormonal contraception, are particularly important [30].

Chronic sleep disorders, in terms of reduced quantity and/or poor quality of sleep, are major and still neglected contributors to HSDD through different pathways, with hyperactivation of the corticotrophin-releasing pathway, hypothalamic dysregulation, and increasing daily distress and fatigue [31].

Box 8.1 Iron Deficient Anemia (IDA): The Most Neglected Non-hormonal Biological Etiology of HSDD in Women

Key Points
- Iron deficiency anemia (IDA) is highly prevalent in women (30–50% in low-income countries) [32].
- IDA doubles the risk of depression, a major contributor to HSDD [33].
- Iron is essential for the synthesis of dopamine, the key neurotransmitter of the "seeking-appetitive lust system" [34].
- Leading etiologies of IDA in women include:

- Low iron intake (poverty, eating disorders, vegan diet, "self-made diet," and aging).
- Reduced intestinal absorption (celiac disease, lactose intolerance, gluten intolerance, irritable bowel syndrome (IBS), and Crohn's disease).
- Increased losses:
   Menstruation: Heavy menstrual bleeding (HMB) occurs in 19–20% of women.
   Delivery with postpartum hemorrhagia.
   Oral-gastro-intestinal: gingivitis, gastritis, IBS, and hemorrhoids.
- Increased needs:
   Adolescence
   Pregnancy
   Athletes
- Reduced availability from storage sites, during chronic inflammatory diseases

Key Clinical Point. Careful clinical history-taking, with a few inexpensive examinations (red blood cell count, hemoglobin, serum iron, ferritin, and transferrin levels), is essential to address IDA, a key and still neglected etiology of HSDD.

The most vulnerable are women with HMB and women after delivery, if iron supplementation was inadequate during pregnancy and/or if delivery caused heavy blood loss.

Box 8.2 Sexual Pain: The Underappreciated Killer of Sex Drive

Feedbacks from the genitals are powerful modulators of sex drive:

- Positive sexual experiences, with fast systemic and genital arousal, intense gorgeous genital congestion (the "orgasmic platform," according to Master and Johnson), and intense orgasm(s) are powerful enhancers that potentiate sexual desire and drive [35].

- Negative sexual experiences, specifically genital pain, may gradually inhibit any sex drive and sexual response. Vulvar pain, recurrent post-coital cystitis, introital and/or deep dyspareunia, vulvovaginal atrophy (VVA), and genitourinary syndrome of menopause (GSM) may all contribute to impaired sex drive, up to a frank aversion of any coital intimacy [36]. Previous sexual abuse can have a long-lasting impact on sex drive through multiple pathophysiological pathways, both biological and psychosexual [37].

Key Clinical Point. A thorough clinical history of comprehensive sexual pain disorders is essential for every woman complaining of HSDD. Every woman should also undergo a competent genital evaluation to diagnose and treat all the clinical conditions that could contribute to her complaints of HSDD. The hyperactive pelvic floor (HPF) should be carefully diagnosed and addressed, as it is a powerful yet neglected etiological contributor to FSDs. HPF can cause reduced genital arousal and lubrication due to pain, sexual pain disorders, genito-pelvic pain penetration disorders (GPPPD), recurrent post-coital cystitis, coital anorgasmia, and painful anal sex.

Psycho-relational factors play a key role in the etiology of HSDD. The most commonly reported are poor self-esteem/body image issues; lifestyle factors (e.g., stress and sleep deprivation); a history of abuse (physical, sexual, and emotional); substance abuse; self-imposed pressure for sex; religious, personal, cultural, or family values; beliefs and taboos; relational conflicts; and sexual factors (e.g., inadequate stimulation and sexual dysfunction in the partner) [22].

8.2.4 Diagnostic Algorithms and Tools

Conventionally, an accurate diagnosis of HSDD requires a time-consuming and extensive diagnostic interview performed by a clinician with expertise in FSD. The key aspects to address when assessing low desire are as follows: (a) whether the disorder is generalized (occurring with every partner and in every situation) or situational; in fact, situational problems often exclude medical factors; (b) the onset and duration, that is, whether the symptoms are lifelong or have been acquired after months/years of satisfying sexual function, and in this case, which are the factors that the woman feels contributes to or precipitates the symptoms; and (c) her level of distress and bother, which defines the mild, moderate, or severe impact of the dysfunction on her personal life [24].

It is crucial to distinguish sexual distress from nonsexual distress and depression. From a couple's perspective, a discrepancy in the level of desire between two partners is common and does not qualify the person with the lower desire to have HSDD per se. The patient should be diagnosed with HSDD only if the discrepancy causes her personal distress [22].

Although obtaining a detailed description of a woman's problem is important to establish the diagnosis and guide treatment, many women with HSDD are at risk of remaining undiagnosed because of limited access to experts trained in FSD. Screening tools play a pivotal role in this context. For example, the brief profile of female sexual function (B-PFSF) [38] and the decreased sexual desire screener (DSDS) [39] are both sensitive and easy-to-use brief diagnostic instruments that help identify HSDD in women who present with a complaint of decreased sexual desire.

The Female Sexual Function Index (FSFI) [40] is considered the gold standard for the measurement of sexual function in women and provides different scores for several sexual domains, including desire. In fact, the two-item desire domain is the only one that can be used independently, with women with scores of ≤ 5 being likely to meet the diagnostic criteria for HSDD [41]. However, the FSFI does not examine distress, a key diagnostic component included in both the DSM and ICD diagnostic systems [42]. For this reason, it is recommended that a validated scale assessing distress be administered along with the FSFI desire domain when making clinical inferences, such as the female sexual distress scale—revised (FSDS-R) or the FSDS-R item 13, a specific question that addresses the level of distress related to low sexual desire [43].

8.2.5 Key Therapeutic Approaches

The ISSWSH process of care for the management of HSDD in women suggests that first-line therapeutic strategies are represented by sexual education and modification of potential biological and psychological contributing factors [22]. For example, sexual pain or arousal disorders should be addressed *before* a specific treatment for HSDD is considered, as relieving these symptoms may improve desire per se. In the case of generalized acquired HSDD persisting, the key therapeutic approaches include psychological sex therapy, testosterone treatment, and centrally acting drugs based on the menopausal status [22]. Due to the multifactorial origin of HSDD, it is crucial that its treatment is planned from a patient- and couple-centered, multidimensional perspective, sequencing options that target either the suspected primary contributing component or the more distressing component for that individual woman to that individual woman [44].

The most common psychological therapies are behavior therapy (i.e., sensate focus exercises), cognitive behavior therapy (CBT), and mindfulness-based CBT [45–47]. Although these are based on a strong rationale, there is a paucity of clinical trials and a lack of adequate control groups to clearly establish the efficacy of these interventions [44].

As physiological and pathological changes in androgen levels influence sexual function in women, they represent a potential target for therapeutic strategies for HSDD. Specifically, systemic transdermal testosterone has been recommended for women with HSDD not primarily related to modifiable factors or comorbidities [48]. A 1% (10 mg/mL) cream is currently approved in Australia, whereas this approach is currently off-label worldwide. A recent Global Position Statement, endorsed by several international societies, suggests that treatment should be administered to naturally or surgically postmenopausal women, with or without concurrent estrogen therapy, in doses that approximate physiological testosterone concentrations for reproductive age [49]. This was mainly based on a meta-analysis of randomized controlled trials supporting the moderate therapeutic benefit, increase in desire (standardized mean difference 0.36, 95% CI 0.22–0.50) and reduction in sexual caused by transdermal testosterone compared to the effects of placebo/comparator therapy [50]. No serious adverse events to testosterone therapy have emerged [50], although long-term safety has not yet been established. Owing to the lack of efficacy and safety data, compounded products should not be used, and government-approved transdermal male formulations may be prescribed cautiously in doses appropriate for women [49]. Expert opinion reports usually suggest one-tenth of the daily dose prescribed to men undergoing replacement therapy for hypogonadism (300-μg/24-h testosterone) [51]. Limited evidence supports the use of testosterone in premenopausal women of late reproductive age [48]. The key messages regarding testosterone treatment are summarized in Table 8.1.

Regarding other androgen-based options for HSDD, a meta-analysis conducted in 2014 showed that dehydroepiandrosterone (DHEA) administration did not significantly impact sexual symptoms in postmenopausal women with normal adrenal function [52].

The centrally acting drugs for HSDD are flibanserin and bremelanotide, which focus on the inhibitory and excitatory pathways linked to the regulation of sexual desire (see Sect. 8.2.1). Flibanserin is a 5-HT1A receptor agonist and 5-HT2A receptor antagonist that has been approved as an oral therapy (once daily, at bedtime) against acquired, generalized HSDD in premenopausal women in the United States (US),

Table 8.1 Key practical points for systemic testosterone therapy, off-label in most countries, according to the "International Society for the Study of Women's Sexual Health Clinical Practice Guideline for the Use of Systemic Testosterone for Hypoactive Sexual Desire Disorder in Women" [48]

Systemic testosterone therapy for women
Who: postmenopausal (natural or surgical) women with HSDD (± other FSDs), with or w/o estrogen replacement
When: after/during appropriate management of other conditions that may contribute to low desire
How: intramuscular injections and oral preparations are not recommended. Transdermal dosing should be targeted to achieve T concentrations in the physiologic premenopausal range
How long: on an average, efficacy emerges after 6–8 weeks; maximal at about 12 weeks. Discontinue after 6 months if no improvement; no safety data >24 months
Formulations: compounded products lack evidence for efficacy and safety. It is reasonable to prescribe off-label approved male formulation at approximately 1/10th of the male dose
T levels monitoring: no blood level as a treatment goal. Total T levels should be measured before initiating therapy to exclude women with midrange to high baseline concentrations, 3–6 weeks after initiating therapy and after 6 weeks if dosing is increased to exclude over-dosing; every 4–6 months once stable levels are achieved

HSDD hypoactive sexual desire disorder, *FSD* female sexual dysfunctions, *T* testosterone

and in naturally postmenopausal women aged 60 years or younger in Canada [53]. Bremelanotide is a melanocortin receptor (MCR) agonist administered via subcutaneous injection on demand before sexual activity. By binding to presynaptic MC4R, bremelanotide has been suggested to stimulate the release of dopamine in key brain regions and has been approved in the US for acquired, generalized HSDD in premenopausal women only [54]. Finally, an off-label CNS agent that has been reported to improve HSDD symptoms is bupropion, a dopamine, and serotonin reuptake inhibitor [55].

Sexual Interest/Desire Disorders: Key Points

- Low desire reflects a dynamic imbalance between excitatory and inhibitory central mechanisms, in favor of the latter.
- Hypoactive sexual desire disorder (HSDD) is characterized by a reduced or absent, spontaneous or responsive desire for several months, associated with clinically significant distress.
- HSDD is the most common form of female sexual dysfunction (10–50%).
- Risk factors for HSDD include the following:
  - Systemic conditions, such as aging, menopause (+ surgical), general medical diseases, pathologic, and physio-

logic (i.e., puerperium) conditions associated with the loss of fluctuations in ovarian hormones, depression and other psychiatric diseases, and medications (i.e., psychotropic drugs)
  - Negative feedbacks from the genitals such as vaginal dryness, sexual pain, vulvar pain, inadequate or absent orgasm, hyperactive pelvic floor, post-coital cystitis, and the genitourinary syndrome of the menopause (GSM)
  - Psycho-relational factors
- Screening tools: B-PFSF, DSDS, and FSFI-D + FSDS-R.
- First-line therapeutic strategies: Sexual education and modifications of contributing factors (i.e., sexual pain, hyperactive pelvic floor, loss of sexual hormones, and treatment of iron-deficient anemia).
- Second-line strategies: Psychological sex therapy (behavior therapy and CBT), testosterone treatment, and centrally acting drugs (flibanserin and bremelanotide).
- Short-term transdermal testosterone treatment in post-menopausal women with HSDD, aimed at restoring premenopausal levels, has proved to be safe and effective.

8.3 Arousal Disorders

8.3.1 Pathophysiology of Genital Arousal Disorders

"Arousal" refers to the physiologic responses that occur during an anticipatory period before and during sexual activity, up to the moment of climax. These encompass both cognitive/emotional and physical components, involving genital (swelling and vaginal lubrication) and nongenital manifestations (increased heart rate, sweating, and hardening of the nipples).

Genital arousal depends on the anatomical and functional integrity of the complex neural, endocrine, and vascular mechanisms, ultimately resulting in increased blood flow. This clinically translates into the engorgement of erectile tissue, such as the clitoral, vestibular, and periurethral corpora cavernosa (homologous to their penile counterpart), and the production of a fluid transudate in the vagina, known as "lubrication." Female genital tissues are rich in arterial vascularization, supplied by branches of the internal pudendal and femoral arteries (labia), ileo-hypogastric pudendal bed (clitoris), branches of the uterus (upper vagina), hypogastric arteries (middle vagina), and middle hemorrhoidal and clitoral arteries (distal vagina) [56]. Briefly, immediately after sexual stimulation, parasympathetic pathways (via the pelvic nerves) lead to the release of vasodilator neurotransmitters in the genital tissues, mainly nitric oxide (NO). NO induces the formation of cyclic guanosine monophosphate (cGMP), which in turn stimulates cGMP-dependent protein kinase (protein kinase G), leading to the relaxation of the vascular smooth muscle cells [57]. The subsequent increase in blood flow and pressure results in the formation of a plasma ultrafiltrate within the vaginal epithelial cells, accumulating at the vaginal surface as a clear, smooth fluid that moistens the vaginal walls, allowing painless penile penetration [56]. It is important to emphasize that it has never been demonstrated that glandular secretion in the human vagina determines its lubrication during arousal.

In the late 1990s, following pivotal experiments performed in female animal models of aortoiliac atherosclerosis, Park et al. theorized that an abnormal arterial circulation or endothelial function within the hypogastric-cavernosal vascular bed could interfere with physiologic arousal processes and manifest with diminished or delayed vaginal lubrication and sensation, pain or discomfort during intercourse, and diminished clitoral sensation or orgasm [58]. These hypotheses have been confirmed by subsequent studies in animal models [59] and humans [60], and observational data have suggested an association between cardiovascular risk factors (e.g., diabetes mellitus) and poor genital arousal [61]. However, adequate studies aimed at establishing a cause-and-effect relationship between FGAD and cardiovascular diseases in women have not been conducted, and currently, there are no conclusive data to support that FGAD is a predictor of future cardiovascular events [62].

Among the lifestyle-related factors, smoking and cycling may significantly impair genital arousal in women. In a laboratory study, acute nicotine use has been shown to reduce genital arousal by 30% in women [63]. Cigarette smoking, both active and passive, is the strongest modifiable predictor of FSD, including genital arousal disorders, in women [64]. Bicycle seat pressure on the perineum may impair arousal and clitoral erection, likely contributing to the genital pain and numbness experienced by female cyclists, similar to the genital and sexual symptoms affecting male cyclists. A survey of female cyclists indicated that 53.9%, 58.1%, and 69.1% of female cyclists had FSD, genital numbness, and genital pain, respectively. After adjusting for age, body mass index, relationship status, smoking history, comorbidities, and average time spent cycling per week, women who reported experiencing genital numbness half the time or more were more likely to have FSD (adjusted odds ratio [aOR], 6.0; 95% CI, 1.5–23.6; $P = 0.01$), especially if localized to the clitoris (aOR, 2.5; 95% CI, 1.2–5.5; $P = 0.02$) [65].

More genital numbness and urinary tract infections (UTIs) were confirmed in another, larger survey, which does not confirm the increased arousal vulnerability reported in the former study. From a clinical point of view, it is important to ask women complaining of female sexual arousal disorder (FSAD) about leisure activities, bicycling particularly, and comorbid complaints of genital numbness, UTIs, and/or saddle sores [66].

8.3.2　Nosology and Current Definitions

The definitions of altered arousal have varied greatly over the years. The DSM-IV-TR identified "female sexual arousal disorder" (FSAD) focusing solely on the lack of an "adequate lubrication-swelling response to sexual excitement," [3] failing to mention non-vaginal responses. As previously reported in the DSM-V, arousal disorder was not described as a distinct diagnostic entity, but rather merged with HSDD, to create the combined diagnostic category of FSIAD (female sexual interest/arousal disorder) [6]. This combination was driven mainly by studies suggesting that FSAD and HSDD are often comorbid and that many women are unable to differentiate desire from arousal [5]. However, the cumulative evidence has not only shown that desire and arousal may be disconnected, but also that a dramatic between-person variability exists in the concordance between "subjective" (positive mental engagement during sexual activity) and "physiological arousal" (vaginal lubrication and other genitals and non-genitals sensations) [67]. In this context, a recent line of research has highlighted the notion that some women are mentally aroused by perceived genital cues, whereas for others, the two types of arousal are asynchronous [68]. These aspects may have clinical implications in the diagnosis and treatment of arousal disorders.

Ultimately, the updated and revised nomenclature proposed by the ISSWSH differentiates female genital arousal disorder (FGAD) from female cognitive arousal disorder (FCAD) [69]. FGAD is characterized by "the distressing difficulty or inability to attain or maintain adequate *genital response*, including vulvovaginal lubrica-tion, engorgement of the genitalia, and sensitivity of the genitalia associated with sexual activity, for 6 months" (grade B) [69]. On the other hand, the diagnosis of FCAD is based on "the distressing difficulty or inability to attain or maintain adequate *mental excitement* associated with sexual activity as manifested by problems with feeling engaged or mentally turned on or sexually aroused for 6 months" (expert opinion) [69]. Both disorders may induce mild, moderate, or severe distress and may be experienced independently or in different combinations.

8.3.3　Prevalence and Leading Etiologies of Female Genital Arousal Disorder

The lack of a clear definition and standardized diagnostic tools has severely limited epidemiological studies on female sexual arousal disorders. In the PRESIDE study, previously mentioned regarding the prevalence of low desire, the overall, unadjusted prevalence of low sexual arousal (without distress), and low sexual arousal inducing distress were 26.1% and 5.4%, respectively. The age bracket displaying the highest prevalence of 7.5% was the middle-aged group (45–64 years) [23]. No data are available on the prevalence of FGAD and FCAD according to the most recent nomenclature.

The current definition of FGAD underlines the importance of organic insults which disrupt the neurovascular mechanism underpinning the genital response to sexual stimuli; in fact, it has been reported that the etiology of FGAD is related to vascular and neurologic injury or dysfunction [69]. Among cardiometabolic diseases potentially causing FSD, diabetes mellitus is probably the one showing the strongest correlations; the more heavily impaired sexual domains in diabetic women are arousal and lubrication [70]. Some studies have indicated that age, duration of disease, metabolic control, and microangiopathic complications, in particular, neuropathy [71], are independently associated with sexual difficulties in women with diabetes [61]. Based on limited evidence, obesity, metabolic syndrome, dyslipidemia, and hypertension may also increase the risk of vasculogenic FSD; however, this effect appears milder than that in men [62].

Regarding neurological integrity, arousal difficulties are common in women with disorders affecting both the central and peripheral nervous systems. Sexual symptoms are often underdiagnosed in patients with spinal cord injury or multiple sclerosis [72]. Pudendal neuropathy (i.e., following childbirth) and radiculopathy of the sacral spinal nerve roots due to sacral or lumbar spinal pathologies, such as disc impingement or spinal stenosis, can also result in genital arousal disorders [73]. Pelvic irradiation and surgery (i.e., hysterectomy or pelvic organ prolapse surgery) are other commonly neglected causes of possible damage to small blood vessels and nerve endings in genital tissues [74]. Interestingly, vaginal delivery has been associated with significantly decreased scores in the sexual arousal domain of the FSFI [75].

A hyperactive pelvic floor, lifelong, or acquired in response to inflammation and/or pain, which reduces the vaginal opening and causes pain during penetration attempts, may cause reflex inhibition of both mental and genital arousal, contributing to poor or absent lubrication [73].

Furthermore, estrogens and androgens seem to play a synergistic role as regulators of the contractile-relaxant machinery underlying peripheral arousal, both in the vagina [76] and in the clitoris [77]. Therefore, low sex steroids levels may contribute to poor vaginal lubrication and clitoral tumescence. However, concerning the effect of estrogen and androgen deficiency, vulvovaginal atrophy, and/or the genitourinary syndrome of menopause (GSM), along with vulvovaginal infections and inflammatory disorders, are considered as *exclusion criteria* for FGAD [69]. However, the exclusion of leading biological etiologies of impaired genital arousal, such as the post-menopausal loss of sexual hormones, deprives women of a very simple and appropriate treatment for vaginal dryness, dyspareunia, and/or other comorbid symptoms of GSM. Since biological/organic etiological factors such as diabe-

tes or radiotherapeutic damage are considered, GSM and the associated loss of sex hormones should also be considered.

In addition, modifiable lifestyle-related factors, such as smoking or bicycling, that could contribute to the onset and maintenance of genital arousal disorders in women should be actively investigated and appropriately treated.

Finally, psycho-relational factors are believed to affect both cognitive and genital arousals. Depression, anxiety, body image concerns, eating disorders, environmental stressors, cultural attitudes, history of sexual abuse, poor sexual stimulation, low relationship satisfaction, communication issues, and sexual dysfunction in the partner (in particular, male premature or delayed ejaculation) should always be evaluated in women complaining of arousal difficulties [78].

The interdependence between the different phases of the sexual response is almost the rule in clinical practice. Different biological etiologies may contribute to different FSDs. To create rigid boundaries, defining a specific disorder more clearly may become a boomerang in clinical practice if the relevant predisposing, precipitating, or maintaining factors of genital arousal impairment are excluded.

8.3.4 Diagnostic Tools for Arousal Disorders

One of the major flaws in the study of female arousal is the lack of a universal, objective, and feasible approach aimed at diagnosing a state of impaired genital blood flow, unlike in men. Penile color Doppler ultrasound performed in nonstimulated conditions is considered the gold standard for the investigation of erectile dysfunction of suspected vascular origin and is commonly performed in clinical practice [79]. Most importantly, assessing the hemodynamic parameters of the penile arteries can provide important information on cardiovascular risk, especially in young and low-risk men [79]. A homologous technique in women has not yet been validated, and the vast majority of data on alterations of female genital arousal have been based on self-report measures, a methodology flawed by a great susceptibility to response bias.

In laboratory settings, the most well-established method for measuring genital blood flow is vaginal photoplethysmography (VPP), which uses a device that emits and reabsorbs light. The rationale of this method is that the amount of backscattered light depends on the transparency of the vaginal tissue, reflecting its variable vasocongestion [80]. The provided measure, known as the vaginal pulse amplitude (VPA), has been found to be a sensitive and reliable marker of genital sexual arousal.

Clitoral artery Doppler ultrasound has been proposed as a noninvasive and objective approach to measuring genital blood flow and is easier to use in clinical settings compared to VPP [81, 82]. However, this technique has not been fully validated, and the most reproducible hemodynamic parameters (peak systolic velocity, resistance index, pulsatility index, and volume flow) and their normative values have yet to be established. Other methods include indirect measures of heat dissipation (i.e., vaginal and labial thermistors and heated oxygen electrodes), thermal imaging cameras, and laser Doppler perfusion imaging [80]. Finally, Schirmer tear test strips have recently been suggested as an objective measure of vaginal lubrication [83].

Arousal-related items in the common female sexual health questionnaires are as follows: Brief Index of Sexual Functioning (BISF-W): 5,13,14; Sexual Function Questionnaire (SFQ): 7,8,9,10,11,12,13,14; female arousal and desire inventory (FADI) (all items); Sexual Interest and Desire Inventory (SIDI): 11,12; Female Sexual Function Index (FSFI): 3,4,5,6 [78].

8.3.5 Key Therapeutic Approaches

The primary strategy to alleviate FGAD symptoms is to address modifiable causes such as poor vascularization due to atherosclerosis and neuropathy due to sacral and lumbar pathologies. In clinical practice, topical sexual hormones (when not contraindicated) are very effective in improving both vascular and neurogenic responses, in addition to addressing the mucosal component of FGAD. The reported subjective improvement correlates well with the objective trophism improvement at the vulvovaginal examination and the lowering of the vaginal pH from 7 to 4.00–4.5 in postmenopausal women complaining of FGAD. Women should be informed that this is an off-label treatment option. The clinical results reported by women are more satisfactory when a co-present hyperactive pelvic floor, lifelong or defensively acquired because of FGAD, is treated with appropriate physiotherapy.

According to the literature, in the absence of drugs with this specific indication, women with FGAD may benefit from vaginal moisturizers and lubricants as a symptomatic approach. In fact, a minimalistic, although in-label approach, plays a role when even topical hormones are contraindicated or not desired by the individual woman. Moisturizers are intended to be used regularly and act by rehydrating mucosal tissue and trapping moisture. On the other hand, lubricants are based on water, silicone, minerals, or plant oil, and are applied as needed to reduce friction during sexual activity. When considering these products, the ideal parameters are body-similar pH (3.5–5) and osmolality (200–600 mOsmol/kg), and a lack of parabens, chlorhexidine, and polyquaternium-15, to reduce the risk of endothelial irritation and side effects [84].

Vibrators, devices that combine vibration and clitoral vacuum suction, and other mechanical devices may provide useful treatment options [85]. Those containing phthalates, polyvinyl chloride, vinyl, and jelly rubber should be avoided.

The most widely studied topical vasodilating agent in women is alprostadil, a synthetic form of prostaglandin E1 that can induce genital smooth muscle relaxation by increasing protein kinase A activity. It has been reported that alprostadil increases genital temperature, arousal [86], and clitoral peak systolic velocity [87] with no significant adverse events. Several promising data are also available for visnadine, a principle extracted from the plant *Ammi Visnaga*, capable of inhibiting smooth muscle contractile responses mediated by calcium entry. A 1% visnadine vulvar spray seems to improve sexual performance in women with arousal disorders [88]. Regarding systemic vasodilators, the evidence is less convincing, with meta-analytic data showing an overall improvement in sexual function compared to that with a placebo, but with some studies have reported negative findings [89]. Significantly higher rates of headache, flushing, and changes in vision have emerged in phosphodiesterase type 5 inhibitor (PDE5i)-treated patients than in those treated with placebos [89].

Women suffering from FGAD associated with vulvovaginal atrophy (VVA) and/or GSM are candidates for the use of approved local estrogen treatments and DHEA. Local prasterone (DHEA) is indicated for moderate-to-severe VVA in postmenopausal women and has been consistently reported to improve several sexual domains, including arousal [90]. The efficacy of local DHEA, a precursor of both estrogen and androgens, appears to be mediated by the activation of androgenic signaling within the vaginal smooth muscle layer [91]. Systemic testosterone treatment in menopausal women with HSDD [49] and intravaginal testosterone [92] have also been reported to enhance arousal measures; however, both are considered off-label.

A comprehensive biopsychosocial treatment plan is advisable to provide women with the most holistic approach to ameliorate FGAD/FCAD. Psychological management options include sensate focus therapy, cognitive behavioral therapy, and mindfulness therapy [78].

Arousal Disorders: Key Points
- Female genital arousal disorder (FGAD) is characterized by the distressing, persistent impairment in the genital sexual response, including vulvovaginal lubrication and engorgement of the genitalia. The prevalence is around 5–10%.
- Female cognitive arousal disorder (FCAD) is a recently proposed diagnostic category characterized by the distressing, persistent impairment in mental excitement during sexual activity.
- Genital arousal depends on the anatomical and functional integrity of neural and vascular mechanisms, resulting in increased blood flow.
- Risk factors for FGAD include all those conditions causing vascular/endothelial and neurologic injury or dysfunction in the genitals, such as cardiometabolic risk factors (i.e., diabetes mellitus), spinal cord injuries, multiple sclerosis, pudendal neuropathy, sacral radiculopathy, pelvic irradiation, or surgery. Low sex steroids levels may contribute to damaging the integrity of small vessels and nerves.
- There is a lack of standardized, reliable, easy-to-use methods to assess genital arousal. Vaginal photoplethysmography (VPP) and clitoral Doppler ultrasound are two of the most studied. Other proposed tools include indirect measures of heat dissipation, thermal imaging cameras, laser Doppler perfusion imaging, and Schirmer tear test strips.
- Therapeutic strategies: No government-approved drugs are available. After addressing modifiable causes, women with FGAD may benefit from vaginal moisturizers and lubricants, vibrators, or topical vasodilating agents (i.e., alprostadil and visnadine). When vulvovaginal atrophy is also present, symptoms may improve with approved (local estrogens and prasterone) or off-label treatments (local or systemic testosterone).
- Sensate focus therapy, cognitive behavioral therapy, and mindfulness therapy are useful for FGAD/FCAD.

8.4 Persistent Genital Arousal Disorder/Genito-Pelvic Dysesthesia

The existence of persistent genital arousal disorder (PGAD) was first postulated in the early 2000s, but systematic characterization has only recently been attempted.

Persistent genital arousal disorder/genito-pelvic dysesthesia (PGAD/GPD) is currently defined as the "persistent or recurrent, unwanted or intrusive, distressing sensations of genital arousal [that occur over a] duration of at least 3 months" [93]. Other types of genito-pelvic dysesthesia (buzzing, tingling, burning, twitching, itching, and pain) may be described. PGAD/GPD is most commonly experienced in the clitoris but may also involve other genito-pelvic regions; the sensations may include being on the verge of an orgasm, experiencing uncontrollable orgasms, and/or having an excessive number of orgasms. The estimated prevalence is approximately 0.6–3% [93]. It is noteworthy that PGAD/GPD is not associated with concomitant sexual desire or fantasies and should not be misdiagnosed as hypersexuality. In fact, it has been reported to have a dramatically detrimental impact on the patient's sexuality, relationships, mental health, and daily functioning [94].

The underlying pathological mechanism has not been clarified; sensory hyperactivity originating in the genitals, pelvic/perineum, cauda equina, spinal cord, or brain has been theorized. Recognized organic risk factors for PGAD/GPD include clitoral, vestibular, vulvar, and vaginal pathology (i.e., vulvodynia, infectious and inflammatory conditions), overactive pelvic floor (PF) dysfunction, pudendal neuropathy, perineal vascular pathology (i.e., pelvic varices or arteriovenous malformations), sacral Tarlov cysts, and lumbar disc disease (i.e., annular tears); CNS organic disorders (i.e., epilepsy); and medications (trazodone, use of or discontinuation of SSRIs/SNRIs) [93].

PGAD/GPD treatment is guided by the identification of the eventual "trigger region," which may be performed through Doppler ultrasound of the clitoral cavernosal artery, local anesthesia testing, neurological testing, electromyography, transperineal ultrasound of the PF muscles, or diagnostic pudendal nerve blocks. If radiculopathy of the lumbosacral nerve roots is suspected, specific neurogenital testing is recommended, with targeted diagnostic injections of local anesthetic at the level suggested by magnetic resonance imaging (MRI) [93].

Psychosocial associated and contributing factors should be addressed, such as anxiety and depressive symptoms, suicidality, obsessive-compulsive symptoms, catastrophization, sexual or emotional trauma, psychiatric comorbidities, sexual functioning, and relationship adjustment [94].

In patients with symptomatic Tarlov cysts or lumbar disc disease, neurosurgical interventions have been reported to be beneficial in the vast majority of cases [95, 96]. Promising results have been obtained by neurolysis of the dorsal nerve to the clitoris, relieving compression of the pudendal nerve [97]. Psychotherapy, sacral/pudendal neuromodulation, and electroconvulsive therapy are other treatment strategies. Off-label pharmacological agents aimed at symptom control may also be considered (anticonvulsants, GABAergic activators, opioid inhibitors of neurotransmission, and SSRI/SNRI) [93].

8.5 Orgasm Disorders

8.5.1 Pathophysiology of Orgasm

Orgasm in women has been defined as "a variable, transient peak sensation of intense pleasure, creating an altered state of consciousness" and inducing a state of "well-being and contentment" [35]. Orgasm may be accompanied by involuntary, rhythmic contractions of the pelvic floor musculature, and uterine and anal contractions [35]. This phenomenon displays wide interpersonal variability in terms of the intensity, duration, and type of required stimulation. In a recent multicenter study conducted on young women in a monogamous stable heterosexual relationship, the stopwatch-measured time to orgasm was approximately 13 min [98]. Although the existence of differently activated organs in women is still debated, evidence suggests many possible triggers: mental, from imagery alone, nipple/breast stimulation, clitoral, vaginal, cervical, anal, etc. [99]. In recent decades, it has been recognized that the vagina and cervix are not insensitive, passive organs, but have a unique and significant sensory cognitive representation, and their stimulation is able to elicit orgasmic sensations [100]. In clinical practice, many women report experiencing orgasm with clitoral stimulation, while others report vaginal penetration, or both. This has been correlated with the anatomical variability of the human clitoris-urethrovaginal complex [99].

Genital sexual stimuli reach the spinal cord mainly in the lumbosacral segments via the pudendal (clitoris), pelvic, and hypogastric nerves (vagina), and are transmitted to supraspinal sites via the spinothalamic and spinoreticular systems; ascending inputs then activate neurons in several areas of the CNS. Recent functional magnetic resonance imaging (fMRI) studies have suggested that, during female orgasm, the activated brain regions include sensory, motor, reward, frontal cortical, and brainstem regions (e.g., nucleus accumbens, insula, anterior cingulate cortex, orbitofrontal cortex, hippocampus, amygdala, hypothalamus, and ventral tegmental area) [101]. The efferent arm of the spinal reflexes is involved in sympathetic, parasympathetic, and somatic activities. Moreover, during orgasm, the concentration of hormones and neurotransmitters related to bonding, such as prolactin and oxytocin, increases.

Multiple mechanisms may be correlated with alterations in orgasmic ability in women. Impairment of the central or peripheral afferent and efferent neural pathways involved in the regulation of the orgasmic response determines orgasmic failure [102]. For example, a spinal cord injury at S2-S4 would blunt the ability to perceive clitoral stimulation, since the pudendal nerves, which convey clitoral sensation, enter the spinal cord at this level.

The pelvic floor seems to play an important role in female orgasmic response. It has been demonstrated that pelvic floor muscles strength, evaluated using perineometer and surface electromyography, is positively correlated with self-reported orgasm ability in healthy volunteers [103]. Overactivity of the PF muscles may impair orgasm by preventing local tissue perfusion and compression of the clitoral, perineal, or rectal branches of the pudendal nerve [104].

Physiological orgasmic responses also depend on the balance between excitatory and inhibitory neurotransmitters in the brain [9], which may be disrupted by medications, drugs, or endocrine alterations (hyperprolactinemia, hypoestrogenism, and hypoandrogenism).

Finally, orgasmic capacity is deeply influenced by psychological and relational factors. Concerning autoerotism, orgasmic difficulty has been associated with young age, low masturbation frequency, low sexual relationship satisfaction, and masturbation practiced "to decrease sexual tension" or "to overcome anxiety" [105]. In another study, lesbian women reported more frequent orgasms than heterosexual women, and women who orgasmed more frequently reported receiving more oral sex, having sex for longer, being more satisfied with their relationships, talking about their sexual fantasies with their partners, and expressing love during sex [106]. Sexual inhibition has been found to act as an independent vulnerability factor for orgasmic difficulties in a large community sample [107]. In partnered sex, variance in orgasmic pleasure was mostly related to partner issues, sexual inhibition, lack of interest, and insufficient experience [108].

8.5.2 Nosology and Current Definitions

The definition of female orgasm disorder (FOD) in the DSM-IV-R was a "persistent or recurrent delay in or absence of orgasm after a normal sexual excitement phase" [3], that evolved in the subsequent edition to a "marked delay in, marked infrequency of, or absence of orgasm and [...] marked reduced intensity of orgasmic sensations," inducing personal distress [6]. The most recent nomenclature proposal has broadened the diagnostic criteria and included the concept of orgasm occurring "too early," as in the male counterpart, and of "orgasm without pleasure." Indeed, the ISSWSH defines FOD as a condition "characterized by a persistent or recurrent, distressing compromise of orgasm frequency, intensity, timing, and/or pleasure associated with sexual activity for a minimum of 6 months" [20].

Specifiers are related to the following: (a) frequency: orgasm occurs with decreased frequency (decreased frequency of orgasm) or is absent (anorgasmia); (b) intensity: orgasm occurs with decreased intensity (muted orgasm); (c) timing: orgasm occurs too late (delayed orgasm) or too early (spontaneous or premature orgasm) than desired by the woman; and (d) pleasure: orgasm occurs with absent or decreased pleasure (anhedonic orgasm or pleasure dissociative orgasmic disorder, PDOD) [20]. Traditional specifiers apply (lifelong vs. situational and generalized vs. situational).

In addition to the new entity PDOD, another provisional diagnosis based on expert opinion has been introduced: female orgasmic illness syndrome (FOIS). This condition is characterized by "peripheral and/or central aversive symptoms that occur before, during, or after orgasm, not related, per se, to a compromise of orgasm quality" [20]. Interestingly, confusion, decreased verbal memory, depression, seizures, and headaches have been reported among these bothersome sensations, as well as gastrointestinal symptoms, muscle aches, and fatigue.

8.5.3 Prevalence and Leading Etiologies of FOD

Orgasmic difficulties are also common. In a random sample of more than 1500 women from the US, 24% reported an inability to achieve orgasm for months in the previous year [109]. The prevalence of DSM-based FOD diagnoses, including distress, is approximately 5% [23].

Neurogenic FOD can be a consequence of CNS lesions, spinal cord injury, diabetic neuropathy, pudendal neuropathy, radiculopathy of the sacral spinal nerve roots due to herniation/compression by intervertebral discs, or other condi-

tions. In women with multiple sclerosis, anorgasmia or hyporgasmia has been reported in up to 37.1% of cases [110].

Psychotropic medications, specifically mood stabilizers, antipsychotics, and antidepressants, often cause delayed or pleasure-less orgasm as a side effect, even after discontinuation [111]. A full history of medication use should be obtained in women with FOD.

A disordered function of the PF muscles that determines either increased activity (hypertonicity), diminished activity (hypotonicity), or inappropriate coordination may be associated with orgasm difficulties [112].

Vascular alterations in the genital bed and related risk factors (diabetes mellitus, obesity, smoking, and peripheral vascular disease) have been correlated with FOD because of the critical role of genital blood flow in peripheral sexual response [62]. Similarly, hormonal alterations that are known to undermine the anatomical and functional integrity of the genital tissue, especially low levels of androgens and estrogens, are potentially correlated with low sexual responsiveness and FOD. Furthermore, all inflammatory, infectious, and immunological conditions that determine dyspareunia (See Chap. 25) can indirectly affect the orgasmic function.

Pathological orgasm may also be experienced in the context of psychosocial issues. Poor body and genital image issues, negative emotions associated with sex, cultural background, shame or embarrassment due to religious beliefs, or familial inhibitions can contribute to anorgasmia or delayed orgasm [113]. Relationship issues should always be addressed; the lack of proper communication with the partner has been described as a key factor in women's orgasmic experience, as well as the partner's sexual dysfunction, such as premature ejaculation or erectile dysfunction [114].

8.5.4 Diagnostic Tools for Orgasm Disorders

Diagnosis requires complete pharmacological, psychosocial, and relational assessment. Genital physical examination is mandatory to assess the sensitivity and integrity of the structures involved.

Vulvoscopy, Q-tip testing, and smear testing are useful for identifying dermatological, inflammatory, and infectious conditions that may interfere with the peripheral sexual response. Laboratory testing is aimed at identifying women with low androgen levels, low estradiol levels, elevated prolactin, or dysthyroidism, who may benefit from replacement treatments or require further diagnostic workup to exclude endocrine diseases contributing to FOD.

In cases of specific clinical suspicion (i.e., vascular or neurological pathology), additional testing is advised. This may include pelvic floor physical therapy assessment, neurophysiological tests (i.e., evoked potentials of the pudendal nerve), MRI of the spine, clitoral/vulvar Doppler ultrasonography, or thermography.

The most commonly used psychometric measures for the evaluation of the subjective experience of the orgasm are the Orgasm Rating Scale [115] and the Orgasm domain of the Female Sexual Function Index [40]. A visual analog scale (VAS) named Orgasmometer-F has been validated in women to assess perceived orgasmic intensity [116]. Other recently developed tools include the Orgasm Beliefs Inventory [117] and the Bodily Sensations of Orgasm questionnaire [118].

8.5.5 Key Therapeutic Approaches

The modification of any reversible risk factors for FOD is recommended prior to considering any symptomatic intervention for desire and orgasm problems. The literature on symptomatic therapies for FOD is limited and contradictory, and there are no government-approved pharmacological treatments for this indication.

Specific randomized controlled trials on the effect of testosterone therapy on the orgasm domain of sexual function have not yet been published. However, a recent meta-analysis showed that compared to a placebo or comparator, testosterone significantly increased orgasms (SMD 0.25, 95% CI 0.18–0.32) in postmenopausal women [50]. Therefore, systemic testosterone treatment, which is off-label in most countries, may be an option for improving FOD in postmenopausal patients with comorbid HSDD.

Off-label agents including flibanserin and bremelanotide (both approved for HSDD in premenopausal women) and the antidepressant bupropion act on the balance of excitatory/inhibitory neurotransmitters, thus potentially facilitating the orgasmic response [119]. Vasodilating agents, such as sildenafil, have been suggested to improve orgasm measures in premenopausal women affected by sexual arousal disorder [120], whereas a less clear effect has been found in estrogenized postmenopausal women [121]; these data need to be confirmed.

Medical devices that provide vibratory stimulation or cause clitoral vascular engorgement by a vacuum system, ultimately enhancing arousal and orgasm, have been proposed as treatment approaches for FOD [122].

Compared with sexual pain disorders, very few studies have addressed the effect of physical therapy (i.e., Kegel exercises) on orgasm [123]. Therefore, conclusive evidence for a specific beneficial effect of FOD cannot be drawn. However, it has been suggested that in patients with hyperactivity of the PF muscles, a reduction in tone may improve orgasmic function [104]. In the clinical setting, appropriate relaxation training of the pelvic floor muscles in synergy with diaphragmatic breathing facilitates genital arousal, with improved genital congestion and lubrication, and can facilitate a more rapid and intense orgasm.

Psychological and behavioral treatments for FOD with the most consistent data include directed masturbation, sensate focus, and psychotherapy [124]. For example, directed masturbation is a cognitive-behavioral and mindfulness-based technique centered on stepwise exposure to genital stimulation. Available studies have demonstrated the efficacy of this type of therapy in FOD [124]. Other proposed approaches with little evidence include sex education, systematic desensitization, bibliotherapy, and coital alignment technique training; however, they may represent beneficial adjuncts [124].

Orgasm Disorders: Key Points
- Female Orgasm Disorder (FOD) is characterized by "a persistent or recurrent, distressing compromise of orgasm frequency, intensity, timing, and/or pleasure associated with sexual activity for a minimum of 6 months."
- Other recently proposed conditions relative to orgasm alterations are the pleasure dissociative orgasmic disorder (PDOD) and the female orgasmic illness syndrome (FOIS).
- The prevalence of orgasmic dysfunction including distress is around 5%.
- Leading etiologies of FOD are as follows: neurogenic conditions (secondary to CNS lesions, spinal cord injury, diabetic neuropathy, pudendal neuropathy, and radiculopathy of the sacral spinal nerve roots); use of medications disrupting the excitation/inhibition balance (i.e., mood stabilizers, antipsychotics, and antidepressants); pelvic floor muscles dysfunction (i.e., hyperactivity); vascular alterations in the genital bed and related risk factors (diabetes mellitus, obesity, smoking, and peripheral vascular disease); hormonal alterations (hypoestrogenism, hypoandrogenism, and hyperprolactinemia); psychosocial issues (sexual inhibition, poor body image, shame, or embarrassment due to cultural background); and poor communication with the partner or partner's sexual dysfunction.
- Diagnostic tools: pharmacological, psychosocial, and relational assessment; genital physical examination; and laboratory testing. Clinically-driven additional investigations include pelvic floor strength assessment; neurophysiological tests; MRI of the spine; and clitoral/vulvar Doppler ultrasonography or thermography.
- Psychometric questionnaires: Orgasm Rating Scale, Orgasm Domain of the Female Sexual Function Index, Orgasmometer-F, Orgasm Beliefs Inventory, and Bodily Sensations of Orgasm questionnaire.
- First-line treatment strategy: modification of any reversible risk factors. Off-label pharmacological therapies: systemic testosterone treatment in postmenopausal patients with comorbid HSDD, flibanserin and bremelanotide in premenopausal patients with comorbid HSDD, or bupropion; vasodilating agents. Medical devices (i.e., vibrators or vacuum systems) and pelvic floor physical therapy may be considered.
- Psychological and behavioral treatments for FOD with the most consistent data on efficacy are: directed masturbation, sensate focus, and psychotherapy.

8.6 Conclusion

The conceptualization, classification, and definition of FSDs are highly dynamic. The complexity of definitions is aimed at describing in the most comprehensive way the many differences and nuances of FSDs in different women and clusters of women. The purpose was to share definitions to standardize the frames and goals of research and investigations.

However, definitions are often difficult to translate into wording that is easy to use with colleagues who are not trained in sexual medicine and, even more importantly, with patients. The difficulty is greater when English definitions must be translated into other languages.

Therefore, the challenge is to find the optimal wording, matching the most comprehensive definition with words that are easier to understand, and best fitting the daily experience of women with sexual disorders. However, this challenge remains to be addressed.

References

1. Parish SJ, Cottler-Casanova S, Clayton AH, McCabe MP, Coleman E, Reed GM. The evolution of the female sexual disorder/dysfunction definitions, nomenclature, and classifications: a review of DSM, ICSM, ISSWSH, and ICD. Sex Med Rev. 2021;9(1):36–56.
2. American Psychiatric Association, editor. Diagnostic and statistical manual of mental disorders. 4th ed. Washington, DC: American Psychiatric Association; 1994.
3. American Psychiatric Association, editor. Diagnostic and statistical manual of mental disorders. 4th rev. ed. Washington, DC: American Psychiatric Association; 2000.
4. Basson R, Leiblum S, Brotto L, Derogatis L, Fourcroy J, Fugl-Meyer K, Graziottin A, Heiman JR, Laan E, Meston C, Schover L, van Lankveld J, Schultz WW. Revised definitions of women's sexual dysfunction. J Sex Med. 2004;1(1):40–8.
5. Brotto LA. The DSM diagnostic criteria for hypoactive sexual desire disorder in women. Arch Sex Behav. 2010;39(2):221–39.
6. American Psychiatric Association, editor. Diagnostic and statistical manual of mental disorders. 5th ed. Washington, DC: American Psychiatric Association; 2013.
7. Giraldi A, Kristensen E, Sand M. Endorsement of models describing the sexual response of men and women with a sexual partner: an online survey in a population sample of Danish adults ages 20-65 years. J Sex Med. 2015;12(1):116–28.
8. Perelman MA. Why the sexual tipping point® model? Curr Sex Health Rep. 2016;8:39–46.
9. Pfaus JG. Pathways of sexual desire. J Sex Med. 2009;6:1506–33.
10. Georgiadis JR, Kringelbach ML, Pfaus JG. Sex for fun: a synthesis of human and animal neurobiology. Nat Rev Urol. 2012;9(9):486–98.
11. Graham MD, Gardner Gregory J, Hussain D, Brake WG, Pfaus JG. Ovarian steroids alter dopamine receptor populations in the medial preoptic area of female rats: implications for sexual motivation, desire, and behaviour. Eur J Neurosci. 2015;42(12):3138–48.
12. Young E, Becker JB. Perspective: sex matters: gonadal steroids and the brain. Neupsychopharmacology. 2009;34(3):537–8.
13. Pfaus JG, Jones SL, Flanagan-Cato LM, Blaustein JD. Female sexual behaviour. In: Plant TM, Zeleznik AJ, Knobil E, Neil JD, editors. Knobil and Neill's physiology of reproduction. 4th ed. Amsterdam: Elsevier; 2015. p. 2287–370.
14. Maseroli E, Vignozzi L. Are endogenous androgens linked to female sexual function? A systemic review and meta-analysis. J Sex Med. 2022;S1743-6095(22):00548-3.
15. Jones SL, Rosenbaum S, Gardner Gregory J, Pfaus JG. Aromatization is not required for the facilitation of appetitive sexual behaviors in ovariectomized rats treated with estradiol and testosterone. Front Neurosci. 2019;13:798.
16. Maseroli E, Santangelo A, Lara-Fontes B, Quintana GR, Mac Cionnaith CE, Casarrubea M, Ricca V, Maggi M, Vignozzi L, Pfaus JG. The non-aromatizable androgen dihydrotestosterone (DHT) facilitates sexual behavior in ovariectomized female rats primed with estradiol. Psychoneuroendocrinology. 2020;115:104606.
17. Clayton AH, DeRogatis LR, Rosen RC, Pyke R. Intended or unintended consequences? The likely implications of raising the bar for sexual dysfunction diagnosis in the proposed DSM-V revisions: 1. For women with incomplete loss of desire or sexual receptivity. J Sex Med. 2012;9(8):2027–39.
18. McCabe MP, Sharlip ID, Atalla E, Balon R, Fisher AD, Laumann E, Lee SW, Lewis R, Segraves RT. Definitions of sexual dysfunctions in women and men: a consensus statement from the fourth international consultation on sexual medicine 2015. J Sex Med. 2016;13(2):135–43.
19. Derogatis LR, Sand M, Balon R, Rosen R, Parish SJ. Toward a more evidence-based nosology and nomenclature for female sexual dysfunctions—part I. J Sex Med. 2016;13(12):1881–7.
20. Parish SJ, Goldstein AT, Goldstein SW, Goldstein I, Pfaus J, Clayton AH, Giraldi A, Simon JA, Althof SE, Bachmann G, Komisaruk B, Levin R, Spadt SK, Kingsberg SA, Perelman MA, Waldinger MD, Whipple B. Toward a more evidence-based nosology and nomenclature for female sexual dysfunctions—part II. J Sex Med. 2016;13(12):1888–906.
21. World Health Organization. International statistical classification of diseases and related health problems. 11th ed. World Health Organization; 2019.
22. Clayton AH, Goldstein I, Kim NN, Althof SE, Faubion SS, Faught BM, Parish SJ, Simon JA, Vignozzi L, Christiansen K, Davis SR, Freedman MA, Kingsberg SA, Kirana PS, Larkin L, McCabe M, Sadovsky R. The International Society for the Study of Women's Sexual Health process of care for management of hypoactive sexual desire disorder in women. Mayo Clin Proc. 2018;93(4):467–87.
23. Shifren JL, Monz BU, Russo PA, Segreti A, Johannes CB. Sexual problems and distress in United States women: prevalence and correlates. Obstet Gynecol. 2008;112(5):970–8.
24. Graziottin A, Serafini A, Palacios S. Aetiology, diagnostic algorithms and prognosis of female sexual dysfunction. Maturitas. 2009;63(2):128–34.
25. Janse F, Tanahatoe SJ, Eijkemans MJ, Fauser BC. Testosterone concentrations, using different assays, in different types of ovarian insufficiency: a systematic review and meta-analysis. Hum Reprod Update. 2012;18(4):405–19.
26. Graziottin A, Koochaki PE, Rodenberg CA, Dennerstein L. The prevalence of hypoactive sexual desire disorder in surgically menopausal women: an epidemiological study of women in four European countries. J Sex Med. 2009;6(8):2143–53.

27. Di Stasi V, Verde N, Maseroli E, Scavello I, Cipriani S, Todisco T, Maggi M, Vignozzi L. Female sexual dysfunction as a warning sign of chronic disease development. Curr Sex Health Rep. 2019;11:307–19.

28. Atlantis E, Sullivan T. Bidirectional association between depression and sexual dysfunction: a systematic review and meta-analysis. J Sex Med. 2012;9(6):1497–507.

29. Buster JE. Managing female sexual dysfunction. Fertil Steril. 2013;100(4):905–15.

30. Davis SR, Wahlin-Jacobsen S. Testosterone in women—the clinical significance. Lancet Diabetes Endocrinol. 2015;3(12):980–92.

31. Kalmbach DA, Kingsberg SA, Roth T, Cheng P, Fellman-Couture C, Drake CL. Sexual function and distress in postmenopausal women with chronic insomnia: exploring the role of stress dysregulation. Nat Sci Sleep. 2019;11:141–53.

32. Camaschella C. Iron-deficiency anemia. N Engl J Med. 2015;372:1832–43.

33. Vahdat Shariatpanaahi M, Vahdat Shariatpanaahi Z, Moshtaaghi M, Shahbaazi SH, Abadi A. The relationship between depression and serum ferritin level. Eur J Clin Nutr. 2007;61:532–5.

34. Toxqui L, Vaquero MP. Chronic iron deficiency as an emerging risk factor for osteoporosis: a hypothesis. Nutrients. 2015;7:2324–44.

35. Meston CM, Levin RJ, Sipski ML, Hull EM, Heiman JR. Women's orgasm. Annu Rev Sex Res. 2004;15:173–257.

36. Simon JA, Goldstein I, Kim NN, Davis SR, Kellogg-Spadt S, Lowenstein L, Pinkerton JV, Stuenkel CA, Traish AM, Archer DF, Bachmann G, Goldstein AT, Nappi RE, Vignozzi L. The role of androgens in the treatment of genitourinary syndrome of menopause (GSM): International Society for the Study of Women's Sexual Health (ISSWSH) expert consensus panel review. Menopause. 2018;25(7):837–47.

37. Maseroli E, Scavello I, Campone B, Di Stasi V, Cipriani S, Felciai F, Camartini V, Magini A, Castellini G, Ricca V, Maggi M, Vignozzi L. Psychosexual correlates of unwanted sexual experiences in women consulting for female sexual dysfunction according to their timing across the life span. J Sex Med. 2018;15(12):1739–51.

38. Rust J, Derogatis L, Rodenberg C, Koochaki P, Schmitt S, Golombok S. Development and validation of a new screening tool for hypoactive sexual desire disorder: the brief profile of female sexual function (B-PFSF). Gynecol Endocrinol. 2007;23:638–44.

39. Clayton AH, Goldfischer E, Goldstein I, DeRogatis L, Nappi R, Lewis-D'Agostino DJ, Kimura T, Hebert A, Pyke R. Validity of the decreased sexual desire screener for diagnosing hypoactive sexual desire disorder. J Sex Marital Ther. 2013;39(2):132–43.

40. Rosen R, Brown C, Heiman J, Leiblum S, Meston C, Shabsigh R, Ferguson D, D'Agostino R Jr. The Female Sexual Function Index (FSFI): a multidimensional self-report instrument for the assessment of female sexual function. J Sex Marital Ther. 2000;26(2):191–208.

41. Gerstenberger EP, Rosen RC, Brewer JV, Meston CM, Brotto LA, Wiegel M, Sand M. Sexual desire and the female sexual function index (FSFI): a sexual desire cutpoint for clinical interpretation of the FSFI in women with and without hypoactive sexual desire disorder. J Sex Med. 2010;7(9):3096–103.

42. Meston CM, Freihart BK, Handy AB, Kilimnik CD, Rosen RC. Scoring and interpretation of the FSFI: what can be learned from 20 years of use? J Sex Med. 2020;17(1):17–25.

43. Derogatis L, Clayton A, Lewis-D'Agostino D, Wunderlich G, Fu Y. Validation of the female sexual distress scale-revised for assessing distress in women with hypoactive sexual desire disorder. J Sex Med. 2008;5(2):357–64.

44. Goldstein I, Kim NN, Clayton AH, DeRogatis LR, Giraldi A, Parish SJ, Pfaus J, Simon JA, Kingsberg SA, Meston C, Stahl SM, Wallen K, Worsley R. Hypoactive sexual desire disorder: International Society for the Study of Women's Sexual Health (ISSWSH) expert consensus panel review. Mayo Clin Proc. 2017;92(1):114–28.

45. Trudel G, Marchand A, Ravart M, Aubin S, Turgeon L, Fortier P. The effect of a cognitive-behavioral group treatment program on hypoactive sexual desire in women. Sex Relation Ther. 2001;16(2):145–64.

46. Pyke RE, Clayton AH. Psychological treatment trials for hypoactive sexual desire disorder: a sexual medicine critique and perspective. J Sex Med. 2015;12(12):2451–8.

47. Brotto LA, Basson R. Group mindfulness-based therapy significantly improves sexual desire in women. Behav Res Ther. 2014;57:43–54.

48. Parish SJ, Simon JA, Davis SR, Giraldi A, Goldstein I, Goldstein SW, Kim NN, Kingsberg SA, Morgentaler A, Nappi RE, Park K, Stuenkel CA, Traish AM, Vignozzi L. International Society for the Study of Women's Sexual Health clinical practice guideline for the use of systemic testosterone for hypoactive sexual desire disorder in women. J Sex Med. 2021;18(5):849–67.

49. Davis SR, Baber R, Panay N, Bitzer J, Perez SC, Islam RM, Kaunitz AM, Kingsberg SA, Lambrinoudaki I, Liu J, Parish SJ, Pinkerton J, Rymer J, Simon JA, Vignozzi L, Wierman ME. Global consensus position statement on the use of testosterone therapy for women. J Clin Endocrinol Metab. 2019;104(10):4660–6.

50. Islam RM, Bell RJ, Green S, Page MJ, Davis SR. Safety and efficacy of testosterone for women: a systematic review and meta-analysis of randomised controlled trial data. Lancet Diabetes Endocrinol. 2019;7(10):754–66.

51. Scavello I, Maseroli E, Di Stasi V, Vignozzi L. Sexual health in menopause. Medicina (Kaunas). 2019;55(9):559.

52. Elraiyah T, Sonbol MB, Wang Z, Khairalseed T, Asi N, Undavalli C, Nabhan M, Altayar O, Prokop L, Montori VM, Murad MH. Clinical review: the

benefits and harms of systemic dehydroepiandrosterone (DHEA) in postmenopausal women with normal adrenal function: a systematic review and meta-analysis. J Clin Endocrinol Metab. 2014;99(10):3536–42.

53. Simon JA, Clayton AH, Kim NN, Patel S. Clinically meaningful benefit in women with hypoactive sexual desire disorder treated with flibanserin. Sex Med. 2022;10(1):100476.

54. Edinoff AN, Sanders NM, Lewis KB, Apgar TL, Cornett EM, Kaye AM, Kaye AD. Bremelanotide for treatment of female hypoactive sexual desire. Neurol Int. 2022;14(1):75–88.

55. Segraves RT, Clayton A, Croft H, Wolf A, Warnock J. Bupropion sustained release for the treatment of hypoactive sexual desire disorder in premenopausal women. J Clin Psychopharmacol. 2004;24(3):339–42.

56. Graziottin A, Giraldi A. Anatomy and physiology of women's sexual function. In: Porst H, Buvat J, editors. ISSM (International Society of Sexual Medicine) standard committee book, standard practice in sexual medicine. Oxford: Blackwell; 2006. p. 289–304.

57. Traish AM, Botchevar E, Kim NN. Biochemical factors modulating female genital sexual arousal physiology. J Sex Med. 2010;7(9):2925–46.

58. Park K, Goldstein I, Andry C, Siroky MB, Krane RJ, Azadzoi KM. Vasculogenic female sexual dysfunction: the hemodynamic basis for vaginal engorgement insufficiency and clitoral erectile insufficiency. Int J Impot Res. 1997;9(1):27–37.

59. Angulo J, Hannan JL. Cardiometabolic diseases and female sexual dysfunction: animal studies. J Sex Med. 2022;S1743-6095(21):00829-8.

60. Caruso S, Cianci A, Malandrino C, Cavallari L, Gambadoro O, Arena G, Pispisa L, Agnello C, Romano M, Cavallari V. Ultrastructural and quantitative study of clitoral cavernous tissue from living subjects. J Sex Med. 2011;8(6):1675–85.

61. Maseroli E, Scavello I, Vignozzi L. Cardiometabolic risk and female sexuality-part I. risk factors and potential pathophysiological underpinnings for female vasculogenic sexual dysfunction syndromes. Sex Med Rev. 2018;6(4):508–24.

62. Miner M, Esposito K, Guay A, Montorsi P, Goldstein I. Cardiometabolic risk and female sexual health: the Princeton III summary. J Sex Med. 2012;9(3):641–51; quiz 652.

63. Harte CB, Meston CM. The inhibitory effects of nicotine on physiological sexual arousal in nonsmoking women: results from a randomized, double-blind, placebo-controlled, cross-over trial. J Sex Med. 2008;5:1184–97. https://doi.org/10.1111/J.1743-6109.2008.00778.X.

64. Ju R, Ruan X, Xu X, Yang Y, Cheng J, Zhang L, Wang B, Qin S, Dou Z, Mueck AO. Importance of active and passive smoking as one of the risk factors for female sexual dysfunction in Chinese women. Gynecol Endocrinol. 2021;37:541–5. https://doi.org/10.1080/09513590.2021.1913115.

65. Greenberg DR, Khandwala YS, Breyer BN, Minkow R, Eisenberg ML. Genital pain and numbness and female sexual dysfunction in adult bicyclists. J Sex Med. 2019;16:1381–9. https://doi.org/10.1016/J.JSXM.2019.06.017.

66. Gaither TW, Awad MA, Murphy GP, Metzler I, Sanford T, Eisenberg ML, Sutcliffe S, Osterberg CE, Breyer BN. Cycling and female sexual and urinary function: results from a large, multinational, cross-sectional study. J Sex Med. 2018;15:510–8. https://doi.org/10.1016/J.JSXM.2018.02.004.

67. Handy AB, Freihart BK, Meston CM. The relationship between subjective and physiological sexual arousal in women with and without arousal concerns. J Sex Marital Ther. 2020;46(5):447–59.

68. Meston CM, Stanton AM. Understanding sexual arousal and subjective-genital arousal desynchrony in women. Nat Rev Urol. 2019;16(2):107–20.

69. Parish SJ, Meston CM, Althof SE, Clayton AH, Goldstein I, Goldstein SW, Heiman JR, McCabe MP, Segraves RT, Simon JA. Toward a more evidence-based nosology and nomenclature for female sexual dysfunctions-part III. J Sex Med. 2019;16(3):452–62.

70. Pontiroli AE, Cortelazzi D, Morabito A. Female sexual dysfunction and diabetes: a systematic review and metaanalysis. J Sex Med. 2013;10:1044–51.

71. Braffett B, Wessells H, Sarma AV. Urogenital autonomic dysfunction in diabetes. Curr Diabetes Rep. 2016;16:119.

72. Drulovic J, Kisic-Tepavcevic D, Pekmezovic T. Epidemiology, diagnosis and management of sexual dysfunction in multiple sclerosis. Acta Neurol Belg. 2020;120(4):791–7.

73. Goldstein I. Pathophysiology and medical management of female genital arousal disorder. In: Goldstein I, Clayton AH, Goldstein AT, Kim NN, Kingsberg SA, editors. Textbook of female sexual function and dysfunction: diagnosis and treatment. 1st ed. Wiley; 2018.

74. Aerts L, Komisaruk B, Bianco-Demichelli F, Pluchino N, Goldstein I. Sexual life after hysterectomy: still a neglected topic? Sex Med Rev. 2020;8(2):181–2.

75. Eid MA, Sayed A, Abdel-Rehim R, Mostafa T. Impact of the mode of delivery on female sexual function after childbirth. Int J Impot Res. 2015;27:118–20.

76. Cellai I, Filippi S, Comeglio P, Cipriani S, Maseroli E, Di Stasi V, Todisco T, Marchiani S, Tamburrino L, Villanelli F, Vezzani S, Corno C, Fambrini M, Guarnieri G, Sarchielli E, Morelli A, Rastrelli G, Maggi M, Vignozzi L. Testosterone positively regulates vagina NO-induced relaxation: an experimental study in rats. J Endocrinol Investig. 2022;45:1161–72.

77. Comeglio P, Cellai I, Filippi S, Corno C, Corcetto F, Morelli A, Maneschi E, Maseroli E, Mannucci E, Fambrini M, Maggi M, Vignozzi L. Differential effects of testosterone and estradiol on clitoral function: an experimental study in rats. J Sex Med. 2016;13(12):1858–71.

78. Segnini I, Kukkonen TM. Psychological management of arousal disorders. In: Goldstein I, Clayton AH, Goldstein AT, Kim NN, Kingsberg SA, editors. Textbook of female sexual function and dysfunction: diagnosis and treatment. 1st ed. Wiley; 2018.

79. Corona G, Rastrelli G, Isidori AM, Pivonello R, Bettocchi C, Reisman Y, Sforza A, Maggi M. Erectile dysfunction and cardiovascular risk: a review of current findings. Expert Rev Cardiovasc Ther. 2020;18(3):155–64.

80. Kukkonen TM. Devices and methods to measure female sexual arousal. Sex Med Rev. 2015;3(4):225–44.

81. Cipriani S, Maseroli E, Di Stasi V, Scavello I, Todisco T, Rastrelli G, Fambrini M, Sorbi F, Petraglia F, Jannini EA, Maggi M, Vignozzi L. Effects of testosterone treatment on clitoral haemodynamics in women with sexual dysfunction. J Endocrinol Investig. 2021;44(12):2765–76.

82. Fernández Pérez M, Fernández Agís I, La Calle Marcos P, Campos Caballero R, Molero Rodríguez F, González Fernández M, Rodríguez Torreblanca C. Validation of a sagittal section technique for measuring clitoral blood flow. Volume flow: a new parameter in clitoral artery Doppler. J Sex Med. 2020;17(6):1109–17.

83. Handy AB, Meston CM. An objective measure of vaginal lubrication in women with and without sexual arousal concerns. J Sex Marital Ther. 2021;47(1):32–42.

84. Potter N, Panay N. Vaginal lubricants and moisturizers: a review into use, efficacy, and safety. Climacteric. 2021;24(1):19–24.

85. Herbenick D, Reece M, Sanders S, Dodge B, Ghassemi A, Fortenberry JD. Prevalence and characteristics of vibrator use by women in the United States: results from a nationally representative study. J Sex Med. 2009;6(7):1857–66.

86. Goldstein SW, Gonzalez JR, Gagnon C, Goldstein I. Peripheral female genital arousal as assessed by thermography following topical genital application of alprostadil vs placebo arousal gel: a proof-of-principle study without visual sexual stimulation. Sex Med. 2016;4(3):e166–75.

87. Becher EF, Bechara A, Casabe A. Clitoral hemodynamic changes after a topical application of alprostadil. J Sex Marital Ther. 2001;27(5):405–10.

88. Caruso S, Mauro D, Cariola M, Fava V, Rapisarda AMC, Cianci A. Randomized crossover study investigating daily versus on-demand vulvar Visnadine spray in women affected by female sexual arousal disorder. Gynecol Endocrinol. 2018;34(2):110–4.

89. Gao L, Yang L, Qian S, Li T, Han P, Yuan J. Systematic review and meta-analysis of phosphodiesterase type 5 inhibitors for the treatment of female sexual dysfunction. Int J Gynaecol Obstet. 2016;133(2):139–45.

90. Bouchard C, Labrie F, Derogatis L, Girard G, Ayotte N, Gallagher J, Cusan L, Archer DF, Portman D, Lavoie L, Beauregard A, Côté I, Martel C, Vaillancourt M, Balser J, Moyneur E, VVA Prasterone Group. Effect of intravaginal dehydroepiandrosterone (DHEA) on the female sexual function in postmenopausal women: ERC-230 open-label study. Horm Mol Biol Clin Investig. 2016;25(3):181–90.

91. Cellai I, Di Stasi V, Comeglio P, Maseroli E, Todisco T, Corno C, Filippi S, Cipriani S, Sorbi F, Fambrini M, Petraglia F, Scavello I, Rastrelli G, Acciai G, Villanelli F, Danza G, Sarchielli E, Guarnieri G, Morelli A, Maggi M, Vignozzi L. Insight on the intracrinology of menopause: androgen production within the human vagina. Endocrinology. 2021;162(2):bqaa219.

92. Davis SR, Robinson PJ, Jane F, White S, White M, Bell RJ. Intravaginal testosterone improves sexual satisfaction and vaginal symptoms associated with aromatase inhibitors. J Clin Endocrinol Metab. 2018;103(11):4146–54.

93. Goldstein I, Komisaruk BR, Pukall CF, Kim NN, Goldstein AT, Goldstein SW, Hartzell-Cushanick R, Kellogg-Spadt S, Kim CW, Jackowich RA, Parish SJ, Patterson A, Peters KM, Pfaus JG. International Society for the Study of Women's Sexual Health (ISSWSH) review of epidemiology and pathophysiology, and a consensus nomenclature and process of care for the management of persistent genital arousal disorder/genito-pelvic dysesthesia (PGAD/GPD). J Sex Med. 2021;18(4):665–97.

94. Pease ER, Ziegelmann M, Vencill JA, Kok SN, Collins CS, Betcher HK. Persistent genital arousal disorder (PGAD): a clinical review and case series in support of multidisciplinary management. Sex Med Rev. 2022;10(1):53–70.

95. Feigenbaum F, Boone K. Persistent genital arousal disorder caused by spinal meningeal cysts in the sacrum; successful neurosurgical treatment. Obstet Gynecol. 2016;126:839–43.

96. Kim C, Blevins J, Goldstein S, Komisaruk B, Goldstein I. Neurogenic persistent genital arousal disorder (PGAD) secondary to radiculopathy of sacral spinal nerve roots (SSNR): treatment outcomes following minimally invasive spine surgery (MISS). J Sex Med. 2020;17:S52.

97. Klifto K, Dellon AL. Persistent genital arousal disorder: treatment by neurolysis of dorsal branch of pudendal nerve. Microsurgery. 2020;40(2):160–6.

98. Bhat GS, Shastry A. Time to orgasm in women in a monogamous stable heterosexual relationship. J Sex Med. 2020;17(4):749–60.

99. Jannini EA, Rubio-Casillas A, Whipple B, Buisson O, Komisaruk BR, Brody S. Female orgasm(s): one, two, several. J Sex Med. 2012;9(4):956–65.

100. Komisaruk BR, Whipple B, Crawford A, Liu WC, Kalnin A, Mosier K. Brain activation during vaginocervical self-stimulation and orgasm in women with complete spinal cord injury: fMRI evidence of mediation by the vagus nerves. Brain Res. 2004;1024:77–88.

101. Wise NJ, Frangos E, Komisaruk BR. Brain activity unique to orgasm in women: an fMRI analysis. J Sex Med. 2017;14(11):1380–91.

102. Azadzoi KM, Siroky MB. Neurologic factors in female sexual function and dysfunction. Korean J Urol. 2010;51(7):443–9.

103. Sartori DVB, Kawano PR, Yamamoto HA, Guerra R, Pajolli PR, Amaro JL. Pelvic floor muscle strength is correlated with sexual function. Investig Clin Urol. 2021;62(1):79–84.

104. Brandon K. Musculoskeletal management of orgasm disorders. In: Goldstein I, Clayton AH, Goldstein AT, Kim NN, Kingsberg SA, editors. Textbook of female sexual function and dysfunction: diagnosis and treatment. 1st ed. Wiley; 2018.

105. Rowland DL, Kolba TN, McNabney SM, Uribe D, Hevesi K. Why and how women masturbate, and the relationship to orgasmic response. J Sex Marital Ther. 2020;46(4):361–76.

106. Frederick DA, John HKS, Garcia JR, Lloyd EA. Differences in orgasm frequency among gay, lesbian, bisexual, and heterosexual men and women in a U.S. national sample. Arch Sex Behav. 2018;47(1):273–88.

107. Tavares IM, Laan ETM, Nobre PJ. Sexual inhibition is a vulnerability factor for orgasm problems in women. J Sex Med. 2018;15(3):361–72.

108. Hevesi K, Gergely Hevesi B, Kolba TN, Rowland DL. Self-reported reasons for having difficulty reaching orgasm during partnered sex: relation to orgasmic pleasure. J Psychosom Obstet Gynaecol. 2020;41(2):106–15.

109. Simons JS, Carey MP. Prevalence of sexual dysfunctions: results from a decade of research. Arch Sex Behav. 2001;30:177–219.

110. Zorzon M, Zivadinov R, Bosco A, Bragadin LM, Moretti R, Bonfigli L, Morassi P, Iona LG, Cazzato G. Sexual dysfunction in multiple sclerosis: a case-control study. I. Frequency and comparison of groups. Mult Scler. 1999;5:418–27.

111. Bala A, Nguyen HMT, Hellstrom WJG. Post-SSRI sexual dysfunction: a literature review. Sex Med Rev. 2018;6(1):29–34.

112. Omodei MS, Marques Gomes Delmanto LR, Carvalho-Pessoa E, Schmitt EB, Nahas GP, Petri Nahas EA. Association between pelvic floor muscle strength and sexual function in postmenopausal women. J Sex Med. 2019;16(12):1938–46.

113. Ishak WW, Bokarius A, Jeffrey JK, Davis MC, Bakhta Y. Disorders of orgasm in women: a litera-

ture review of etiology and current treatments. J Sex Med. 2010;7(10):3254–68.

114. Burri A, Graziottin A. Cross-cultural differences in women's sexuality and their perception and impact of premature ejaculation. Urology. 2015;85(1):118–24.

115. Mah K, Binik YM. Do all orgasms feel alike? Evaluating a two-dimensional model of the orgasm experience across gender and sexual context. J Sex Res. 2002;39:104–13.

116. Mollaioli D, Di Sante S, Limoncin E, Ciocca G, Gravina GL, Maseroli E, Fanni E, Vignozzi L, Maggi M, Lenzi A, Jannini EA. Validation of a Visual Analogue Scale to measure the subjective perception of orgasmic intensity in females: the Orgasmometer-F. PLoS One. 2018;13(8):e0202076.

117. Séguin LJ, Blais M. The development and validation of the orgasm beliefs inventory. Arch Sex Behav. 2021;50(6):2543–61.

118. Dubray S, Gérard M, Beaulieu-Prévost D, Courtois F. Validation of a self-report questionnaire assessing the bodily and physiological sensations of orgasm. J Sex Med. 2017;14(2):255–63.

119. Modell JG, May RS, Katholi CR. Effect of bupropion-SR on orgasmic dysfunction in nondepressed subjects: a pilot study. J Sex Marital Ther. 2000;26(3):231–40.

120. Caruso S, Intelisano G, Lupo L, Agnello C. Premenopausal women affected by sexual arousal disorder treated with sildenafil: a double-blind, cross-over, placebo-controlled study. BJOG. 2001;108(6):623–8.

121. Basson R, Brotto LA. Sexual psychophysiology and effects of sildenafil citrate in oestrogenised women with acquired genital arousal disorder and impaired orgasm: a randomised controlled trial. BJOG. 2003;110(11):1014–24.

122. Billups KL. The role of mechanical devices in treating female sexual dysfunction and enhancing the female sexual response. World J Urol. 2002;20(2):137–41.

123. Nazarpour S, Simbar M, Ramezani Tehrani F, Alavi Majd H. Effects of sex education and Kegel exercises on the sexual function of postmenopausal women: a randomized clinical trial. J Sex Med. 2017;14(7):959–67.

124. Marchand E. Psychological and behavioral treatment of female orgasmic disorder. Sex Med Rev. 2021;9(2):194–211.

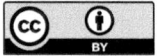

Penile Diseases and Dysmorphisms (Phimosis, Frenulum, Micropenis, and Buried Penis)

Marco Spilotros and Fabio Michele Ambruoso

9.1 Foreskin Disease: Balanitis and Balanoposthitis

9.1.1 Definition and Epidemiology

Balanitis is an inflammation of the glans penis, fairly common, affecting approximately 3–11% of males during their life time, if the inflammatory process involves even the prepuce the condition is termed balanoposthitis [1, 2]. Balanoposthitis involves both the glans and the foreskin and occurs in approximately 6% of uncircumcised males. Balanoposthitis occurs only in uncircumcised males. Balanitis and posthitis could present infectious and noninfectious etiologies, and they are not age related. Approximately 1 in 30 uncircumcised are affected by balanoposthitis, and phimosis represents a risk factor for this kind of condition. Circumcision has a protective role estimated in a 68% lower prevalence of balanitis than uncircumcised males [1, 2].

9.1.2 Pathophysiology

The most common cause of these condition is related to poor local hygiene, since the moist environment under the penile foreskin promotes the growth of organisms that could be the cause of balanitis. Between the normal flora of the foreskin and glans, Candida albicans is the most common yeast causing infection in certain circumstances especially when the patient has underlying pathological conditions such as diabetes, tumors of the glans and foreskin, immunodeficiency, or changes in the Ph baseline [3]. Other infectious causes of balanitis are sexually transmitted diseases (STDs such as gonorrhea, Chlamydia, herpes virus, human papillomavirus, syphilis, and trichomoniasis), Group B and A beta-hemolytic streptococci, and Gardnerella vaginalis infection [4]. Several skin conditions may also trigger balanitis such as psoriasis. Among noninfectious etiologies of balanitis, there are poor hygiene, chemicals irritants (detergent and spermicides) drug allergies, morbid obesity, allergic reaction, and local traumas [5].

9.1.3 Skin Conditions

Between the skin condition that could cause balanitis is important to highlight circinate balanitis (associated with reactive arthritis and HLA-B27), pseudo-epitheliomatous keratotic and micaceous balanitis and zoon balanitis (the latter three have been linked to skin cancer) [6, 7]. Balanitis xerotica obliterans (BXO) is an infiltrative chronic penile skin condition which is histologically

M. Spilotros (✉) · F. M. Ambruoso
Department of Emergency and Organ Transplantation-Urology, Andrology and Kidney Transplantation Unit, University of Bari, Bari, Italy

© The Author(s) 2023
C. Bettocchi et al. (eds.), *Practical Clinical Andrology*,
https://doi.org/10.1007/978-3-031-11701-5_9

identical to lichen sclerosus (hyperkeratosis, atrophy of the stratum spinosum Malpighii associated with hydropic degeneration of the basal cells associated with inflammatory infiltration of the mild dermis and edema), macroscopically characterized by hardened whitish tissue, and edema at the tip of the penis involving foreskin, glans of the penis, and often even the urethral meatus and urethra, leading to phimosis, strictures, and micturition discomfort. Treatment for BXO includes medical options such as topical steroid and surgical procedures including circumcision [8–10].

9.1.4 Clinical Findings and Diagnosis

Penile pain irradiating to the glans, redness, and itchiness are frequent symptoms of balanitis. At physical examination, signs frequently found are tight shiny skin on the glans, redness of the glans penis mucosa, swelling, soreness, and a thick white discharge under the foreskin commonly associated with an unpleasant smell. Painful micturition and phimosis could result in case of severe and chronic inflammation [11].

Essentially balanitis is a clinical diagnosis related to history and physical findings. Additional testing are justified by clinical presentation such as purulent discharge (bacterial culture is indicated), vesicular lesions (herpes simplex virus testing), ulcer (syphilis testing), and urethritis (testing for mycoplasma and trichomonas) [6].

9.1.5 Treatment

The strategy to manage a balanitis is to exclude STI, improve, or achieve a proper hygiene with frequent washing and drying off the prepuce. Topical antifungals are the first-line treatment in patients with balanoposthitis for 1–3 weeks with clotrimazole 1% twice daily or miconazole 1%. Nystatin cream is an alternative in patients allergic to imidazoles. Treatment of the partners of patients with balanitis is recom-

mended. In serious case of inflammation, Fluconazole 150 mg orally should be combined with topical imidazole and low potency steroids. If identified and involvement of subcutaneous tissue, a first generation cephalosporin should be administered. In recurrent episodes of balanoposthitis, especially in diabetic and immunocompromised patients, circumcision is recommended [3, 6, 11].

9.2 Foreskin Disease: Phimosis and Paraphimosis

9.2.1 Definition and Epidemiology

Prepuce, or foreskin, is the skin surrounding the glans penis which is at birth physiologically adherent until the 3–4 years of life (physiologic phimosis). As the penis grows, epithelial debris accumulates under the prepuce and produces a progressive separation between the foreskin and the glans forming the preputial sac. Less than 5% of newborns have a completely retractable prepuce, and this condition progressively changes with growth. At 3 years of life, about 90% of child have a fully retractable foreskin [12]. Phimosis is defined as the condition in which the prepuce cannot be retracted over the glans penis. Phimosis can persist over 3 years of age and in this case may be considered pathological; its incidence among 7-year-olds is 8% and progressively decrease to 1% at 17-year-old boys [13, 14].

9.2.2 Pathophysiology

Risk factors for phimosis are trauma (attempt to retraction), recurrent or chronic balanoposthitis, chronic inflammatory conditions like balanitis xerotica obliterans (BXO), a condition characterized by a sclerotic constricting ring in the distal end of the prepuce associated to edema, causing persistent non-retractability of the foreskin (Fig. 9.1). Its definitive diagnosis is based on histological features: hyperkeratosis with follicular atrophy of the spongiosa with

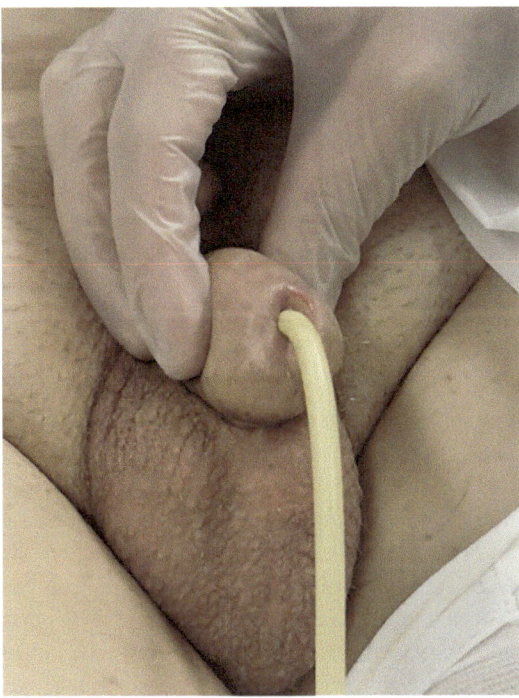

Fig. 9.1 Unretractable phimosis in catheterized patient

hydropic degeneration of basal cell, band-like chronic inflammatory cell infiltration with homogenization of collagen. BXO has an incidence of 0.6%; common onset is characterized by local infection, bleeding before phimosis, meatal stenosis that could cause urinary retention [8, 15].

9.2.3 Clinical Findings and Diagnosis

Generally, the unretractable foreskin shows inelastic scar tissue that prevent glans penis exposure; whitish color at the tip of the foreskin and edema are typical findings of BXO. In case of severe tightness of the foreskin, acute urinary retention is not a rare complication. Itchiness and redness of the glans penis in frequent when underlying balanitis is present. Diagnosis is related to history and physical findings. Histopathology of the foreskin removed is mandatory to confirm BXO as cause of phimosis.

9.2.4 Treatment

The treatment of choice to manage pathological phimosis is circumcision. In adults, circumcision is undertaken in operating room under local or general anesthesia. With the sleeve technique, a circumferential incision is made overlying the coronal impression of the glans through the skin. On the ventral surface, the skin incision should be in a V-shape opposite the frenulum. Once the foreskin is retracted, a second circumferential incision is made 0.5 cm below the coronal sulcus. On the dorsal surface, a plane superficial to Buck's fascia between the two circumferential incisions is created through blunt dissection. The ring of the prepuce is incised along this plane and then removed circumferentially. The circumcision is completed reapproximating the skin and the dartos of the inner prepuce with absorbable sutures in separate layers. In those cases, when severe tightness of the foreskin make it impossible to retract it on in case of paraphimosis, a dorsal slit is performed from the tip of the prepuce extending from the circumferential outer skin incision to the inner prepuce below the coronal sulcus [16].

Other options to treat phimosis (not indicated in BXO) are designed to achieve a fully retractile foreskin and can be pharmacological and surgical. Topical steroids such as clobetasol propionate and hydrocortisone together with regular attempts of prepuce retraction can achieve high success rates in 4–8 weeks of therapy, thanks to the anti-inflammatory and immunodepressive action associated to foreskin thinning [17]. Between surgical option, preputioplasty is an attempt to achieve a loosening of the scar tissue through its longitudinal incision which is then sutured in a transverse way [18]. Several preputioplasty techniques have been described: Welsh reported a triple full thickness incision across the stenotic ring followed by transvers suturing. In Wåhlin preputioplasty, three rhomboid incisions along the scarring ring are performed and closed by oblique suturing while Hoffman reported the use of multiple V-Y plasty along the constricting ring [19, 20].

Disposable circumcision suture device has been recently introduced, and it has gained increasing popularity. Shorter operation time, standardization of the technique, better cosmetic appearance, and fewer complications have been reported compared to classic cirumcision [21, 22]. Different disposable devices in different sizes are available and generally consist of a bell-shaped glans pedestal, ring blade, handle, shell, and suture staple. During the procedure, the glans lies under the glans pedestal and the foreskin is wrapped around the rod of the circumcision device. Once the knob is triggered, the foreskin is cut by the ring-shaped blade and staples are placed [22].

9.3 Paraphimosis

9.3.1 Definition, Epidemiology, and Treatment

Paraphimosis is an urological/andrological emergency whose clinical manifestation is a foreskin left retracted due to entrapment of a tight of the tissue proximal to the corona, leading to venous and lymphatic congestion. Signs in a patient with paraphimosis are glans engorgement, edema, and erythema of the prepuce; if the condition persist for few hours, bluish discoloration, tears, and necrosis of the superficial tissue may happen. Firstly, a manual reduction should be attempted, pushing forcefully the glans and retracting the foreskin in the natural position; in case of severe edema, multiple punctures to the edematous tissue before manual reduction are recommended. If manual reduction is achieved, some authors advise circumcisions because of paraphimosis tendency to recur; whereas when manual resolution is not possible, a dorsal slit is mandatory [23, 24].

9.4 Short Frenulum

9.4.1 Definition, Epidemiology, and Treatment

Frenulum breve, or short frenulum, is a dysmorphism in which the frenulum of the penis, which is an elastic band of tissue under the glans penis

that connects to the foreskin and helps contract it over the glans, is too short and thus hinders the movement of the foreskin, preventing full retraction of the foreskin.

The presence of a frenulum breve is a common cause for dyspareunia in males, often resulting in painful intercourse and trauma to the frenulum. Frenuloplasty is commonly performed under local anesthesia (either in day surgery or in an outpatient setting) as an alternative to circumcision for frenular pain and scarring, very effective procedure giving excellent functional results and patient satisfaction. Commonly, frenuloplasty is performed through a transverse incision of the frenulum which is then suture longitudinally with interrupted sutures. Careful hemostasis is mandatory due to the risk of severe bleeding from the frenula artery and its branches. Alternative techniques include the V-Y plasty and Z-plasty. The "pull and burn" technique described by Gyftopoulous is a sutureless approach involving the diathermy applied to the point of maximum tension of the frenulum followed by a controlled vertical tear [25, 26].

9.5 Micropenis

9.5.1 Definition and Epidemiology

Micropenis is a specific genitalia disorder whose incidence is about 1.5 per 10,000 newborns diagnosed through a thorough physical examination. The definition of micropenis is based on the stretched penile length (SPL; Fig. 9.2) measured from the pubis to the tip of the stretched penis (Table 9.1). 2.5 standard deviations less than the mean for the age without other pathological conditions of the penile shaft and distal urethra (i.e., hypospadias) [27, 28].

9.5.2 Pathophysiology

Micropenis is a result of a hormonal abnormality occurring after 12 weeks of gestation. Sexual male differentiation is linked to the presence of SRY gene (sex-determining region Y) on the Y chromosome. The gonadal differentiation into

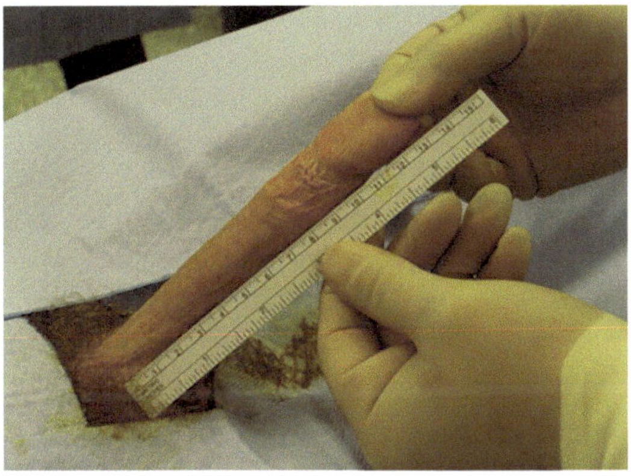

Fig. 9.2 Stretched penile length measured from the pubis to the tip of the stretched penis. (Picture by Mr. David Ralph, St. Peters Andrology Centre, London, UK)

Table 9.1 Normal SPL according to age and the corresponding 2.5 standard deviation defining micropenis [27, 28]

Age	Age mean ± SD mean (cm)	−2.5 SD (cm)
Newborn, 30-week gestation	2.5 ± 0.4	1.5
Newborn, 34-week gestation	3.0 ± 0.4	2.0
0–5 months	3.9 ± 0.8	1.9
6–12 months	4.3 ± 0.8	2.3
1–2 years	4.7 ± 0.8	2.6
2–3 years	5.1 ± 0.9	2.9
3–4 years	5.5 ± 0.9	3.3
4–5 years	5.7 ± 0.9	3.5
5–6 years	6.0 ± 0.9	3.8
6–7 years	6.1 ± 0.9	3.9
7–8 years	6.2 ± 1.0	3.7
8–9 years	6.3 ± 1.0	3.8
9–10 years	6.3 ± 1.1	3.8
10–11 years	6.4 ± 1.2	3.7

testicular tissue mediated by SRY gene involves three hormones: AMH (anti-Mullerian hormone), testosterone, and DHT (dihydrotestosterone). AMH induces regression of the paramesonephric ducts; testosterone stimulates the development of the mesonephric ducts (Wolffian ducts) into seminal vesicle, vas deferens, and epididymis; dihydrotestosterone supplies growth to male sexual characteristics including scrotal sac maturation, penile, and testicular size [29]. At 8 weeks of gestation, gonadotropin from placenta stimulates the

fetal Leydig cells to produce testosterone, thus inducing differentiation of genital tubercle, genital folds, and genital swelling into glans penis, shaft of the penis, and the scrotum, respectively. During the second and the third trimester, the growth of the penis occurs through fetal androgens, produced under stimulation by fetal pituitary gonadotropin. In the postnatal period, further growth takes place under the influence of the hypothalamic-pituitary axis leading to an high androgen levels between the first and the third month of life, then these levels reduce to the lowest until puberty [28].

Micropenis can be a result of a disturbance of the process started before, although true micropenis is considered to occur only from hormonals abnormality arising after 12 weeks of gestation (Table 9.2). The etiologies can be divide into five groups: deficient testosterone secretion (hypogonadotropic hypogonadism and hypergonadotropic hypogonadism), incomplete form of 5 alpha reductase deficiency or androgen receptor defects, idiopathic and associated with

Table 9.2 Common cause of micropenis

Hypogonadotropic hypogonadism (secondary hypogonadism)
1. Kallmann syndrome
2. Rudd syndrome
3. Bardet-Biedl syndrome
4. Laurence-Moon syndrome
5. Prader-Willi syndrome
Hypergonadotropic hypogonadism (primary or peripheral/gonadal hypogonadism)
1. Anorchia and testicular dysgenesis
2. Poly-X syndromes including Klinefelter syndrome
3. LH receptor mutation
4. Defects in androgen biosynthesis
5. Trisomy 21
6. Autosomal disorders (Robinow's syndrome, Noonan's syndrome, Laurence-Moon syndrome)
Defects in testosterone action
1. Androgen receptor defects
2. 5-α reductase deficiency
3. Growth hormone/insulin-like growth factor-I deficiency
Congenital disorders
1. Cloacal exstrophy
2. Associated to other malformations
Idiopathic

other congenital abnormalities [30]. In hypogonadotropic hypogonadism or secondary hypogonadism, the gonadal failure is due to abnormal pituitary gonadotropin levels related to absent or inadequate hypothalamic GnRH secretion or failure of pituitary gonadotropin secretion. Kallmann syndrome associated with anosmia or Prader-Willi syndrome associated with low height, hyperphagia and hypotonia can be diagnosed in patients with micropenis. In hypergonadotropic hypogonadism, the primary testicular defect is due to gonadal dysgenesis or associated with poly Y syndromes such as Klinefelter's syndrome. Consanguinity or drugs used during pregnancy in particular anti-androgen medications (flutamide, testolactone, enzalutamide, and spironolactone) are possible cause of Idiopathic micropenis [28, 31].

9.5.3 Diagnosis

Physical examination is essential to produce an accurate diagnosis: in the first instance, the clinicians must have a clear definition of micropenis and how to measure the penis properly, hence to exclude confounding condition such as webbed penis and hidden penis.

Stretched penile length measurement is taken from the pubic bone, taking care to compress the suprapubic fat pad, to the distal tip of the penis which is put on maximal stretch with retracted foreskin. Assessment of the penile shaft circumference, volume of the testicles, and size of the scrotum are also recommended to rule out hypoplastic corpora cavernosa, cryptorchidism or small volume testicle and hypoplastic scrotum particularly in pediatric and adolescent population. Location of the urethral meatus and curvature of the penile shaft are other important characteristics to investigate. Endocrinological evaluation is recommended and a baseline measurement of gonadotropin releasing hormone (GnRH), luteinizing hormone (LH), and follicle stimulating hormone (FSH) are mandatory in case of clinical suspicion of hypogonadotropic hypogonadism which can be associated to adrenocorticotropic and growth hormone deficiency.

Levels of prolactin help to understand the level of the defect in the hypothalamus-pituitary axis: high level is linked to hypothalamic defects whereas low level of prolactin is related to the pituitary glans [31]. Testicular function may also be assessed through serum testosterone levels and dihydrotestosterone. When abnormal laboratory findings are shown, ultrasound of the testis and brain MRI to evaluate the pituitary glands are indicated [32].

9.5.4 Treatment

Treatment can be divided in medical and surgical, and its aim is to achieve normal sexual and urinary function in the standing position. Regarding medical therapy, it is important to highlight that testosterone treatment of child on masculinization during puberty is still not fully clear and better long-term data are needed to fully understand the effects of treatment. Testosterone is available as intramuscular (IM) and topical: IM testosterone enanthate 25 mg is recommended every 3 weeks for 3 months, topical 5% testosterone cream in children and infants who are less than 8 years of age. Significant increase in penile length is reported but, if an unsatisfactory response is achieved after a short period of treatment, repeated administration for short periods may be performed. Dihydrotestosterone has been reported some efficacy especially in infants with 5 alpha reductase deficiency with an estimated 150% increase in penile length [33, 34]. Human recombinant FSH and LH treatment has been reported in children with micropenis in hypogonadotropic hypogonadism with a significant increase only in testicular volume and not satisfactory increase in penile size [35]. Surgical therapy is an alternative in the management of micropenis in those patients who proved unsatisfactory achievement with endocrinological therapy. Sex reassignment surgery in case of absence of testicular tissue was reported in the late 70th but more recently, this approach has been taken into consideration less frequently due to the psychological impact of gender reassignment [36, 37]. Taking into consideration the

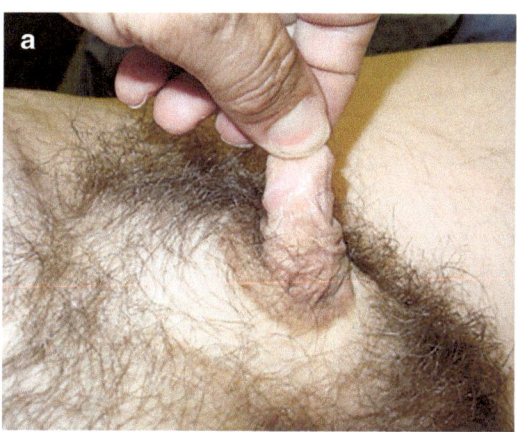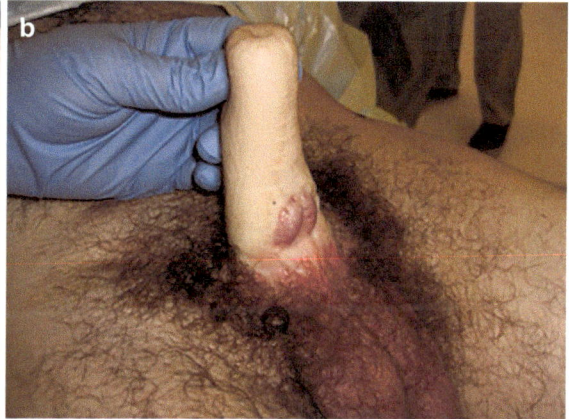

Fig. 9.3 (**a**) Pre-operative appearance of micropenis; (**b**) post-operative results in patients with micropenis underwent to radial forearm flap; the native glans penis is pre-served and left ventrally to keep erogenous sensation. (Picture by Mr. David Ralph, St. Peters Andrology Centre, London, UK)

significant psychosexual problems in those adults who underwent sex reassignment surgery and the conflicting data regarding this kind of surgery, it should be undertaken with extreme caution in high volume centers [38, 39]. Reconstructive surgery is nowadays a challenging but valid option for the treatment of micropenis. The first series was reported in the early 1970s, and in the following decades, advances in penile reconstruction surgery have been described [40]. The harvesting of a fasciocutaneous neophallus on a free flap on the radial artery or anterolateral thigh flap (ALT) has been reported with satisfactory outcomes, and more recently, the osteocutaneous fibula flap, the free scapular flap, the suprapubic abdominal wall flap, and the vertical rectus abdominis flap have been proposed as surgical options for the treatment of micropenis [41, 42]. The radial forearm free flap is the gold standard site to penile reconstruction surgery, mostly applied in female to male transsexualism, which consists in a microsurgical dissection of a radial forearm flap, possibly the nondominant arm should be chosen for flap harvest, and construction of a tube-within-a-tube phallus while the flap is still pedicled to the forearm [41, 43, 44] (Fig. 9.3a, b). It is a versatile flap because it is possible also to transfer tactile sensation through incorporation of the medial or lateral antebrachial cutaneous nerve. A small skin flap and a full thickness skin graft is sutured proximally to the glans area to create the balanopreputialis sulcus. The receptor vessels are to the common femoral artery and the greater saphenous vein. The antebrachial cutaneous nerve is anastomosed to the ilio-inguinal nerve for protective sensation and the median nerve to one of the dorsal penile/clitoral nerves for erogenous sensation. Three months after surgery, the glans can be tattooed in order to create a more realistic glans appearance; the patient can undergo to implantation prosthesis surgery after a 12-month period when protective sensation has returned to the tip of the penis. The most common complications are related urinary fistulas, urethral strictures wound closure of the harvest site, flap anastomosis. Cosmetic and functional results are acceptable especially when a prosthesis is implanted but complications are frequent, and for this reason, a multidisciplinary team approach in high volume centers is recommended [41, 43, 44].

9.6 Buried Penis

9.6.1 Definition and Epidemiology

Buried penis is a penile abnormality in which the penis of normal corporal size and length barely protrudes from the body since it can be partially or completely hidden below the surface of the skin (Fig. 9.4). The penis can be located beneath

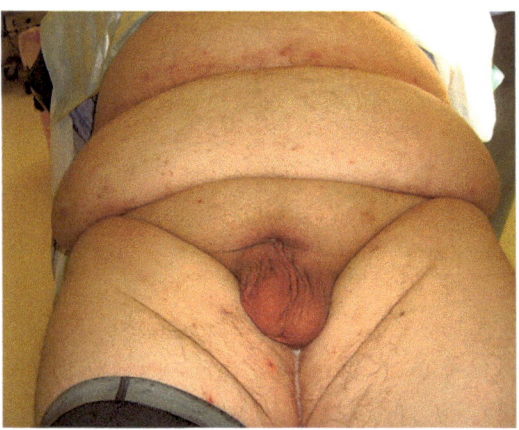

Fig. 9.4 Buried penis in obese patient. (Picture by Mr. David Ralph, St. Peters Andrology Centre, London, UK)

the abdomen or the scrotum while in the most complex cases, it can lie beneath skin of the thigh. The differential diagnosis with micropenis lies in the normal size of the phallus which is affected by poor exposure [45]. Some authors use the term concealed penis as it allows a further sub-classification of the disease into trapped buried and complex penis. Buried penis was first classified by Crawford into partial and complete types in 1977: the partial type is characterized by the proximal half of the penile shaft buried in the subcutaneous tissue and gives rise to a "stumpy-looking" penis; whereas the complete type, the phallus is completely invisible and the glans is covered only by foreskin buried below the abdominal wall [46].

9.6.2 Pathophysiology

Buried penis can be caused by congenital or acquired conditions. Whereas acquired type of buried penis, in which the phallus is normal sized encompassed by skin, subcutaneous tissue and fat in the prepubic area, is often associated with other pathological conditions including obesity, balanitis xerotica obliterans (BXO), lymphedema, and complication of penile surgery. In case of obesity, the overexpression of the central abdominal and suprapubic fat pad can be respon-

sible of buried penis; particularly, the fat in the suprapubic area can be difficult to loose and surgery represents the only option in these patients. This aspect is highlighted by the rate of patients surgically treated for buried penis who are obese in the 87% of the cases [47]. Balanitis xerotica obliterans (BXO) and recurrent infection in diabetic patients can cause sclerosis of the glans, urethra and foreskin can result in a scar of the skin of the penile shaft and prepuce with consequent entrapment of the penis below the suprapubic skin. Complications following circumcision could be responsible of buried penis in case of excessive foreskin removed or scarring of the suture line that can trap the penis and push it below the suprapubic area. A telescope mechanism of the penile shaft to the surrounding dartos and skin is at the base of the dysgenic dartos as cause of buried penis. In these patients, dartos fascia does not fix the penile skin to the deep fascia of the suspensory ligament and the consequent hypermobility of skin and fascia determines the retraction of the corpora and glans penis into the scrotum or below the pubis [47, 48].

9.6.3 Clinical Findings and Diagnosis

Physical examination is essential to establish the stretched penile length and exclude micropenis. The evidence of whitish phimotic skin and glans fusion are suggestive of BXO while abdominal and suprapubic examination often shows overhanging suprapubic fat. Commonly, patients complain of LUTS including straining to void and weak urine flow, post void dribbling and recurrent urinary tract infection. These symptoms are frequently related to coexisting meatal or urethral stricture. Inability to have sexual intercourse or painful erection are often reported by patients. During examination, the penis should be delivered in order to assess the glans, the urethral meatus, and the penile skin. In case of suspect of a urethral stricture, a urethrocystography or urethrocystoscopy is recommended [49, 50].

9.6.4　Treatment

The aim of the treatment of buried penis is to achieve voiding standing and restore sexual and cosmetic function. The authors report about the 87% improvements in voiding and up to the 94% in the sexual function [51]. In case of obesity, weight loss should be the first step with bariatric surgery for patients with a BMI >40 or over. In obese patients, surgical options include fat removal from the lower abdomen a suprapubic area. Panniculectomy, abdominoplasty, and suprapubic lipectomy are common surgical techniques used to reduce the amount of fat causing buried penis. During panniculectomy, which is indicated for the removal of subcutaneous fat and excessive skin following weight loss or bariatric surgery, a V-shaped incision is performed above the mons pubis from the skin level down to the rectus fascia. The suprapubic lipectomy includes the removal of the suprapubic fat through a W-shaped incision starting a couple of centimeters from the base of the penis. The amount of tissue removed can be linked to the intraoperative bleeding that can be significant in case of large panniculi. Abdominoplasty involves removal of the fat and skin in excess below the umbilicus and tightening (plication of the rectus abdominus) of the fascia of the abdominal wall with relocation of the umbilicus. Following fat removal, tacking suture from tunica albuginea to the ventral dartos is recommended in order to prevent retraction on the penile shaft [49, 50] and grafting of the penile shaft previously buried may be necessary (Fig. 9.5).

In case of buried penis related to BXO, iatrogenic loss of penile skin or scarring and lymphedema, the approach is based on first instance on the removal of the skin affected by the disease and grafting in case of skin deficiency. If primary closure is not feasible, techniques used to correct the defects are flaps or autografting. When autografting, the surgeon has to deal with two choices: thickness of the skin graft and the harvest site suitable for the recipient site; commonly used harvest sites are the abdomen, lateral thigh, and in selected patients supraclavicular and postauricular skin; split thickness skin grafts (0.003 mm)

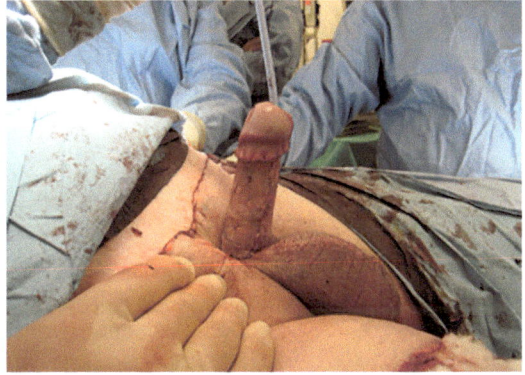

Fig. 9.5 Post-operative appearence following suprapubic lipectomy and split thickness skin grafts to the penile shaft in obese patient. (Picture by Mr. David Ralph, St. Peters Andrology Centre, London, UK)

are often used due to their good survival rated, the lack or hair follicle and good aesthetic match and no need for a local flap or subsequent grafting for the donor site, a compressive dressing is required; however, thick split graft tends to provide more mechanical resistance and less shrinkage rates at the cost of a major donor site care. In the first 24–48 h, the graft is without blood supply and appears white (nutrient and oxygen passively diffuse to the graft), then formation of vascular anastomose between the graft and the host begins producing capillary refill leading to a cyanotic appearance, finally the revascularization occurs. The graft over time may become hypopigmented or hyperpigmented. Following the harvest, the skin graft is placed on the recipient site, with quilting suture, or bolster and negative pressure wound dressing to prevent mobilization of the graft; in order to prevent hematomas and seromas, a graft's healing disruptors, if using a not meshed skin graft, "pie crusting technique" is required, this technique entails creating perforation in the graft with blade [49, 52].

References

1. Edwards S. Balanitis and balanoposthitis: a review. Genitourin Med. 1996;72(3):155–9. [PMC free article] [PubMed].
2. Vohra S, Badlani G. Balanitis and balanoposthitis. Urol Clin North Am. 1992;19(1):143–7. [PubMed].

3. Lisboa C, Ferreira A, Resende C, Rodrigues AG. Infectious balanoposthitis: management, clinical and laboratory features. Int J Dermatol. 2009;48(2):121–4. [PubMed].
4. Kyriazi NC, Cistenbader CL. Group A beta-hemolytic streptococcal balanitis: it may be more common than you think. Pediatrics. 1991;88:154–6.
5. Morris BJ, Krieger JN. Penile inflammatory skin disorders and the preventive role of circumcision. Int J Prev Med. 2017;8:32. [PMC free article] [PubMed].
6. Borelli S, Lautenschlager S. [Differential diagnosis and management of balanitis]. Hautarzt. 2015;66(1):6–11.
7. English JC, Laws RA, Keough GC, Wilde JL, Foley JP, Elston DM. Dermatoses of the glans penis and prepuce. J Am Acad Dermatol. 1997;37(1):1–24; quiz 25–6. [PubMed].
8. Chalmers RJ, Burton PA, Bennett RF, Goring CC, Smith PJ. Lichen sclerosus et atrophics. A common and distinctive cause of phimosis in boys. Arch Dermatol. 1984;120:1025–7.
9. Bale PM, Lochhead A, Martin HC, Gollow I. Balanitis xerotica obliterans in children. Pediatr Pathol. 1987;7:617–27.
10. Kiss A, Csontai A, Pirot L, Nyirady P, Merksz M, Kiraly L. The response of balanitis xerotica obliterans to local steroid application compared with placebo in children. J Urol. 2001;165:219–20.
11. Escala JM, Rickwood AM. Balanitis. Br J Urol. 1989;63:196–7.
12. Gardiner D. The fate of the foreskin: a study of circumcision. Br Med. 1949;J.2:1433–7.
13. Hsieh TF, Chang CH, Chang SS. Foreskin development before adolescence in 2149 schoolboys. Int J Urol. 2006;13:968–70.
14. Yang C, Liu X, Wei GH. Foreskin development in 10 421 Chinese boys aged 0-18 years. World J Pediatr. 2009;5:312–5.
15. Morris BJ, Krieger JN, Klausner JD. CDC's male circumcision recommendations represent a key public health measure. Glob Health Sci Pract. 2017;5(1):15.
16. Hayashi Y, Kojima Y, Mizuno K, Kohri K. Prepuce: phimosis, paraphimosis, and circumcision. ScientificWorldJournal. 2011;11:289–301.
17. Palmer LS, Palmer JS. The efficacy of topical betamethasone for treating phimosis: a comparison of two treatment regimens. Urology. 2008;72:68–71.
18. Cuckow PM, Rix G, Mouriquand PDE. Preputialplasty: a good alternative to circumcision. J Pediatr Surg. 1994;29:561–3.
19. Wåhlin N. "Triple incision plasty". A convenient procedure for preputial relief. Scand J Urol Nephrol. 1992;26:107–10.
20. Hoffman S, Metz P, Ebbehøj J. A new operation for phimosis: prepuce-saving technique with multiple Y-V-plasties. Br J Urol. 1984;56:319–21.
21. Huo ZC, Liu G, Li XY, et al. Use of a disposable circumcision suture device versus conventional circumcision: a systematic review and meta-analysis. Asian J Androl. 2017;19(3):362–7. https://doi.org/10.4103/1008-682X.174855.

22. Lv BD, Zhang SG, Zhu XW, et al. Disposable circumcision suture device: clinical effect and patient satisfaction. Asian J Androl. 2014;16(3):453–6. https://doi.org/10.4103/1008-682X.127816.
23. Reynard JM, Barua JM. Reduction of paraphimosis the simple ways—the Dundee technique. BJU Int. 1999;83:859–60.
24. DeVries CR, Miller AK, Packer MG. Reduction of paraphimosis with hyaluronidase. Urology. 1996;48:464–5.
25. Gyftopoulos K. Male dyspareunia due to short frenulum: the suture-free, "pull and burn" method. J Sex Med. 2009;6(9):2611–4.
26. Whelan P. Male dyspareunia due to short frenulum: an indication for adult circumcision. Br Med J. 1977;2(6103):1633–4.
27. Aaronson IA. Micropenis: medical and surgical implications. J Urol. 1994;152(1):4–14.
28. Wiygul J, Palmer LS. Micropenis. ScientificWorldJournal. 2011;11:1462–9.
29. Lee PA, Mazur T, Danish R, Amrhein J, Blizzard RM, Money J, Migeon CJ. Micropenis. I. Criteria, etiologies and classification. Johns Hopkins Med J. 1980;146(4):156–63.
30. Ludwig G. Micropenis and apparent micropenis—a diagnostic and therapeutic challenge. Andrologia. 1999;31(Suppl 1):27.
31. Grumbach MM. A window of opportunity: the diagnosis of gonadotropin deficiency in the male infant. J Clin Endocrinol Metab. 2005;90(5):3122–7.
32. Hamilton J, Blaser S, Daneman D. MR imaging in idiopathic growth hormone deficiency. AJNR Am J Neuroradiol. 1998;19(9):1609–15.
33. Choi SK, Han SW, Kim DH, de Lignieres B. Transdermal dihydrotestosterone therapy and its effects on patients with microphallus. J Urol. 1993;150(2 Pt 2):657–60.
34. Ben-Galim E, Hillman RE, Weldon VV. Topically applied testosterone and phallic growth. Its effects in male children with hypopituitarism and microphallus. Am J Dis Child. 1980;134(3):296–8.
35. Bougnères P, François M, Pantalone L, Rodrigue D, Bouvattier C, Demesteere E, Roger D, Lahlou N. Effects of an early postnatal treatment of hypogonadotropic hypogonadism with a continuous subcutaneous infusion of recombinant follicle-stimulating hormone and luteinizing hormone. J Clin Endocrinol Metab. 2008;93(6):2202–5.
36. Kogan SJ, Williams DI. The micropenis syndrome: clinical observations and expectations for growth. J Urol. 1977;118(2):311–3.
37. Jones HW Jr, Park IJ, Rock JA. Technique of surgical sex reassignment for micropenis and allied conditions. Am J Obstet Gynecol. 1978;132(8):870–7.
38. Reilly JM, Woodhouse CR. Small penis and the male sexual role. J Urol. 1989;142(2 Pt 2):569–71.
39. Lee PA, Houk CP. Outcome studies among men with micropenis. J Pediatr Endocrinol Metab. 2004;17(8):1043–53.
40. Hinman F Jr. Microphallus: characteristics and choice of treatment from a study of 20 cases. J Urol. 1972;107(3):499–505.

41. Monstrey S, Hoebeke P, Selvaggi G, Ceulemans P, Van Landuyt K, Blondeel P, Hamdi M, Roche N, Weyers S, De Cuypere G. Penile reconstruction: is the radial forearm flap really the standard technique? Plast Reconstr Surg. 2009;124(2):510–8.

42. Sinatti C, Wolff D, Buncamper M, Verla W, Claes K, Lumen N, Waterloos M, Monstrey S, Hoebeke P, Spinoit AF. Phalloplasty in biological men with penile insufficiency. J Pediatr Urol. 2020;16(3):404–5. https://doi.org/10.1016/j.jpurol.2020.04.015. Epub 2020 Jun 4. PMID: 32507564.

43. Leriche A, Timsit MO, Morel-Journel N, Bouillot A, Dembele D, Ruffion A. Long-term outcome of forearm flee-flap phalloplasty in the treatment of transsexualism. BJU Int. 2008;101:1297–300.

44. Garaffa G, Spilotros M, Christopher NA, Ralph DJ. Total phallic reconstruction using radial artery based forearm free flap phalloplasty in patients with epispadias-exstrophy complex. J Urol. 2014;192(3):814–20. https://doi.org/10.1016/j.juro.2014.03.105. Epub 2014 Apr 1. PMID: 24704015.

45. Ho TS, Gelman J. Evaluation and management of adult acquired buried penis. Transl Androl Urol. 2018;7(4):618–27.

46. Crawford BS. Buried penis. Br J Plast Surg. 1977;30(1):96–9. https://doi.org/10.1016/s0007-1226(77)90046-7. PMID: 836989.

47. Higuchi TT, Yamaguchi Y, Wood HM, et al. Evaluation and treatment of adult concealed penis. Curr Urol Rep. 2012;13:277–84.

48. Alter GJ, Ehrlich RM. A new technique or correction of the hidden penis in children and adults. J Urol. 1999;161:455.

49. Anandan L, Mohammed A. Surgical management of buried penis in adults. Cent European J Urol. 2018;71(3):346–52. https://doi.org/10.5173/ceju.2018.1676. Epub 2018 Sep 22. PMID: 30386659; PMCID: PMC6202613.

50. Stephen JR, Burks FN. Buried penis repair: tips and tricks. Int Braz J Urol. 2020;46(4):519–22.

51. Theisen KM, Fuller TW, Rusilko P. Surgical management of adult-acquired buried penis: impact on urinary and sexual quality of life outcomes. Urology. 2018;116:180–4.

52. Thakar HJ, Dugi DD III. Skin grafting of the penis. Urol Clin North Am. 2013;40(3):439–48.

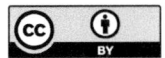

Fabrizio Palumbo, Francesco Sebastiani,
Fabio Crocerossa, and Nicola Mondaini

10.1 Introduction

Fabrizio Palumbo, Francesco Sebastiani

Acute genital injuries are a peculiar occurrence which demands specific attentions from the specialist in both the diagnostic and therapeutic approach to the patient.

Thorough history taking is mandatory when first assessing the patient, but it is important to keep in mind several important aspects pertaining to the high emotional impact usually associated with such afflictions. Sensibility is required when discussing the issue with the patient, especially when there is the possibility of permanent functional consequences in relation to sexual function and fertility. Furthermore, in some cases, a psychiatric origin of the event can be considered.

The physical examination should take place in a quiet, reserved office, and should always include a complete evaluation of penis and testicles, as well as the abdominal and perineal area. Potential concomitant injury to other relevant organs should be taken into consideration, and therefore, the physical examination can be extended accordingly.

There are situations in which photographic documentation and forensic material acquisition may be advisable, for example, in the case of potential sexual abuse or violence. The specialist should refer to local legal protocols when assessing possible victims.

Key points of the assessment of an andrological emergency patient are listed in Table 10.1.

The aim of this chapter is to review the clinical and therapeutic aspects of major andrological emergencies.

Table 10.1 Key points when assessing an andrological emergency patient

High emotional impact	Sensibility
	Psychological support
	Potential psychiatric origin
Privacy and intimacy	Separate from other patients
	Adequate place for physical examination
Legal concerns	Consider potential abuse/ violence
	Legal protocol if needed
	Photographic documentation
	Forensic material acquisition
Genital evaluation	Penis and testicles
	Genital skin loss
Potential concomitant injury	Microscopic/macroscopic haematuria
	Extend general examination as needed

F. Palumbo (✉) · F. Sebastiani
Department of Urology, Di Venere Hospital,
Bari, Italy

F. Crocerossa · N. Mondaini
Department of Urology, Magna Graecia University of Catanzaro, Catanzaro, Italy
e-mail: crocerossa@unicz.it; n.mondaini@unicz.it

C. Bettocchi et al. (eds.), *Practical Clinical Andrology*,
https://doi.org/10.1007/978-3-031-11701-5_10

10.2 Paraphimosis

Fabrizio Palumbo, Francesco Sebastiani

10.2.1 Clinical Presentation

Paraphimosis is defined by the entrapment of the foreskin behind the corona of the glans penis, with consequent impossibility to restore its usual anatomic position by moving it distally to cover the glans [1]. It is considered a true andrological emergency because if the retracted foreskin remains trapped behind the coronal sulcus for a significant amount of time, venous and lymphatic drainage can be gradually impaired, as well as arterial blood flow—though the latter usually occurs in a matter of hours to days. The end result is glans ischemia and consequent necrosis which may also affect the distal portion of the urethra [2, 3].

Clinical presentation is typical: the patient complains of distal penile swelling with or without pain. Engorgement of the foreskin, in which a tight ring of constrictive tissue is usually detectable, is another distinctive finding. It is advisable to pay close attention to the colour of the glans penis, since pale or dark hues may be indicative of ischemia or even imminent necrosis. The diagnosis is confirmed when manual retraction of the foreskin proves to be difficult or impossible [4]. The history of the patient also aids in completing the diagnosis, since catheterization, intercourse, cleaning manoeuvres, and penile instrumentation are typically found to be triggering events, as well as the presence of genital piercings and dermatologic afflictions [5].

Paraphimosis usually affects uncircumcised males, even though it is still a possible occurrence in circumcised patients if removal of the foreskin was incomplete [6]. The most affected age groups are children (0.2%), teenagers, and the elderly (1%) [7]: this is thought to be due to the lower frequency of physiologically occurring preputial dilation in the case of lacking daily hygiene and regular sexual activity. In general, every male for whom genital hygiene presents difficulties attributable to a poor elasticity of the foreskin is at risk of developing paraphimosis [4].

10.2.2 Management

Immediate action must be taken to restore the foreskin to its normal position and prevent ischemia and necrosis of the glans penis. Various techniques have been described to minimize the oedema of the skin before attempting the reduction manoeuvre.

Simple manual compression of the oedematous foreskin while gently pulling the penile shaft upwards is the most commonly used approach. The compression can be carried out for several minutes before attempting foreskin reduction, and can be repeated. If the swelling has subsided, the thumbs can be pressed on the tip of the glans while the other fingers gently pull the foreskin upwards. Lubrication can be applied as needed [8].

Other methods are described in the literature, though often reported in small case series. Some authors obtain compression by means of applying gauze pad and an elastic bandage to the distal portion of the penis for 10 to 20 min in order to reduce the swelling before the manual reduction manoeuvre [9]. A "sleeve" obtained by cutting the thumb of a surgical glove and filled with local anaesthetic cream can be placed over the penis for about 30 min with the intent of softening the oedematous skin and providing analgesia [10].

Osmotic methods have also been described: the rationale is to create a gradient to allow fluids to leave the oedematous areas through the skin. This is achieved with the application of granulated sugar or gauze soaked in mannitol solution around the skin [11, 12].

Injection of hyaluronidase directly in the swollen foreskin has been described to disperse the trapped fluids within the constrictive foreskin, allowing easy resolution of the paraphimosis [13]. Some practitioners have also described a technique involving multiple punctures of the foreskin to decrease the oedema [14].

It should be noted that the patient may not always be compliant to reduction manoeuvres because of discomfort and pain, especially when managing a prolonged, severe paraphimosis with multiple attempts at reduction. Local anaesthesia with a standard penile block can be considered in selected cases [15].

If manual reduction attempts are unsuccessful, surgical treatment of the paraphimosis is necessary. A dorsal slit or full circumcision provides resolution of the emergency and prevention of future recurrences [16].

10.3 Penile Strangulation Injury

Fabrizio Palumbo, Francesco Sebastiani

10.3.1 Clinical Presentation

Penile strangulation occurs as a compartment syndrome in which the penile shaft is circumferentially constricted and trapped by an object, resulting in venous and arterial flow impairment and consequent vasculogenic damage to the corpora cavernosa [17]. Prolonged and unresolved strangulation may lead to oedema, ischemia, urethrocutaneous fistula, and tissue necrosis with penile amputation [18].

Penile strangulation injury is a rare clinical entity, not commonly encountered during daily practice, but it can be challenging to manage for the treating specialist. In infants, the causing object is often identified to be maternal hair. This is also known as "hair tourniquet syndrome" and usually occurs between 2 and 6 months of age. Hormonal post-partum changes in the mother are linked to increased hair loss. During hygiene manoeuvres, it is possible that this excess hair accidentally coils around the infant's penis (or other appendages as well) without the parent noticing, especially in the presence of skin folds [19]. Hair tourniquet syndrome is rarer in children, for whom toys or other house objects are more likely to cause injury. Adolescent and adults often report penile strangulation injuries due to various kinds of rings employed for sexual gratification or even sexual abuse: wedding rings, rubber bands, metallic plumbing, bottle necks, etc [20]. Due to the social stigma, it is possible that medical attention-seeking is delayed in this age group, potentially worsening the clinical presentation.

Bhat et al. proposed a detailed classification of severity for penile strangulation injury clinical presentation and symptoms [21]:

- Grade 1: Oedema of distal penis. No evidence of skin ulceration or urethral injury.
- Grade 2: Injury to skin and constriction of corpus spongiosum but no evidence of urethral injury. Distal penile oedema with decreased penile sensation.
- Grade 3: Injury to skin and urethra but no urethral fistula. Loss of distal penile sensation.
- Grade 4: Complete division of corpus spongiosum leading to urethral fistula and constriction of corpus cavernosum with loss of distal penile sensation.
- Grade 5: Gangrene, necrosis, or complete amputation of distal penis.

It should be noted that strangulation injury may also lead to acute retention of urine [22].

The diagnosis of this condition is of course visual, but a complete assessment of damage extent may require further investigation—such as a urethral methylene blue test or voiding urography—after immediate removal of the offending object [23].

10.3.2 Management

Every attempt to remove the constricting object must be made promptly and with an appropriate method in order to preserve the integrity of the involved anatomical structures. Since the object to be removed may be of differing size and material, and equipment available at the time of the emergency may vary, there is no standard technique for removal and every treatment choice must be made on a case-by-case basis [24].

Depending on the severity of the injury and the grade of constriction, local anaesthesia may be necessary. This can be achieved with a standard penile block. In the case of acute urinary retention, emptying the bladder may be required by transurethral (when possible) or suprapubic catheterization [25].

As a first approach, manual removal with traction can be attempted by previously lubricating the area [26]. If the object is non-metallic or somewhat thin, it can be susceptible to being severed with relatively simple tools such as a cutter. Larger and sturdier object may require cutting with instruments commonly used in orthopaedic or orthodontic surgery, and even industrial tools such as saws and drills. Special precautions must be taken in order to avoid further damage to the penis, for example, by applying bandages, laryngoscopes, or tongue depressors for protection [27].

Of course, the immediate availability of heavy-duty cutting instruments is not to be taken for granted in a general hospital setting. On the other hand, a severely swollen penile shaft may not permit sufficient access for a large tool. Several authors describe a fairly atraumatic removal method known as the "thread" or "string" technique. A silk or similarly composed thread is passed under the constricting object with one of its ends. The other end is tightly wound around the length of the penile shaft, starting from the position of the object and proceeding distally. This causes the girth of the swollen penis to gradually decrease as the coils wound. Then, the string is unwound, starting from the proximal end and so the object is made to slip off [28]. Modifications to this technique account for excessive swelling of the glans by incision or positioning of a Medicut needle in the glans to continuously draw blood and reduce engorgement during the procedure [27]. Other authors advocate for the aspiration of corporal blood from the glans or the lateral aspects of the penile shaft to manage oedema and congestion [29].

When all possible attempts at removing the object fail, surgery is the only remaining option. Degloving of the penile shaft is followed by penile reconstruction techniques ranging from skin grafting to total phallic reconstruction, depending on the extent of the injury [25].

Long-term consequences of a penile strangulation injury mostly depend on the timing of resolution. Rates of lasting sequelae range from 13% to 30% in the literature, mainly involving penile amputation and the developing of urethrocutane-ous fistulae, so it is safe to say that more than two-thirds of patients usually achieve a full recovery when treated [30, 31].

10.4 Penile Blunt Trauma

Fabrizio Palumbo, Francesco Sebastiani

10.4.1 Clinical Presentation

Penile trauma deriving from an external force is a fairly uncommon occurrence: rates of incidence in emergency departments approximate one every 175,000 patients. The anatomical disposition of male genitalia makes injury relatively unlikely, but sexual activity, traffic, work, and sports accidents can nevertheless pose a risk of blunt trauma. From the diagnostic and pathophysiologic point of view, it is important to distinguish between a trauma occurring in an erect penis and one occurring in a flaccid penis, since the resulting injuries usually vary [32].

Blunt penile trauma in a flaccid penis is usually a consequence of perineal or general lower-body trauma, such as those occurring in traffic accidents. This usually results in the crushing of the cavernosal crura against the pelvic bones with consequential extratunical or cavernosal haematoma without rupturing of the tunica albuginea. Infrequently, there can be rupture of the cavernosal artery with formation of an arterial-lacunar fistula which can manifest as high-flow priapism [33]. If pelvic bone fracture is present, there is a 5–10% chance of posterior urethral lesions: in fact, the posterior urethra is linked to the pelvis bone by means of the puboprostatic ligaments as well as the perineal membrane [34].

When it comes to trauma involving an erect penis, penile fracture deriving from tunica albuginea rupturing is the most likely consequence. The tunica albuginea presents a two-part structure composed of collagen and elastin: the inner layer is circularly arranged, while the outer layer is longitudinally arranged. The tensile resistance of the tunica depends on the outer layer, which has a typically variable thickness and it is thinnest in its ventrolateral aspect, especially during erection. In this situation, the tunica albuginea thins from 2 mm to 0.5–0.25 mm [35]. Even though the tunica albuginea can support fairly high intracavernosal pressures without rupturing, the sudden increase caused by abnormal bending of the erect penis can exceed the resistance of the albuginea, causing it to tear. This is defined as a penile fracture. Urethral injury may also be present in 10–20% of cases [36]. Of note, the albuginea ruptures are usually unilateral, and when bilateral, they tend to be more frequently associated with urethral injury. The tears in the albuginea are usually transverse and located on the ventral and proximal aspect of the shaft [37].

Aside from the previously cited traffic, work, and sports accidents, the vast majority of penile traumata occurs to an erect penis in the act of sexual intercourse (80% of patients) according to a recent metanalysis [37]. This usually is attributable to a buckling injury sustained while accidentally striking the perineum or pubic bone during vigorous sexual activity or, according to some authors, because some sexual positions pose a greater risk than others ("woman on top" or "doggy-style") [38]. Aetiology of the trauma may also vary according to geographical region of origin and ethnicity: in Africa and Middle East, nearly 50% of penile fracture events are attributable to a manoeuvre known as "Taghaandan," which is the act of abruptly bending the erect penile shaft to facilitate immediate detumescence and is derived from local habits [39]. Other known causes are excessive force during masturbation, rolling over in bed with an erect penis, and micturition attempts with an erect penis [37]. In terms of age group, this seems to be an injury that mostly occurs in sexually active young adults and adults, with an average age of 36 years [37].

Penile blunt trauma without fracture usually presents with pain and local haematoma, with high-flow priapism possibly following [32]. Penile fracture has a more peculiar clinical presentation. It is typical that the patient recalls being engaged in sexual intercourse when suddenly hearing a "snapping" or "popping" noise, followed by sudden detumescence [40]. The patient then presents with haematoma and penile swelling, rarely penile deviation. Haematoma is the most common finding, and its distribution and extension depends on the integrity of the Buck's fascia: in the case of breaching, it can extend beyond the penile shaft and reach the perineum (with the peculiar "butterfly" disposition) or the abdomen [41]. Urethral injury is suspected in the case of haematuria, acute urinary retention, or other voiding symptoms [42].

Diagnosis is frequently apparent just from patient history and clinical signs [43]. Ultrasound examination, although operator-dependent, is frequently used in this context to detect the presence and location of cavernosal rupturing, which usually appears as an irregular hypoechoic or hyperechoic defect in the albuginea. Colour-Doppler US may also be used as an adjunct procedure in the suspect of concomitant vascular abnormalities [32]. Magnetic Resonance Imaging (MRI) has shown a 100% sensitivity and 77.8% specificity in detecting tunical rupture, and fairly lower but acceptable results for detection of urethral injury. It could theoretically help avoid unnecessary surgery in border-line cases, but it is not a substitute of clinical assessment and may not be readily available in emergency situations so it is not considered part of routine assessment [44]. The suspected presence of urethral injury may require further diagnostic procedures such as cystourethrography or cystoscopy [45].

10.4.2 Management

Conservative management with compression bandages, cooling, anti-inflammatory, antibiotic, and analgesic therapy is usually only viable for contusions without fracture or cases with documented minimal damage to the albuginea and corpora [46]. In all other cases involving penile fracture, immediate or minimally delayed surgical exploration is considered to be the best approach to minimize long-term sequelae [47].

Since timing affects later outcomes, most surgeons perform surgery within a few hours after the trauma, especially in the presence of detectable urethral injury. However, if the latter can be excluded based on diagnostics, surgical intervention can safely be delayed to a maximum of 48 h [48].

Surgical treatment of penile fracture involves the evacuations of blood clots and the repair of the tunica albuginea defect. The usual incision is sub-coronal with consequent full degloving of the penile shaft, but since most tunical tears are located in the proximal segment of the shaft, alternative accesses such as penoscrotal have been adopted to avoid the possible complications associated with degloving (haematoma, skin necrosis, infections, and oedema). Of course, fairly accurate pre-operative detection of tunical defects is required in order to correctly plan the surgical approach [48].

The tunical tears are usually repaired with slow absorbable sutures to avoid the formation of palpable knots which usually follow the utilization of non-absorbable sutures [49]. Identification of urethral injury requires immediate intraoperative repair, preferably in two layers and using small sutures, with a Foley catheter positioned afterwards [47].

Regarding long-term consequences, conservative management of penile fracture has proven to be more associated with negative sequelae than immediate surgical repair. Corporeal fibrosis, plaque formation, and secondary penile curvature occur in roughly 50% of non-surgically treated penile fractures and require subsequent surgical correction in up to 16% of cases. Erectile dysfunction is also more frequent than with surgical treatment [50].

After repair, long-term complications are less frequent and include indurated scars at the site of repair, penile deformity, erectile dysfunction, and urethral stricture [37].

10.5   Penile Open Trauma

Fabrizio Palumbo, Francesco Sebastiani

10.5.1   Clinical Presentation

As with penile blunt trauma, occurrence of penetrating injuries to the male genitalia is fairly uncommon due to its anatomical location. Most of the reported cases of open trauma to the penis are derived from wartime reports, traffic accidents, crime, and industrial machinery. Therefore, oftentimes and depending on the cause, an open wound which involves the penis is part of a complex condition which may involve several other organs and anatomical regions [51].

Stabbing and bullet wounds to male genitalia involve the penile shaft in 80–90% of cases, followed in frequency by the scrotum and the urethra: the latter sustains injury in up to 22% of cases [52]. Aside from visually apparent damage to the shaft, it is therefore important to immediately assess eventual damage done to the urethra, which can be signalled by the presence of blood in the urethral meatus, haematuria, and voiding symptoms [53]. Diagnostic evaluation of urethral injury is strongly recommended and can be performed with urine analysis, retrograde urography, cystoscopy, or intraoperative application of methylene blue [54].

Biting injury to the male genitalia have been described, deriving both from humans and animals. This occurrence is rare even if bites in general make for about 1% of all emergency department consultations [55]. Aside from the obvious damage to the skin, soft tissues and possible urethral involvement, the main danger in biting wounds is infection, which occurs in about 10–20% of cases. Animal bites more often pose the risk of transmitting rabies, tetanus, *Staphylococcus*, *Streptococcus*, *E. coli*, and anaerobes infection, while human bites bear the additional risk of potential sexually transmitted diseases such as syphilis, hepatitis, HIV, and herpes [56].

Burning wounds to male external genitalia are extremely rare in isolation and, for the most part, are a component of larger body burns. About 5–13% of burn victims report burns of the penis and perineum, mainly in the context of daily life, traffic and industrial accidents by flame, scalding, and chemical burns [57]. Clinical assessment of burn depth is paramount to choosing the correct managing options, but can be challenging and may require a specialist consultation [58].

Trouser zips-related injury has been described to account for a significant portion of penile injuries, especially in the paediatric population. This is thought to be due to the location of trouser zippers, which is close to the male genitalia [59]. However, it seems to be not entirely uncommon an injury also in the male adult population: an epidemiological research carried out in the United States found that 29.8% of all penile injuries presenting in an emergency department occurred while using a trouser zip, making it the most common aetiology of adult penile injury in the emergency departments [60]. Most commonly, the penile skin is the part that becomes entrapped between the locked teeth or within the buckle of the fastener, while involvement of the scrotum is much rarer [60].

Traumatic amputation of the penis can be partial or complete, depending on the severity of the cause. Main causes are self-infliction by patients with psychiatric disorders, bizarre autoerotic acts, daily life, traffic or industrial accidents, wartime wounds, or uncontrolled surgical practices such as clandestine ritual circumcisions [61, 62]. Clinical assessment should include a close evaluation of the extent of the amputation to define which anatomical structures have been damaged, prior to attempting surgical treatment.

10.5.2 Management

Treatment of penile open trauma may be multifaceted and complex. Aside from primary wound treatment, there are multiple other factors to be considered. Functional recovery entails the possibility for the patient to restore erection and sexual activity, fertility, and regular micturition. Cosmetic results may also be of importance. Since aetiologies and causative factors can be diverse, as well as the extent of damage sustained, no single strategy can be considered effective and treatment must be planned on a case-by-case basis [51].

Stabbing and bullet wounds require immediate surgical exploration. Objectives are wound cleaning, control of bleeding, eventual removal of foreign bodies and debridement of necrotic tissue, with scrupulous antibiotics and tetanus prophylaxis. In the case of urethral injury, urinary diversion by means of a suprapubic catheter guarantees micturition without further damage to the urethra [51]. Reconstruction of affected anatomical structures is necessary. In the case of urethral injury, repair procedures can be performed immediately in the first approach if the damage is minimal. Authors have reported approaches ranging from open surgery primary repair to endoscopic realignment over a stenting urethral catheter. In the case of extensive damage, it is preferrable to defer to a staged uretroplasty. Long-term sequelae depend on the original injury and include penile curvature, urethral stricture, and erectile dysfunction though outcomes are usually acceptable [63].

Biting wounds treatment revolves mainly around antibiotic, rabies, and tetanus prophylaxis with the surgical approach consisting primarily of wound irrigation, tissue debridement, and closure or repair of defects. Depending on the extent of damage, reconstructive techniques such as skin flaps, immediate or staged urethroplasty, or even phalloplasty may be required. Complications stem mainly from the contaminated nature of the wound and include infection and necrosis [64].

In the case of burns affecting the genitalia, treatment depends strictly on the extent of damage. In most cases, the approach is conservative, with local irrigation, topical antibiotics, and covering medication. Debridement of non-viable tissue may be performed immediately or during the process of secondary healing, if needed. Skin graft and plastic reconstructive surgery are kept as a last resort for severe conditions or to deal with late-stage disfiguring scarring [57].

Trouser zip-related entrapment of penile skin requires removal of the zip lock, which can be achieved in various ways. Lubrication and careful unzipping can be attempted. Further methods involve the incision of the fabric component of the zip lock between each tooth, the cutting of the slider buckle with a suitable severing tool, or the excision of the trapped portion of skin, which involves circumcision if the prepuce is affected [60].

Amputation management, as in other traumata of the genitalia, depends on the timing of medical attention-seeking on behalf of the patient and on the extent of the injury. In the literature, penile reimplantation has been shown to be successful if performed within a maximum of 7–15 h after the event. Other factors which can be beneficial to a penile reattachment attempt are the availability of a surgical microscope to locate and utilize viable veins, arteries and nerves, team expertise, severity of the injury, and the condition of the severed distal segment of the shaft. Even in the case of immediate apparent technical success of the operation, sequelae such as infection, loss of penile sensation, erectile dysfunction, urethral stricture, skin necrosis, and penile implant failure are well documented, although less common with microvascular repair [65].

10.6   Testicular Trauma

Fabrizio Palumbo, Francesco Sebastiani

10.6.1   Clinical Presentation

Scrotal trauma includes blunt and penetrating injuries along with burns, bites, and skin avulsions as already seen above regarding penile trauma. The anatomical location and morphology of the scrotum apparently makes it vulnerable to traumatic injury, though the incidence of scrotal trauma is actually quite low due to the presence of somewhat protective elements such as the tunica albuginea surrounding the testicles and the mobility of the scrotal sac [51]. Blunt trauma to the testicles is the most frequent and may result in testicular contusion, scrotal haematoma, testicular dislocation, haematocele, and testicular rupture. The latter two are respectively represented by the accumulation of blood in the tunica vaginalis and the disruption of the tunica albuginea [66]. Testicular dislocation or migration is quite rare, with the testis migrating along the length of the inguinal canal, towards the abdomen and suprapubic region, or in a subcutaneous aberrant position [67]. The testis has a higher risk of damage when the dynamics of the trauma force it to be pressed against hard structures such as the inferior pubic ramus or the pubic symphy-

sis. It has been demonstrated that the structure of the testis can withstand a maximum force of 50 kg, beyond which testicular rupture ensues [68]. Of all possible kinds of testicular trauma, penetrating trauma and testicular rupture are the most severe forms which constitute true scrotal emergencies and require immediate surgical treatment, while low-grade traumas are often reported days later by patients showing signs of self-limiting traumatic epididymitis [69].

Regarding possible aetiologies, sports-associated trauma seems by far the most common occurrence at over 50% of cases, while traffic accidents (especially concerning motorbikes), falls, and violent injury make for the rest [70].

Clinical and instrumental examination should be aimed at investigating the eventual presence of major testicular injury such as rupture and penetrating wounds. Anamnestic history of recent trauma and clinical examination are the first steps to a correct diagnosis. The patient usually presents with scrotal pain and a swelling which can be tender or firm at palpatory evaluation and can be indicative of the internal accumulation of blood: transillumination is negative in the case of haematocele. Scrotal skin may show signs of aberrant discoloration referrable to haematoma. Conversely, if the affected hemiscrotum appears to be empty at palpation, a testicular dislocation may be suspected [69]. General symptoms of testicular trauma range from nausea, vomit, and giddiness to syncope or fainting.

It is important to note that no matter how accurate the physical examinations, findings may be discordant with the extent of the internal injury. Ultrasonography is the first-line imaging method to evaluate scrotal trauma, especially when adjunct colour Doppler is performed. Findings coherent with testicular rupture are heterogeneous parenchymal echostructure and irregular margins of the tunica albuginea. US colour-Doppler imaging can also contribute to the evaluation of the presence of parenchymal blood flow, scrotal wall thickening due to haematoma, and the presence of haematocele within the tunica vaginalis. Despite being operator-dependent and open to the possibility of false-negative descriptions, sensitivity, and specificity in ruling out testicular rupture has consistently been reported to be over 90% in various case series, making US the most useful diagnostic tool in scrotal trauma [71]. Magnetic Resonance Imaging has proved to be even more reliable in diagnosing testicular rupture, especially in uncertain cases, but the costs and possible lack of ready availability in the emergency settings are to be considered important drawbacks to its first-line employment [72]. When it comes to traumatic testicular dislocation, although rare, the diagnosis may be fairly challenging and require accurate US or even Computed Tomography scans to locate the testis [73].

10.6.2 Management

The objective of a correct treatment of testicular injury is the protection of testicular function and the prevention of long-term sequelae such as impaired fertility, hypogonadism, and chronic pain, which are fortunately infrequent if timely treatment is administered [74].

Minor trauma can be conservatively managed as long as the diagnostic workup has ruled out all serious conditions. A testicular contusion or scrotal haematoma limited to the skin wall can be safely managed without surgical intervention, as well as haematoma or haematocele which is less than three times larger than the contralateral testis [75]. Conservative management consists in cooling therapy, anti-inflammatory drugs, and scrotal elevation support [69]. Even so, large haematoceles initially treated with conservative intent may demand delayed surgical treatment due to the developing of infection or persistent pain: in these cases, outcomes are often poorer and the operation results more frequently in orchiectomy [76].

Major trauma, such as testicular rupture, large haematoma, and haematocele, as well as penetrating injuries, require prompt surgical intervention. Exploration allows for evacuation of blood clots, haemostasis, removal of necrotic tissue, and repair of the tunica albuginea, usually with an absorbable suture. In the case of extensive and irreparable damage, orchiectomy can be necessary [77]. Penetrating trauma requires removal of non-viable tissue and reconstruction of damaged structures. This can involve the spermatic cord with consequent vasovasostomy, the tunica albuginea, and scrotal skin with reconstruction techniques which can also be multi-staged when damage is extensive [78]. Testicular dislocation may rarely be approached under anaesthesia with US-guided reduction, but most of the times, it requires surgical intervention. It has been observed that adherence phenomena readily ensue in the victim, so careful dissection, relocation, and fixation of the testis in the scrotal sac is the correct approach [73].

Overall, timely and on-point treatment of testicular trauma yields favourable outcomes: if surgical treatment is performed within 48–72 h from the injury, up to 80% of patients manage to avoid orchiectomy [51].

10.7 Testicular Torsion

Fabrizio Palumbo, Francesco Sebastiani

10.7.1 Clinical Presentation

Testicular torsion is a true urologic emergency which demands immediate intervention from the specialist in order to prevent testicular loss. It occurs because of a twisting of the spermatic cord which causes venous congestion, impairment of arterial blood flow, and eventual ischemia of the testis [69].

There are two pathophysiologic categories of testicular torsion. Intravaginal torsion occurs because the tunica vaginalis of the testicle is not perfectly adherent to the posterolateral side of the testicle, as it physiologically should be, but it is instead attached in a higher position surrounding the epididymis and the spermatic cord. This causes the testicle to hang more freely than normal in the tunica vaginalis, which enables torsion. This anatomical situation is known as the clapper-bell deformity [79]. Extravaginal torsion is more typical of the perinatal stages of life, when the tunica vaginalis has not yet adhered to the gubernaculum testis, enabling the whole testicle along with the spermatic cord and the tunica vaginalis to become twisted [80].

The twisting of the spermatic cord leads to impairment of venous outflow and arterial inflow, which consequently causes ischemia. If the torsion is complete, the viability of the testis deteriorates rapidly; therefore, it has been documented that salvage is frequently possible if detorsion is performed in less than 8 h, but it is rare after 24 h from the event [81]. Ischemia onset is reported to be generally happening at 4–8 h after torsion [82].

Testicular torsion is not a rare occurrence: about 0.5% of emergency department visits involve some kind of scrotal complaint, of which roughly a quarter end up being attributable to this condition [83]. It can happen at any age, but the most common age groups are infants in the perinatal stage and adolescents aged between 12 and 18 years [84]. A familial link and predisposition have been recently suggested among risk factors [85]. Other predisposing factors cited in the literature are hyperactive cremasteric reflex in cold weather [86], as well as the presence of the clapper-bell deformity described above [79]. The onset may be spontaneous, consequent to physical activity, or associated with trauma to the scrotum [80].

Patient history and examination are important in guiding the diagnosis, which is sometimes challenging due to multiple possible differential diagnoses. Testicular torsion may be suspected especially in the presence of susceptible age and abrupt appearance of single-sided testicular pain with less than 24-h duration— even if pain lasting more than 24 h does not put testicular torsion out of question. The patient may present with nausea, vomiting, scrotal enlargement, testicular pain on palpation, redness and retraction of scrotal skin, proximal dislocation of the testicle with or without aberrant positioning. Alterations of cremasteric reflex and the Prehn's sign—with a lack of pain relief when elevating the testicle—may be present but are not to be considered fully reliable [87].

Certain clinical presentations may be challenging because of vagueness of the symptoms or overlap with other differential diagnoses. The pain may not always be referred to the affected testicle, but rather to the inguinal or lower abdominal area. The pain can also be intermittent, or rather the symptoms can be mimicked by a number of other conditions. Such is the case with torsion of cryptorchid testicles, torsion of testicular appendages, epididymo-orchitis, hernia, neoplasms, and many others [88].

In the face of these challenges, various clinical decision tools and nomograms have been designed to aid the clinician. The Testicular Workup for Ischemia and Suspected Torsion (TWIST) [89] defines five criteria to grade a suspect of testicular torsion. Each criterion gets a score:

- Testicular swelling: 2 points.
- Hard testicle: 2 points.
- Absence of cremasteric reflex: 1 point.
- Nausea or vomiting: 1 point.
- High-riding testicle: 1 point.

A total score of 0–2 is considered low risk with 100% negative predictive value for torsion. No further diagnostics is needed. A score of 3–4 is considered intermediate and requires Ultrasonography for further investigation. A score of 5 or more is considered high risk with 100% positive predictive value for torsion: immediate surgical exploration is suggested.

The diagnostic workup of suspect testicular torsion can strongly benefit from Ultrasonography with colour Doppler evaluation. Although operator-dependent, the ready availability, low costs, and lack of ionizing radiation far outweigh its drawbacks. Standard US can help in diagnosis by visualizing pathognomonic findings such as the scrotal whirlpool sign of the spermatic cord or the redundant spermatic cord sign. The testicle may also be found in an abnormal horizontal lie [90]. On the other hand, colour Doppler evaluation helps in establishing the presence of macrovascular blood flow: in complete testicular torsion, vascularization is typically absent [91]. However, when testicular torsion is incomplete or the patient is young with small volume testicles, false negatives can occur [92]. High-resolution colour Doppler US should be used if available, and some authors advocate for advanced US techniques such as Contrast-Enhanced US which, however, may not always be readily available [93].

Other imaging techniques with high detection rates of testicular torsion are Computed Tomography, Magnetic Resonance Imaging, and Nuclear Imaging, but all are severely limited by availability in the emergency setting, costs, and exposure to ionizing radiation. They can be useful in dubious situations, but delay surgical exploration which, in and of itself, is the gold standard in the diagnosis of testicular torsion and also allows treatment [94].

10.7.2 Management

As stated before, testicular salvage in the case of torsion is strictly time-dependent. In particular, salvage rate approximate 100% if detorsion is achieved within 4 h of the event, and decreases to 90% if delayed by 4–8 h [95].

Manual detorsion can be attempted; however, it should not be intended as a means to avoid surgical exploration rather than a way to limit the consequences of prolonged ischemia while preparations for intervention are underway. For the left testicle, manual rotation should be performed in a clockwise fashion from the point of view of the practitioner; while for the right testicle, it should be performed counterclockwise. The manoeuvre can be repeated to account for the usual range of testicular torsion which may vary from 180 to 1080 degrees. Generally speaking, resolution of pain and restoration of blood flow on US are to be considered indicative of a successfully performed manoeuvre, which are nevertheless to be followed by surgical exploration and testicular fixation since residual torsion may still be present. Manual detorsion can be difficult or impossible to carry out in the presence of encumbering scrotal wall thickening, hydrocele, or intense local inflammation [96].

Surgical exploration under anaesthesia is the gold standard to confirm or rule out a diagnosis of testicular torsion and constitutes the treatment of choice. The incision is usually transverse hemiscrotal or performed in the midline. After gaining access to the scrotal sac, the number of cord rotation can be identified and detorsion can be carried out. Testicular viability is then intraoperatively assessed: depending on the age of the patient and duration of ischemia, clinical signs of re-establishment of blood flow can appear in the form of improvement in colour. Furthermore, intraoperative Colour Doppler US or fluorescent dye may be of help in making the decision. Fixation of a salvaged testis is mandatory, as is fixation of the contralateral testis to prevent recurrence of torsion and metachronous torsion on the other side. On the other hand, it is important to perform orchiectomy in the case of a non-salvageable testis to prevent the formation of anti-sperm antibodies that could potentially hamper functionality of the contralateral testis [97].

The main long-term concerns in patients who suffered from testicular torsion are subfertility and infertility. Unilateral torsion has been shown to importantly affect spermiogenesis in 50% of cases and to produce borderline impairment in 20% [98]. Though research in the field has not yet fully clarified, if there are precise correlations, it has been noted that high levels of anti-sperm antibodies are usually found in testicular torsion patients, regardless of whether an orchiectomy or orchidopexy with testicular salvage have been performed. Sperm motility has been shown to be usually higher after orchiectomy than after orchidopexy. The hypothesis is that maintenance of a compromised, ischemic testis may impair testicular function [99]. Other sequelae include infection and delayed atrophy of the salvaged testis. Case series have been reported in which the rate of atrophy in the salvaged testis can reach 41%, so the topic of prolonged follow-up, its relevancy and significance after testicular torsion is a matter of debate [100]. Cosmetic concerns regarding an empty hemiscrotum after orchiectomy are sometimes expressed by the patient; however, it should be noted that the actual acceptance rate of testicular prosthesis placement is relatively low and amounts to about one-third of the patients who are offered this possibility by the surgeon. It has to be said that modern testicular prostheses exhibit low complication rates and high patient satisfaction [101].

10.8   Penile Abscess

Fabrizio Palumbo, Francesco Sebastiani

10.8.1   Clinical Presentation

Corpus cavernosum abscess is a very rare, urgent condition which poses the risk of sepsis, loss of function of the penis and eventual penectomy if left untreated [102]. The most frequently detected causative agents are Neisseria gonorrhoeae, coagulase-negative Staphylococcus aureus, Trichomonas vaginalis, along with polymicrobial infection occurrences [103].

The literature on the subject is mainly derived from case reports and very small case series. Triggering events reported as-of yet include penile trauma, cavernosography, intracavernosal injections, Winter procedures for priapism and undetermined causes [102–107].

The entity and severity of presentation presents wide variation. Local symptoms include penile swelling and discoloration, abnormal consistency of the corpora, pain, voiding symptoms, cutaneous or urethral discharge in the case of rupturing or fistula. Systemic signs include fever, elevated white cells count and sepsis, although they are not always present [102].

Though there is no standardized approach to instrumental diagnosis, imaging techniques may be required to fully assess the extent of tissue damage before planning a treatment strategy. Standard US may show subcutaneous tissue swelling, inhomogeneous hypoechoic areas in the corpora cavernosa, and interruptions in the tunica albuginea. Contrast-enhanced US, when available, may document avascular areas wrapped in hyperperfused rims and may help define a suspicion of fistula [108]. CT scan may be required for a correct staging of abscess extent and for assessing the eventual involvement of other organs [109].

10.8.2   Management

Treatment should be early and aggressive in order to avoid potential sepsis and loss of the organ. Antibiotic prophylaxis is of course necessary and should take account of culture-isolated pathogens when possible [103].

Although puncture drainages of the corpora are often described as an early approach with the aim of pus excretion and microbiological sample collection, they have rarely shown to be a definitive and effective treatment. Most of the cases reported in the literature ultimately required some kind of surgical exploration of the corpora cavernosa with cavernotomy and debridement of non-viable tissue. This has a high chance of resulting in fibrosis and erectile dysfunction, although these sequelae can be treated with penile vacuum pump therapy and eventual penile prosthesis implantation provided the infection is fully resolved [102].

Penectomy is considered the last-resort treatment when conservative approaches fail due to untimely management or uncontrollable infection [104].

10.9   Fournier's Gangrene

Fabrizio Palumbo, Francesco Sebastiani

10.9.1   Clinical Presentation

First described by French physician Jean Alfred Fournier in 1883, Fournier's gangrene is a form of necrotizing fasciitis of the genital and perineal region with concomitant thrombosis of local arteries. It results in gangrene of the skin and subcutaneous tissue, sepsis, and multiple organ failure [110]. Its prognosis is poor and time-dependent as untimely treatment can be fatal in over 90% of cases [111].

Fournier's gangrene is rare: 1.6 cases per 100,000 men per year are reported in the literature. Men are notably far more at risk than women, and the average reported age is 50.9 years [112]. Most cases arise from localized infectious processes of the genitals, perineal, or anorectal area—which on their part can derive from poor hygiene, trauma, iatrogenic instrumentation or surgery, intestinal afflictions, etc.—in the presence of predisposing conditions. The latter are thought to include immunodepression, alcoholism, obesity, and cancer [113].

The pathogenetic origin of Fournier's gangrene is due to the necrosis of fascial structures prompted by bacteriemia. Infections lead to a cytokine-induced process of endothelial damage and abnormal activation of the coagulation cascade leading to thrombosis of the vessels which provide vascularization to the fascia. Concomitant endothelium extravasation, swelling, and white blood cells recruitment contribute to furthering the ischemia and necrosis process [113].

Patient history can help in suspecting this diagnosis when predisposing factors are noted. It is not unusual that medical attention-seeking on behalf of the patient is not immediate, especially if the patient presents concomitant situations that prevent him from noticing early symptoms, e.g., morbid obesity, poor hygiene, impairments in self-care ability, and low socio-economic status. When observed, local signs and symptoms range from discoloration and ulceration of genital and perianal skin to full-on tissue necrosis with palpable crepitus, purulent discharge, and swelling, usually appearing and worsening during the course of 3–5 days. There can be voiding symptoms and micturition impairment. General signs and symptoms correlate with the degree of sepsis: fever, white blood cells alterations such as leucocytosis or leukopenia, alterations in platelet count, elevated C-reactive protein, dysproteinaemia, alterations in indexes of renal or hepatic function indicative of multi-organ failure [114].

Beside clinical assessment, it is important to obtain imaging documentation in order to correctly define the extent of the infection, its source and possible spreading pathways [115]. US easily detects the presence of fluid and gas in subcutaneous tissues and may be useful for better orienting the clinical diagnosis; however, its major drawback is the impossibility to precisely stage the extent of the disease. In fact—aside for evaluation of the scrotum—deep assessment of the perineum or the ischioanal fossa is often impractical or impossible to perform with an US probe, depending on the anatomy of the patient and the severity of the condition. CT scan is the imaging modality of choice in Fournier's gangrene, especially when contrast-enhanced, because of its complete assessment of the abdominal and pelvic area in which it detects affected areas showing gas and fluid collection. Precise research of possible sources of infection in the abdomen increases the chance of planning optimal surgical treatment [116]. Technically speaking, MRI should yield a superior degree of precision in the assessment of soft tissues, but its reports in the literature are limited by the lower availability in emergency clinical settings [117].

10.9.2 Management

Fournier's gangrene requires immediate emergency treatment upon presentation and detection in order to avoid a fatal outcome. Broad-spectrum antibiotics accounting for Gram-positive, Gram-negative, and anaerobic bacteria are suggested as a means to reduce systemic toxicity and limit the circulation of the causative microorganism. In the case of subsequent successful microbic isolation via cultures, the choice of drugs can be adjusted accordingly. Patient resuscitation may be in order in the case of severe sepsis [118].

Surgical debridement with removal of necrotic and infected tissue is the crucial step to halt progression of the disease. Even a few hours delay has been shown to significantly increase the risk of death [119]. Extensive removal of all nonviable tissue, including a slim window of healthy adjacent tissue, is recommended. It is important to note that patients require daily wound care and possibly repeated surgical operations during the course of the hospital stay in order to fully excise all affected tissue. An average of 3.5 surgical operations per patient has been reported in the literature [120]. Depending on the extent of tissue necrosis, it could be necessary to consider a faecal and/or urinary diversion, respectively, via colostomy and cystostomy [121].

In regards to reconstructive procedures after successful and complete removal of necrotic tissues, various options are described. Vacuum-assisted closure (VAC) is a method which exposes the open wound to negative pressure, with the intent to reducing oedema and promoting blood flow to enhance second-intention healing. When available and suitable to the extent and location of tissue defects, it has proved advantageous over conventional wound management [122]. In the case of larger defects, various plastic reconstruction techniques such as scrotal advancement flaps, split thickness skin grafts, fascio-cutaneous, and myo-cutaneous flaps have been considered. They are reported to have satisfactory results, but as complex surgical procedures, there exists the possibility of further complications [117].

10.10 Penile Prosthesis Complications

Nicola Mondaini, Luca Crocerossa

10.10.1 Clinical Presentation

Penile prosthesis implantation is the gold standard in treatment of ED when medical therapy either fails or is contraindicated or unwanted by the patient. Despite improvements in surgical technique and implanted materials, IPP surgery retains a substantial complication rate. Complications of IPP implantation, while infrequent, can become serious and may be accompanied by severe morbidity and decreased satisfaction. These complications can be intraoperative or postoperative. Intraoperative complications include perforation of the tunica albuginea during dilatation of the corpora or perforation of the septum, with or without urethral injury [123]. The most frequent and severe postoperative complication is infection. Other major postoperative complications include mechanical failure: erosion and protrusion of cylinders; "S-shaped" deformity of the penis; and glans deflection; reservoir dislocation or acute abdomen due to bowel injury. The scro-

tum is the most common location for haematoma formation and this is due to an absence of compressive forces to abate any local bleeding. Haematomas can present in the immediate postoperative period or in a delayed fashion [124].

The recognition of urethral perforation can be difficult, so it is recommended that clinicians take extra caution to look for potential signs such as urethral bleeding, a visible dilator on the urethral meatus or prosthesis cylinder, or leakage of irrigation solution out of the urethra after instilling the corpora through the corporotomy [125, 126].

Penile prosthesis infections can be divided into clinically apparent and subclinical penile prosthesis infections. Clinically apparent penile prostheses can be diagnosed from symptoms such as new onset of penile pain, erythema, and induration overlying a prosthesis part, fever, drainage, and ultimately device extrusion. While most of these infections occur in the early perioperative period, late device infections have been documented. Subclinical prosthetic infections occur more frequently. These infections, which most often manifest by chronic prosthesis-associated pain, are difficult to diagnose and even more challenging to treat [127]. The complications of surgery can have economic ramifications (hospital admissions and revision surgery) and also negatively impact patient satisfaction and quality of life as there is a risk of penile length loss [124].

Cylinder erosion typically presents with the prosthesis protruding through the glans, urethral meatus, or distal penile shaft. Urethral erosion is characterized by dysuria, urethral discharge, early prosthetic infection, and glans necrosis [125].

10.10.2 Management

Almost all of these, postoperative complications require surgical repair. In case of urethral injury, depending on the size and location of perforation, the surgeon must determine whether continuation or cessation of the operation is appropriate. If there is a proximal perforation, immediate urethral repair accompanied by primary implantation and urinary diversion with a suprapubic catheter is suggested and abandoning the procedure should be considered if the injury is closer to the urethral meatus. However, when a urethral injury occurs and one or both corpora are dilated, abandoning the procedure may end in irreversible corporal fibrosis and penile shortening. Consequently, some clinicians have advocated for the insertion of a temporary malleable prosthesis after salvage washout and later a definitive inflatable prosthesis [125, 126].

Infection requires removal of the prosthesis and antibiotic administration. Alternatively, removal of the infected device with immediate replacement with a new prosthesis has been described using a washout protocol with successful salvages achieved in >80% of cases [128]. In case of reservoir dislocation, surgical reposition is mandatory. In case of acute abdomen due to bowel injury, removal of the reservoir and colostomy are necessary. The management of haematomas is usually conservative, and scrotal exploration is seldom required.

10.11 Priapism

Nicola Mondaini, Luca Crocerossa

10.11.1 Clinical Presentation

Priapism is defined as a penile erection lasting longer than 4 h in absence of sexual stimulation [129]. Incidence of priapism ranges between 0.3 and 5.4 per 1,00,000 males per year. Based on patient history and pathophysiology, two variants of priapism can be defined: ischaemic or low-flow priapism (IP) and non-ischaemic or high-flow priapism (NIP). IP is the most common type of priapism, accounting for 95% of cases; it is characterized by a minimal or no arterial inflow associated to complete occlusion of venous outflow of the corpora cavernosa; the resulting state of acidosis, glucose deficiency and hypoxia induces oedema, inflammation, and progressive necrotic degeneration of smooth muscle cells.

Stuttering or intermittent priapism is a subtype of IP characterized by an history of recurrent self-resolving painful erections lasting less than 4 h and usually occurring in patients with sickle cell disease (SCD) or other hematologic diseases. The most frequent causes of IP are the recreational use of erectile agents (intracavernous injection of alprostadil, papaverine, phentolamine or, rarely, oral PDE-5 inhibitors) and the use of antipsychotics or trazodone. Hereditary hematologic pathologies or blood cancers can cause IP by altering blood viscosity. Rarer aetiologies include amyloidosis, pelvic tumours, spinal cord, or peripheral nerve injuries. NIP is caused by the disruption of cavernous tissues almost invariably due to pelvic or genital trauma (straddle injury) resulting in an arteriolar-sinusoidal fistula leading to excessive corpora blood flow.

Clinical presentation of IP is characterized by a fully rigid erection often associated to penile pain. Glans and corpus spongiosum of the urethra are often flaccid. Contrarywise, NIP typically manifests as a painless, incomplete erection that occurs after days to weeks from a pelvic trauma. A natural erection during sexual stimulation or for nocturnal penile tumescence can be the trigger for both.

10.11.2 Management

The goal of emergency management of priapism is the resolution of the acute episode in order to preserve the long-term erectile function. Management should include at least patient's medical history, physical examination, corporal aspiration, and penile blood gas analysis [123]. History should focus on the onset and duration of the erection, presence of concomitant diseases and medications, use of recreational drugs, history of traumas and previous episodes of priapism. Physical examination must also include the evaluation of the abdomen and perineum.

Penile blood aspiration is performed by inserting a large bore (19-gauge or higher) butterfly needle in one or both of corpora cavernosa; regional anaesthesia before the procedure is achieved by infiltration at 2 and 10 o'clock at the base of the penis shaft which ensures sufficient block of the dorsal penile nerves to relieve pain and increase patient compliance. One drain puncture is enough for detumescence since corpora usually communicate through an incomplete midline septum; needle can be inserted either into corpora tip, through the glans, or into the middle of the shaft; in this case, 3 or 9 o'clock positions are preferred to not damage the urethra and the dorsal neurovascular bundle.

Initial aspirated blood will help differentiation between priapism types, being dark red in IP and bright red in NIP. Blood gas analysis is necessary for confirmation: in IP, blood gas values are typical of hypoxemic acidotic blood, with a P_{O2} lower than 30 mmHg, a P_{CO2} higher than 60 mmHg and a pH lower than 7.25. in NIP, blood gas analysis reveals systemic oxygenated blood, having a P_{O2} higher than 90 mmHg, a P_{CO2} lower than 40 mmHg and a pH around 7.4. Colour duplex Doppler ultrasonography of the penis can be used in conjunction with or as an alternative to penile blood gas analysis to differentiate between IP and NIP.

NIP must be promptly recognized and distinguished from IP owing its relative low risk in developing ED and the tendency to spontaneous resolution; moreover, NIP cannot be managed with any of the therapies for IP; NIP should be treated conservatively with ice and pelvic compression and/or angioembolization of the arterial-sinusoidal fistula after 1–2 months after onset. NIP is therefore not a medical emergency and will not be discussed further.

The treatment of stuttering priapism coincides with that of IP which is described below; however, a supportive therapy for the underlying haematological condition should be added, including hydration, oxygen administration, and blood transfusions as well as a long-term therapy for the prevention of future episodes.

In IP, corporal aspiration should be continued until arterial blood is seen through the syringe and complete detumescence is reached; restoration of oxygenated blood is required for preventing smooth muscle necrosis, fibrotic degeneration, and long-term ED. Cold saline irrigation with 0.9 NaCl is often associated to aspiration to promote evacuation of blood clots. Aspiration is resolutive in 30% of IP cases [130]. In case of failure, injection of sympathomimetic agents should be initiated. Phenylephrine is the most commonly used agent, given its high selectivity of α1-adrenoreceptors with low systemic cardiovascular effects. A dose of 100 to 200 μg of phenylephrine must be injected at intervals of 3–5 min until detumescence. A cumulative dose of 1000 μg is considered the maximum to avoid significant adverse events (hypertension or bradycardia) in adults [131]. Pulse and blood pressure sequential monitoring is required during administration and for at least 1 h afterwards. The efficacy of aspiration/irrigation and sympathomimetic injection is reported to be around 80% [132].

In case of failure of the above measures, surgical management of IP should be considered. Surgical procedures for IP are divided in shunting procedures and penile prothesis implantation (PPI). Shunting is the first-line treatment after aspiration/injection and are distinguished in proximal and distal shunting; goal of both is the drainage on hypoxic blood and restoration of venous outflow of the corpora cavernosa by the creation of an iatrogenic fistula with other structures.

Proximal shunts restore the venous outflow by creating communication between the corpus cavernosum and corpus spongiosum at the base of the penis or between the corpus cavernosum and the saphenous vein; proximal shunts have now fallen into disuse due to the risk of serious complications such as urethral damage, local thrombosis, and pulmonary embolism.

Distal shunting aims to create a fistula between the tip of corpora and the glans. Several percutaneous procedures have been described; however, there is insufficient evidence to draw definitive conclusions on which to choose for efficacy, safety, and prevention of relapse or long-term ED. The three most common techniques obtain this result by inserting a biopsy needle (Winter's technique) or a No. 11 blade scalpel (Ebbehoj's technique) or by inserting and rotating a No. 10 blade scalpel (T-shunt) through the glans into the corpora cavernosa. These procedures are usually performed unilaterally, but they can be repeated on the contralateral side if erection is not resolved. Corporoglanular dilation by an Hegar dilator can be added to increase the blood flow through the shunt (tunnelling).

Shunt procedures must be reserved to patients with IP lasting less than 24 h. Within this time limit, the changes in smooth muscle are still reversible and men who have achieved detumescence recover their potency in nearly all cases [133]. On the other side, patients with IP lasting longer than 48 h are bound to develop ED and must be treated with PPI. PPI is usually performed between 2 and 3 weeks after IP onset. This time window seems to balance the risks associated to an early implantation (including high rates of infections and penile prosthetic erosions, especially in patients treated with distal shunting) and the risks associated with a delayed PPI (including a high complication rate and poor patient satisfaction due to foreshortening and narrowing of the corpora cavernosa caused by penile fibrosis) [134]. In patients with IP lasting longer than 24 h but less than 48 h, the decision on the type of procedure to perform can be guided by a contrast-enhanced penile MRI, that has been shown to have an extremely high sensitivity in detecting necrosis/fibrosis of the smooth muscle.

References

1. Choe JM. Paraphimosis: current treatment options. Am Fam Physician. 2000;62(12):2623–8.
2. Palmisano F, Gadda F, Spinelli MG, Montanari E. Glans penis necrosis following paraphimosis: a rare case with brief literature review. Urol Case Rep. 2018;16:57–8.
3. Sato Y, Takagi S, Uchida K, Shima M, Tobe M, Haga K, Honama I, Hirobe M. Long-term follow-up of penile glans necrosis due to paraphimosis. IJU Case Rep. 2019;2(4):171–3.
4. Offenbacher J, Barbera A. Penile Emergencies. Emerg Med Clin North Am. 2019;37(4):583–92. https://doi.org/10.1016/j.emc.2019.07.001.
5. Kessler CS, Bauml J. Non-traumatic urologic emergencies in men: a clinical review. West J Emerg Med. 2009;10(4):281–7.
6. Fuenfer MM, Najmaldin A. Emergency reduction of paraphimosis. Eur J Pediatr Surg. 1994;4(6):370–1. https://doi.org/10.1055/s-2008-1066138.
7. Herzog LW, Alvarez SR. The frequency of foreskin problems in uncircumcised children. Am J Dis Child. 1986;140(3):254–6.
8. Manjunath AS, Hofer MD. Urologic emergencies. Med Clin North Am. 2018;102(2):373–85.
9. Pohlman GD, Phillips JM, Wilcox DT. Simple method of paraphimosis reduction revisited: point of technique and review of the literature. J Pediatr Urol. 2013;9(1):104–7.
10. Khan A, Riaz A, Rogawski KM. Reduction of paraphimosis in children: the EMLA® glove technique. Ann R Coll Surg Engl. 2014;96(2):168.
11. Cahill D, Rane A. Reduction of paraphimosis with granulated sugar. BJU Int. 1999;83(3):362.
12. Anand A, Kapoor S. Mannitol for paraphimosis reduction. Urol Int. 2013;90(1):106–8.
13. Hayashi Y, Kojima Y, Mizuno K, Kohri K. Prepuce: phimosis, paraphimosis, and circumcision. ScientificWorldJournal. 2011;3(11):289–301.
14. Kumar V, Javle P. Modified puncture technique for reduction of paraphimosis. Ann Roy Coll Surg. 2001;83:126–7.
15. Flores S, Herring AA. Ultrasound-guided dorsal penile nerve block for ED paraphimosis reduction. Am J Emerg Med. 2015;33(6):863.e3-5.
16. Samm BJ, Dmochowski RR. Urologic emergencies. Postgrad Med. 1996;100:187–200.
17. Sarkar D, Gupta S, Maiti K, Jain P, Pal DK. Penile strangulation by different objects and its removal by the modified string method: Management of four cases with review of literature. Urol Ann. 2019;11(1):1–5. https://doi.org/10.4103/UA.UA_178_17.
18. Hussain HM. A hair tourniquet resulting in strangulation and amputation of penis: case report and literature review. J Paediatr Child Health. 2008;44(10):606–7. https://doi.org/10.1111/j.1440-1754.2008.01394.x.
19. Hussin P, Mawardi M, Masran MS, Ganaisan P. Hair tourniquet syndrome: revisited. G Chir. 2015;36(5):219–21. https://doi.org/10.11138/gchir/2015.36.5.219.
20. Monib S, Amr B. Penile rings: no innovation without evaluation. Eur J Case Rep Intern Med. 2019;7(1):001292. https://doi.org/10.12890/2019_001292.
21. Bhat AL, Kumar A, Mathur SC, Gangwal KC. Penile strangulation. Br J Urol. 1991;68(6):618–21. https://doi.org/10.1111/j.1464-410x.1991.tb15426.x.
22. Nuhu A, Edino ST, Agbese GO, Kallamu M. Penile gangrene due to strangulation by a metallic nut: a case report. West Afr J Med. 2009;28(5):340–2. https://doi.org/10.4314/wajm.v28i5.55018.
23. Shaeer O. Methylene blue-guided repair of fractured penis. J Sex Med. 2006;3(2):349–54. https://doi.org/10.1111/j.1743-6109.2005.00155.x.
24. Detweiler MB. Penile incarceration with metal objects--a review of procedure choice based on penile trauma grade. Scand J Urol Nephrol. 2001;35(3):212–7. https://doi.org/10.1080/003655901750291980.

25. Ivanovski O, Stankov O, Kuzmanoski M, Saidi S, Banev S, Filipovski V, Lekovski L, Popov Z. Penile strangulation: two case reports and review of the literature. J Sex Med. 2007;4(6):1775–80. https://doi.org/10.1111/j.1743-6109.2007.00601.x.

26. Puvvada S, Kasaraneni P, Gowda RD, Mylarappa P, T M, Dokania K, Kulkarni A, Jayakumar V. Stepwise approach in the management of penile strangulation and penile preservation: 15-year experience in a tertiary care hospital. Arab J Urol. 2019 17(4):305-313. doi: https://doi.org/10.1080/20905 98X.2019.1647677.

27. Noh J, Kang TW, Heo T, Kwon DD, Park K, Ryu SB. Penile strangulation treated with the modified string method. Urology. 2004;64(3):591. https://doi.org/10.1016/j.urology.2004.04.058.

28. Vähäsarja VJ, Hellström PA, Serlo W, Kontturi MJ. Treatment of penile incarceration by the string method: 2 case reports. J Urol. 1993;149(2):372–3. https://doi.org/10.1016/s0022-5347(17)36088-3.

29. Talib RA, Canguven O, Al Ansari A, Shamsodini A. Treatment of penile strangulation by the rotating saw and 4-needle aspiration method: two case reports. Arch Ital Urol Androl. 2014;86(2):138–9. https://doi.org/10.4081/aiua.2014.2.138.

30. Tash JA, Eid JF. Urethrocutaneous fistula due to a retained ring of condom. Urology. 2000;56(3):508. https://doi.org/10.1016/s0090-4295(00)00665-8.

31. Carney JDD, McAninch JW. Retained penile constriction devices: management and complications. J Urol. 2001;165:83.

32. Dell'Atti L. The role of ultrasonography in the diagnosis and management of penile trauma. J Ultrasound. 2016;19(3):161–6. https://doi.org/10.1007/s40477-016-0195-4.

33. Bertolotto M, Calderan L, Cova MA. Imaging of penile traumas--therapeutic implications. Eur Radiol. 2005;15(12):2475–82. https://doi.org/10.1007/s00330-005-2900-0.

34. Velarde-Ramos L, Gómez-Illanes R, Campos-Juanatey F, Portillo-Martín JA. Traumatic lesions of the posterior urethra. Actas Urol Esp. 2016;40(9):539–48. https://doi.org/10.1016/j.acuro.2016.03.011.

35. Hsu GL, Brock G, von Heyden B, Nunes L, Lue TF, Tanagho EA. The distribution of elastic fibrous elements within the human penis. Br J Urol. 1994;73(5):566–71. https://doi.org/10.1111/j.1464-410x.1994.tb07645.x.

36. De Stefani S, Stubinski R, Ferneti F, Simonato A, Carmignani G. Penile fracture and associated urethral injury. ScientificWorldJournal. 2004;7(4 Suppl 1):92–9. https://doi.org/10.1100/tsw.2004.52.

37. Falcone M, Garaffa G, Castiglione F, Ralph DJ. Current Management of Penile Fracture: an up-to-date systematic review. Sex Med Rev. 2018;6(2):253–60. https://doi.org/10.1016/j.sxmr.2017.07.009.

38. Reis LO, Cartapatti M, Marmiroli R, de Oliveira Júnior EJ, Saade RD, Fregonesi A. Mechanisms predisposing penile fracture and long-term outcomes on erectile and voiding functions. Adv Urol. 2014;2014:768158. https://doi.org/10.1155/2014/768158.

39. Majzoub AA, Canguven O, Raidh TA. Alteration in the etiology of penile fracture in the Middle East and Central Asia regions in the last decade; a literature review. Urol Ann. 2015;7(3):284–8. https://doi.org/10.4103/0974-7796.157973.

40. Ory J, Bailly G. Management of penile fracture. Can Urol Assoc J. 2019;13(6 Suppl 4):S72–4. https://doi.org/10.5489/cuaj.5932.

41. Pavan N, Tezzot G, Liguori G, Napoli R, Umari P, Rizzo M, Chiriacò G, Chiapparrone G, Vedovo F, Bertolotto M, Trombetta C. Penile fracture: retrospective analysis of our case history with long-term assessment of the erectile and sexological outcome. Arch Ital Urol Androl. 2014;86(4):359–70. https://doi.org/10.4081/aiua.2014.4.359.

42. Barros R, Ribeiro JGA, da Silva HAM, de Sá FR, Fosse AM Jr, Favorito LA. Urethral injury in penile fracture: a narrative review. Int Braz J Urol. 2020;46(2):152–7. https://doi.org/10.1590/S1677-5538.IBJU.2020.99.02.

43. Kasaraneni P, Mylarappa P, Gowda RD, Puvvada S, Kasaraneni D. Penile fracture with urethral injury: our experience in a tertiary care hospital. Arch Ital Urol Androl. 2019;90(4):283–7. https://doi.org/10.4081/aiua.2018.4.283.

44. Sokolakis I, Schubert T, Oelschlaeger M, Krebs M, Gschwend JE, Holzapfel K, Kübler H, Gakis G, Hatzichristodoulou G. The role of magnetic resonance imaging in the diagnosis of penile fracture in real-life emergency settings: comparative analysis with intraoperative findings. J Urol. 2019;202(3):552–7. https://doi.org/10.1097/JU.0000000000000211.

45. Garg M, Goel A, Dalela D, Patil S. Penile fracture with urethral injury: evaluation by contrast imaging. BMJ Case Rep. 2013;2013:bcr2013010318. https://doi.org/10.1136/bcr-2013-010318.

46. Ouellette L, Hamati M, Hawkins D, Bush C, Emery M, Jones J. Penile fracture: surgical vs. conservative treatment. Am J Emerg Med. 2019;37(2):366–7. https://doi.org/10.1016/j.ajem.2018.06.051.

47. Rees RW, Brown G, Dorkin T, Lucky M, Pearcy R, Shabbir M, Shukla CJ, Summerton DJ, Muneer A, BAUS. Section of andrology and Genitourethral surgery (AGUS). British Association of Urological Surgeons (BAUS) consensus document for the management of male genital emergencies - penile fracture. BJU Int. 2018;122(1):26–8. https://doi.org/10.1111/bju.14167.

48. De Luca F, Garaffa G, Falcone M, Raheem A, Zacharakis E, Shabbir M, Aljubran A, Muneer A, Holden F, Akers C, Christopher N, Ralph DJ. Functional outcomes following immediate repair of penile fracture: a tertiary referral Centre experience with 76 consecutive patients. Scand J Urol.

2017;51(2):170–5. https://doi.org/10.1080/2168180 5.2017.1280532.

49. Pandyan GV, Zaharani AB, Al RM. Fracture penis: an analysis of 26 cases. ScientificWorldJournal. 2006;6:2327–33. https://doi.org/10.1100/ tsw.2006.363.

50. Gamal WM, Osman MM, Hammady A, Aldahshoury MZ, Hussein MM, Saleem M. Penile fracture: long-term results of surgical and conservative management. J Trauma. 2011;71(2):491–3. https://doi. org/10.1097/TA.0b013e3182093113.

51. van der Horst C, Martinez Portillo FJ, Seif C, Groth W, Jünemann KP. Male genital injury: diagnostics and treatment. BJU Int. 2004;93(7):927–30. https:// doi.org/10.1111/j.1464-410X.2003.04757.x.

52. Goldman HB, Dmochowski RR, Cox CE. Penetrating trauma to the penis: functional results. J Urol. 1996;155(2):551–3.

53. Mohr AM, Pham AM, Lavery RF, Sifri Z, Bargman V, Livingston DH. Management of trauma to the male external genitalia: the usefulness of American Association for the Surgery of Trauma organ injury scales. J Urol. 2003;170(6 Pt 1):2311–5. https://doi. org/10.1097/01.ju.0000089241.71369.fa.

54. Phonsombat S, Master VA, McAninch JW. Penetrating external genital trauma: a 30-year single institution experience. J Urol. 2008;180(1):192–5.; ; discussion 195-6. https://doi. org/10.1016/j.juro.2008.03.041.

55. Gomes CM, Ribeiro-Filho L, Giron AM, Mitre AI, Figueira ER, Arap S. Genital trauma due to animal bites. J Urol. 2001;165(1):80–3. https://doi. org/10.1097/00005392-200101000-00020.

56. Rothe K, Tsokos M, Handrick W. Animal and Human Bite Wounds. Dtsch Arztebl Int. 2015;112(25):433–42; quiz 443. https://doi. org/10.3238/arztebl.2015.0433.

57. Michielsen D, Van Hee R, Neetens C, LaFaire C, Peeters R. Burns to the genitalia and the perineum. J Urol. 1998;159(2):418–9. https://doi.org/10.1016/ s0022-5347(01)63937-5.

58. Yoshino Y, Ohtsuka M, Kawaguchi M, Sakai K, Hashimoto A, Hayashi M, Madokoro N, Asano Y, Abe M, Ishii T, Isei T, Ito T, Inoue Y, Imafuku S, Irisawa R, Ohtsuka M, Ogawa F, Kadono T, Kawakami T, Kukino R, Kono T, Kodera M, Takahara M, Tanioka M, Nakanishi T, Nakamura Y, Hasegawa M, Fujimoto M, Fujiwara H, Maekawa T, Matsuo K, Yamasaki O, Le Pavoux A, Tachibana T, Ihn H. Wound/burn guidelines committee. The wound/burn guidelines—6: guidelines for the management of burns. J Dermatol. 2016;43(9):989–1010. https:// doi.org/10.1111/1346-8138.13288.

59. Yip A, Ng SK, Wong WC, Li MK, Lam KH. Injury to the prepuce. Br J Urol. 1989;63:535–8.

60. Bagga HS, Tasian GE, McGeady J, Blaschko SD, McCulloch CE, McAninch JW, Breyer BN. Zip-related genital injury. BJU Int. 2013;112(2):E191–4. https://doi.org/10.1111/bju.12009.

61. Aboseif S, Gomez R, McAninch JW. Genital self-mutilation. J Urol. 1993;150(4):1143–6. https://doi. org/10.1016/s0022-5347(17)35709-9.

62. Djordjevic ML, Bizic M, Stojanovic B, Joksic I, Bumbasirevic UV, Ducic S, Mugabe H, Krstic Z, Bumbasirevic MZ. Outcomes and special techniques for treatment of penile amputation injury. Injury. 2019;50(Suppl 5):S131–6. https://doi.org/10.1016/j. injury.2019.10.064.

63. Tausch TJ, Cavalcanti AG, Soderdahl DW, Favorito L, Rabelo P, Morey AF. Gunshot wound injuries of the prostate and posterior urethra: reconstructive armamentarium. J Urol. 2007;178(4 Pt 1):1346–8. https://doi.org/10.1016/j.juro.2007.05.141.

64. Bertozzi M, Appignani A. The management of dog bite injuries of genitalia in paediatric age. Afr J Paediatr Surg. 2013;10(3):205–10. https://doi. org/10.4103/0189-6725.120875.

65. Raheem OA, Mirheydar HS, Patel ND, Patel SH, Suliman A, Buckley JC. Surgical management of traumatic penile amputation: a case report and review of the world literature. Sex Med. 2015;3(1):49–53. https://doi.org/10.1002/sm2.54.

66. Morey AF, Broghammer JA, Hollowell CMP, McKibben MJ, Souter L. Urotrauma Guideline 2020: AUA Guideline. J Urol. 2021;205(1):30–5. https://doi.org/10.1097/JU.0000000000001408.

67. Naseer A, King D, Lee H, Vale J. Testicular dislocation: the importance of scrotal examination in a trauma patient. Ann R Coll Surg Engl. 2012;94(2):e109–10. https://doi.org/10.1308/00358 8412X13171221502266.

68. Wasko R, Goldstein AG. Traumatic rupture of the testicle. J Urol. 1966;95(5):721–3. https://doi. org/10.1016/s0022-5347(17)63527-4.

69. Bourke MM, Silverberg JZ. Acute scrotal emergencies. Emerg Med Clin North Am. 2019;37(4):593–610. https://doi.org/10.1016/j. emc.2019.07.002.

70. Haas CA, Brown SL, Spirnak JP. Penile fracture and testicular rupture. World J Urol. 1999;17(2):101–6. https://doi.org/10.1007/s003450050114.

71. Wang Z, Yang JR, Huang YM, Wang L, Liu LF, Wei YB, Huang L, Zhu Q, Zeng MQ, Tang ZY. Diagnosis and management of testicular rupture after blunt scrotal trauma: a literature review. Int Urol Nephrol. 2016;48(12):1967–76. https://doi.org/10.1007/ s11255-016-1402-0.

72. Kim SH, Park S, Choi SH, Jeong WK, Choi JH. The efficacy of magnetic resonance imaging for the diagnosis of testicular rupture: a prospective preliminary study. J Trauma. 2009;66(1):239–42. https://doi. org/10.1097/TA.0b013e318156867f.

73. Gómez RG, Storme O, Catalán G, Marchetti P, Djordjevic M. Traumatic testicular dislocation. Int Urol Nephrol. 2014;46(10):1883–7. https://doi. org/10.1007/s11255-014-0736-8.

74. Patil MG, Onuora VC. The value of ultrasound in the evaluation of patients with blunt scrotal

trauma. Injury. 1994;25(3):177–8. https://doi.org/10.1016/0020-1383(94)90157-0.

75. Tiguert R, et al. Management of shotgun injuries to the pelvis and lower genitourinary system. Urology. 2000;55:193.

76. Etabbal AM, et al. War-related penile injuries in Libya: single-institution experience. Arab J Urol. 2018;16:250.

77. Dalton DM, Davis NF, O'Neill DC, Brady CM, Kiely EA, O'Brien MF. Aetiology, epidemiology and management strategies for blunt scrotal trauma. Surgeon. 2016;14(1):18–21. https://doi.org/10.1016/j.surge.2014.06.006.

78. Hudak SJ, et al. Operative management of wartime genitourinary injuries at Balad air force theater hospital, 2005 to 2008. J Urol. 2009;182:180.

79. Dogra V. Bell-clapper deformity. Am J Roentgenol. 2003;180(4):1176–7.

80. Schick MA, Sternard BT. Testicular Torsion. Treasure Island (FL): StatPearls Publishing; 2020.

81. Mellick LB, Sinex JE, Gibson RW, Mears K. A systematic review of testicle survival time after a Torsion event. Pediatr Emerg Care. 2019;35(12):821–5.

82. Sharp VJ, Kieran K, Arlen AM. Testicular torsion: diagnosis, evaluation, and management. Am Fam Physician. 2013;88(12):835–40.

83. Naouar S, Braiek S, El Kamel R. Testicular torsion in undescended testis: a persistent challenge. Asian J Urol. 2017;4(2):111–5.

84. Ogunyemi OI. Testicular Torsion; Published 2018. Available from: https://emedicine.medscape.com/article/2036003-overview#a7. Accessed February17 2020.

85. Shteynshlyuger A, Yu J. Familial testicular torsion: a meta analysis suggests inheritance. J Pediatr Urol. 2013;9(5):683–90. https://doi.org/10.1016/j.jpurol.2012.08.002.

86. Mabogunje OA. Testicular torsion and low relative humidity in a tropical country. Br Med J (Clin Res Ed). 1986;292(6517):363–4. https://doi.org/10.1136/bmj.292.6517.363.

87. Srinivasan A, Cinman N, Feber KM, Gitlin J, Palmer LS. History and physical examination findings predictive of testicular torsion: an attempt to promote clinical diagnosis by house staff. J Pediatr Urol. 2011;7(4):470–4. https://doi.org/10.1016/j.jpurol.2010.12.010.

88. Fehér ÁM, Bajory Z. A review of main controversial aspects of acute testicular torsion. J Acute Dis. 2016;5(1):1–8. https://doi.org/10.1016/j.joad.2015.06.017.

89. Sheth KR, Keays M, Grimsby GM, Granberg CF, Menon VS, DaJusta DG, Ostrov L, Hill M, Sanchez E, Kuppermann D, Harrison CB, Jacobs MA, Huang R, Burgu B, Hennes H, Schlomer BJ, Baker LA. Diagnosing testicular Torsion before urological consultation and imaging: validation of the TWIST

90. Bandarkar AN, Blask AR. Testicular torsion with preserved flow: key sonographic features and value-added approach to diagnosis. Pediatr Radiol. 2018;48(5):735–44. https://doi.org/10.1007/s00247-018-4093-0.

91. Blaivas M, Brannam L. Testicular ultrasound. Emerg Med Clin North Am. 2004;22(3):723–48. https://doi.org/10.1016/j.emc.2004.04.002.

92. Karaca L, Oral A, Kantarci M, Sade R, Ogul H, Bayraktutan U, Okur A, Yüce I. Comparison of the superb microvascular imaging technique and the color doppler techniques for evaluating children's testicular blood flow. Eur Rev Med Pharmacol Sci. 2016;20(10):1947–53.

93. Selim YARM, Albroumi SA. Acute torsion of the testis in children and young adults: role of high resolution and color doppler ultrasonography. Egypt J Radiol Nucl Med. 2015;46(1):151–7. https://doi.org/10.1016/j.ejrnm.2014.11.018.

94. Gotto GT, Chang SD, Nigro MK. MRI in the diagnosis of incomplete testicular torsion. Br J Radiol. 2010;83(989):e105–7. https://doi.org/10.1259/bjr/95900989.

95. Watkin NA, Reiger NA, Moisey CU. Is the conservative management of the acute scrotum justified on clinical grounds? Br J Urol. 1996;78(4):623–7. https://doi.org/10.1046/j.1464-410x.1996.16321.x.

96. Demirbas A, Demir DO, Ersoy E, Kabar M, Ozcan S, Karagoz MA, Demirbas O, Doluoglu OG. Should manual detorsion be a routine part of treatment in testicular torsion? BMC Urol. 2017;17(1):84. https://doi.org/10.1186/s12894-017-0276-5.

97. Thakare N, O'Flynn KJ, Pearce I. Testicular torsion: a urological emergency. Trends Urol Men's Heal. 2010;1(1):31–4. https://doi.org/10.1002/tre.161.

98. Visser AJ, Heyns CF. Testicular function after torsion of the spermatic cord. BJU Int. 2003;92(3):200–3. https://doi.org/10.1046/j.1464-410x.2003.04307.x.

99. Arap MA, Vicentini FC, Cocuzza M, Hallak J, Athayde K, Lucon AM, Arap S, Srougi M. Late hormonal levels, semen parameters, and presence of antisperm antibodies in patients treated for testicular torsion. J Androl. 2007;28(4):528–32. https://doi.org/10.2164/jandrol.106.002097.

100. He M, Li M, Zhang W. Prognosis of testicular torsion orchiopexy. Andrologia. 2020;52(1):e13477. https://doi.org/10.1111/and.13477.

101. Hayon S, Michael J, Coward RM. The modern testicular prosthesis: patient selection and counseling, surgical technique, and outcomes. Asian J Androl. 2020;22(1):64–9. https://doi.org/10.4103/aja.aja_93_19.

102. Paladino JR Jr, Nascimento FJ, Gromatsky C, Pompeo AC. Corpus cavernosum abscess after Winter procedure performance. BMJ Case Rep. 2014, 2014:bcr2013202089. https://doi.org/10.1136/bcr-2013-202089.

103. Sagar J, Sagar B, Shah DK. Spontaneous penile (cavernosal) abscess: case report with discussion of aetiology, diagnosis, and management with review of literature. ScientificWorldJournal. 2005;21(5):39–41. https://doi.org/10.1100/tsw.2005.4.

104. Ehara H, Kojima K, Hagiwara N, et al. Abscess of the corpus cavernosum. Int J Infect Dis. 2007;11:553–4.

105. Velcek D, Evans JA. Cavernosography. Radiology. 1982;144:781–5.

106. Orvis BR, Lue TF. New therapy for impotence. Urol Clin North Am. 1987;14:569–81.

107. Koksal T, Kadioglu A, Tefekli A, et al. Spontaneous bacterial abscess of bilateral cavernosal bodies. BJU Int. 1999;84:1107–8.

108. Roberto L, Silvestro C, Lucia D, Umberto B, Antonella C, Daniele M. A rare case of a spontaneous abscess of the corpus cavernosum: the role of contrast-enhanced ultrasound in diagnosis and post-therapeutic follow-up. J Ultrasound. 2021;24(4):567–72. https://doi.org/10.1007/s40477-020-00473-8.

109. Dugdale CM, Tompkins AJ, Reece RM, Gardner AF. Cavernosal abscess due to streptococcus anginosus: a case report and comprehensive review of the literature. Curr Urol. 2013;7(1):51–6. https://doi.org/10.1159/000343555.

110. Aliev SA, Rafiev SF, Rafiev FS, Aliev ES. Furnier's disease in surgeon practice. Khirurgiia (Mosk). 2008;11:58–63.

111. Ephimenko NA, Privolnee VV. Furnier's gangrene. Clin Microbiol Antimicrob Chemother. 2008;10:25–34.

112. Prohorov AV. Furnier's gangrene. Kazan Med J. 2016;97:256–61.

113. Chernyadyev SA, Ufimtseva MA, Vishnevskaya IF, Bochkarev YM, Ushakov AA, Beresneva TA, Galimzyanov FV, Khodakov VV. Fournier's gangrene: literature review and clinical cases. Urol Int. 2018;101(1):91–7. https://doi.org/10.1159/000490108.

114. Doluoğlu ÖG, Karagöz MA, Kılınç MF, Karakan T, Yücetürk CN, Sarıcı H, et al. Overview of different scoring systems in Fournier's gangrene and assessment of prognostic factors. Turk J Urol. 2016;42:190–6.

115. Levenson RB, Singh AK, Novelline RA. Fournier gangrene: role of imaging. Radiographics. 2008;28(2):519–28. https://doi.org/10.1148/rg.282075048.

116. Avery LL, Scheinfeld MH. Imaging of penile and scrotal emergencies. Radiographics. 2013;33(3):721–40. https://doi.org/10.1148/rg.333125158.

117. Singh A, Ahmed K, Aydin A, Khan MS, Dasgupta P. Fournier's gangrene. A clinical review. Arch Ital Urol Androl. 2016;88(3):157–64. https://doi.org/10.4081/aiua.2016.3.157.

118. Burch DM, Barreiro TJ, Vanek VW. Fournier's gangrene: be alert for this medical emergency. JAAPA. 2007;20(11):44–7. https://doi.org/10.1097/01720610-200711000-00020.

119. Thwaini A, Khan A, Malik A, Cherian J, Barua J, Shergill I, Mammen K. Fournier's gangrene and its emergency management. Postgrad Med J. 2006;82(970):516–9. https://doi.org/10.1136/pgmj.2005.042069.

120. Chawla SN, Gallop C, Mydlo JH. Fournier's gangrene: an analysis of repeated surgical debridement. Eur Urol. 2003;43(5):572–5. https://doi.org/10.1016/s0302-2838(03)00102-7.

121. Korkut M, Içöz G, Dayangaç M, Akgün E, Yeniay L, Erdoğan O, Cal C. Outcome analysis in patients with Fournier's gangrene: report of 45 cases. Dis Colon Rectum. 2003;46(5):649–52. https://doi.org/10.1007/s10350-004-6626-x.

122. Assenza M, Cozza V, Sacco E, Clementi I, Tarantino B, Passafiume F, Valesini L, Bartolucci P, Modini C. VAC (vacuum assisted closure) treatment in Fournier's gangrene: personal experience and literature review. Clin Ter. 2011;162(1):e1–5.

123. Salonia A, Bettocchi C, Boeri L, et al. European Association of Urology guidelines on sexual and reproductive health—2021 update: male sexual dysfunction. Eur Urol. 2021;80(3):333–57. https://doi.org/10.1016/J.EURURO.2021.06.007.

124. Cayetano-Alcaraz AA, Yassin M, Desai A, Tharakan T, Tsampoukas G, Zurli M, Minhas S. Penile implant surgery-managing complication. Fac Rev. 2021;10:73.

125. Minhas S. Urethral perforation during penile implant surgery: what to do? J Sex Med. 2017;14(7):867–9. https://doi.org/10.1016/j.jsxm.2017.05.003.

126. Carlos EC, Sexton SJ, Lentz AC, et al. Urethral injury and the penile prosthesis. Sex Med Rev. 2019;7(2):360–8. https://doi.org/10.1016/j.sxmr.2018.06.003.

127. Carson CC. Diagnosis, treatment and prevention of penile prosthesis infection. Int J Impot Res. 2003;15(Suppl 5):S139–46.

128. Chandrapal J, Harper S, Davis LG, Lentz AC. Penile implant infection: experience with expanded salvage criteria and a shortened course of postoperative antibiotics. Sex Med. 2020;8(3):383–7.

129. Montague DK, Jarow J, Broderick GA, et al. American urological association guideline on the management of priapism. J Urol. 2003;170(4 Pt 1):1318–24. https://doi.org/10.1097/01.ju.0000087608.07371.ca.

130. Ateyah A, Rahman El-Nashar A, Zohdy W, Arafa M, Saad E-DH. Intracavernosal irrigation by cold saline as a simple method of treating iatrogenic prolonged erection. J Sex Med. 2005;2(2):248–53. https://doi.org/10.1111/j.1743-6109.2005.20235.x.

131. Ericson C, Baird B, Broderick GA. Management of Priapism: 2021 update. Urol Clin North Am. 2021;48(4):565–76. https://doi.org/10.1016/j.ucl.2021.07.003.

132. Broderick GA, Kadioglu A, Bivalacqua TJ, Ghanem H, Nehra A, Shamloul R. Priapism: pathogenesis, epidemiology, and management. J Sex Med. 2010;7(1 Pt 2):476–500. https://doi.org/10.1111/j.1743-6109.2009.01625.x.

133. Zacharakis E, Raheem AA, Freeman A, et al. The efficacy of the T-shunt procedure and intracavernous tunneling (snake maneuver) for refractory ischemic priapism. J Urol. 2014;191(1):164–8. https://doi.org/10.1016/j.juro.2013.07.034.

134. Johnson MJ, Kristinsson S, Ralph O, Chiriaco G, Ralph D. The surgical management of ischaemic priapism. Int J Impot Res. 2020;32(1):81–8. https://doi.org/10.1038/s41443-019-0197-9.

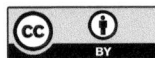

Giuseppe Carrieri, Ugo Falagario, Marco Recchia, and Marco Finati

11.1 Penile Cancer

11.1.1 Epidemiology, Etiology, and Pathology

Worldwide incidence of penile cancer (PC) is affected by race, ethnicity, and prevalence of HPV, resulting in an extreme variability through different geographic areas. In South America, Eastern Asia, and some parts of Africa, PC can account up to 2% of all male tumors. In USA, the higher incidence is reported in white Hispanics, followed by Native and African Americans, respectively [1–3]. Risk of PC increases with age, with a peak in the sixth decade. HPV infections are responsible for approximately one out of three cases [4, 5].

HPV has been found in 7–100% of intraepithelial cancer and 30–40% of invasive penile tumor. Subtypes 16 and 18 are the most common cofactors involved in the carcinogenesis of penile squamous cell carcinoma (SCC) [6–8]. Other anatomical conditions, such as phimosis and chronic penile inflammation, may play a role in the tumor genesis. Smoking habit and multiple sexual partners increased the risk three to five times, although the last factor may be correlated to higher risk of sexually transmitted infections, including Papillomavirus.

HPV is responsible both for penile and cervical cancer. However, female sexual partners of penile cancer patients do not have an increased risk of developing cervical malignancy [9–12].

About 95% of PC are SCC (or variants) and usually originate from a premalignant lesion, as shown in Table 11.1.

SCC could exhibit a variety of growth patterns and HPV associations, resulting in different aggressiveness and prognosis [13–15]. Histological subtype, perineural invasion, lymphovascular invasion, depth of invasion, and grade of the primary tumor are recognized as the major pathological predictors of metastasis and prognosis of PC [16]. According to these findings, SCC should be classified into three risk groups:

Table 11.1 Penile cancer premalignances

Lesions sporadically associated with squamous cell carcinoma (SCC) of the penis
• Bowenoid papulosis of the penis (HPV related)
• Lichen sclerosis
Premalignant lesions (up to one-third transform to invasive SCC)
• Penile intraepithelial lesions
• Giant condylomata (Buschke-Lowenstein)
• Bowen's disease
• Paget's disease (intradermal ADK)

Supplementary Information The online version contains supplementary material available at [https://doi.org/10.1007/978-3-031-11701-5_11].

G. Carrieri (✉) · U. Falagario · M. Recchia
M. Finati
Department of Urology and Organ Transplantation, University of Foggia, Foggia, Italy
e-mail: giuseppe.carrieri@unifg.it

11.1.2 Diagnostic Evaluation

Penile cancer can be cured in over 80% of cases if diagnosed early but is a life-threatening disease when lymphatic metastasis occurs.

Physical examination is in most of cases sufficient for a clinical diagnosis, however penile carcinoma may be hidden under a phimosis [17]. Palpation of the penis to assess the extent of local invasion and palpation of both groins to assess the lymph node status should always be performed. Local staging to provide information about infiltration of the corpora may be performed with Ultrasound (US) or magnetic resonance imaging (MRI). The sensitivity and specificity of MRI in predicting corporal or urethral invasion was reported as 82.1% and 73.6%, and 62.5% and 82.1%, respectively [18]. Penile Doppler US has been reported to have a higher staging accuracy than an MRI in detecting corporal infiltration [19]. Staging for systemic metastases using abdomino-pelvic CT and chest X-ray is recommended in patients with positive inguinal nodes [20–22]. PET/CT is an option [23].

11.1.3 Treatment of the Primary Tumor

The aims of the treatment of the primary tumor are complete tumor removal with as much organ preservation as possible, without compromising oncological control. Surgical treatment can be mutilating and devastating for the patient's psychological well-being, and since local recurrence has little influence on long-term survival, organ preservation strategies are justified [24].

11.2 Treatment of Superficial Non-invasive Disease (PeIN)

Treatment of superficial non-invasive disease (PeIN) includes topical chemotherapy with imiquimod or 5-fluorouracil and laser treatment with a neodymium:yttrium-aluminum-garnet (Nd:YAG) or carbon dioxide (CO_2) laser [25–30]. Circumcision is advisable prior to the use of topical agents. Due to high persistence/recurrence rates, treatment must be assessed by biopsy, and long-term surveillance is warranted. Glans resurfacing, total or partial, can be a primary treatment for PeIN or a secondary option in case of failure of the above mentioned. Additionally, patients and physician should be aware that up to 20% of patients undergoing glans resurfacing for presumed PeIN were found to have invasive disease on histopathological examination [31].

11.3 Treatment of Invasive Disease Confined to the Glans (T1–T2)

In patients with invasive penile cancer confined to the glans (T1–T2), treatment choice depends on tumor size, histology, localization (if urethral meatus is involved), and patient preference.

Small and localized invasive lesions should receive organ-sparing treatment. Additional circumcision, local excision, partial glansectomy, or total glansectomy with reconstruction are surgical options. External beam radiotherapy or brachytherapy as well as laser therapy may be an option but the risk of more invasive disease must be recognized. For a general recommendation, 3–5 mm can be considered a safe maximum [20, 32]. Conservative surgery may be performed safely in well-selected patients with discrete tumors by intraoperative frozen-section analysis.

11.4 Organ-Preserving Treatments

Organ-sparing surgery offers better outcomes in terms of quality of life (QoL) but have higher risk of local recurrence. Three years local recurrence rates range from 18% after organ-sparing surgery to 4% after amputation surgery (partial or radical) [33]. Amputation of recurrent disease may be necessary, although survival appears to be unaffected if early diagnosis and treatment are achieved. For these reasons, organ-sparing surgery should only be offered to patients compliant with a strict follow-up schedule.

11.4.1 Laser Therapy

The two most widely used laser energy sources are the CO_2 and Nd:YAG, lasers. Although the CO_2 laser has been widely used previously, the superficial depth of penetration (limited to 0.1 mm) makes it less than optimal for the treatment of penile carcinoma in situ or small T1 tumors.

Conversely, the Nd:YAG laser has a wavelength of 1064 nm and results in protein denaturation at a depth of up to 6 mm. Reported local recurrence rates after Nd:YAG laser treatment of T1 tumors range from 10% to 48% [27, 28]. Inguinal nodal recurrence has been reported in 21% of patients [28] and 7 years overall survival range from 85 to 95% [30].

11.4.2 Moh's Micrographic Surgery

Moh's micrographic surgery is a historical technique consisting of layer-by-layer resection of penile lesion with intraoperative microscopic examination of histological margins. Nowadays, Moh's micro-surgery has been replaced by surgical excision with intraoperative frozen-section assessment of margin status.

11.4.3 Glans Resurfacing

Glans resurfacing has been proposed over the last years for management of carcinoma in situ of the glans penis. In this technique, subdermal dissection of the skin and subepithelial connective tissue of the underlying corpora spongiosa is performed. Reconstruction is then performed with a graft (split skin or buccal mucosa). Few studies have reported results of glans resurfacing in patients with PeIN or T1 with local recurrence rates of 0% and 6% respectively at a median follow-up of 30 months [34].

11.4.4 Glansectomy

Up to 80% of penile lesions are confined to the glans or prepuce [35]. Therefore, glansectomy combined with split-skin graft reconstruction of a neoglans is the preferred treatment for T1–T3 penile cancer of the glans. The skin is incised at the subcoronal level and deepened onto Buck's fascia. Dissection is performed over or under Buck's fascia according to clinical or MRI suspicion of tunical involvement, or when the disease is of high volume with high-risk features. The glans is excised, and the urethra is sutured to the corpora. Finally, a neoglans is created using a split-thickness skin graft. In a recent report on 172 patients undergoing glansectomy, the local recurrence rate was 9% at a median follow-up of 41.4 m [36].

11.4.5 Radiotherapy

External bean radiotherapy with a minimum dose of 60 Gy combined with brachytherapy or brachytherapy alone is a safe organ-preserving approach with good results in selected patients with T1–2 lesions <4 cm in diameter [37, 38].

11.5 Treatment Recommendations for Invasive Penile Cancer (T2–T4)

Total glansectomy with or without corpora cavernosa transection to achieve negative surgical margins is an option if patients with T2 tumors without gross cavernosum involvement [39]. Partial or total amputation is the first-line treatment in patients with T3 disease or patients with T2 disease and adverse features for organ preservation. These includes a tumors of size 4 cm or more, grade 3 lesions, and invasion into the glans urethra. Radiotherapy is an option. Partial and total amputation should also be considered in patients unfit for reconstructive surgery or non-compliant to follow-up [40].

Penile amputation remains the standard therapy for patients with deeply invasive or high-grade cancers. Partial or total penectomy should be considered in patients exhibiting adverse features for cure by organ preservation strategies such as tumors size ≥ 4 cm, grade 3 lesions, and invasion of the glans urethra or corpora cavernosa.

11.6 Management of Regional Lymph Nodes

11.6.1 Lymphadenectomy

Lymphatic spread of penile cancer starts with superficial and deep inguinal lymph nodes followed by the pelvic lymph nodes [24]. Pelvic nodal disease without ipsilateral inguinal lymph node metastasis and contralateral metastatic spread have never been reported. Further lymphatic spread from the pelvic nodes to retroperitoneal nodes (para-aortic and para-caval) is classified as systemic metastatic disease.

Following these rules, treatment of regional lymph nodes is performed step by step based on the clinical inguinal lymph node status. If clinical lymph nodes appear negative on palpation and are not enlarged (cN0), micro-metastatic disease occurs in up to 25% of cases and invasive lymph node staging is required since no imaging technique can reliably detect or exclude micro-metastatic disease. In clinically positive lymph nodes (cN1/cN2), metastatic disease is highly likely and lymph node surgery with histology is required.

Enlarged fixed inguinal lymph nodes (cN3) require neoadjuvant chemotherapy and surgery.

11.7 Andrological Aspects of Penile Cancer

11.7.1 Consequences after Penile Cancer Treatment

Over the last 15 years, the management of penile cancer shifted from a model based on oncologic control to a more balanced approach, taking into account patients' quality of life in terms of sexual function, voiding while standing up, and cosmesis.

Few comparative studies in the literature reported that local excision led to better sexual out-comes than glansectomy. Similarly, men after partial penectomy reported significantly more problems with orgasm, cosmesis, life interference, and urinary function than those who had undergone penile-sparing surgery (83% vs. 43%, $p < 0.0001$). Interestingly, there were no differences in erectile function, sexual desire, intercourse satisfaction, or overall sexual satisfaction [41].

11.7.2 Sexual Activity and Quality of Life After Treatment for Penile Cancer

Laser and topical treatments have no impact on quality of life and sexuality [42]. Similarly, patients undergoing glans resurfacing reported that the sensation at the tip of their penis was no different or better after surgery [34]. In patients undergoing glansectomy, spontaneous erection, rigidity, and penetrative capacity decline in up to 21% with 25% of patients unable to orgasm [43, 44]. Patients' satisfaction after partial and total penectomy is much lower. Indeed, only 55.6% of patients had erectile function that allowed sexual intercourse after partial penectomy and only 33.3% were satisfied with their sex life. After total amputation, a significant effect on sexual life and overall QoL, although there were no negative implications in terms of partner relationships, self-assessment or the evaluation of masculinity [45]. Even if the evidence is very limited, total phallic reconstruction following full or near-total penile amputation is possible, with cosmetically acceptable results [46–48].

11.8 Testicular Cancer

11.8.1 Epidemiology, Etiology, and Pathology

With an estimated worldwide incidence of 75,000 new cases per year [49], testicular cancer (TC) represents 1% of all neoplasms and 5% of urological tumors. Its incidence is constantly increasing, especially in Western Countries, with a peak in the third and fourth decade of life.

Table 11.2 The 2016 World Health Organization (WHO) histological classification of TC and the 2016 TNM classification

2016 World Health Organization (WHO) histological classification	2016 TNM classification
Germ cell tumors • Germ cell neoplasia in situ (GCNIS)	Stage Ia Primary tumor limited to the testis and epididymis, with no evidence of microscopic vascular or lymphatic invasion and normal tumor marker levels
Derived from GCNIS • Seminoma • Embryonal carcinoma • Yolk sac tumor, post-pubertal type • Trophoblastic tumors • Teratoma, post-pubertal type • Teratoma with somatic malignant components • Mixed germ cell tumors Germ cell tumors unrelated to GCNIS • Spermatocytic tumor • Yolk sac tumor, pre-pubertal type • Mixed germ cell tumor, pre-pubertal type	Stage Ib Locally invasive TC, with no sign of distant metastasis Stage IS Persistently elevated serum tumor marker levels after orchidectomy Stage II Lymph node invasion
Sex cord/stromal tumors • Leydig cell tumor • Sertoli cell tumor • Granulosa cell tumor • Thecoma/fibroma group of tumors • Other sex cord/gonadal stromal tumors • Tumors containing both germ cell and sex cord/gonadal stromal	Stage III Presence of at least one distant metastasis and/or persistently highly elevated tumor marker levels
Miscellaneous non-specific stromal tumors • Ovarian epithelial tumors • Tumors of the collecting ducts and rete testis	

Germ cell tumor is the predominant histotype which can be found in 90–95% of all TCs. At diagnosis, 1–2% of tumors are bilateral and 5% of GCTs have a primary extragonadal location [50, 51].

TC recognizes a series of morphological and functional risk factors enclosed in the so-called "Testicular dysgenesis syndrome," including cryptorchidism, hypospadias, sub- or infertility, and hypogonadism. Other risk factors include a familiar history of TC and presence of contralateral tumor [52, 53]. A genetic predisposition is often responsible for advanced stage tumors. Specifically, an isochromosome found on the short arm of chromosome 12 (i12p) is overexpressed in the GCT related to germ cell neoplasia in situ (GCNIS), while a cKIT mutations is often present in seminoma. These mutations play a major role in pathological upgrade and invasiveness [54].

The 2016 World Health Organization (WHO) histological classification of TC [55, 56] and the 2016 TNM classification [57], are presented in Table 11.2. About 75–80% of seminoma and 55–64% non-seminoma patients exhibit stage I at diagnosis [58]. Serum tumor marker levels are strong predictors of metastasis and prognosis representing an essential selection tool for adjuvant therapies.

11.8.1.1 Diagnostic Evaluation

Testicular cancer usually present as a scrotal mass or diffuse enlargement detected by patient's self-examination or it may be an incidental finding during testicular ultrasonography (US) [59] (Fig. 11.1). Physical examination may reveal bulky retroperitoneal disease or supraclavicular, scalene and inguinale nodes involvement. Gynecomastia may be present [60]; back and flank plain can be reported because of retroperitoneal metastasis.

Valuation of symptoms is also important. Urethral and irritative symptoms and testicular pain of acute onset may help in differential diagnosis with epididymitis or epididymitis-related orchitis.

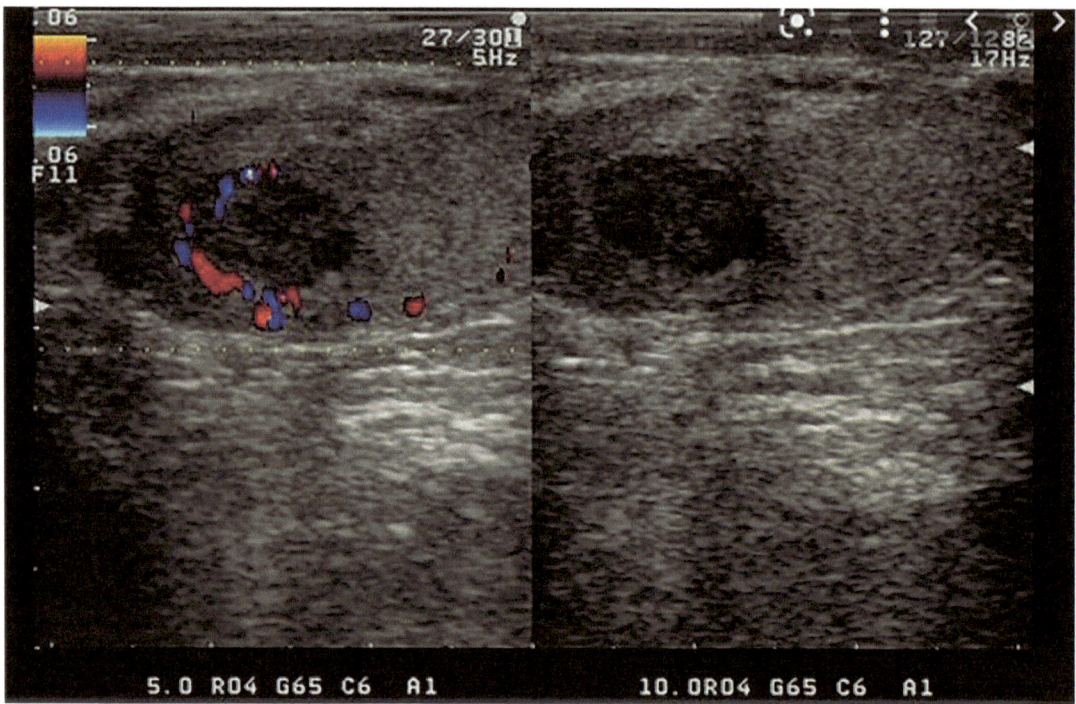

Fig. 11.1 Testicular cancer detected by US: you may see the hypervascular testicular lesion

Transillumination of scrotum may reveal the presence of hydrocele. Even if testicular cancer is evident by testicular examination, high frequency US is mandatory. Other differential diagnosis includes spermatocele, hematocele, granulomatous orchitis, and varicocele. International guidelines recommend chest, abdomen, and pelvis computerized tomography (TC) for M staging.

Finally, serum tumor markers are of pivotal for diagnosis and treatment of testicular cancer. AFP (alpha-fetoprotein), β-HCG (human chorionic gonadotropin), and lactic acid dehydrogenase (LDH) should always be determined before and during follow-up after orchidectomy. Normal serum markers may not exclude tumor, while persistence of high levels after surgical treatment indicates a probability of disease progression.

11.8.1.2 Disease Management

Gold standard for management of testicular tumor is inguinal exploration with cross-clamping of spermatic cord vasculature and eventual orchifunicolectomy. Scrotal approaches and open biopsy of testis must be avoided. If testicular cancer cannot be excluded, radical orchiectomy must be performed [61]. *Testing sparing surgery* must be considered for small tumors, in case of solitary testis, when benign pathology is suspected or in patients with synchronous/metachronous tumor [62]. Further treatments depends on histology of tumor and its clinical stage.

11.8.2 GCNIS (Germinal Cell Neoplasia In Situ)

If GCNIS is diagnosed and contralateral testis is healthy, we can perform the following:

- Radical orchiectomy.
- Close observation (as the 5-years risk of developing TC is 50%) if patient is compliant [63].
- Radiotherapy (18–20 Gy in fractions of 2 Gy), which is the gold standard in case solitary testis. It can turn out in infertility and Leydig cells insufficiency.

11.8.2.1 Stage I Germ Cell Tumors

Seminoma: Clinical Stage I

After radical orchiectomy, the options for management are as follows:

- Surveillance: low-stage seminoma has a very positive survival rate (almost 90%) and can be treated with radical orchiectomy alone. Surveillance is the preferred option, because radiotherapy and chemotherapy are associated with important morbidity and risk of secondary malignancy [64]. It consists of 10-years follow-up, which includes physical examination, serum markers (every 3–6 months for year 1, 6–12 months for years 2–3, then annually until year 10). Imaging includes abdominal and pelvic TC, chest X-ray.
- Radiotherapy (usually 2500–3000 cGy): this low dose of radiation is well-tolerated [65], and can be offered to patients that cannot make surveillance, and with contraindications to perform chest-abdomen CT.
- Carboplatin chemotherapy: adjuvant therapy with carboplatin must be taken in consideration as a salvage therapy after irradiation or if risk of occult metastasis is present (tumor >4 cm; involvement of testis).

11.8.2.2 NSGCT (Non-seminoma Germ Cell Tumors): Clinical Stage I

NSGCT: CS I tumors are classified according to risk of development of occult metastasis. All treatment options must be discussed with individual patients, to let them make an informed decision about further treatment. The risk-adapted strategy takes into consideration the lymphovascular probability of invasion:

- **Low risk (no vascular invasion):**
  - Standard option: surveillance.
  - If patients cannot agree surveillance protocol: 1 cycle of BEP (bleomycin, etoposide, and cisplatin) as *adjuvant* therapy [66].
  - If remains conditions against surveillance or chemotherapy is not proposed: *nerve-sparing retroperitoneal lymph node dissection* [67].
- **High risk (vascular invasion present):**
  - Standard option: 1 cycle of BEP (bleomycin, etoposide, and cisplatin) as *adjuvant therapy*.
  - If chemotherapy is not chosen, *nerve-sparing retroperitoneal lymph node dissection* or surveillance (the last option, if any other curative option is unavailable) (Fig. 11.2).

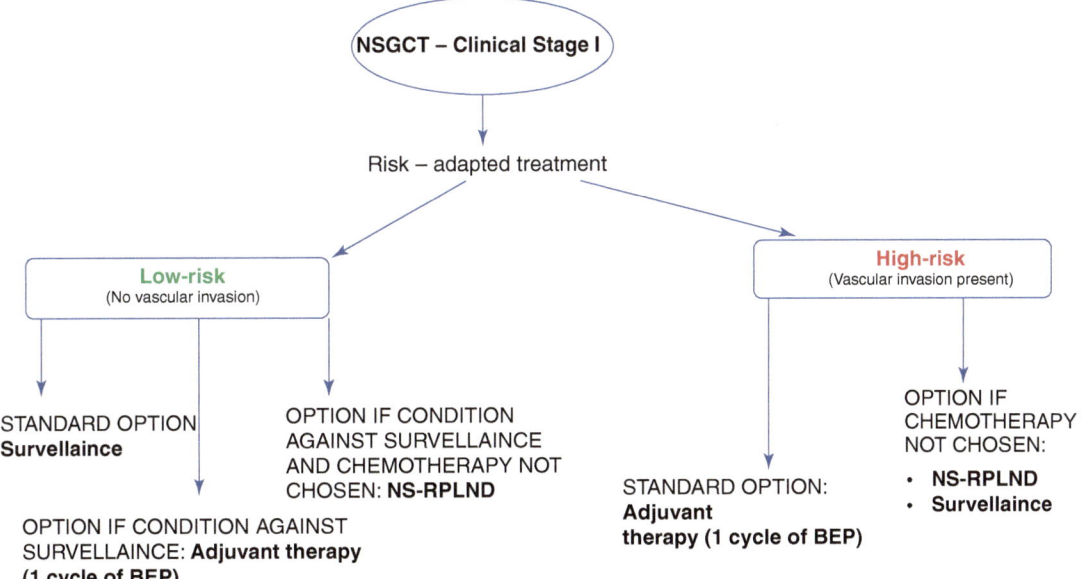

Fig. 11.2 NSGCT CS I—treatment according to the EAU guidelines 2021©

In patients with elevated serum markers or relapsing during surveillance, according to the IGCCC Group Classification of prognosis, the therapy may include 3–4 cycles of BEP followed by resection in case of residual tumour [67].

11.8.2.3 Metastatic Germ Cell Cancer (Stage IIA–IIB)

Stage IIA-IIB Seminoma

Nowadays, chemotherapy is the preferred alternative to radiotherapy for stage II seminoma. It consists of three cycles of BEP or four cycles of EP (etoposide and cisplatin) in case of contraindications to bleomycin for older patients. Radiotherapy may be considered in elderly selected patients who difficulty tolerate systemic therapy [68]. Acute toxicity is reported almost exclusively from chemotherapy, while long-term toxicity derives

from the irradiation following RT, with bowel damage and risk for secondary tumors [69].

Stage IIA-IIB NSGCT

All patients with elevated serum markers (Marker +) at Stage IIA-IIB NGCS tumors require three cycles of primary chemotherapy (BEP) according to IGCCCG risk-group. Nerve-sparing (NS) retroperitoneal lymph node resection (RPLND) can be performed in patients with II A NGCS stage (Marker -) in specialized centers by an experienced surgeon. Surveillance may be considered in the same stage in patients with normal markers and lymph nodes <2 cm in greatest axial diameter, and re-evaluation after six weeks is mandatory.

Relapse of tumor occurs in almost 30% of patients with pathological stage II treated with RPLND, with specifical further therapy according to prognosis risk-group (Fig. 11.3).

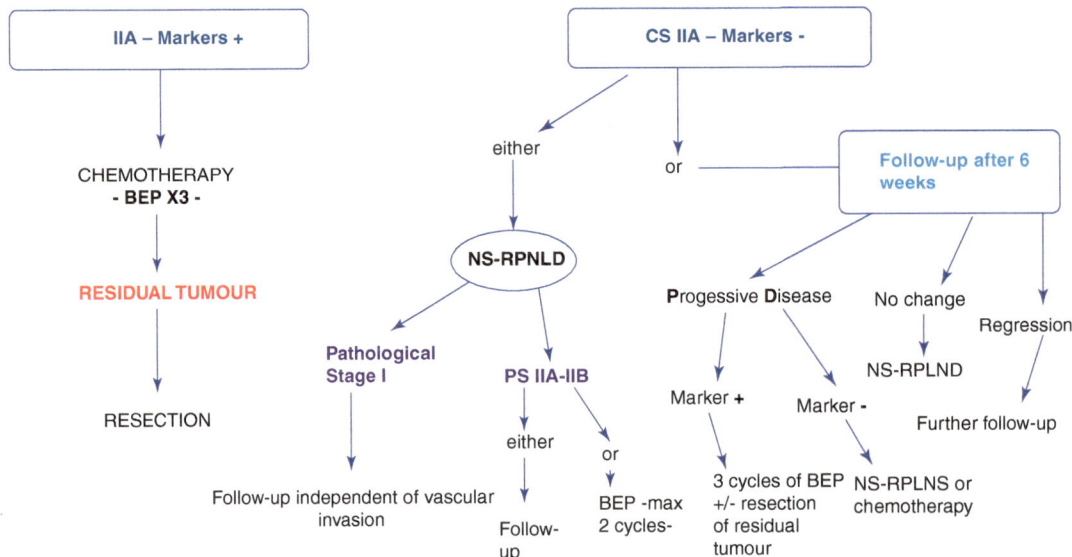

Fig. 11.3 NSGCT CS IIA-IIB—treatment according to the EAU guidelines 2021©

11.9 Andrological Aspects of Testicular Cancer

11.9.1 Testicular Cancer and Gonadal Function

Sperm abnormalities and Leydig cell's dysfunction in patient with testicular cancer are very common before orchidectomy. Histopathological studies have shown a very high incidence of abnormalities in the contralateral testis of patients with unilateral TC. These abnormalities result in poor semen quality [70]. Additionally, reproductive function may decrease after treatment [71]; for this reason, semen preservation should be offered to all patients [61].

The association between testicular cancer, cryptorchidism/small testis, endocrine, and andrological aspects has been widely investigated.Lower sperm concentration and total sperm count, and increased levels of FSH were found in patients with testicular cancer before treatment. No differences were found in the level of testosterone and estradiol, while man with testicular cancer who had increased level of HCG had very low LH levels [72]. A possible explanation for the lower LH-levels could be the altered secretion of LH-RH by hypothalamus because of the cancer. The increased levels of HCG in some patients could explain the normal level of testosterone and estradiol, and the lower LH-level too (in fact, HCG may stimulate production of testosterone and estradiol by Leydig cells, exerting LH-like effects) [70].

11.9.2 Fertility and Sexual Disfunction After Treatment for Testicular Cancer

Because of the high cure rate of patients with testicular cancer, their quality life after treatment is an important point to discuss. Fertility and sexual aspects are known to condition QoL.

Previous studies have confirmed the impairment of fertility in these patients even before orchidectomy and diagnosis; moreover, gonadal function is affected by surgical treatment, radiotherapy, and chemotherapy in patients with TC.

Leydig cells are more resistant than germinal cells to chemotherapy; however, endocrine disfunction commonly happen during follow-up [72]. Postoperative serum measurement of LH and testosterone must be performed, and the patients might be asked about symptoms and signs of androgen deficiency, to assess the need of androgen therapy. High postoperative FSH levels ($\geq$24 IU/l) are associated with persistent infertility.

Even if a new pregnancy is unlike during cytotoxic treatment and the first year after treatment, contraception is recommended in this period because of the high risk of teratogenic effects induced by radio-chemotherapy. This risk is higher during the first period after treatment, because the patient may still have some sperm exposed to DNA damage.

Additionally, adjuvant therapies and the associated psychological distress may lead to sexual disfunction affecting partner relationship. Orchidectomy itself do not impact erectile function but nerve-sparing retroperitoneal lymph node dissection that may be necessary in some advanced cases may lead to dry ejaculation.

In this scenario, it is very important to counsel patients about cryopreservation, eventual testicular sperm extraction, fertility after treatment, and need for androgen replacement therapies.

Every patient with testicular cancer should be managed by a multidisciplinary team including urologist, oncologist, radiologist, endocrinologist, pathologist, phycologist, and fertility experts. Patients should not be encouraged with false hopes, and alternative plans should be discussed. Indeed, although modern techniques of assisted fecundation (e.g., ICSI-*intracytoplasmic sperm injection*) can be performed even in a very poor quality, semen [73] and the benefits of cryopreservation are clear, outcomes of fertility treatments are in most of cases unpredictable.

References

1. Backes DM, Kurman RJ, Pimenta JM, Smith JS. Systematic review of human papillomavirus prevalence in invasive penile cancer. Cancer Causes Control. 2009;20(4):449–57. https://doi.org/10.1007/s10552-008-9276-9.
2. Chaux A, Netto GJ, Rodríguez IM, et al. Epidemiologic profile, sexual history, pathologic features, and human papillomavirus status of 103 patients with penile carcinoma. World J Urol. 2013;31(4):861–7. https://doi.org/10.1007/s00345-011-0802-0.
3. Parkin DM, Bray F. Chapter 2: the burden of HPV-related cancers. Vaccine. 2006;24(Suppl 3):S3/11–25. https://doi.org/10.1016/j.vaccine.2006.05.111.
4. Barnholtz-Sloan JS, Maldonado JL, Pow-sang J, Giuliano AR, Guiliano AR. Incidence trends in primary malignant penile cancer. Urol Oncol. 2007;25(5):361–7. https://doi.org/10.1016/j.urolonc.2006.08.029.
5. Hartwig S, Syrjänen S, Dominiak-Felden G, Brotons M, Castellsagué X. Estimation of the epidemiological burden of human papillomavirus-related cancers and non-malignant diseases in men in Europe: a review. BMC Cancer. 2012;12:30. https://doi.org/10.1186/1471-2407-12-30.
6. Stankiewicz E, Kudahetti SC, Prowse DM, Ktori E, Cuzick J, Ambroisine L, Zhang X, Watkin N, Corbishley C, Berney DM. HPV infection and immunochemical detection of cell-cycle markers in verrucous carcinoma of the penis. Mod Pathol. 2009;22(9):1160–8. Accessed October 27, 2021. https://pubmed.ncbi.nlm.nih.gov/19465901/
7. Kayes O, Ahmed HU, Arya M, Minhas S. Molecular and genetic pathways in penile cancer. Lancet Oncol. 2007;8(5):420–9. Accessed October 27, 2021. https://pubmed.ncbi.nlm.nih.gov/17466899/
8. Muñoz N, Castellsagué X, Berrington de González A, Gissmann L. Chapter 1: HPV in the etiology of human cancer. Vaccine. 2006;24(Suppl 3):S3/1-10. Accessed October 27, 2021. https://pubmed.ncbi.nlm.nih.gov/16949995/
9. Dillner J, von Krogh G, Horenblas S, Meijer CJ. Etiology of squamous cell carcinoma of the penis. Scand J Urol Nephrol Suppl. 2000;205:189–93. https://doi.org/10.1080/00365590050509913.
10. Maden C, Sherman KJ, Beckmann AM, Hislop TG, Teh CZ, Ashley RL, Daling JR. History of circumcision, medical conditions, and sexual activity and risk of penile cancer. J Natl Cancer Inst. 1993;85(1):19–24. https://doi.org/10.1093/jnci/85.1.19.
11. Van Howe RS, Hodges FM. The carcinogenicity of smegma: debunking a myth. J Eur Acad Dermatol Venereol. 2006;20(9):1046–54. https://doi.org/10.1111/j.1468-3083.2006.01653.x.
12. de Bruijn RE, Heideman DAM, Kenter GG, van Beurden M, van Tinteren H, Horenblas S. Patients with penile cancer and the risk of (pre)malignant cervical lesions in female partners: a retrospective cohort analysis. BJU Int. 2013;112(7):905–8. https://doi.org/10.1111/bju.12237.
13. Velazquez EF, Barreto JE, Rodriguez I, Piris A, Cubilla AL. Limitations in the interpretation of biopsies in patients with penile squamous cell carcinoma. Int J Surg Pathol. 2004;12(2):139–46. https://doi.org/10.1177/106689690401200207.
14. Renaud-Vilmer C, Cavelier-Balloy B, Verola O, et al. Analysis of alterations adjacent to invasive squamous cell carcinoma of the penis and their relationship with associated carcinoma. J Am Acad Dermatol. 2010;62(2):284–90. https://doi.org/10.1016/j.jaad.2009.06.087.
15. EAU Guidelines: Penile Cancer | Uroweb. Accessed October 27, 2021. https://uroweb.org/guideline/penile-cancer/
16. Winters BR, Mossanen M, Holt SK, Lin DW, Wright JL. Predictors of Nodal Upstaging in Clinical Node Negative Patients With Penile Carcinoma: A National Cancer Database Analysis. Urology. 2016;96:29–34. Accessed October 27, 2021. https://pubmed.ncbi.nlm.nih.gov/27450944/
17. Afonso LA, Cordeiro TI, Carestiato FN, Ornellas AA, Alves G, Cavalcanti SMB. High risk human papillomavirus infection of the foreskin in asymptomatic men and patients with phimosis. J Urol. 2016;195(6):1784–9. https://doi.org/10.1016/j.juro.2015.12.096.
18. Hanchanale V, Yeo L, Subedi N, et al. The accuracy of magnetic resonance imaging (MRI) in predicting the invasion of the tunica albuginea and the urethra during the primary staging of penile cancer. BJU Int. 2016;117(3):439–43. https://doi.org/10.1111/bju.13041.
19. Bozzini G, Provenzano M, Romero Otero J, Margreiter M, Garcia Cruz E, Osmolorskij B, Verze P, Pavan N, Sanguedolce F, Buffi N, Ferrucio GG, Taverna G. Role of Penile Doppler US in the Preoperative Assessment of Penile Squamous Cell Carcinoma Patients: Results From a Large Prospective Multicenter European Study. Urology. 2016;90:131–5. Accessed October 31, 2021. https://pubmed.ncbi.nlm.nih.gov/26776562/
20. Ornellas AA, Seixas AL, Marota A, Wisnescky A, Campos F, de Moraes JR. Surgical treatment of invasive squamous cell carcinoma of the penis: retrospective analysis of 350 cases. J Urol. 1994;151(5):1244–9. https://doi.org/10.1016/s0022-5347(17)35222-9.
21. Horenblas S, van Tinteren H, Delemarre JF, Moonen LM, Lustig V, van Waardenburg EW. Squamous cell carcinoma of the penis. III. Treatment of regional lymph nodes. J Urol. 1993;149(3):492–7. Accessed October 31, 2021. https://pubmed.ncbi.nlm.nih.gov/8437253/
22. Zhu Y, Zhang SL, Ye DW, Yao XD, Jiang ZX, Zhou XY. Predicting pelvic lymph node metastases in penile cancer patients: a comparison of computed tomography, Cloquet's node, and disease burden of inguinal lymph nodes. Onkologie. 2008;31(1–2):37–41. https://doi.org/10.1159/000112462.

23. Graafland NM, Lam W, Leijte JAP, et al. Prognostic factors for occult inguinal lymph node involvement in penile carcinoma and assessment of the high-risk EAU subgroup: a two-institution analysis of 342 clinically node-negative patients. Eur Urol. 2010;58(5):742–7. https://doi.org/10.1016/j.eururo.2010.08.015.

24. Leijte JA, Kirrander P, Antonini N, Windahl T, Horenblas S. Recurrence patterns of squamous cell carcinoma of the penis: recommendations for follow-up based on a two-centre analysis of 700 patients. Eur Urol. 2008;54(1):161–8. Accessed October 31, 2021. https://pubmed.ncbi.nlm.nih.gov/18440124/

25. Bandieramonte G, Colecchia M, Mariani L, et al. Peniscopically controlled CO2 laser excision for conservative treatment of in situ and T1 penile carcinoma: report on 224 patients. Eur Urol. 2008;54(4):875–82. https://doi.org/10.1016/j.eururo.2008.01.019.

26. Colecchia M, Nicolai N, Secchi P, et al. pT1 penile squamous cell carcinoma: a clinicopathologic study of 56 cases treated by CO2 laser therapy. Anal Quant Cytol Histol. 2009;31(3):153–60.

27. Meijer RP, Boon TA, van Venrooij GEPM, Wijburg CJ. Long-term follow-up after laser therapy for penile carcinoma. Urology. 2007;69(4):759–62. https://doi.org/10.1016/j.urology.2007.01.023.

28. Frimberger D, Hungerhuber E, Zaak D, Waidelich R, Hofstetter A, Schneede P. Penile carcinoma. Is Nd:YAG laser therapy radical enough? J Urol. 2002;168(6):2418–21. Accessed October 31, 2021. https://pubmed.ncbi.nlm.nih.gov/12441930/

29. Piva L, Nicolai N, Di Palo A, Milani A, Merson M, Salvioni R, Stagni S, Vecchio D, Zanoni F, Ferri S, Pizzocaro G. Therapeutic alternatives in the treatment of class T1N0 squamous cell carcinoma of the penis: indications and limitations. Arch Ital Urol Androl. 1996;68(3):157–61. Accessed October 31, 2021. https://pubmed.ncbi.nlm.nih.gov/8767503/

30. Rothenberger KH, Hofstetter A. Laser therapy of penile carcinoma. Urologe A. 1994;33(4):291–4.

31. Shabbir M, Muneer A, Kalsi J, Shukla CJ, Zacharakis E, Garaffa G, Ralph D, Minhas S. Glans resurfacing for the treatment of carcinoma in situ of the penis: surgical technique and outcomes. Eur Urol. 2011;59(1):142–7. Accessed October 31, 2021. https://pubmed.ncbi.nlm.nih.gov/21050658/

32. Philippou P, Shabbir M, Malone P, et al. Conservative surgery for squamous cell carcinoma of the penis: resection margins and long-term oncological control. J Urol. 2012;188(3):803–8. https://doi.org/10.1016/j.juro.2012.05.012.

33. Veeratterapillay R, Teo L, Asterling S, Greene D. Oncologic Outcomes of Penile Cancer Treatment at a UK Supraregional Center. Urology. 2015;85(5):1097–103. Accessed October 31, 2021. https://pubmed.ncbi.nlm.nih.gov/25769781/

34. Hadway P, Corbishley CM, Watkin NA. Total glans resurfacing for premalignant lesions of the penis: initial outcome data. BJU Int. 2006;98(3):532–6. https://doi.org/10.1111/j.1464-410X.2006.06368.x.

35. Guyatt GH, Oxman AD, Kunz R, et al. Going from evidence to recommendations. BMJ. 2008;336(7652):1049–51. https://doi.org/10.1136/bmj.39493.646875.AE.

36. Parnham AS, Albersen M, Sahdev V, et al. Glansectomy and Split-thickness skin graft for penile cancer. Eur Urol. 2018;73(2):284–9. https://doi.org/10.1016/j.eururo.2016.09.048.

37. Crook J, Jezioranski J, Cygler JE. Penile brachytherapy: technical aspects and postimplant issues. Brachytherapy. 2010;9(2):151–8. https://doi.org/10.1016/j.brachy.2009.05.005.

38. de Crevoisier R, Slimane K, Sanfilippo N, et al. Long-term results of brachytherapy for carcinoma of the penis confined to the glans (N- or NX). Int J Radiat Oncol Biol Phys. 2009;74(4):1150–6. https://doi.org/10.1016/j.ijrobp.2008.09.054.

39. Smith Y, Hadway P, Biedrzycki O, Perry MJ, Corbishley C, Watkin NA. Reconstructive surgery for invasive squamous carcinoma of the glans penis. Eur Urol. 2007;52(4):1179–85. Accessed October 31, 2021. https://pubmed.ncbi.nlm.nih.gov/17349734/

40. Azrif M, Logue JP, Swindell R, Cowan RA, Wylie JP, Livsey JE. External-beam radiotherapy in T1-2 N0 penile carcinoma. Clin Oncol (R Coll Radiol). 2006;18(4):320–5. https://doi.org/10.1016/j.clon.2006.01.004.

41. Kieffer JM, Djajadiningrat RS, van Muilekom EA, Graafland NM, Horenblas S, Aaronson NK. Quality of life for patients treated for penile cancer. J Urol. 2014;192(4):1105–10. Accessed October 31, 2021. https://pubmed.ncbi.nlm.nih.gov/24747092/

42. Skeppner E, Windahl T, Andersson SO, Fugl-Meyer KS. Treatment-seeking, aspects of sexual activity and life satisfaction in men with laser-treated penile carcinoma. Eur Urol. 2008;54(3):631–9. Accessed October 31, 2021. https://pubmed.ncbi.nlm.nih.gov/18788122/

43. Austoni E, et al. Reconstructive surgery for penile cancer with preservation of sexual function. Eur Urol Suppl. 2008;7:116. https://www.eusupplements.europeanurology.com/article/S1569-9056(08)60182-7/pdf

44. Ayres B, et al. Glans resurfacing – a new penile preserving option for superficially invasive penile cancer. Eur Urol Suppl. 2011;10:340. http://www.eusupplements.europeanurology.com/article/S1569-9056(11)61084-1/abstract.

45. Sosnowski R, Kulpa M, Kosowicz M, et al. Quality of life in penile carcinoma patients - post-total penectomy. Cent Eur J Urol. 2016;69(2):204–11. https://doi.org/10.5173/ceju.2016.828.

46. Garaffa G, Raheem AA, Christopher NA, Ralph DJ. Total phallic reconstruction after penile amputation for carcinoma. BJU Int. 2009;104(6):852–6. https://doi.org/10.1111/j.1464-410X.2009.08424.x.

47. Gerullis H, Georgas E, Bagner JW, Eimer C, Otto T. Construction of a penoid after penectomy using a transpositioned testicle. Urol Int. 2013;90(2):240–2. https://doi.org/10.1159/000341555.

48. Hage JJ. Simple, safe, and satisfactory secondary penile enhancement after near-total oncologic amputation. Ann Plast Surg. 2009;62(6):685–9. https://doi.org/10.1097/SAP.0b013e3181835ae1.

49. Cancer Today. Accessed October 27, 2021. http://gco.iarc.fr/today/home

50. Park JS, Kim J, Elghiaty A, Ham WS. Recent global trends in testicular cancer incidence and mortality. Medicine (Baltimore). 2018;97(37):e12390. https://doi.org/10.1097/MD.0000000000012390.

51. Oosterhuis JW, Looijenga LHJ. Testicular germ-cell tumours in a broader perspective. Nat Rev Cancer. 2005;5(3):210–22. https://doi.org/10.1038/nrc1568.

52. Lip SZL, Murchison LED, Cullis PS, Govan L, Carachi R. A meta-analysis of the risk of boys with isolated cryptorchidism developing testicular cancer in later life. Arch Dis Child. 2013;98(1):20–6. https://doi.org/10.1136/archdischild-2012-302051.

53. Jørgensen N, Rajpert-De Meyts E, Main KM, Skakkebaek NE. Testicular dysgenesis syndrome comprises some but not all cases of hypospadias and impaired spermatogenesis. Int J Androl. 2010;33(2):298–303. https://doi.org/10.1111/j.1365-2605.2009.01050.x.

54. Looijenga L, Van der Kwast TH, Grignon D, Egevad L, Kristiansen G, Kao CS, Idrees MT. Report from the International Society of Urological Pathology (ISUP) Consultation Conference on Molecular Pathology of Urogenital Cancers: IV: Current and Future Utilization of Molecular-Genetic Tests for Testicular Germ Cell Tumors. Am J Surg Pathol. 2020;44(7):e66–79. Accessed October 27, 2021. https://www.ncbi.nlm.nih.gov/pmc/articles/PMC7289140/

55. Williamson SR, Delahunt B, Magi-Galluzzi C, Algaba F, Egevad L, Ulbright TM, Tickoo SK, Srigley JR, Epstein JI, Berney DM. The World Health Organization 2016 classification of testicular germ cell tumours: a review and update from the International Society of Urological Pathology Testis Consultation Panel. Histopathology. 2017;70(3):335–46. Accessed October 27, 2021. https://pubmed.ncbi.nlm.nih.gov/27747907/

56. EAU Guidelines: Testicular Cancer [Internet]. Uroweb. [citato 1 novembre 2021]. Disponibile su: https://uroweb.org/guideline/testicular-cancer/

57. TNM Classification of Malignant Tumours, 8th Edition | Wiley. Accessed October 27, 2021. https://www.wiley.com/en-ru/TNM+Classification+of+Malignant+Tumours%2C+8th+Edition-p-9781119263579

58. Klepp O, Flodgren P, Maartman-Moe H, Lindholm CE, Unsgaard B, Teigum H, Fosså SD, Paus E. Early clinical stages (CS1, CS1Mk+ and CS2A) of nonseminomatous testis cancer. Value of pre- and postorchiectomy serum tumor marker information in prediction of retroperitoneal lymph node metastases. Swedish-Norwegian Testicular Cancer Project (SWENOTECA). Ann Oncol. 1990;1(4):281–8. Accessed October 27, 2021. https://pubmed.ncbi.nlm.nih.gov/1702312/

59. Germà-Lluch J. Clinical pattern and therapeutic results achieved in 1490 patients with germ-cell Tumours of the testis: the experience of the Spanish germ-cell cancer group (GG). Eur Urol. 2002;42(6):553–63. https://doi.org/10.1016/S0302-2838(02)00439-6.

60. Mieritz MG, Christiansen P, Jensen MB, et al. Gynaecomastia in 786 adult men: clinical and biochemical findings. Eur J Endocrinol. 2017;176(5):555–66. https://doi.org/10.1530/EJE-16-0643.

61. Brydøy M, Fosså SD, Klepp O, et al. Paternity and testicular function among testicular cancer survivors treated with two to four cycles of cisplatin-based chemotherapy. Eur Urol. 2010;58(1):134–41. https://doi.org/10.1016/j.eururo.2010.03.041.

62. Fizazi K, Pagliaro L, Laplanche A, et al. Personalised chemotherapy based on tumour marker decline in poor prognosis germ-cell tumours (GETUG 13): a phase 3, multicentre, randomised trial. Lancet Oncol. 2014;15(13):1442–50. https://doi.org/10.1016/S1470-2045(14)70490-5.

63. Hoei-Hansen CE, Rajpert-De Meyts E, Daugaard G, Skakkebaek NE. Carcinoma in situ testis, the progenitor of testicular germ cell tumours: a clinical review. Ann Oncol. 2005;16(6):863–8. https://doi.org/10.1093/annonc/mdi175.

64. Petersen PM, Giwercman A, Daugaard G, Rørth M, Petersen JH, Skakkeb NE. Effect of Graded Testicular Doses of Radiotherapy in Patients Treated for Carcinoma-In-Situ in the Testis. J Clin Oncol. 2002;20(6):1537–43.

65. Jones WG, Fossa SD, Mead GM, et al. Randomized trial of 30 versus 20 Gy in the adjuvant treatment of stage I testicular seminoma: a report on Medical Research Council trial TE18, European organisation for the research and treatment of cancer trial 30942 (ISRCTN18525328). J Clin Oncol. 2005;23(6):1200–8. https://doi.org/10.1200/JCO.2005.08.003.

66. Böhlen D, Burkhard FC, Mills R, Sonntag RW, Studer UE. Fertility and sexual function following orchiectomy and 2 cycles of chemotherapy for stage I high risk NONSEMINOMATOUS germ cell cancer. J Urol. 2001;165(2):441–4. https://doi.org/10.1097/00005392-200102000-00022.

67. Krege S, Beyer J, Souchon R, et al. European consensus conference on diagnosis and treatment of germ cell cancer: a report of the second meeting of the European germ cell cancer consensus group (EGCCCG): part I. Eur Urol. 2008;53(3):478–96. https://doi.org/10.1016/j.eururo.2007.12.024.

68. Culine S, Kerbrat P, Kramar A, et al. Refining the optimal chemotherapy regimen for good-risk metastatic nonseminomatous germ-cell tumors: a randomized trial of the Genito-urinary Group of the French Federation of cancer centers (GETUG T93BP). Ann Oncol. 2007;18(5):917–24. https://doi.org/10.1093/annonc/mdm062.

69. Giannatempo P, Greco T, Mariani L, et al. Radiotherapy or chemotherapy for clinical stage IIA and IIB seminoma: a systematic review and meta-analysis of

patient outcomes. Ann Oncol. 2015;26(4):657–68. https://doi.org/10.1093/annonc/mdu447.

70. Berthelsen JG, Skakkebaek NE. Gonadal function in men with testis cancer**supported by grants from the Danish Cancer Society and the Danish Medical Research Council. Fertil Steril. 1983;39(1):68–75. https://doi.org/10.1016/S0015-0282(16)46760-9.

71. Rives N, Perdrix A, Hennebicq S, et al. The semen quality of 1158 men with testicular cancer at the time of cryopreservation: results of the French national CECOS network. J Androl. 2012;33(6):1394–401. https://doi.org/10.2164/jandrol.112.016592.

72. Hansen PV, Hansen SW. Gonadal function in men with testicular germ cell cancer:the influence of cisplatin-based chemotherapy. Eur Urol. 1993;23(1):153–6. https://doi.org/10.1159/000474585.

73. Fritz K, Weissbach L. Sperm parameters and ejaculation before and after operative treatment of patients with germ-cell testicular cancer. Fertil Steril. 1985;43(3):451–4. https://doi.org/10.1016/S0015-0282(16)48448-7.

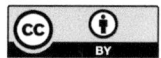

Male Reproduction: From Pathophysiology to Clinical Assessment

12

Giuseppe Grande and Carlo Foresta

Couple infertility, defined as the lack of conception after at least 12 months of regular unprotected sexual intercourse aimed at pregnancy [1], is a common clinical condition.

It is a multifactorial disorder affecting one out of six couples in Western countries, and male factor infertility is implicated in about 50% of cases [2].

Male infertility may depend by pre-testicular (for example, hypothalamic or pituitary diseases), testicular, and post-testicular (for example, obstructive pathologies of seminal ducts) causes.

The pathophysiology and the clinical assessment, including treatment strategies, of these situations will be discussed in the next chapters of this book.

However, a large proportion (30–60%) of infertile males does not receive a clear diagnosis. In these cases, generally reported as idiopathic infertility, there is a strong suspicion of genetic factors yet to be discovered, and research in this field will probably reduce the proportion of unexplained infertility in the next years [3].

Furthermore, male fertility may be influenced by a host of lifestyle risk factors such as environ-

ment, nutrition, exposure to infections, and smoking. Therefore, lifestyle and environment risk factors may have a role in many cases of idiopathic male infertility.

In this chapter, we will focus our attention on these risk factors, discussing three paradigmatic situations of interference between environment/lifestyle and male fertility, thus providing the pathophysiological basis of their detrimental impact on male fertility: exposure to environmental endocrine disruptors, such as perfluoroalkyl substances (PFAS); exposure to viruses, such as HPV; effect of nutritional status and obesity.

12.1 PFAS Pollution and Male Fertility

PFAS are a class of organic molecules characterized by fluorinated hydrocarbon chains, widely used in industry and consumer products including oil and water repellents, coatings for cookware, carpets, and textiles. PFAS have unique physical chemical properties due to their amphiphilic structures and their strong carbon–fluorine bonds. Consequently, long-chain PFAS are non-biodegradable and bioaccumulate in the environment [4]. PFAS have been found in humans and in the global environment and their toxicity, environmental fate, and sources of human exposure have been a major subject of research. PFAS have

G. Grande · C. Foresta (✉)
Unit of Andrology and Reproductive Medicine & Centre for Male Gamete Cryopreservation, Department of Medicine, University of Padova, Padova, Italy
e-mail: carlo.foresta@unipd.it

© The Author(s) 2023
C. Bettocchi et al. (eds.), *Practical Clinical Andrology*,
https://doi.org/10.1007/978-3-031-11701-5_12

risen many concerns for their bioaccumulation in body tissues and potential harmful effects in humans [4]. In fact, inhalation of air particles and/or ingestion of contaminated food products and drinking water have been claimed as major routes of exposure to PFAS. Accordingly, PFAS have been found in several human tissues, such as the brain, placenta, semen, and testis even in the presence of acknowledged blood/tissue barriers [5, 6]. Exposure to PFAS has been widely described in several countries, with considerable differences in terms of geographical distribution, ethnicity, molecular weight (long-chain or short-chain PFAS), and degree of fluorination [7–9]. On this matter, perfluorooctanoic acid (PFOA) and perfluorooctanesulfonic acid (PFOS) are the most common and most studied PFAS in toxicological terms.

Epidemiological studies have focused not only on their impact on foetal development, but also on the relationship between PFAS and human fertility, although studies have been focused mostly on female fertility. However, both in vitro and animal studies on PFAS toxicity have shown a negative effect of PFOA and PFOS on testicular function, by the alteration of steroidogenic machinery and subsequent defect of spermatogenesis [10, 11].

Exposure to high levels of PFOS, and of PFOA and PFOS combined, are associated with a reduction in the concentration of morphologically normal spermatozoa in adult men [12, 13]. Furthermore, Raymer et al. reported, in a study of men attending an in-vitro fertilization clinic, that luteinizing hormone (LH) and free testosterone were significantly positively correlated with plasma PFOA [14]. Although conclusive data have not still provided, preliminary data seem to suggest moreover an increased sperm DNA fragmentation in exposed men [15, 16].

Among the endocrine effects of PFOS, it should be underlined that it affects the hypothalamic–pituitary axis activity [17, 18]. A testicular toxicity of PFOS has been demonstrated in rats [18]. High doses of PFOS orally administered in rats for 28 days modify the relative gene and protein receptor expressions of several hormones of the hypothalamus-pituitary-testicular axis (GnRH, LH, FSH, and testosterone) [19].

In humans, in utero exposure to PFOA was associated later in adult life with lower sperm concentration and total sperm count and with higher levels of luteinizing hormone and follicle-stimulating hormone [20]. In infertile male patients, PFOS levels were higher than fertile subjects. Furthermore, in these patients, a higher gene expression of estrogen receptor (ER) α, Erβ, and androgen receptor (AR) has been reported [21, 22], thus suggesting that PFAS activity might be linked also to the genetic expression of sex hormones nuclear receptors.

Regarding androgen receptor (AR), PFOS and PFOA cause a reduction in its protein expression in hypothalamus, pituitary gland, and testis. This inhibition might reflect PFOS action on post-transcriptional processes of the AR synthesis. AR-dependent gene expression is indeed crucial for male sexual differentiation in utero and male reproductive function and development in adults, including spermatogenesis [23].

Three compounds (PFHxS, PFOS, and PFOA) act as ER agonists in vitro, and five PFAS (PFHxS, PFOS, PFOA, PFNA, and PFDA) act as AR antagonists. Their combined action, as observed in PFCs mixture, induces a synergistic impact on AR function [24]. These findings clearly suggest an antiandrogenic potential of PFAS.

In a recent study, we investigated the possible association between the exposure to PFOA and PFOS and endocrine disruption through the evaluation of developmental alterations and reproductive disorders in a group of 212 young males from the Veneto region, a wide area in the northeast of Italy featured by high environmental exposure to these chemicals [11]. Compared to 171 age-matched controls residing outside of the exposed area, subjects from the contaminated area showed increased levels of circulating testosterone (T) and LH, pointing toward an antagonistic action of PFOA on the binding of T to its natural AR.

Interestingly, most of the exposed male population showed a reduction in testicular volume, penile length, and anogenital distance but not anthropometric measures. These findings could be explained by considering that anogenital distance and anthropometric measures are differentially determined during fetal and prepubertal development, respectively [25]. Pre-natal exposure to androgens during the "masculinization programming window," a critical window during testicular development, is positively associated with anogenital distance in mammals [26]. On these bases, anogenital distance has been suggested as a putative marker of prenatal exposure to chemicals with a known antiandrogenic effect, or endocrine disruptors in general. As the first report on water contamination of PFAS goes back to 1977 [27], the dimension of the problem is alarming as it affects entire generations of individuals, from 1978 onward.

It has been moreover demonstrated that PFOS has the ability to cross the blood brain barrier [28] and the placenta [29], although the exact mechanism has not been yet clarified. In the same way, PFOS may disrupt the Sertoli cell tight junction-permeability barrier, which ultimately might induce a dysfunction in blood-testis barrier, associated with infertility [30].

In semen of exposed subjects PFOA is more represented than PFOS, despite the pattern of serum concentrations is essentially reversed. In detail, average PFOA levels retrieved in semen samples from exposed subjects were 0.67 ng/mL, ranging from 0 to nearly 6 ng/mL [11]. Furthermore, seminal PFOA levels correlate with seminal pH, thus suggesting a putative interference of PFOA at a prostatic level [11]. The presence of PFAS in seminal plasma suggests either a possible involvement of prostate, that might explain a weak association between PFOS exposure and prostate cancer [31].

Moreover, semen levels of PFOA are significantly correlated with the presence of altered sperm parameters, and namely of motility. This evidence is suggestive of a direct effect of PFOA on gamete function. More recently, we have demonstrated that incubation of sperm cells with PFOA is associated with negative effects on sperm viability, independently from the exposure time and concentration [32]. Progressive motility is significantly impaired by PFOA exposure even at the lowest concentration of 0.1 ng/mL, as reported in Fig. 12.1.

The direct influence of PFOA on sperm motility is related to the impaired metabolic performance associated with a decreased mitochondrial respiratory activity.

Furthermore, it has been demonstrated that PFOA accumulates in sperm membrane, thus dis-

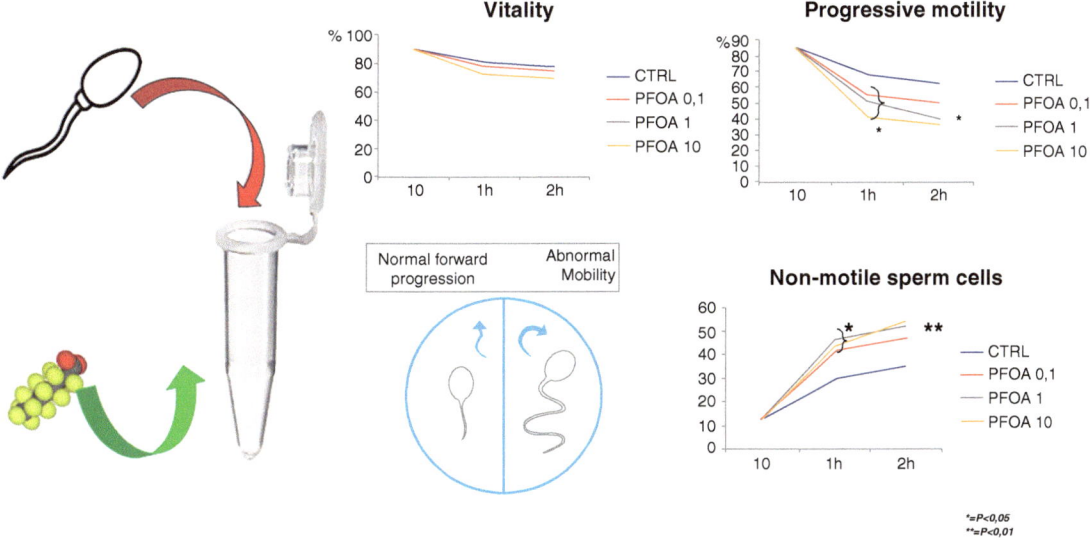

Fig. 12.1 Incubation of sperm cells with PFOA reduces sperm vitality and progressive motility and increases the percentage of non-motile cells

rupting membrane fluidity. Membrane fluidity, acknowledged as a major determinant of sperm motility and fertilization potential, is associated with decreased packing order of phospholipids in the outer layer of the plasma membrane. Plasma membrane is a key organelle, with a pivotal role in sperm physiology and the fine modulation of its composition, from ejaculation to fecundation, has critically effect on the overall efficacy of the fertilization process [33]. During the transit of sperm cell through the female reproductive tract, there is an increase in membrane fluidity, due to cholesterol deprivation by sterols acceptors like albumin of HDL, which is associated with the gain of progressive motility and fusogenic properties [34, 35]. Because of its high hydrophobicity, PFOA might randomly accumulate in sperm membranes, thus altering local pH and permeability to ionic species and, in turn, membrane potential as recently observed also in somatic cell models [36]. Accordingly this model, the local perturbation of membrane composition, may also induce in the production of free radicals, as recently demonstrated for other chemical species such as graphene-oxide [37], possibly explaining the association between PFAS exposure and sperm-DNA damage.

Finally, it can be hypothesized that sperm cells may be exposed to PFAS not only in seminal plasma of exposed males but also in genital secretion of exposed females. It has been in fact demonstrated that cervical mucus from women resident in highly exposed areas have higher levels of PFOA in cervical mucus, compared to control sub-jects [29].

Taken together, these data underline the multi-faced role of pollutants, such as PFAS, in male infertility. PFAS exposure acts at different levels impairing the reproductive system: through a modulation of AR expression, both in utero and after the birth; through the alteration of the Sertoli cell tight junction-permeability barrier, which ultimately changes destabilized Sertoli cell BTB integrity; directly altering sperm cell function, causing an impairment of sperm motility, likely relied on the alteration of plasma-membrane potential due to a disruption of membrane fluidity; inducing and increase in sperm DNA frag-

mentation, which might be due to increased ROS levels; and finally by a putative impairment of prostate function.

12.2 HPV Infection and Male Infertility

A large spectrum of viruses may infect the testis and other male genital organs, thereby impairing male fertility [38]. Human Papillomavirus (HPV) is the etiological agent of the most common sexually transmitted infection worldwide, with an estimated 6.2 million new cases annually [39]. HPV comprises a group of small non-enveloped epitheliotropic viruses with a double-stranded circular DNA genome made- up of 8000 bp. Its virion has an icosahedral shape, of 55 nm diameter, constructed of 52 capsomeres, each containing five molecules of the major capsid protein L1 and a smaller number of the minor capsid protein L2 [40]. HPV consists of more than 200 genotypes, adapted to specific epithelial tissues, such as anogenital skin and mucosa [41]. According to the basis of oncogenic potential, HPV can be divided into two different groups: high-risk (HR-HPV) and low-risk (LR-HPV). The former ones, that include the well-known 16 and 18 types, have been classified as oncogenic to humans according to the International Agency for Research on Cancer [42], and may cause neoplastic transformations in the following epithelial areas: cervix, vagina, vulva, anus, penis, and oropharynx [43]. The latter ones, such as 6 and 11 types, are responsible of benign diseases such as genital warts [44]. HPV infections are primarily contracted by direct contact of the skin or mycoses with an infected lesion. Genital HPV infection is largely transmitted through sexual intercourse, mostly insertive intercourses, although non-penetrative types of contact (i.e., genital-genital, oral-genital, and manual-genital) represent possible routes of transmission [45].

Recently, it has been clearly confirmed that, in addition to the well-known external genital areas, HPV virions may also be detected inside the male reproductive tract. In detail, it has been detected in male accessory glands, where it can represent a possible cause of male accessory gland infection [46]. This localization in accessory gland is reflected in changes in seminal parameters such as an increase of pH and viscosity and a reduction of seminal volume [47, 48].

Finally, HPV was found in semen, both in exfoliated cells and even bound to spermatozoa [49] as reported in Fig. 12.2.

Several studies have underlined the possible role of HPV in causing male infertility [50]. In fact, several authors have confirmed the presence of the virus in the seminal fluid of men suffering from idiopathic infertility [47, 51]. These data, combined with the higher prevalence of sperm HPV-infection in infertile subjects compared to general population [52], suggested a role for HPV as a cause of sperm damage and, consequently, of male infertility.

Several studies reported that HPV infection is related with a reduction in seminal parameters. Five studies reported a relation between HPV seminal infection and a reduction in sperm motility [49, 53–56]. Moreover, Piroozmand showed also a significant reduction of the sperm count [53]. An increased sperm DNA fragmentation index has been moreover reported by Boeri et al.

when semen infections involved high-risk HPV genotypes [57] while Yang et al. demonstrated that HPV seminal infection is associated with a reduction in sperm normal morphology [58].

More recently, Moghimi et al., observed a significantly higher prevalence of high-risk HPV in infertile men, compared to fertiles, associated with an impairment of sperm morphology and motility [59].

HPV infection in semen represents moreover a risk factor for the development of anti-sperm antibodies (ASAs). In fact, the prevalence of ASAs is higher in infected infertile patients compared to non-infected infertiles and general population. Moreover, in infected infertile subjects, presence of antibodies is associated with a further reduction of sperm motility [60]. In detail, more than 40% of HPV infected infertile patients had ASAs on the sperm surface. Moreover, infected patients had a higher mean percentage of ASAs compared with non-infected ones [55]. These findings suggested that sperm autoimmunity could probably be HPV-dependent. In order to confirm this finding, Garolla et al. documented the presence of both viral proteins and immunoglobulins in the same sperm cells of samples with positive sperm-mixed antiglobulin

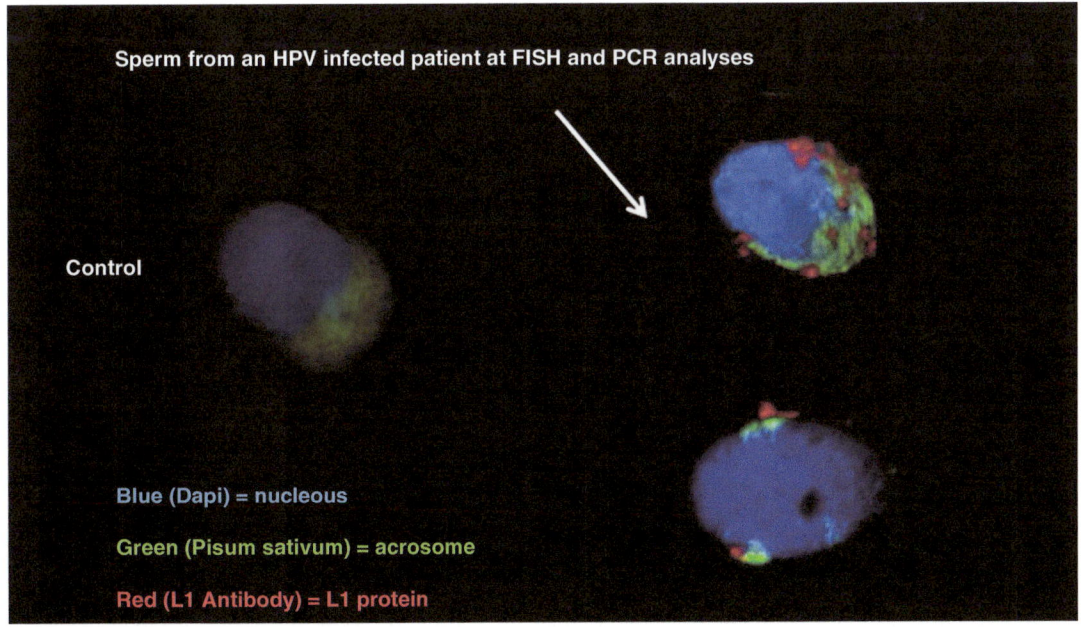

Fig. 12.2 Immunofluorescence for HPV L1 capsid protein (red) in sperm cells

reaction (Mar) test results. Notably, when immuno-fluorescence for HPV 16-L1 was present on the sperm surface, they observed co-staining for IgA and IgG. This observation suggests that semen infection represents a new clinical condition associated with the presence of ASAs. In infected males, a significant viral clearance (approximately 85.3%) is obtained after 24 months of follow-up and the reduction in sperm infection paralleled the disappearance of ASAs and with the progressive improvement of sperm motility [55].

Several studies have analyzed the effect of semen HPV infection, in terms of reduction of fertility both in natural [61] and in assisted reproduction [61–64]. An increase in miscarriage rate has been moreover reported by Garolla et al. [61].

To understand the pathophysiological role of HPV in fertilization, we performed an in vitro study evaluating the ability of the virus-infected sperm to transfer HPV DNA and capsid proteins to oocyte during fertilization. After transfecting a human sperm with a plasmidic episome containing HPV E6 and E7 proteins, the hamster egg-human sperm penetration test has been performed to show the ability of infected sperm to transfer the capsid protein L1 to oocyte and the expression of E6 and E7 viral protein in the fertilized oocyte [65]. We may therefore conclude that both spermatozoa transfected with E6 and E7 genes and exposed to HPV L1 capsid protein are able to penetrate the oocyte. These laboratory data, combined with the observation that HPV DNA is found in a larger proportion of abortions rather than voluntary termination of pregnancy [62], may suggest an active role for HPV (which is carried to the egg by the spermatozoa) in the etiology of premature term gestation. This phenomenon could lead to an increase in the fragmentation of embryonic DNA, thus resulting in alteration and apoptosis of the embryo [65].

On the basis of these evidences, we recommend testing for HPV in the male partner of the infertile couples in the following cases: male affected by unexplained couple infertility (not related to known male or female factors), asthenozoospermia, presence of ASA, positive medical history for HPV infection or evidence of ongoing HPV-related diseases [50].

When HPV is detected in at least one of the members of an infertile couple, it is important to provide careful counselling. A 2014 controlled study showed the effectiveness of this strategy. Couples in which both partners had HPV infection at genital site were carefully counselled to follow some strict advices aimed to clear the virus (such as hygiene of both of their reproductive tract and their hand; using personal underwear and personal towels only; avoiding oral and anal sex) and monitored at 6, 12, 18, and 24 months. Counselled couples had a significantly higher clearance rate and shorter time of viral persistence, compared to non-counselled infected controls [66].

Recent evidence has moreover suggested that HPV vaccination is a valid tool even in patients who have already contracted the infection. In fact, it has been demonstrated that HPV infected patients receiving vaccination have a faster rate of seroconversion and greater viral clearance compared to infected patients who did not receive vaccination [67]. In detail, vaccinated patients showed a higher viral clearance that paralleled an improvement of sperm motility and a reduction in the percentage of anti-sperm antibodies. Furthermore, couples where the male partner received vaccination recorded higher pregnancy and delivery rates and a lower miscarriage rate [68].

In addition to counselling and adjuvant vaccination, different techniques of sperm selection (centrifugation, discontinuous density gradient, and direct Swim-up) have been tested aimed to remove HPV from the sperm surface. However, all techniques had very poor or even absent effect in the complete removal of the virus. Very recently, our group tested a modified swim-up technique with the addiction of hyaluronidase enzyme obtaining the complete elimination of HPV from infected samples [69]. The rationale of this treatment was to cleave the binding of HPV to its putative ligand, Syndecan-I, located on the sperm surface. Compared to normal swim-up technique, the modified swim-up with hyaluronidase was able to abolish the binding between HPV and sperm in 100% cases of infected sperm, confirmed by negative fluorescent in-situ hybridization

(FISH) for HPV, without any significant impairment of either motility or DNA fragmentation in the spermatozoa.

12.3 Obesity and Male Infertility

Obesity is defined as an abnormal or excessive accumulation of fat. According to the World Health Organization (WHO), a body mass index (BMI) that is greater than or equal to 25 kg/m^2 is classified as overweight, a BMI greater than 30 kg/m^2 is considered obesity, and a BMI greater than 40 kg/m^2 is considered severe obesity [70].

The worldwide prevalence of obesity has risen dramatically in the last decades, so that 1.9 billion adults worldwide are overweight and around 650 million have obesity [71].

Couples with an obese male partner have a significantly higher risk of infertility than couples with normal-weight male partners [72]. Moreover, male obesity negatively affects the success of assisted reproductive technology (ART) [72]. Mushtaq et al. reported in 2018 that male obesity is associated with a significant reduction in pregnancy and live birth rates in intracytoplasmic sperm injection cycles [73].

Previous population-based studies reported a reduction of semen parameters in overweight and obese men [72, 74, 75]. Further studies demonstrated the association between obesity and asthenozoospermia or teratozoospermia [76]. A systematic review and meta-analysis performed by Sermondade et al. in 2013 reported the association between obesity and azoospermia/oligozoospermia [77].

Several mechanisms have been hypothesized to explain obesity-induced sperm dam- age [78].

A pivotal role is played by heat-induced damage. Testicular thermal stress increases in obese men and is mainly due to fat accumulation in the suprapubic region and around the pampiniform plexus. Spermatogenesis is a temperature-dependent process, and an increase in scrotal temperature can disrupt its progression. In detail, obese men have both right and left scrotal temperatures that are significantly higher than control subjects. Healthy controls had a mean scrotal temperature of 34.738 °C, about two degrees below core body temperature. Moreover, in these subjects, fluctuations of scrotal temperature were characterized by a pattern similar to a circadian rhythm, with high fluctuations between day and night, between daily activities, and between different body postures. In contrast, obese men showed continuously increased mean scrotal temperatures (35.388 °C), with temperature fluctuations reduced in number and amplitude, and circadian patterns less evident or even absent, as reported in Fig. 12.3.

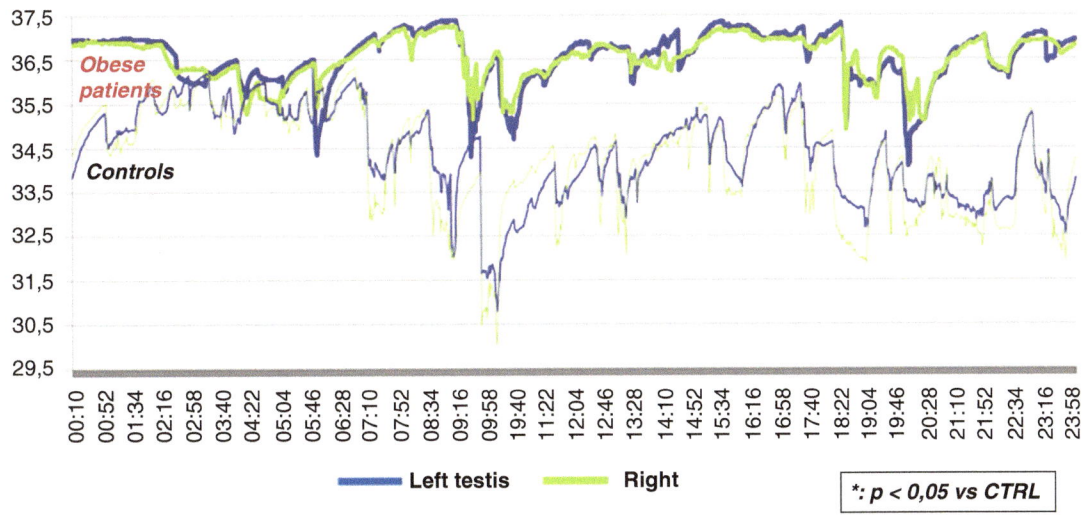

Fig. 12.3 Scrotal temperature in obese subjects and controls

These data underline that in obese men, the spermatogenic alteration is primarily related to hyperthermia due to the excess of adipose tissue [79].

Furthermore, several hormonal alterations have been described and contribute to impairing spermatogenesis in obese patients.

Most obese males have impaired reproductive hormonal profiles compared to normal-weight men. The excessive visceral fat decreases the serum sex hormone-binding globulin (SHBG), total and free T, and inhibin B levels and increases the conversion of T into 17ß-estradiol due to greater aromatase activity [80].

We have recently demonstrated in explants of subcutaneous adipose tissue (SAT) from obese males the presence of higher levels of intracellular T and E2, compared with lean subjects. In addition, after adrenergic stimulation, T release is reduced in obese SAT. Testosterone accumulation resulted in even lower expression in androgen-responsive genes, further contributing to adipose tissue dysfunction and to systemic hypogonadism, as evidenced by higher estrogens determined by increased aromatase expression in obese SAT [81]. Aromatase activity indeed increases with the body fat mass and further increases fat accumulation, creating a vicious cycle [82]. In obese male patients, the higher aromatase activity leads to a decreased T/E2 ratio [83].

Furthermore, obesity is associated with higher serum SHBG, so furtherly reducing free testosterone levels [84]. In addition, the associated hyperinsulinemia has a direct inhibitory effect on spermatogenesis, increasing nuclear and mitochondrial DNA damage [85].

12.4   Conclusions

In conclusion, exposure to environmental risk factors, such as pollutants or infections, or adverse lifestyle, i.e., causing obesity, may interfere at different levels with male fertility, and might play a major role in situations of idiopathic infertility. We have provided three examples, describing their role as a cause of male infertility,

from pathophysiology to clinical assessment. As a consequence, their role should be considered in the clinical workflow of male infertility.

References

1. Zegers-Hochschild F, Adamson GD, Dyer S, Racowsky C, de Mouzon J, Sokol R, et al. The international glossary on infertility and fertility care, 2017. Fertil Steril. 2017;108(3):393–406. Available from: https://pubmed.ncbi.nlm.nih.gov/28760517/
2. de Kretser DM. Male infertility. Lancet. 1997;349(9054):787–90. Available from: https://pubmed.ncbi.nlm.nih.gov/9074589/
3. Rocca MS, Msaki A, Ghezzi M, Cosci I, Pilichou K, Celeghin R, et al. Development of a novel next-generation sequencing panel for diagnosis of quantitative spermatogenic impairment. J Assist Reprod Genet. 2020;37(4):753. Available from: /pmc/articles/PMC7183017/
4. Steenland K, Fletcher T, Savitz DA, et al. Environ Health Perspect. 2010;118(8):1100–8. Available from: https://ehp.niehs.nih.gov/doi/abs/10.1289/ehp.0901827
5. Li N, Mruk DD, Chen H, Wong CKC, Lee WM, Cheng CY. Rescue of perfluorooctanesulfonate (PFOS)-mediated Sertoli cell injury by overexpression of gap junction protein connexin 43. Sci Rep. 2016;6(1):1–14. Available from: https://www.nature.com/articles/srep29667
6. Inoue K, Okada F, Ito R, Kato S, Sasaki S, Nakajima S, et al. Perfluorooctane sulfonate (PFOS) and related perfluorinated compounds in human maternal and cord blood samples: Assessment of PFOS exposure in a susceptible population during pregnancy. Environ Health Perspect. 2004;112(11):1204–7.
7. Fromme H, Tittlemier SA, Völkel W, Wilhelm M, Twardella D. Perfluorinated compounds – exposure assessment for the general population in western countries. Int J Hyg Environ Health. 2009;212(3):239–70.
8. Alexander J, Atli Auðunsson G, Benford D, Cockburn A, Cravedi J-P, Dogliotti E, et al. Perfluorooctane sulfonate (PFOS), perfluorooctanoic acid (PFOA) and their salts Scientific Opinion of the Panel on Contaminants in the Food chain. EFSA J. 2008;6(7):653. Available from: https://onlinelibrary.wiley.com/doi/full/10.2903/j.efsa.2008.653
9. Calafat AM, Wong LY, Kuklenyik Z, Reidy JA, Needham LL. Polyfluoroalkyl chemicals in the U.S. population: Data from the national health and nutrition examination survey (NHANES) 2003-2004 and comparisons with NHANES 1999-2000. Environ Health Perspect. 2007;115(11):1596–602. Available from: http://www.ehponline.org/docs/
10. Foresta C, Tescari S, di Nisio A. Impact of perfluorochemicals on human health and reproduction: a male's perspective. J Endocrinol Invest. 2017;41(6):639–

45. Available from: https://link.springer.com/article/10.1007/s40618-017-0790-z

11. di Nisio A, Sabovic I, Valente U, Tescari S, Rocca MS, Guidolin D, et al. Endocrine disruption of androgenic activity by perfluoroalkyl substances: clinical and experimental evidence. J Clin Endocrinol Metab. 2019;104(4):1259–71. Available from: https://academic.oup.com/jcem/article/104/4/1259/5158211

12. Toft G, Jönsson BAG, Lindh CH, Giwercman A, Spano M, Heederik D, et al. Exposure to perfluorinated compounds and human semen quality in arctic and European populations. Hum Reprod. 2012;27(8):2532–40. Available from: https://academic.oup.com/humrep/article/27/8/2532/711152

13. Joensen UN, Bossi R, Leffers H, Jensen AA, Skakkebæk NE, Jørgensen N. Do Perfluoroalkyl compounds impair human semen quality? Environ Health Perspect. 2009;117(6):923–7.

14. Raymer JH, Michael LC, Studabaker WB, Olsen GW, Sloan CS, Wilcosky T, et al. Concentrations of perfluorooctane sulfonate (PFOS) and perfluorooctanoate (PFOA) and their associations with human semen quality measurements. Reprod Toxicol. 2012;33(4):419–27.

15. Specht IO, Hougaard KS, Spanò M, Bizzaro D, Manicardi GC, Lindh CH, et al. Sperm DNA integrity in relation to exposure to environmental perfluoroalkyl substances – a study of spouses of pregnant women in three geographical regions. Reprod Toxicol. 2012;33(4):577–83.

16. Louis GMB, Chen Z, Schisterman EF, Kim S, Sweeney AM, Sundaram R, et al. Perfluorochemicals and human semen quality: the LIFE study. Environ Health Perspect. 2015;123(1):57–63. https://doi.org/10.1289/ehp.1307621.

17. Pereiro N, Moyano R, Blanco A, Lafuente A. Regulation of corticosterone secretion is modified by PFOS exposure at different levels of the hypothalamic–pituitary–adrenal axis in adult male rats. Toxicol Lett. 2014;230(2):252–62.

18. López-Doval S, Salgado R, Pereiro N, Moyano R, Lafuente A. Perfluorooctane sulfonate effects on the reproductive axis in adult male rats. Environ Res. 2014;134:158–68.

19. López-Doval S, Salgado R, Lafuente A. The expression of several reproductive hormone receptors can be modified by perfluorooctane sulfonate (PFOS) in adult male rats. Chemosphere. 2016;155:488–97.

20. Vested A, Ramlau-Hansen CH, Olsen SF, Bonde JP, Kristensen SL, Halldorsson TI, et al. Associations of in Utero exposure to perfluorinated alkyl acids with human semen quality and reproductive hormones in adult men. Environ Health Perspect. 2013;121(4):453–8. https://doi.org/10.1289/ehp.1205118.

21. la Rocca C, Tait S, Guerranti C, Busani L, Ciardo F, Bergamasco B, et al. Exposure to endocrine disruptors and nuclear receptors gene expression in infertile and fertile men from italian areas with different environmental features. Int J Environ Res Public Health.

2015;12:12426–45. Available from: https://www.mdpi.com/1660-4601/12/10/12426/htm

22. la Rocca C, Alessi E, Bergamasco B, Caserta D, Ciardo F, Fanello E, et al. Exposure and effective dose biomarkers for perfluorooctane sulfonic acid (PFOS) and perfluorooctanoic acid (PFOA) in infertile subjects: preliminary results of the PREVIENI project. Int J Hyg Environ Health. 2012;215(2):206–11.

23. Gao W, Bohl CE, Dalton JT. Chemistry and structural biology of androgen receptor. Chem Rev. 2005;105(9):3352–70. Available from: https://pubs.acs.org/doi/abs/10.1021/cr020456u

24. Kjeldsen LS, Bonefeld-Jørgensen EC. Perfluorinated compounds affect the function of sex hormone receptors. Environ Sci Pollut Res Int. 2013;20(11):8031–44. Available from: https://link.springer.com/article/10.1007/s11356-013-1753-3

25. Petak SM, Nankin HR, Spark RF, Swerdloff RS, Rodriguez-Rigau LJ, American Association of Clinical Endocrinologists. American Association of Clinical Endocrinologists Medical Guidelines for clinical practice for the evaluation and treatment of hypogonadism in adult male patients--2002 update. Endocr Pract. 2020;8(6):440–56. Available from: https://pubmed.ncbi.nlm.nih.gov/15260010/

26. Mitchell RT, Mungall W, McKinnell C, Sharpe RM, Cruickshanks L, Milne L, et al. Anogenital distance plasticity in adulthood: implications for its use as a biomarker of fetal androgen action. Endocrinology. 2015;156(1):24–31. Available from: https://pubmed.ncbi.nlm.nih.gov/25375036/

27. ARPAV (The Regional Agency of Environmental Protection of Veneto Region). Stato dell'inquinamento da sostanze perfluoroalchilice (PFAS) in provincial di Vicenza, Padova, Verona [in Italian]. 2013. http://www.arpa.veneto.it/temi-ambientali/acqua/file-e-allegati/documenti/acque-interne/pfas/Nota Tecnica PFAS.pdf.

28. Austin ME, Kasturi BS, Barber M, Kannan K, MohanKumar PS, SMJ MK. Neuroendocrine effects of perfluorooctane sulfonate in rats. Environ Health Perspect. 2003;111(12):1485–9. Available from: https://pubmed.ncbi.nlm.nih.gov/12948888/

29. Kim S, Choi K, Ji K, Seo J, Kho Y, Park J, et al. Trans-placental transfer of thirteen perfluorinated compounds and relations with fetal thyroid hormones. Environ Sci Technol. 2011;45(17):7465–72. Available from: https://pubs.acs.org/doi/abs/10.1021/es202408a

30. Li N, Mruk DD, Chen H, Wong CKC, Lee WM, Cheng CY. Rescue of perfluorooctanesulfonate (PFOS)-mediated Sertoli cell injury by overexpression of gap junction protein connexin 43. Sci Rep. 2016;6:29667. Available from: https://pubmed.ncbi.nlm.nih.gov/27436542/

31. Eriksen KT, Sørensen M, McLaughlin JK, Lipworth L, Tjønneland A, Overvad K, et al. Perfluorooctanoate and perfluorooctanesulfonate plasma levels and risk of cancer in the general Danish population. J Natl

Cancer Inst. 2009;101(8):605–9. Available from: https://pubmed.ncbi.nlm.nih.gov/19351918/

32. Šabović I, Cosci I, de Toni L, Ferramosca A, Stornaiuolo M, di Nisio A, et al. Perfluoro-octanoic acid impairs sperm motility through the alteration of plasma membrane. J Endocrinol Invest. 2020;43(5):641–52. Available from: https://pubmed.ncbi.nlm.nih.gov/31776969/

33. Flesch FM, Gadella BM. Dynamics of the mammalian sperm plasma membrane in the process of fertilization. Biochim Biophys Acta. 2000;1469(3):197–235.

34. Toshimori K. Maturation of mammalian spermatozoa: modifications of the acrosome and plasma membrane leading to fertilization. Cell Tissue Res. 1998;293(2):177–87. Available from: https://link.springer.com/article/10.1007/s004410051110

35. Haidl G, Opper C. Changes in lipids and membrane anisotropy in human spermatozoa during epididymal maturation. Hum Reprod. 1997;12(12):2720–3. Available from: https://academic.oup.com/humrep/article/12/12/2720/660460

36. Kleszczyński K, Składanowski AC. Mechanism of cytotoxic action of perfluorinated acids.: I. alteration in plasma membrane potential and intracellular pH level. Toxicol Appl Pharmacol. 2009;234(3):300–5.

37. Arbo MD, Altknecht LF, Cattani S, Braga W, Peruzzi CP, Cestonaro L, et al. In vitro cardiotoxicity evaluation of graphene oxide. Mutat Res Genet Toxicol Environ Mutagen. 2019;1(841):8–13.

38. Dejucq N, Jégou B. Viruses in the mammalian male genital tract and their effects on the reproductive system. Microbiol Mol Biol Rev. 2001;65(2):208–31. Available from: https://journals.asm.org/doi/abs/10.1128/MMBR.65.2.208-231.2001

39. Dunne EF, Nielson CM, Stone KM, Markowitz LE, Giuliano AR. Prevalence of HPV infection among men: A systematic review of the literature. J Infect Dis. 2006;194(8):1044–57. Available from: https://pubmed.ncbi.nlm.nih.gov/16991079/

40. Doorbar J, Quint W, Banks L, Bravo IG, Stoler M, Broker TR, et al. The biology and life-cycle of human papillomaviruses. Vaccine. 2012;30(Suppl 5):F55-70. Available from: https://pubmed.ncbi.nlm.nih.gov/23199966/

41. Bouvard V, Baan R, Straif K, Grosse Y, Secretan B, el Ghissassi F, et al. A review of human carcinogens--Part B: biological agents. Lancet Oncol. 2009;10(4):321–2. Available from: https://pubmed.ncbi.nlm.nih.gov/19350698/

42. IARC Working Group on the Evaluation of Carcinogenic Risks to Humans. Human papillomaviruses. IARC Monogr Eval Carcinog Risks Hum. 2007;90:1–636. Available from: https://pubmed.ncbi.nlm.nih.gov/18354839/

43. Cubie HA. Diseases associated with human papillomavirus infection. Virology. 2013;445(1–2):21–34. Available from: https://pubmed.ncbi.nlm.nih.gov/23932731/

44. de Sanjosé S, Brotons M, Pavón MA. The natural history of human papillomavirus infection. Best Pract Res Clin Obstet Gynaecol. 2018;47:2–13.

45. Dunne EF, Park IU. HPV and HPV-associated diseases. Infect Dis Clin North Am. 2013;27(4):765–78. Available from: https://pubmed.ncbi.nlm.nih.gov/24275269/

46. la Vignera S, Vicari E, Condorelli RA, Franchina C, Scalia G, Morgia G, et al. Prevalence of human papilloma virus infection in patients with male accessory gland infection. Reprod Biomed Online. 2015;30(4):385–91. Available from: https://pubmed.ncbi.nlm.nih.gov/25684094/

47. MAM R, Grénman SE, Pöllänen PP, JJO S, Syrjänen SM. Detection of high-risk HPV DNA in semen and its association with the quality of semen. Int J STD AIDS. 2004;15(11):740–3. Available from: https://journals.sagepub.com/doi/10.1258/0956462042395122

48. Damke E, Kurscheidt FA, Balani VA, Takeda KI, Irie MMT, Gimenes F, et al. Male partners of infertile couples with seminal infections of human papillomavirus have impaired fertility parameters. Biomed Res Int. 2017;2017:4684629. Available from: https://pubmed.ncbi.nlm.nih.gov/28835893/

49. Foresta C, Pizzol D, Moretti A, Barzon L, Pal G, Garolla A. Clinical and prognostic significance of human papillomavirus DNA in the sperm or exfoliated cells of infertile patients and subjects with risk factors. Fertil Steril. 2010;94(5):1723–7. Available from: https://pubmed.ncbi.nlm.nih.gov/20056213/

50. Muscianisi F, de Toni L, Giorato G, Carosso A, Foresta C, Garolla A. Is HPV the novel target in male idiopathic infertility? A systematic review of the literature. Front Endocrinol (Lausanne). 2021;12:643539. Available from: https://pubmed.ncbi.nlm.nih.gov/25270519/

51. Nielson CM, Flores R, Harris RB, Abrahamsen M, Papenfuss MR, Dunne EF, et al. Human papillomavirus prevalence and type distribution in male anogenital sites and semen. Cancer Epidemiol Biomarkers Prev. 2007;16(6):1107–14. Available from: https://pubmed.ncbi.nlm.nih.gov/17548671/

52. Foresta C, Noventa M, de Toni L, Gizzo S, Garolla A. HPV-DNA sperm infection and infertility: from a systematic literature review to a possible clinical management proposal. Andrology. 2015;3(2):163–73. Available from: https://pubmed.ncbi.nlm.nih.gov/25270519/

53. Piroozmand A, Nasab SDM, Erami M, Hashemi SMA, Khodabakhsh E, Ahmadi N, et al. Distribution of human papillomavirus and Antisperm antibody in semen and its association with semen parameters among infertile men. J Reprod Infertil. 2020;21(3):183.

54. Lai YM, Lee JF, Huang HY, Soong YK, Yang FP, Pao CC. The effect of human papillomavirus infection on sperm cell motility. Fertil Steril. 1997;67(6):1152–5.

55. Garolla A, Pizzol D, Bertoldo A, de Toni L, Barzon L, Foresta C. Association, prevalence, and clearance of human papillomavirus and antisperm antibodies in infected semen samples from infertile patients.

Fertil Steril. 2013;99(1):125–131.e2. Available from: https://pubmed.ncbi.nlm.nih.gov/23043686/

56. Foresta C, Garolla A, Zuccarello D, Pizzol D, Moretti A, Barzon L, et al. Human papillomavirus found in sperm head of young adult males affects the progressive motility. Fertil Steril. 2010;93(3):802–6. Available from: https://pubmed.ncbi.nlm.nih.gov/19100537/

57. Boeri L, Capogrosso P, Ventimiglia E, Pederzoli F, Cazzaniga W, Chierigo F, et al. High-risk human papillomavirus in semen is associated with poor sperm progressive motility and a high sperm DNA fragmentation index in infertile men. Hum Reprod. 2019;34(2):209–17. Available from: https://pubmed.ncbi.nlm.nih.gov/30517657/

58. Yang Y, Jia CW, Ma YM, Zhou LY, Wang SY. Correlation between HPV sperm infection and male infertility. Asian J Androl. 2013;15(4):529–32. Available from: https://pubmed.ncbi.nlm.nih.gov/23603919/

59. Moghimi M, Zabihi-Mahmoodabadi S, Kheirkhah-Vakilabad A, Kargar Z. Significant Correlation between High-Risk HPV DNA in Semen and Impairment of Sperm Quality in Infertile Men. Int J Fertil Steril. 2019;12(4):306–9. Available from: https://pubmed.ncbi.nlm.nih.gov/30291691/

60. Heidenreich A, Bonfig R, Wilbert DM, Strohmaier WL, Engelmann UH. Risk factors for antisperm antibodies in infertile men. Am J Reprod Immunol. 1994;31(2–3):69–76. Available from: https://pubmed.ncbi.nlm.nih.gov/8049027/

61. Garolla A, Engl B, Pizzol D, Ghezzi M, Bertoldo A, Bottacin A, et al. Spontaneous fertility and in vitro fertilization outcome: new evidence of human papillomavirus sperm infection. Fertility and Sterility [Internet]. 2016;105(1):65–72.e1. Available from: http://www.fertstert.org/article/S0015028215019354/fulltext

62. Perino A, Giovannelli L, Schillaci R, Ruvolo G, Fiorentino FP, Alimondi P, et al. Human papillomavirus infection in couples undergoing in vitro fertilization procedures: impact on reproductive outcomes. Fertil Steril. 2011;95(5):1845–8. Available from: https://pubmed.ncbi.nlm.nih.gov/21167483/

63. Depuydt CE, Donders GGG, Verstraete L, vanden Broeck D, JFA B, Salembier G, et al. Infectious human papillomavirus virions in semen reduce clinical pregnancy rates in women undergoing intra-uterine insemination. Fertility and sterility [Internet]. 2019;111(6):1135–44. Available from: https://pubmed.ncbi.nlm.nih.gov/31005311/

64. Depuydt CE, Donders G, Verstraete L, Vanden Broeck D, Beert J, Salembier G, et al. Time has come to include human papillomavirus (HPV) testing in sperm donor banks. Facts Views Vis Obgyn. 2018;10(4):201.

65. Foresta C, Patassini C, Bertoldo A, Menegazzo M, Francavilla F, Barzon L, et al. Mechanism of human papillomavirus binding to human spermatozoa and fertilizing ability of infected spermatozoa. PLoS One.

2011;6(3):e15036. Available from: https://pubmed.ncbi.nlm.nih.gov/21408100/

66. Garolla A, Pizzol D, Vasoin F, Barzon L, Bertoldo A, Foresta C. Counseling reduces HPV persistence in coinfected couples. J Sex Med. 2014;11(1):127–35. Available from: https://pubmed.ncbi.nlm.nih.gov/24165376/

67. Foresta C, Garolla A, Parisi SG, Ghezzi M, Bertoldo A, di Nisio A, et al. HPV prophylactic vaccination in males improves the clearance of semen infection. EBioMedicine. 2015;2(10):1487–93. Available from: https://pubmed.ncbi.nlm.nih.gov/26629543/

68. Garolla A, de Toni L, Bottacin A, Valente U, de Rocco PM, di Nisio A, et al. Human papillomavirus prophylactic vaccination improves reproductive outcome in infertile patients with HPV semen infection: a retrospective study. Sci Rep. 2018;8(1):912. Available from: https://pubmed.ncbi.nlm.nih.gov/29343824/

69. de Toni L, Cosci I, Carosso A, Barzon L, Engl B, Foresta C, et al. Hyaluronidase-based swim-up for semen selection in patients with human papillomavirus semen infection. Biol Reprod. 2021;104(1):211–22. Available from: https://pubmed.ncbi.nlm.nih.gov/33164043/

70. Obesity and overweight [Internet]. [cited 2022 Jan 31]. Available from: https://www.who.int/en/news-room/fact-sheets/detail/obesity-and-overweight

71. Pasquali R, Casanueva F, Haluzik M, van Hulsteijn L, Ledoux S, Monteiro MP, et al. European Society of Endocrinology Clinical Practice Guideline: Endocrine work-up in obesity. Eur J Endocrinol. 2020;182(1):G1–32. Available from: https://pubmed.ncbi.nlm.nih.gov/31855556/

72. Campbell JM, Lane M, Owens JA, Bakos HW. Paternal obesity negatively affects male fertility and assisted reproduction outcomes: a systematic review and meta-analysis. Reprod Biomed Online. 2015;31(5):593–604. Available from: https://pubmed.ncbi.nlm.nih.gov/26380863/

73. Mushtaq R, Pundir J, Achilli C, Naji O, Khalaf Y, El-Toukhy T. Effect of male body mass index on assisted reproduction treatment outcome: an updated systematic review and meta-analysis. Reprod Biomed Online. 2018;36(4):459–71. Available from: https://pubmed.ncbi.nlm.nih.gov/29452915/

74. Le W, Su SH, Shi LH, Zhang JF, Wu DL. Effect of male body mass index on clinical outcomes following assisted reproductive technology: a meta-analysis. Andrologia. 2016;48(4):406–24. Available from: https://pubmed.ncbi.nlm.nih.gov/26276351/

75. Eisenberg ML, Kim S, Chen Z, Sundaram R, Schisterman EF, Buck Louis GM. The relationship between male BMI and waist circumference on semen quality: data from the LIFE study. Hum Reprod. 2014;29(2):193–200. Available from: https://pubmed.ncbi.nlm.nih.gov/24306102/

76. la Vignera S, Condorelli RA, Vicari E, Calogero AE. Negative effect of increased body weight on sperm conventional and nonconventional flow cyto-

metric sperm parameters. J Androl. 2012;33(1):53–8. Available from: https://pubmed.ncbi.nlm.nih.gov/21273503/

77. Sermondade N, Faure C, Fezeu L, Shayeb AG, Bonde JP, Jensen TK, et al. BMI in relation to sperm count: an updated systematic review and collaborative meta-analysis. Hum Reprod Update. 2013;19(3):221–31. Available from: https://pubmed.ncbi.nlm.nih.gov/23242914/

78. Barbagallo F, Condorelli RA, Mongioì LM, Cannarella R, Cimino L, Magagnini MC, et al. Molecular mechanisms underlying the relationship between obesity and male infertility. Metabolites. 2021;11(12):840. Available from: https://pubmed.ncbi.nlm.nih.gov/34940598/

79. Garolla A, Torino M, Miola P, Caretta N, Pizzol D, Menegazzo M, et al. Twenty-four-hour monitoring of scrotal temperature in obese men and men with a varicocele as a mirror of spermatogenic function. Hum Reprod. 2015;30(5):1006–13. Available from: https://academic.oup.com/humrep/article/30/5/1006/591060

80. Chavarro JE, Toth TL, Wright DL, Meeker JD, Hauser R. Body mass index in relation to semen quality, sperm DNA integrity, and serum reproductive hormone levels among men attending an infertility clinic. Fertil Steril. 2010;93(7):2222–31. Available from: https://pubmed.ncbi.nlm.nih.gov/19261274/

81. di Nisio A, Sabovic I, de Toni L, Rocca MS, Dall'Acqua S, Azzena B, et al. Testosterone is sequestered in dysfunctional adipose tissue, modifying androgen-responsive genes. Int J Obes (Lond). 2005;44(7):1617–25. Available from: https://pubmed.ncbi.nlm.nih.gov/32203110/

82. Xu X, Sun M, Ye J, Luo D, Su X, Zheng D, et al. The effect of aromatase on the reproductive function of obese males. Horm Metab Res. 2017;49(8):572–9. Available from: https://pubmed.ncbi.nlm.nih.gov/28679145/

83. Hajshafiha M, Ghareaghaji R, Salemi S, Sadegh-Asadi N, Sadeghi-Bazargani H. Association of body mass index with some fertility markers among male partners of infertile couples. Int J Gen Med. 2013;6:447–51. Available from: https://pubmed.ncbi.nlm.nih.gov/23785240/

84. Davidson LM, Millar K, Jones C, Fatum M, Coward K. Deleterious effects of obesity upon the hormonal and molecular mechanisms controlling spermatogenesis and male fertility. Hum Fertil (Camb). 2015;18(3):184–93. Available from: https://pubmed.ncbi.nlm.nih.gov/26205254/

85. Agbaje IM, Rogers DA, McVicar CM, McClure N, Atkinson AB, Mallidis C, et al. Insulin dependant diabetes mellitus: implications for male reproductive function. Hum Reprod. 2007;22(7):1871–7. Available from: https://pubmed.ncbi.nlm.nih.gov/17478459/

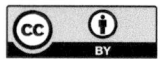

Clinical Interpretation of Semen Analysis

13

Csilla Krausz and Ginevra Farnetani

13.1 Introduction

Semen analysis is a key step in the evaluation of the fertility potential of the male partner of a couple, as it reflects not only the efficiency of spermatogenesis, but also the integrity of post-testicular structures necessary for sperm transport and anterograde ejaculation. The WHO reference values of sperm parameters are based on the analysis of 3500 men (from 12 countries) in couples with time to pregnancy of one year or less. The current thresholds refer to the one-sided lower reference limit of the fifth percentile and are shown in Table 13.1 together with the 50th percentile [1, 2]. It should be stressed that these reference values are applicable only if the analysis is performed according to the recommended standardized procedures. The WHO manual is freely accessible at the following link: https://www.who.int/publications/i/item/9789240030787. The majority of fertile men is expected to have their parameters within the range of the 50th percentile. However, fertility is a "couple-concept" and even severe alterations of semen parameters (much below the fifth percentile) can be compatible with the induction

of pregnancy, provided that the female partner's fertility status is optimal. Vice versa, exceptionally good sperm count does not always imply natural conception. In fact, there is a substantial overlap of semen examination results between fertile and infertile men [3].

Table 13.1 Principal semen parameters and their distribution corresponding to 5th and 50th percentile according to the WHO sixth edition guidelines [1]

Semen parameter	Lower reference value (5th percentile)	50th percentile
Macroscopic parameters		
Appearance	Grey-opalescent	
Viscosity	Forms small discrete drops (thread <2 cm long)	
Volume	1.4 ml	2.3 ml
pH	7.2	
Microscopic parameters		
Sperm concentration	16×10^6/ml	66×10^6/ml
Total sperm count	39×10^6/ejaculate	210×10^6/ejaculate
Total motility	42%	64%
Progressive motility	30%	55%
Normal forms	4%	14%
Vitality	54%	78%
Peroxidase-positive leucocytes	$<1 \times 10^6$/ml	
MAR test	<50%	

C. Krausz (✉) · G. Farnetani
Department of Experimental and Clinical Biomedical Sciences "Mario Serio", Centre of Excellence DeNothe, University of Florence, Florence, Italy
e-mail: csilla.krausz@unifi.it;
ginevra.farnetani@unifi.it

C. Bettocchi et al. (eds.), *Practical Clinical Androlology*,
https://doi.org/10.1007/978-3-031-11701-5_13

13.2   Semen Analysis: General Concepts

Semen evaluation is divided into two parts: macroscopic and microscopic analysis (Fig. 13.1). It is essential that the laboratory performs the analysis according to the current WHO guidelines and participate at an external quality control (EQC) program. In fact, wide discrepancies in the assessments of sperm count, motility, and morphology can result when comparing semen analysis outcomes from different laboratories [4, 5]. Together with EQC programs, participating in periodical teaching courses improves the experience of the laboratory and allows to maximize the probability of obtaining the established standards of quality [6]. In consideration of the above, when interpreting a semen analysis report, it is important that the clinician ascertains whether a given laboratory participates in EQC programs with success.

For each part of the analysis, different parameters are considered and depending on their alteration, different clinical conditions can be suspected. In case of normozoospermia, a second analysis is not mandatory. On the contrary, if one or more semen parameters are altered, repetition is necessary in order to rule out potential pre-analytical and analytical factors, together with biological variability. Among pre-

analytical factors, inappropriate abstinence time, incomplete collection of the ejaculate, inadequate transport of the semen sample would request a short-term repetition. Analytic variables can derive from casual and systematic errors during the procedures. Endogenous factors such as high fever or medications may interfere with spermatogenesis during its entire length (approx. 72 days), therefore the repetition should take place after the completion of the entire spermatogenic cycle.

13.3   Macroscopic Evaluation of Semen

Macroscopic evaluation refers to the chemical and physical parameters of the ejaculate including fluidification, viscosity, appearance, odor, volume, and pH. The main macroscopic alterations are summarized in Table 13.2.

13.3.1 Liquefaction, Viscosity, and Appearance

Liquefaction of the semen needs 15–30 min, and this process is regulated by the prostatic secretion, which is rich in citric acid acting in synergy with proteolytic enzymes (lysozyme, α-amylase, and β-glucuronidase) and prostatic specific antigen (PSA), a trypsin-like protease, that cleaves the semenogelin proteins. PSA may be altered due to congenital or acquired (for instance, prostatitis) factors.

Viscosity is the characteristic of an ejaculate specimen to exhibit a homogeneous stickiness, which may be reduced or increased due to various conditions reported in Table 13.2. A normally liquefied sample will have an opalescent appearance, with a cream/grey color. This parameter is influenced by the concentration of spermatozoa: a transparent ejaculate might indicate an extreme reduction in the number of spermatozoa, while a highly concentrated specimen will be opaque. High viscosity may indicate prostatitis. A red-brown appearance of the ejaculate should alert the clinician for the presence

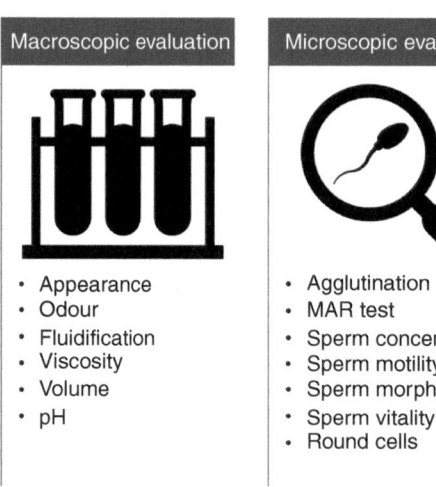

| Macroscopic evaluation | Microscopic evaluation |

- Appearance
- Odour
- Fluidification
- Viscosity
- Volume
- pH

- Agglutination
- MAR test
- Sperm concentation
- Sperm motility
- Sperm morphology
- Sperm vitality
- Round cells

Fig. 13.1 Principal parameters evaluated during semen analysis

Table 13.2 Summary of the main semen alterations and related suspected clinical conditions

Semen parameter	Reason for higher values	Reason for lower values
Fluidification	–	Reduction or absence of PSA
Viscosity	Accessory sex glands dysfunction	Azoo/ cryptozoospermia
	Infections or inflammation of the genitourinary tract (prostatitis)	
Volume	Exudate due to inflammation of accessory sex glands	Distal obstruction or CBAVD
		Partial retrograde ejaculation
		Androgen deficiency
		Prostatis/ vesciculitis or both
		Incomplete collection
pH	Prostatitis	Agenesis of seminal vesicles or their obstruction
	Delay in analysis	
Agglutination	Autoimmunity	–
MAR test	Autoimmunity	–
Leukocytes	Infections or inflammation of the genitourinary tract	–
Sperm number	–	Hypothalamus-pituitary dysfunctions
		Primary quantitative spermatogenic disturbances
		Urogenital duct obstruction
Sperm motility and morphology	–	Infection/ inflammation of the urogenital tract
		Lifestyle/ environmental factors
		Congenital sperm defects
		Medications

PSA prostate-specific antigen; *MAR test* mixed antiglobulin reaction test; *CBAVD* congenital bilateral absence of vas deferens

of erythrocytes in the semen. This condition is known as hematospermia and based on the age of the patient, it can have different etiology: in younger men (<40 years), it could be due to inflammation or urogenital infections, while in older men (>40 years), it could underlie more serious pathologies, such as prostate cancer [7].

13.3.2 Volume and pH

Seminal plasma is composed mainly by the secretions of the accessory glands (about 90%) whereas the contribution of the epididymis and bulbourethral glands are minimal. *Semen volume* not only expresses the secretory activity of these glands, but also their responses to autonomous nerve stimulation elicited by sexual arousal, which will lead to smooth muscle contractions that empties each gland. Prostate and seminal vesicles are target organs of androgens; therefore, severe androgen deficiency is associated with lower semen volume. In addition, when seminal fluid volume is markedly reduced, the clinician should ask the patient whether the collection was complete.

Both prostate and seminal vesicles contribute to the *semen pH* with their secretions: prostate produces an acidic fluid, while seminal vesicles produce an alkaline fluid leading to the typical neutral pH, around 7.2–7.4. Changes in pH may indicate different pathological conditions, as shown in Table 13.2, even though this parameter is susceptible to analytical biases as well. The pH typically increases with time after ejaculation, so when a highly alkaline specimen is observed, poor sample handling and delay in analysis should be excluded prior interpretation [1].

13.4 Microscopic Evaluation of Semen

Microscopic evaluation refers to the characteristics of the cellular fraction of semen and includes agglutination, aggregation, sperm concentration, motility, vitality, morphology, and round cells. The main microscopic semen alterations are summarized in Table 13.2.

13.4.1 Agglutination and Sperm Antibodies

Aggregation and agglutination are two different parameters. *Aggregation* is the adherence of both motile and immotile spermatozoa to mucus strands or non-sperm cells. *Agglutination*, instead, is the tendency of motile spermatozoa to form clumps and it can be categorized based on the degree of agglutination and the sperm structures involved [1]. This feature could indicate the presence of an immunological cause of infertility, even though the presence of *anti-sperm antibodies* (ASA) should be confirmed by further testing, such as the commercially available mixed antiglobulin reaction test (MAR test). It is important to notice that ASA and agglutination not always come together. Indeed, sperm agglutination can be caused by other factors rather than autoimmunity, as well as antibodies can be present without sperm agglutination.

ASA have been found in several pathological conditions which may lead to the interruption of the blood-testis barrier, such as testicular torsion, testicular carcinoma, and orchitis [8]. The presence of ASA as an isolated abnormality is seen in less than 5% of infertile males and occurs mainly in association with normal sperm counts [8]. In fact, testing for ASA can be requested in case of unexplained couple infertility with normozoospermic male partner [9]. ASA can interfere with physiological reproduction at many levels, affecting sperm number and motility, the ability to transit through cervical mucus, acrosome reaction, and zona pellucida binding [9, 10].

13.4.2 Sperm Number, Motility, Vitality, and Morphology

Sperm number is a quantitative marker of spermatogenesis, whereas sperm motility, vitality, and morphology are qualitative parameters.

Sperm concentration is defined as the number of spermatozoa per unit volume of semen. As stated above, semen volume mainly originates from the accessory sex glands, hence sperm concentration is influenced by their activity and does not represent a direct measure of testicular sperm output. A much better reflection of the capacity of the testis to produce sperm refers to total sperm count (TSC). The fifth percentile reference value for TSC is >39 millions of spermatozoa.

Three quantitative alterations can be distinguished as follows:

- Azoospermia: absence of spermatozoa in the ejaculate and in the pellet after centrifugation.
- Cryptozoospermia: absence of spermatozoa in the ejaculate but present in the pellet after centrifugation.
- Oligozoospermia: sperm concentration or TSC lower than the fifth percentile value (Table 13.1).

Sperm motility is classified based on the direction and velocity of sperm movement into the following categories: (i) progressive motility (rapid and slow); (ii) non-progressive sperm movement; and (iii) immotile spermatozoa [1]. The reduction in sperm motility, called asthenozoospermia (total motility <42% and progressive motility <30%) can be due to congenital or acquired factors. Especially extreme asthenozoospermia, with or without associated teratozoospermia (see below), is due to different genetic anomalies [11]. Sperm motility defects can be present in the context of a syndrome, known as Primary Ciliary Dyskinesia (PCD). PCD is a rare recessive autosomic disorder characterized by defects of motile cilia and flagella, leading to asthenozoospermia, chronic respiratory tract infections, and *situs inversus* [12]. *DNAI1* and *DNAH5* gene mutations account for about 30% of PCD cases, whereas the remaining 70% could be explained by mutations in other 26 genes involved in various ciliary ultrastructural defects [13].

In case the percentage of immotile sperm is higher than 40%, vitality test is indicated in order to distinguish vital and dead cells [1]. The extreme reduction in *sperm vitality* is known as necrozoospermia.

Sperm morphology assessment is aimed at the evaluation of the shape of spermatozoon, which consists of a head and tail, connected through the midpiece, a thicker part of the tail containing mitochondria. The rest of the tail consists of a principal piece (axoneme or ciliary structure surrounded by outer dense fibers), a fibrous sheath with longitudinal columns and an endpiece.

The evaluation of sperm morphology is the most challenging part of semen analysis since its standardization is more complex than the measurement of the other parameters. Human ejaculates contain spermatozoa with a wide range of different morphological appearances. Sperm morphology is assessed by the "strict" criteria and any slight abnormality of the spermatozoa will classify it to have abnormal morphology. In fact, the large majority of spermatozoa does not fulfil the WHO criteria for being considered as "normal" even in the specimen of fertile men [1]. Consequently, the 50th percentile of reference values would correspond to only 14% of typical forms. In the large majority of patients affected by teratozoospermia (normal forms <4%), head, midpiece, tail, and cytoplasmic residue defects are combined, and different spermatozoa may present different types of abnormalities. These mixed morphological defects are usually related to defective spermatogenesis or epididymal inflammation. The presence of excessive cytoplasm around the midpiece is associated with an increased production of ROS and oxidative stress [14]. The WHO guidelines included the calculation of indices of multiple sperm defects among the extended examinations of morphological abnormalities. However, due to the overlapping values between fertile and infertile men, the application of these indices in the clinical practice is still questionable [1].

The opposite of "polymorphic" teratozoospermia are those rare conditions, where all abnormal spermatozoa bear the same specific anomaly. These monomorphic teratozoospermia cases are related to genetic defects and among them, the two typical monomorphic sperm head defects are globozoospermia and macrozoospermia [15]. Both conditions are associated with functional abnormalities leading to severe impairment of fertilizing ability. For instance, macrozoospermia or macrocephalia is characterized by the pres-

ence of spermatozoa with large head and multiple flagella. It is a rare recessive disease due to mutations in *AURKC* gene. Macrozoospermia is typically associated with a high rate of aneuploidy and polyploidy caused by the nondisjunction of chromosomes or defective cytokinesis during meiosis [16]. It has been reported that sulfasalazine treatment may induce transient increase of large headed spermatozoa in the ejaculate with an improvement in sperm morphology and motility after the cessation of the treatment [17]. Therefore, careful medical history taking is essential to rule out iatrogenic teratozoospermia.

An example of extreme astheno/teratozoospermia (AT) are the sperm tail abnormalities. Multiple morphological abnormalities of the sperm flagellum (MMAF) are a rare form of AT, characterized by a mosaic of sperm cells with absent, short, irregular, and coiled flagellum. Routine semen analysis can easily evidence MMAF through optic microscopy, but the transmission electron microscopy and genetic testing are necessary to define the exact ultrastructural defects and their origin, respectively. Besides the major candidate gene *(DNAH1)*, other gene defects have been identified and currently a total of 18 genetic causes are known for being responsible for 30–60% of MMAF cases [18]. There is a growing evidence that mutation in some of these genes *(DNAH17, CFAP65,* and *CEP135)* confers very poor prognosis even for IntraCytoplasmic Sperm Injection (ICSI) pregnancies [18]. It is therefore possible that in the near future, genetic testing in MMAF patients may have also a predictive value for ICSI outcome.

It is well known since many years that sperm centriole alterations are associated with unsuccessful ICSI. Human spermatozoa contain two centrioles: the proximal one (PC), located near the head base, and the distal one (DC), located at the base of the axoneme. Sperm centrioles have many different functions, which are essential not only for flagellum movement but also for normal morphology, cell division, and zygote development [19]. In fact, sperm is the sole contributor of centrioles to the zygote, and is essential for bipolar spindle formation during the first division after fertilization. Therefore, sperm centriole defects may cause failure of embryo development. The spectrum of semen phenotypes associated with centriole defects ranges from azoo/oligozoospermia to astheno/teratozoospermia. For instance, abnormal positioning of centrioles can lead to dysplasia of the fibrous sheath [19]. In addition, centriole defects can also cause acephalic spermatozoa syndrome (ASS). It can be due to the dissociation between PC and DC causing the sperm neck to break, resulting in decapitated sperm heads. To date, seven genes (*SUN5*, *BRDT*, *PFMBP1*, *TSGA10*, *DNAH6*, *HOOK1*, and *CEP112*) have been found mutated in infertile men with acephalic spermatozoa [20].

13.4.3 How to Interpret the Three Principal Sperm Parameters

Sperm number, motility, and morphology should not be considered individually but in combination. In fact, the main clinical question is, how many progressively motile and normal spermatozoa are present in an ejaculate. For instance, in semen presenting all three parameters corresponding to the WHO lowest reference value, there are 11.7 million of progressively motile and 1.56 million morphologically normal spermatozoa. However, a moderately oligozoospermic man (for instance, 25 million spermatozoa) showing 50% of progressive motility and 7% of typical morphology would have a higher number of total progressive (12.5 million spermatozoa) and normal spermatozoa (1.75 million spermatozoa) in his ejaculate in respect to a man defined as "normozoospermic" based on the fifth percentile of each of the three parameters. Therefore, the clinical consequence of isolated oligozoospermia in this man remains questionable. Similar scenarios can occur when sperm number is very high whereas motility and morphology is slightly below the fifth percentile. On the other hand, it is also clear that when the three parameters are lower than the defined thresholds, i.e., oligoas-

thenoteratozoospermia (OAT), the odds of subfertility sharply increase [3]. Some authors propose to calculate the total motile sperm count (TMSC) which correlates better with spontaneous pregnancy than individual parameters [21].

13.4.4 Round Cells

Apart from spermatozoa, epithelial and round cells can be observed in the ejaculate. Epithelial cells are derived from the genitourinary tract, while round cells refer to either leukocytes or immature germ cells [1].

Leukocytospermia (LCS) is defined as the presence of more than 1×10^6 leukocytes (white blood cells, WBC) per ml of semen. The relationship between WBCs concentration and semen quality is questioned in men asymptomatic for a genital tract infection [22]. The presence of a high number of WBCs and a reduced ejaculated volume has been proposed as an indicator for infections and inflammations of the genitourinary tract [23]. However, the association of LCS with fertility potential is controversial [22].

13.5 From Semen Analysis to Diagnosis

Semen analysis, together with medical history and physical exam, represents the first step of the diagnostic work-up of infertile men. In some instances, the result of semen analysis is suggestive for specific forms of reproductive impairments, which then will be confirmed by subsequent laboratory and instrumental exams (e.g., additional semen microbiological examinations in case of suspected infections or inflammations; transrectal ultrasound exam in case of suspected distal obstruction; genetic exams in case of monomorphic teratozoospermia, etc.). In this paragraph, we are going to briefly describe informative semen analysis's outcomes.

13.5.1 General Considerations on Azoospermia/ Cryptozoospermia

Azoospermia, affecting about 1% of the general male population, is incompatible with natural pregnancy. It is extremely important that the laboratory performs the analysis of semen sediment after centrifugation, allowing to differentiate between azoospermia and cryptozoospermia. Although the likelihood of spontaneous fertilization remains extremely unlikely even in case of cryptozoospermia, the importance in distinguishing between these two conditions refers to different in vitro fertilization options, i.e., in azoospermia testicular sperm extraction (TESE) must precede ICSI. As stated above, when sperm parameters are abnormal, semen analysis must be repeated. Therefore, the diagnosis of azoospermia must be confirmed in at least two semen analysis (possibly after the whole spermatogenic cycle) because it could be a temporary disorder, or it could alternate with cryptozoospermia.

Azoospermia can be divided into obstructive (OA) and non-obstructive (NOA) forms. In OA, spermatogenesis is unaffected, and the absence of spermatozoa in the ejaculate is due to bilateral distal or proximal obstruction of the urogenital tract. NOA is a symptom that can be associated with three different testis histology: Sertoli cell-only syndrome (SCOS), maturation arrest at different stages of germ cell maturation (MA), or hypospermatogenesis. The differential diagnosis is fundamental as the patient management and treatment options are different [24]. The definition of the etiology is also relevant, since NOA due to primary spermatogenic failure cannot be treated with medical therapy, whereas if the cause is a hypothalamus-pituitary dysfunction, the treatment with gonadotropin is effective in about 90% of cases [25]. In the large majority of OA cases and in primary testicular failure, TESE is the most viable treatment option.

13.5.1.1 Which Parameters May Help Clinicians to Distinguish Between NOA and OA?

In Table 13.3, we report five examples of seminal analysis output that are suggestive for a specific etiology. As stated above, when no spermatozoa is present in the ejaculate, it is important to evaluate the sediment after centrifugation, as their presence is indicative of cryptozoospermia (scenario A).

When azoospermia is confirmed by examining the sediment, three parameters are useful to distinguish between OA and NOA: semen volume, pH, and the presence of immature germ cells. When semen volume is reduced, different pH may indicate different etiology. For instance, an acidic pH indicates the absence of the seminal vesicles secretions, which together with the absence of spermatozoa could strongly suggest congenital bilateral absence of the vas deferens (CBAVD) associated to the agenesis of seminal vesicles (scenario B). Reduced semen volume with normal pH, instead, can be seen in case of severe hypoandrogenism (scenario C). When semen volume and pH are normal, the analysis of the pellet smears for the presence of spermatogenetic cells is useful [9]. If they are present, a maturation arrest can be suspected (scenario D), while if they are absent, a proximal obstruction can be the cause (scenario E).

13.5.1.2 Which Sperm Parameters are Informative in Quantitative and Qualitative Impairment of Spermatogenesis?

In Table 13.4, we report some examples of oligo/astheo/teratozoospermia. The reduction in sperm concentration, especially $<5 \times 10^6$/ml, is rarely a stand-alone condition, as it is typically associated with other semen alterations. However, isolated oligozoospermia can be found in case of patients with congenital hypogonadotropic hypogonadism treated with gonadotropins (scenario A). In such cases, all semen parameters are normal except for the sperm number which in the majority of cases remains below the reference value.

Table 13.3 Examples of routine semen analysis outputs in azoospermia

Semen parameters	A	B	C	D	E
Volume (ml)	2,5	1	1	2,5	2,5
pH	7,4	6	7,4	7,4	7,4
Viscosity	N	N	N	N	N
Agglutination	No	No	No	No	No
Total sperm count ($\times 10^6$)	0	0	0	0	0
Progressive motility (%)	-	-	-	-	-
Non-progressive motility (%)	-	-	-	-	-
Immotile spermatozoa (%)	-	-	-	-	-
Vitality (%)	-	-	-	-	-
Normal forms (%)	-	-	-	-	-
Leukocytes ($\times 10^6$)	0	0	0	0	0
Notes	**Few motile spermatozoa** are present in the sediment	Absence of spermatozoa in the sediment	Absence of spermatozoa in the sediment	**Immature germ cells** are present in the sediment	Absence of spermatozoa in the sediment
Suspected etiology	Crypto	CBAVD	SHA	MA	PO

Altered semen parameters are in red. *N* normal; *CBAVD* congenital absence of vas deference; *MA* maturation arrest; *PO* proximal obstruction; *SHA* severe hypoandrogenism; *Crypto* cryptozoospermia

Regarding combined forms of semen alterations, scenario B reports a man exhibiting oligo-asthenoteratozoospermia (OAT) with other anomalies: agglutination is present, increased viscosity, and leukocytospermia. In this particular patient, the cause of OAT could be an inflammation or infection of the urogenital tract.

Asthenozoospermia is the most frequent sperm defect observed in infertile men, with variable degrees of severity. In case of total sperm immotility, it is mandatory to distinguish between immotile live and dead sperm (necrozoospermia). A large proportion of live but immotile cells, as seen in scenario C, may indicate structural defects in the flagellum [26]. On the other hand, when complete asthenozoospermia is due to a high percentage of dead cells, as seen in scenario D, it can be associated with an epididymal pathology [27, 28], adult polycystic kidney disease or it can be observed often in patients with spinal cord injury [28]. A second ejaculate within a short-term period of approximately 60 min has been shown to improve seminal quality as compared with the first ejaculate in patients with epididymal necrozoospermia [29].

Semen analysis outcomes reported in scenario E exhibit alterations of motility and morphology classified as asthenoteratozoospermia. It is important that the laboratory describes whether the atypical forms have different anomalies or if they are the same. In fact, this is a case of polymorphic teratozoospermia in which defects of the

Table 13.4 Examples of routine semen analysis output showing quantitative and/or qualitative defects

Semen parameters	A	B	C	D	E	F
Volume (ml)	2	1,5	2	2	2	2
pH	7,2	8	7,3	7,3	7,3	7,3
Viscosity	N	++	N	N	N	N
Agglutination	No	Yes	No	No	No	No
Total sperm count ($\times 10^6$)	10	20	45	45	45	45
Progressive motility (%)	40	5	1	0	5	45
Non-progressive motility (%)	30	15	2	2	5	35
Immotile spermatozoa (%)	10	80	97	98	90	20
Vitality (%)	-	40	80	0	60	-
Normal forms (%)	4	2	4	4	1	1
Leukocytes ($\times 10^6$)	0	3	0	0	0	0
Immature germ cells ($\times 10^6$)	0	0	0	0	0	0
Notes	-	MAR test: negative	-	-	Multiple morphological anomalies (tail and head)	Round-headed spermatozoa without acrosome
Definition of the defect	**Isolated oligozoospermia**	**OAT**	**Extreme Asthenozoospermia**	**Necrozoospermia**	**AT**	**Globozoospermia**
Examples of potential etiologies	Hypo Hypo after hormonal treatment	inflammation or infection of the urogenital tract	Ultrastructural defects of the sperm tail	Epididymal pathologies, polycystic kidney, spinal cord injury	MMAF	Biallelic deletion of DPY19L2

Semen alterations are in red. *N* normal; *OAT* oligoasthenoteratozoospermia; *AT* asthenoteratozoospermia; *Hypo* hypogonadotropic hypogonadism; *MMAF* multiple morphological abnormalities of the flagellum tail and the head are present. This scenario is compatible with MMAF (see above). Scenario F reports a specific monomorphic teratozoospermia, called globozoospermia. This condition is characterized by the production of spermatozoa with round head without acrosome, hence they are missing PLCζ, an acrosome phospholipase, essential for the activation of the oocyte. Globozoospermia is a rare autosomic recessive disease and the most prevalent genetic defect observed in men with 100% globozoospermia is the complete deletion of *DPY19L2* [16]. In case of complete globozoospermia, ICSI should be followed by artificial oocyte activation [11].

13.6 Value and Limits of the Semen Analysis

Routine semen analysis is a valuable diagnostic test although it has its own limitations. In fact, because infertility involves male and female factors, it will not be possible to predict fertility using parameters from either partner alone, unless there is azoospermia in the man or premature ovarian failure in the woman [30]. While azoospermia undoubtedly causes infertility, the presence of triple defects—reduced sperm number, motility, and morphology—also increases the likelihood of a male factor responsible for couple infertility [3]. On the other hand, in case of normozoospermia, searching for female factors could have more relevance at the initial stages of the diagnostic work-up. Despite many discussions about the clinical importance of semen parameters, semen analysis remains a fundamental step in clinical andrology. This is because it may reveal a series of anomalies, which can guide clinician to further explore the etiology behind these defects. It is therefore important that the report is fully reliable, which implies that semen analysis is performed in specialized laboratories strictly following the WHO guidelines and participating at external quality control programs. Clinicians should also be aware of the fact that semen parameters are susceptible of variations due to pre-analytical, analytical factors, together with intraindividual

biological variability. Therefore, when semen alterations are observed, a second evaluation is mandatory.

Although routine sperm analysis is able to diagnose extreme conditions which are typically associated with functional and genetic defects, microscopic examination does not provide direct information on the functional integrity of the spermatozoa. For instance, it is unable to detect DNA fragmentation, ultrastructural defects, the inability of spermatozoa to undergo acrosome reaction, to bind the zona pellucida or to fertilize the egg. For this reason, the new WHO manual also describes a series of test which are part of the so-called extended examinations. Among them, the evaluation of sperm DNA fragmentation is already introduced in many laboratories all over the world; however, its clinical utility remains still controversial [1, 9]. Another section of the WHO manual deals with advanced functional tests which are aimed at assessing the competence of human spermatozoa to fulfil those processes which are essential to conception. These specialized assays are available mainly in research laboratories and are used to assess the effect of environmental and pharmacological compounds on spermatogenesis. However, since their association with the fertilizing potential of the male gamete is promising, it is possible that these assays will be included among the so-called extended examination procedures in the future.

In conclusion, although routine semen analysis is considered a poor indicator of reproductive outcomes, it remains a valuable diagnostic test in couple infertility. It provides information on whether infertility can be related to the male partner and is able to identify alterations which can guide clinicians towards tailored diagnostic exams.

References

1. WHO laboratory manual for the examination and processing of human semen.
2. Campbell MJ, Lotti F, Baldi E, Schlatt S, Festin MPR, Björndahl L, et al. Distribution of semen examination results 2020—A follow up of data collated for

the WHO semen analysis manual 2010. Andrology. 2021;9(3):817–22.

3. Guzick DS, Overstreet JW, Factor-Litvak P, Brazil CK, Nakajima ST, Coutifaris C, et al. Sperm morphology, motility, and concentration in fertile and infertile men. The New England journal of medicine. N Engl J Med. 2001;345:1388–93.

4. Neuwinger J, Behre HM, Nieschlag E. External quality control in the andrology laboratory: an experimental multicenter trial. Fertil Steril. 1990;54:308–14.

5. Filimberti E, Degl'Innocenti S, Borsotti M, Quercioli M, Piomboni P, Natali I, et al. High variability in results of semen analysis in andrology laboratories in Tuscany (Italy): the experience of an external quality control (EQC) programme. Andrology. 2013;1:401–7.

6. Barratt CLR, Björndahl L, Menkveld R, Mortimer D. ESHRE special interest group for andrology basic semen analysis course: a continued focus on accuracy, quality, efficiency and clinical relevance. Hum Reprod. 2011;26:3207–12.

7. Mulhall JE, Albertsen PC. Hemospermia: diagnosis and management. Urology. 1995;46:463–7.

8. Tournaye H, Krausz C, Oates RD. Novel concepts in the aetiology of male reproductive impairment. Lancet Diabetes Endocrinol. 2017;5:544–53.

9. Ferlin A, Calogero AE, Krausz C, Lombardo F, Paoli D, Rago R, et al. Management of male factor infertility: position statement from the Italian Society of Andrology and Sexual Medicine (SIAMS): Endorsing Organization: Italian Society of Embryology, Reproduction, and Research (SIERR). J Endocrinol Investig. 2022;45:1085–113.

10. Barbonetti A, Castellini C, D'Andrea S, Cordeschi G, Santucci R, Francavilla S, et al. Prevalence of anti-sperm antibodies and relationship of degree of sperm auto-immunization to semen parameters and post-coital test outcome: a retrospective analysis of over 10 000 men. Hum Reprod. 2019;34:834–41.

11. Krausz C, Riera-Escamilla A. Genetics of male infertility. Nat Rev Urol. 2018;15:369–84.

12. Knowles MR, Zariwala M, Leigh M. Primary ciliary dyskinesia. Clin Chest Med. 2016;37:449.

13. Coutton C, Escoffier J, Martinez G, Arnoult C, Ray PF. Teratozoospermia: spotlight on the main genetic actors in the human. Hum Reprod Update. 2015;21:455–85.

14. Aitken J, Buckingham D, Krausz C. Relationships between biochemical markers for residual sperm cytoplasm, reactive oxygen species generation, and the presence of leukocytes and precursor germ cells in human sperm suspensions. Mol Reprod Dev. 1994;39:268–79.

15. Beurois J, Cazin C, Kherraf ZE, Martinez G, Celse T, Touré A, et al. Genetics of teratozoospermia: Back to the head. Best Pract Res Clin Endocrinol Metab. 2020;34:101473.

16. Chianese C, Fino MG, Riera Escamilla A, López Rodrigo O, Vinci S, Guarducci E, et al. Comprehensive investigation in patients affected by sperm macrocephaly and globozoospermia. Andrology. 2015;3:203–12.

17. Cosentino MJ, Chey WY, Takihara H, Cockett ATK. The effects of sulfasalazine on human male fertility potential and seminal prostaglandins. J Urol. 1984;132:682–6.

18. Touré A, Martinez G, Kherraf ZE, Cazin C, Beurois J, Arnoult C, et al. The genetic architecture of morphological abnormalities of the sperm tail. Hum Genet. 2020;140:21–42.

19. Avidor-Reiss T, Carr A, Fishman EL. The sperm centrioles. Molecular and cellular endocrinology. Mol Cell Endocrinol. 2020;518:110987.

20. Mazaheri Moghaddam M, Mazaheri Moghaddam M, Hamzeiy H, Baghbanzadeh A, Pashazadeh F, Sakhinia E. Genetic basis of acephalic spermatozoa syndrome, and intracytoplasmic sperm injection outcomes in infertile men: a systematic scoping review. J Assist Reprod Genet. 2021;38:573–86.

21. Zinaman MJ, Brown CC, Selevan SG, Clegg ED. Semen quality and human fertility: a prospective study with healthy couples. J Androl. 2000;21:145–53.

22. Jungwirth A, Giwercman A, Tournaye H, Diemer T, Kopa Z, Dohle G, et al. European Association of Urology guidelines on male infertility: the 2012 update. Eur Urol. 2012;62:324–32.

23. Calogero AE, Duca Y, Condorelli RA, la Vignera S. Male accessory gland inflammation, infertility, and sexual dysfunctions: a practical approach to diagnosis and therapy. Andrology. 2017;5:1064–72.

24. Tournaye H, Krausz C, Oates RD. Concepts in diagnosis and therapy for male reproductive impairment. Lancet Diabetes Endocrinol. 2017;5:554–64.

25. Young J, Xu C, Papadakis GE, Acierno JS, Maione L, Hietamäki J, et al. Clinical management of congenital hypogonadotropic hypogonadism. Endocr Rev. 2019;40:669–710.

26. Chemes HE, Rawe VY. Sperm pathology: a step beyond descriptive morphology. Origin, characterization and fertility potential of abnormal sperm phenotypes in infertile men. Hum Reprod Update. 2003;9:405–28.

27. Wilton LJ, Temple-Smith PD, Baker HWG, de Kretser DM. Human male infertility caused by degeneration and death of sperm in the epididymis. Fertil Steril. 1988;49:1052–8.

28. Correa-Pérez JR, Fernández-Pelegrina R, Aslanis P, Zavos PM. Clinical management of men producing ejaculates characterized by high levels of dead sperm and altered seminal plasma factors consistent with epididymal necrospermia. Fertil Steril. 2004;81:1148–50.

29. Check JH, Chase JS. Improved semen quality after a short-interval second ejaculation. Fertil Steril. 1985;44:416–8.

30. Wang C, Swerdloff RS. Limitations of semen analysis as a test of male fertility and anticipated needs from newer tests. Fertil Steril. 2014;102:1502.

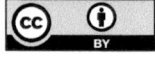

Therapy in Oligozoospermia (Varicocele, Cryptorchidism, Inflammation, and Seminal Tract Infections)

14

Gian Maria Busetto, Ramadan Saleh, Murat Gül, and Ashok Agarwal

14.1 Varicocele

Varicocele is an abnormal dilatation, elongation, and tortuosity of the pampiniform plexus of veins draining the testicles and is associated with venous reflux. Varicocele is diagnosed on ultrasound by the demonstration of venous diameter of >3 mm in the upright position, and during the Valsalva maneuver, and venous reflux duration is >2 s [1, 2]. The prevalence of varicocele is estimated to be approximately 20% in the general population, 40% among men with primary infertility, and 80% among men with secondary infertility [3]. A prevalence trial on 816 infertile men report that 74.6% of them had primary infertility while 25.4% secondary infertility. The overall prevalence of varicocele was 32.0% and varicocele accounted for 32.2% of patients with primary infertile, and 28.5% with secondary infertile [4].

Since the early report by Tulloch [5], extensive research has been done to explore the role of varicocele in male infertility. However, the topic of varicocele remains as one of the most controversial issues among andrologists and reproductive scientists. Several mechanisms have been postulated to explain the pathogenesis of infertility in men with varicocele, including scrotal hyperthermia, testicular hypoxia, hormonal disturbances, and the backflow of toxic metabolites [6] (Fig. 14.1). Elevated scrotal temperature in varicocele patients results from venous stasis and retrograde flow, which compromises the testicular heat exchange system [7, 8]. Testicular hypoxia in patients with varicocele is caused by vasoconstriction of pre-capillary arterioles, a compensatory mechanism to maintain the physiological intra-testicular pressure [9].

Scrotal hyperthermia, testicular hypoperfusion, and reflux of toxic metabolites enhance the generation of reactive oxygen species (ROS) that can overwhelm the antioxidant capacity of the sperm resulting in the status of oxidative stress (OS). The latter is thought to play a central role in the pathogenesis of male infertility in general and in varicocele in particular [10]. A meta-analysis indicated significantly higher levels of seminal ROS and lower antioxidant capacity in varicocele

G. M. Busetto (✉)
Department of Urology, University of Foggia, Policlinico Riuniti, Foggia, Italy
e-mail: gianmaria.busetto@unifg.it

R. Saleh
Department of Dermatology, Venereology and Andrology, Faculty of Medicine, Sohag University, Sohag, Egypt

Ajyal IVF Center, Ajyal Hospital, Sohag, Egypt

M. Gül
Department of Urology, Selcuk University School of Medicine, Konya, Turkey

A. Agarwal
American Center for Reproductive Medicine, Cleveland Clinic, Cleveland, OH, USA
e-mail: agarwaa@ccf.org

© The Author(s) 2023
C. Bettocchi et al. (eds.), *Practical Clinical Andrology*,
https://doi.org/10.1007/978-3-031-11701-5_14

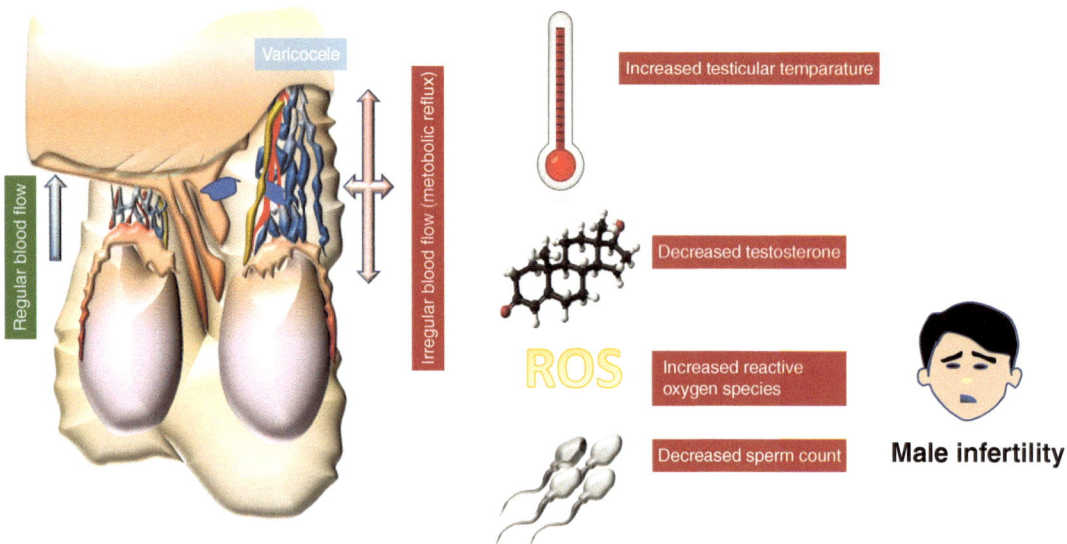

Fig. 14.1 Mechanism of action of varicocele on male infertility

patients compared to healthy controls [11]. High seminal OS in infertile men with varicocele has been associated with low conventional sperm parameters [12, 13] and increased sperm DNA fragmentation (SDF) [12, 14].

Additionally, a lower percentage of sperm DNA methylation and an altered sperm DNA integrity have been observed in varicocele patients compared to fertile controls [15, 16]. Furthermore, the gene variants that cause prot-amine deficiency have been reported at higher frequencies in varicocele patients with abnormal sperm parameters [17]. Recent studies showed altered seminal plasma proteomic profiles of var-icocele patients in association with increased generation of ROS and pro-oxidant proteins, and up-regulation of antioxidant systems [18–20]. Varicocele patients show alteration in the expres-sion of 253 proteins that are involved in sperm functions, including sperm motility, capacitation, hyperactivation, acrosome reaction, and fertiliza-tion [21]. Furthermore, the latter study indicated higher protein alterations among patients with bilateral varicoceles than those with unilateral varicocele.

Experimental animal studies with induced varicoceles indicated progressive decline of semen quality [22], and impairment of the fertil-

izing capacity of the haploid male gamete [23]. In infertile men, varicoceles may be associated with abnormal semen quality [24], or even com-plete azoospermia [25]. The current treatment options for infertile men with varicocele include varicocele repair (VR), empirical therapies, and assisted reproductive technology (ART).

In clinical practice, the decision to conduct VR during the management of infertile men with clinical varicocele is challenging in many aspects. First, the selection of patients that will benefit most from varicocele treatment and the timing of treatment may be difficult [26, 27]. Second, the outcome of VR may be a subject of great vari-ability as it relies on several factors, including patient's age, varicocele grade, testicular volume, pretreatment semen parameters, and reproductive hormone levels [26–28]. Last but not least is the method of VR, as the evidence is not satisfactory enough to suggest the optimum method [1].

In addition, there is no consensus as to the management of infertile men with subclinical varicocele. However, a recent systematic review and meta-analysis found no improvement in pregnancy rate after surgical repair of subclini-cal varicoceles [29]. Moreover, the current guidelines by the European Association of Urology (EAU) offers a "weak" suggestion to not treat varicocele in infertile men who have normal semen analysis or with a sub-clinical varicocele [1]. Once again, EAU guidelines [1] and the American Urological Association (AUA)/the American Society for Reproductive Medicine (ASRM) guidelines [30] do not mention specific measures for the management of varicocele associated with isolated sperm defects such as oligozoospermia, asthenozoospermia, necrozoospermia, or teratozoospermia, and do not determine which technique to choose for the management of recurrent varicoceles.

VR can be either surgical (varicolectomy) or through angiographic embolization. Surgical repair of varicocele includes open non-microsurgical techniques whether inguinal (Ivanissevich) or high retroperitoneal ligation (Palomo), open microsurgical techniques (inguinal or sub-inguinal) or laparoscopic [31, 32]. In a recent systematic review, the highest spontaneous pregnancy rate was found following subinguinal microsurgical VR (41%) as compared to inguinal (26%), retroperitoneal (37%), laparoscopic transperitoneal (26%), and percutaneous embolization (36%) [33]. However, a previous meta-analysis indicated no specific technique to be the most effective in improving the outcome [34]. The EAU guidelines report the microsurgical technique as having the lowest risk of recurrence (evidence level 2a) compared to non-microscopic approaches while highlighting the need for microsurgical training and expertise [1]. Using optical magnification helps avoid postoperative complications such as testicular devascularization or hydrocele with sparing of arteries and lymphatics, and decreased potential of recurrence rates [35]. Additionally, the microsurgical subinguinal VR has the advantage of a short postoperative recovery because no major muscles are dissected [36]. However, microsurgery necessitates the presence of expensive equipment and special surgical skills. Alternative methods for identifying the spermatic artery during VR include the use of intraoperative Doppler or direct visualization of arterial pulsations with or without the use of a vasodilator such as papaverine [37]. Percutaneous embolization of varicoceles may result in less post-procedural pain than

surgical repairs. However, this latter approach is limited by technical difficulties and higher recurrence rates [38, 39].

The accumulating evidence suggests that VR can improve conventional sperm parameters (sperm concentration, motility, and morphology), seminal OS, SDF [40–42], and serum testosterone concentrations [43]. Although the positive impact of VR on semen quality is evident for all surgical techniques [26, 44, 45], the microsurgical approach appears to provide superior results [40]. Studies exploring the impact of VR on spontaneous pregnancy outcomes yielded equivocal results [40, 44, 46–51]. However, a meta-analysis revealed significantly higher clinical pregnancy rates (OR = 1.59) and live birth rates (OR = 2.17) among patients who underwent intracytoplasmic sperm injection (ICSI) following VR [52].

The impact of VR on seminal OS markers and SDF has been extensively investigated over the last two decades with conflicting results. Positive outcome of VR included reduction of 8-hydroxydeoxyguanosine (8-OhdG), a known marker for oxidative DNA damage, as well as an increase in seminal thiols and ascorbic acid (Vitamin C) 6 months after surgery [53]. Similarly, inguinal varicocelectomy with loop magnification resulted in a significant reduction of seminal ROS, and a rise in total antioxidant capacity (TAC) and SDF [54].

Using microsurgical retroperitoneal high ligation technique, a significant reduction in seminal malonaldehyde (MDA), a lipid peroxidation product, was observed at 3 and 6 months following varicocelectomy [55]. Furthermore, spermatic vein ligation caused a significant increase in seminal TAC levels at 3 and 6 months following surgery, particularly in patients with grade II and III varicoceles [56]. However, no significant change was observed in TAC levels at 10 and 24 months post-varicocelectomy, despite a positive impact on TAC regulation and associated improvement of sperm motility [57].

Varicocele repair has also been shown to reduce SDF and enhance the chance of spontaneous pregnancy and ART outcomes [58]. A meta-analysis concluded that VR is associated with a significant reduction of SDF with a mean difference of −3.37% (95% CI −4.09 to −2.65, $p < 0.00001$) [59]. Another recent meta-analysis including 11 studies (a total of 394 patients) demonstrated a significant reduction in SDF levels by 5.79% following VR [60].

A different meta-analysis, including 1070 infertile men with clinical varicocele indicated a significant reduction of SDF rates following VR. The effect was more evident among the patients with elevated pre-operative SDF values [61]. The ASRM 2015 guidelines recommend VR and antioxidants as valuable methods in reducing SDF [62]. The EAU guidelines also recommend VR in infertile men with high SDF and/or unexplained infertility [63].

Given the paramount role of OS in the pathogenesis of varicocele-mediated infertility, there is significant interest in the use of antioxidants in the management of varicocele as a sole therapy or combined with VR [32, 64]. Additionally, the fact that antioxidants are non-invasive and relatively cheap may encourage their prescription by practitioners for the treatment of varicocele prior to surgical intervention or ART [32]. This has been reflected in a recent global survey of clinical practice patterns in which 39% of reproductive specialists stated that they recommend antioxidant therapy for infertile men with varicocele [65].

A recent monocentric, randomized, double-blind, placebo-controlled trial investigated the effect of 6 months of supplementation with L-carnitine, acetyl-L-carnitine, and other micronutrients on sperm quality in infertile men with oligo- and/or astheno- and/or teratozoospermia with or without varicocele [66]. Sperm concentration, total sperm count, progressive motility, and total motility were significantly increased in the patients that received supplementation, and the positive outcome was more evident in those diagnosed with varicocele. Interestingly, 10/12 spontaneous pregnancies were reported in the supplementation group. Therapy with a combination of pentoxifylline, zinc, and folic acid improved sperm morphology in infertile men with varicocele [67]. Also, zinc supplementation in infertile males with or without VR resulted in a significant increase in sperm motility after two months of therapy, particularly in patients with low seminal zinc concentrations [68].

Microsurgical VR resulted in significantly higher sperm concentration and pregnancy outcomes compared to a combination therapy consisting of clomiphene citrate, vitamin A, vitamin E, selenium, L-carnitine, and pentoxifylline [69]. Administration of vitamin C for 6 months following VR improved sperm morphology and motility, but not sperm count [70]. The intake of N-acetylcysteine, post-varicocelectomy, significantly improved SDF and pregnancy rates [71]. A combination of folic acid and zinc sulfate following VR improved sperm parameters and serum inhibin-B levels, compared to surgery alone or the intake of zinc sulfate or folic acid alone [72].

These results indicate that using antioxidants combined with VR in infertile patients may provide additional benefits to the surgery alone [73]. However, administration of L-carnitine for six months following inguinal varicocelectomy did not benefit the sperm parameters or the SDF compared to surgery alone or placebo [74]. The role of antioxidants therapy in infertile men with varicocele is not clear due to the lack of well-designed studies and the absence of guidelines [75–79]. Future studies are warranted to clarify the role of antioxidants in the management of varicocele-associated male infertility, and to answer many queries related to the type, dose, and duration of antioxidants, as well as the potential complications including reductive stress [75].

Finally, ART is an additional option offered to infertile couples with varicocele under certain circumstances such as failure of natural pregnancy following surgery or advanced female partner's age. ART outcomes in infertile men with clinical varicocele may be enhanced by surgical and/or antioxidant treatment [32].

14.2 Cryptorchidism

Cryptorchidism, undescended testis, is a common birth defect of the male genital tract that is usually diagnosed before male puberty. It is defined as the absence of one or both testes in normal scrotal position. During initial clinical evaluation, it may refer to palpable or nonpalpable testes, which are either cryptorchid or absent. Even if cryptorchidism is generally considered congenital, some cases occur beyond the neonatal period (acquired cryptorchidism). Most common risk factors for congenital cryptorchidism are prematurity, low weight at birth, small gestational age size, breech presentation, and maternal diabetes, while for acquired one, the main risk is retractile testis [80]. Genetic studies report a hereditary risk, but the susceptibility is polygenic and multifactorial. Clustering of undescended testis has been observed in some families affecting different individuals in the same generation with variable phenotype [81, 82]. The most studied genes for nonsyndromic cryptorchidism are INSL3, RXFP2, HOXA10, and HOXA11 [83]. Environmental risk factors include maternal excessive alcohol consumption, smoking (the most debated), increased use of anti-inflammatory/painkillers, and endocrine-disrupting chemicals consumption (particularly diethylstilbestrol) [84–87]. Testicular hormones also regulate testicular descent, and a defective production or action may contribute to the pathogenesis of cryptorchidism. Persistent Mullerian duct syndrome, Klinefelter syndrome (47,XXY), central nervous system, and gastrointestinal disorders are even associated with a higher incidence of cryptorchidism [88–90]. It was also postulated that cryptorchidism is a part of testicular dysgenesis syndrome along with hypospadias, testis cancer, and reduced semen quality [91].

The development of gonads starts during the fifth week of gestation, and cells arise from the posterior abdominal wall of the embryo [92]. Cells' differentiation and their organization proceed to create the histologic compartments within the testicle, and at the same time, the scrotum develops together with the connection to the prostate, creating the sperm route [92]. The most common alteration, occurring during the first trimester and resulting in an extra-inguinal localization of testis, is reported during the migration of germ cells from the posterior abdominal wall toward the inguinal canals and the scrotum [92]. Certain regulatory genes have been identified in animal models to drive gonads descent: insulin-like 3 (INSL3), laxin/insulin-like family peptide receptor 2 (LGRF8), anti-Müllerian hormone (AMH), and HOX gene family [93]. All these genes can be involved in testis descent alteration, and infertility due to impaired spermatogenesis can be associated. Even androgens are required to induce regression of the cranial suspensory ligament and allow testis descent [93].

When an alteration in any of these processes is reported, cryptorchidism can occur. Incidence is 4% of newborns, and in the first year of age 1.5%, unilateral cryptorchidism is more common and is almost twice bilateral [94]. Undescended testis is related with male infertility, but there is an important difference between who has unilateral (treated during first years of life) and those with bilateral and treated later. Studies underling this difference, and paternity ranges from 96% between unilateral treated cryptorchidism to 70% in bilateral cryptorchidism. In these patients, inhibin-B levels differed between unilateral and bilateral undescended testis while testosterone levels were almost similar [95]. These differences are significant to underline that fertility is impaired more because of alteration in seminiferous epithelium than Leydig cell steroidogenesis. Even analysis performed with electron microscopy found higher ultrastructural defects in men with bilateral cryptorchidism than in the control group's unilateral ones [96].

The diagnostic process is not often easy and should start with the physical examination performed in supine, upright cross-legged and standing position that are the best to determine the localization of testis. Scrotal asymmetry is a common clinical sign usually reported in unilateral cryptorchidism [97]. More than 75% of undescended testes are palpable and more than 60% are unilateral usually involving the right side [98, 99]. Analyzing metanalysis and biggest single center series, after surgery, 3–34% of testis were localized in the abdomen, 12% near internal ring, 16–63% canalicular, and all the others near to the external ring [98, 100–102]. Undescended testis can be palpable when are localized along the line of normal descent between the abdomen and scrotum or anterior to the rectus abdominus muscle or, more rarely, in a perirenal, prepubic, femoral, peripenile, perineal, or contralateral scrotal position [101] (Figs. 14.2 and 14.3). Nonpalpable testis are reported when localized in abdominal or transinguinal position, in case complete atrophy or vanishing testis, and when an extra abdominal localization is reported [101].

Hypospadias can be associated with cryptorchidism in 12% to 24% of cases and even small penis can be reported when cryptorchidism is due to hypogonadotropic hypogonadism [101].

The dosage of hormones is important in cases of suspected bilateral atrophy or vanishing testes because elevated basal serum gonadotropin lev-

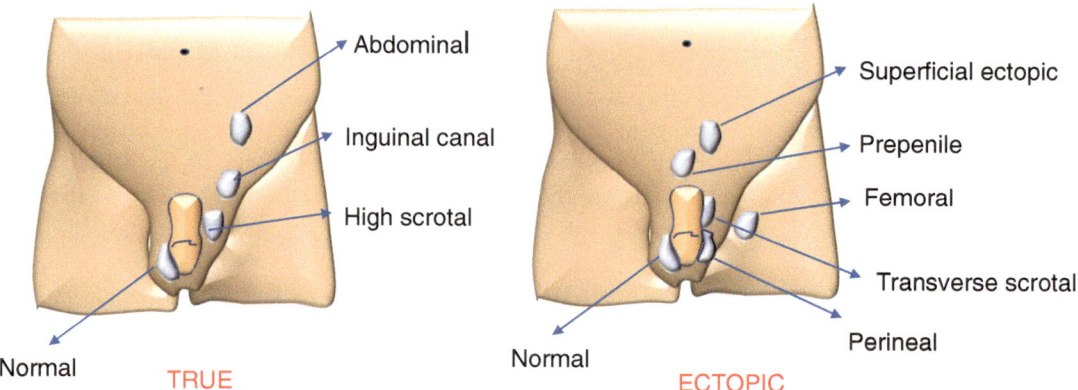

Fig. 14.2 True and ectopic undescended testis localizations

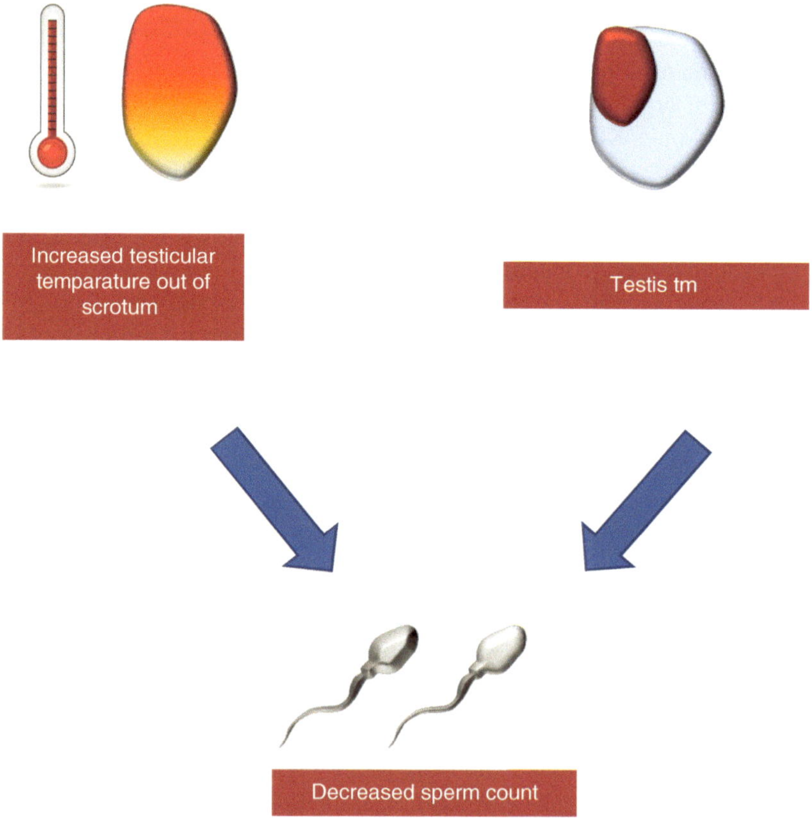

Fig. 14.3 Risks of undescended testis causing infertility

els (FSH and LH), undetectable AMH and inhibin B levels, and no response to hCG stimulation are common [103]. When doubts remain, surgical abdominal exploration is suggested. Diagnostic evaluation often is completed with inguino-scrotal ultrasonography and magnetic resonance imaging, particularly in cases of nonpalpable testis [104, 105]. The first has a sensitivity and specificity of 45% and 78% while the latter of 65% and 100% [104, 106, 107]. There is no specific imaging evaluation for vanishing and atrophic testes that requires initial scrotal exploration because often are near the scrotum, but this approach is useless when a vanishing testis is intraabdominal. Laparoscopy should be performed to confirm or exclude the presence of a viable or remnant abdominal testis, unless a prominent scrotal nubbin is palpable [108, 109]. Usually, diagnostic laparoscopy and contemporary orchidopexy is the preferable approach for all nonpalpable testis [108, 109].

The management of cryptorchism is based on surgical correction. The surgical approach for palpable undescended testis is inguinal orchido-pexy with eventual repair of concomitant hernia [110]. Scrotal surgical approach is a viable alternative [111]. For nonpalpable undescended testis, surgical approach can be open or laparoscopic, in one or two stages and possibly with spermatic vessel transection. In some cases, orchiectomy is required (testis abdominal localization, impossibility of mobilization, or high neoplastic risk) [112]. The surgery is performed to optimize testicular function and cosmesis, prevent testicular malignancy, maintain fertility, and avoid hernia or torsion. After six months of postnatal observation, to allow spontaneous testicular descent, orchidopexy is indicated. This approach is suggested because after six months, spontaneous descent is uncommon, and after the surgery, testis growth is restored [113, 114]. After orchidopexy, studies report that size of the undescended testis is like those of normal contralateral testis [115]. However, final recommendations cannot be made because some series report a difference in size of testes, even if the treatment is performed before puberty [116]. There are not conclusive reports on contralateral fixation of a solitary testis in cases of monarchism. Medical therapy with hormones (hCG or LHRH), to stimulate testes descent and germ cell maturation is no longer suggested because of the lack of conclusive data. The majority of studies report no difference or a slight difference with placebo [117, 118].

Analyzing data regarding fertility in later life, the perfect timing of orchidopexy remains still inconclusive. In general, surgery is suggested before puberty because there is the belief that germ cells development remains quiescent till puberty, causing no remarkable difference if orchidopexy is performed at an earlier age [119]. Negri et al. reported that retrieval of sperm from 30 azoospermic men, affected by undescended bilateral testis and treated with orchidopexy, was not affected by the timing of surgery (overall success rate was 73%) [120]. Another experience with 42 azoospermic patients, once again, does not underline the difference in sperm retrieval success rate if orchidopexy is performed before or after ten years of age (61.9% and 57.1%, respectively) [121]. On the other side, there is a trial with 38 azoospermic men where sperm retrieval success rate was 94% for those who performed orchidopexy up to 10 years of age, 43% between 11 and 20 years, and 44% for those older than 20 years [122]. Finally, in EAU guidelines, it is stated that "paternity in men with unilateral cryptorchidism is almost equal to men without cryptorchidism" (LE:1B). Last but not least, even though it is considered experimental, some centers worldwide offer testicular tissue cryopreservation to children with undescended testis to restore fertility in adulthood [123, 124].

14.3   Inflammation and Seminal Tract Infections

Male accessory gland infections (MAGI) indicate infection and/or inflammation of accessory glands such as the prostate, seminal vesicles, and Cowper's glands. Male genital tract infections (MGTI) is commonly used to indicate the eventual involvement of the complete male genital tract. During MGTI and MAGI, the presence of an elevated number of leukocytes and/or pathogens in semen, together with inflammatory signs, are common.

Male infertility is often linked with MGTIs and is one of the most common cause of male infertility, accounting for approximately 15% of cases. An abnormal leukocyte count is reported in the ejaculate and Chlamydia trachomatis, Escherichia coli, and Neisseria gonorrhoeae are the most common causes of infection [125, 126].

The impaired accessory glands function and genital tract inflammation can affect semen quality, leading to deterioration of spermatogenesis, sperm function alteration, and seminal tract obstruction [127, 128]. Inflammatory response is led by pro-inflammatory cytokines: tumor necrosis factor-α (TNF-α), IL-1α, IL-6 or IL-8 [129, 130].

The most common reported infections are prostatitis and epididymitis, both different between acute and chronic presentation and can lead to seminal tract obstruction. In severe cases, involvement of the testis can cause orchitis with high rates of infertility and sometimes can be a cause of testicular atrophy and spermatogenic impairment [131, 132]. Also, there is a broad spectrum of urethritis caused by both sexually transmitted and non-sexually transmitted pathogens [133, 134].

Usually, pathogens reported for seminal tract infections are bacteria including Chlamydia trachomatis, Urea plasma urealyticum, Neisseria gonorrhoeae, Mycoplasma hominis, and Mycoplasma genitalium [125]. Between Gram negatives, Escherichia coli is the most common and is responsible for most prostatitis and epididymo-orchitis [125]. All pathogens, and especially Chlamydia, can affect semen parameters and sperm function [135–137]. Even if MGTI/MAGI are common, often present asymptomatically (50% of cases) [125], and these silent infections may remain undetected and untreated leading to female partner transmission, severe complications and/or infertility [136–138].

Bacterial prostatitis are classified in accordance with the National Institute of Diabetes, Digestive and Kidney Diseases (NIDDK) of the National Institutes of Health (NIH) and should be distinguished by chronic pelvic pain syndrome (CPPS). The classification include type I—Acute bacterial prostatitis (ABP), type II—Chronic bacterial prostatitis (CBP), type III - Chronic non-bacterial prostatitis (CPPS) divided in IIIA and IIIB (Inflammatory CPPS and Non-inflammatory CPPS), and type IV—Asymptomatic inflammatory prostatitis (histological prostatitis) [139, 140]. Acute bacterial prostatitis is characterized by voiding symptoms and perineal pain that can be associated with malaise and fever. Chronic bacterial prostatitis is defined by symptoms that persist for at least three months. Analyzing prostatitis syndrome, a retrospective trial on more than 1400 patients found that an infectious etiology was found in 74.2% of cases (C. trachomatis 37.2%, T. vaginalis 10.5%, E. coli 6.6%, and U. urealyticum 5%) [141]. Diagnostic evaluation is based on culture of mid-stream urine and the Meares and Stamey test to determine the bacterial strain and choose antibiotic therapies [142, 143]. Further test can include transrectal ultrasound and PSA dosage, and in rare cases prostate biopsy. Therapeutic management is mainly dependent on bacterial strain, inflammation status and symptoms. Fluoroquinolones are the most used antibiotics with second and third generations (ciprofloxacin, levofloxacin, and prulifloxacin) reported to be similarly effective in microbiological eradication [144]. Different antibiotics such doxycycline, azithromycin, and metronidazole have been reported to be effective [144]. Further than antibiotics, phytotherapy or PDE5i can be used in association and may improve symptom relief and quality of life, particularly in patients with chronic prostatitis [145, 146].

Epididymitis, as the second most common MAGI, is characterized by pain, swelling, and increased temperature of the epididymis, which may involve the testis and scrotal skin. The mechanism underlying epididymitis is retrograde reflux of infectious agents. The most common pathogens are C. trachomatis, Enterobacteriaceae (E. coli), and N. gonorrhoeae [147]. Other less commonly seen agents are mumps virus, tuberculosis, or Brucella and Candida spp. Culture of a mid-stream urine is the most used test for diagnosis, while sexually transmitted infections like *C. trachomatis* or *N. gonorrhoeae* should be detected by nucleic acid amplification techniques on first voided urine or urethral swab. The management usually consists of empirical antimicrobial therapy that could be varied when a pathogen is identified. The most commonly used antibiotics are doxycycline and fluoroquinolones. Even azithromycin is effective against *C. trachomatis*. A single high parenteral dose of a third-generation cephalosporin can be used against *N. gonorrhoeae* [148–150]. Rare cases require surgical intervention to drain abscesses or debride tissue.

Urethritis, sometimes involved in male fertility problems, can be divided in infectious or non-infectious, and in gonococcal urethritis (GU) or non-gonococcal urethritis (NGU) if caused by *Neisseria gonorrhoeae* or not. Between non-gonococcal ones, most common pathogens are *Chlamydia trachomatis*, *Mycoplasma genitalium*, *Ureaplasma urealyticum*, and *Trichomonas vaginalis*. Reported symptoms, even useful for correct diagnosis, are mucopurulent or purulent discharge, dysuria, and urethral pruritus. Gram or methylene-blue stain of urethral secretions demonstrate inflammation and the presence of ≥ 10 polymorphonuclear leucocytes per high power field in the sediment from first-void urine sample or a positive leukocyte esterase test are considered positive for urethritis [151, 152]. When a urethritis is suspected, *C. trachomatis*, *M. genitalium*, and *N. gonorrhoea* should be tested with nucleic acid amplification techniques. Usually for gonococcal urethritis, a combination therapy with two antimicrobials is recommended [152]. Ceftriaxone in association with azithromycin should be used as first-line treatment, alternatively ceftriaxone can be substituted with cefixime while doxycycline is an alternative to macrolides [152]. Non-gonococcal urethritis, when a pathogen is not identified, can be treated empirically with doxycycline or alternatively with azithromycin [151]. Moxifloxacine can be used for resistant *M. genitalium* and pristinamycin and josamycin are another alternative [153]. Fluoroquinolones can be considered an alternative to doxycycline and azitromicin when a resistant Clamydia infection is reported [154].

References

1. Minhas S, Bettocchi C, Boeri L, Capogrosso P, Carvalho J, Cilesiz NC, Cocci A, Corona G, Dimitropoulos K, Gül M, Hatzichristodoulou G, Jones TH, Kadioglu A, Martínez Salamanca JI, Milenkovic U, Modgil V, Russo GI, Serefoglu EC, Tharakan T, Verze P, Salonia A, EAU Working Group on Male Sexual and Reproductive Health. European Association of Urology Guidelines on Male Sexual and Reproductive Health: 2021 Update on Male Infertility. Eur Urol. 2021;85:603–20. https://doi.org/10.1016/j.eururo.2021.08.014.
2. Bertolotto M, Freeman S, Richenberg J, Belfield J, Dogra V, Huang DY, Lotti F, Markiet K, Nikolic O, Ramanathan S, Ramchandani P, Rocher L, Secil M, Sidhu PS, Skrobisz K, Studniarek M, Tsili A, Turgut AT, Pavlica P, Derchi LE, Members of the ESUR-SPIWG WG. Ultrasound evaluation of varicoceles: systematic literature review and rationale of the ESUR-SPIWG Guidelines and Recommendations. J Ultrasound. 2020;23(4):487–507. https://doi.org/10.1007/s40477-020-00509-z.
3. Alsaikhan B, Alrabeeah K, Delouya G, et al. Epidemiology of varicocele. Asian J Androl. 2016;18(2):179–81.
4. Shafi H, Esmaeilzadeh S, Agajani Delavar M, Hosseinpour Haydari F, Mahdinejad N, Abedi S. Prevalence of varicocele among primary and secondary infertile men: association with occupation, smoking and drinking alcohol. N Am J Med Sci. 2014;6(10):532–5. https://doi.org/10.4103/1947-2714.143285.
5. Tulloch WS. Consideration of sterility; subfertility in the male. Edinburg Med J. 1952;59:29–34.
6. Agarwal A, Hamada A, Esteves SC. Insight into oxidative stress in varicocele-associated male infertility: part 1. Nat Rev Urol. 2012;9(12):678–90.
7. Goldstein M, Eid JF. Elevation of intratesticular and scrotal skin surface temperature in men with varicocele. J Urol. 1989;142(3):743–5.
8. Green KF, Turner TT, Howards SS. Varicocele: reversal of the testicular blood flow and temperature effects by varicocele repair. J Urol. 1984;131(6):1208–11.
9. Gat Y, Zukerman Z, Chakraborty J, et al. Varicocele, hypoxia and male infertility. Fluid mechanics analysis of the impaired testicular venous drainage system. Hum Reprod. 2005;20(9):2614–9.
10. Smits RM, Mackenzie-Proctor R, Yazdani A, et al. A comprehensive investigation of sperm DNA damage and oxidative stress injury in infertile patients with subclinical, normozoospermic, and astheno/oligozoospermic clinical varicocoele. Andrologia. 2017;49(4):18–27.
11. Agarwal A, Prabakaran S, Allamaneni SSSR. Relationship between oxidative stress, varicocele and infertility: a meta-analysis. Reprod Biomed Online. 2006;12(5):630–3.

12. Saleh RA, Agarwal A, Sharma RK, Said TM, Sikka SC, Thomas AJ Jr. Evaluation of nuclear DNA damage in spermatozoa from infertile men with varicocele. Fertil Steril. 2003;80(6):1431–6. https://doi.org/10.1016/s0015-0282(03)02211-8.

13. Abd-Elmoaty MA, Saleh R, Sharma R, Agarwal A. Increased levels of oxidants and reduced antioxidants in semen of infertile men with varicocele. Fertil Steril. 2010;94(4):1531–4.

14. Zini A, Dohle G. Are varicoceles associated with increased deoxyribonucleic acid fragmentation? Fertil Steril. 2011;96:1283–7.

15. Bahreinian M, Tavalaee M, Abbasi H, et al. DNA hypomethylation predisposes sperm to DNA damage in individuals with varicocele. Syst Biol Reprod Med. 2015;61(4):179–86.

16. Tavalaee M, Bahreinian M, Barekat F, et al. Effect of varicocelectomy on sperm functional characteristics and DNA methylation. Andrologia. 2015;47(8):904–9.

17. Nayeri M, Talebi AR, Heidari MM, et al. Polymorphisms of sperm protamine genes and CMA3 staining in infertile men with varicocele. Rev Int Androl. 2020;18(1):7–13.

18. Samanta L, Agarwal A, Swain N, et al. Proteomic signatures of sperm mitochondria in varicocele: clinical use as biomarkers of varicocele associated infertility. J Urol. 2018;200(2):414–22.

19. Panner Selvam M, Agarwal A, Baskaran S. Proteomic analysis of seminal plasma from bilateral varicocele patients indicates an oxidative state and increased inflammatory response. Asian J Androl. 2019;21(6):544–50.

20. Panner Selvam MK, Samanta L, Agarwal A. Functional analysis of differentially expressed acetylated spermatozoal proteins in infertile men with unilateral and bilateral varicocele. Int J Mol Sci. 2020;21:3155.

21. Agarwal A, Sharma R, Durairajanayagam D, et al. Differential proteomic profiling of spermatozoal proteins of infertile men with unilateral or bilateral varicocele. Urology. 2015;85(3):580–8.

22. Sofikitis N, Miyagawa I. Bilateral effect of varicocele on testicular metabolism in the rat. Int J Fertil. 1994;39:239–47.

23. Sofikitis NV, Miyagawa I, Incze P, Andrighetti S. Detrimental effect of left varicocele on the reproductive capacity of the early haploid male gamete. J Urol. 1996;156(1):267–70.

24. Redmon JB, Carey P, Pryor JL. Varicocele: the most common cause of male factor infertility. Hum Reprod Update. 2002;8(1):53–8.

25. Saleh R, Mahfouz RZ, Agarwal A, Farouk H. Histopathologic patterns of testicular biopsies in infertile azoospermic men with varicocele. Fertil Steril. 2010;94:2482–5.

26. Baazeem A, Belzile E, Ciampi A, Dohle G, Jarvi K, Salonia A, et al. Varicocele and male factor infertility treatment: a new meta-analysis and review of the role of varicocele repair. Eur Urol. 2011;60:796–808.

27. Persad E, O'Loughlin CAA, Kaur S, Wagner G, Matyas N, Hassler-Di Fratta MR, et al. Surgical or radiological treatment for varicoceles in subfertile men. Cochrane Database Syst Rev. 2021;2021:CD000479.

28. Cayan S, Shavakhabov S, Kadioğlu A. Treatment of palpable varicocele in infertile men: a meta-analysis to define the best technique. J Androl. 2009;30:33–40.

29. Kim HJ, Seo JT, Kim KJ, Ahn H, Jeong JY, Kim JH, et al. Clinical significance of subclinical varicocelectomy in male infertility: systematic review and meta-analysis. Andrologia. 2016;48:654–61.

30. Schlegel PN, Sigman M, Collura B, De Jonge CJ, Eisenberg ML, Lamb DJ, Mulhall JP, Niederberger C, Sandlow JI, Sokol RZ, Spandorfer SD, Tanrikut C, Treadwell JR, Oristaglio JT, Zini A. Diagnosis and treatment of infertility in men: **AUA/ASRM** guideline PART II. J Urol. 2021;205(1):44–51.

31. Will MA, Swain J, Fode M, Sonksen J, Christman GM, Ohl D. The great debate: varicocele treatment and impact on fertility. Fertil Steril. 2011;95:841–52.

32. Su JS, Farber NJ, Vij SC. Pathophysiology and treatment options of varicocele: an overview. Andrologia. 2021;53(1):e13576.

33. Lundy SD, Sabanegh ES. Varicocele management for infertility and pain: a systematic review. Arab J Urol. 2018;16:157–70.

34. Ding H, Tian J, Du W, Zhang L, Wang H, Wang Z. Open non-microsurgical, laparoscopic or open microsurgical varicocelectomy for male infertility: a meta-analysis of randomized controlled trials. BJU Int. 2012;110:1536–42.

35. Mehta A, Goldstein M. Microsurgical varicocelectomy: a review. Asian J Androl. 2013;15:56–60.

36. Wang J, Xia SJ, Liu ZH, Tao L, Ge JF, Xu CM, et al. Inguinal and subinguinal micro-varicocelectomy, the optimal surgical management of varicocele: a meta-analysis. Asian J Androl. 2015;17:74–80.

37. Shehata A, Elheny A, El-Sewaify AM. Testicular arterial supply: effect of different varicocelectomy approaches. Egypt J Surg. 2019;38:70–8.

38. Cassidy Dr D, Jarvi K, Grober E, Lo K. Varicocele surgery or embolization: which is better? J Can Urol Assoc. 2012;6:266–8.

39. Practice Committee of the American Society for reproductive medicine and the Society for Male Reproduction and Urology. Report on varicocele and infertility: a committee opinion. Fertil Steril. 2014;102:1556–60.

40. Baazeem A, Belzile E, Ciampi A, et al. Varicocele and male factor infertility treatment: a new meta-analysis and review of the role of varicocele repair. Eur Urol. 2011;60(4):796–808.

41. Jensen CFS, Østergren P, Dupree JM, et al. Varicocele and male infertility. Nat Rev Urol. 2017;14(9):523–33.

42. Smit M, Romijn JC, Wildhagen MF, et al. Decreased sperm DNA fragmentation after surgical varicoce-

lectomy is associated with increased pregnancy rate. J Urol. 2013;189(1 Suppl):S146–50.

43. Hsiao W, Rosoff JS, Pale JR, et al. Varicocelectomy is associated with increases in serum testosterone independent of clinical grade. Urology. 2013;81(6):1213–8.

44. Agarwal A, Deepinder F, Cocuzza M, Agarwal R, Short RA, Sabanegh E, et al. Efficacy of varicocelectomy in improving semen parameters: new meta-analytical approach. Urology. 2007;70:532–8.

45. Schauer I, Madersbacher S, Jost R, Hbner WA, Imhof M. The impact of varicocelectomy on sperm parameters: a meta-analysis. J Urol. 2012;187:1540–7.

46. Nieschlag E, Hertle L, Fischedick A, Abshagen K, Behre HM. Update on treatment of varicocele: counselling as effective as occlusion of the vena spermatica. Hum Reprod. 1998;13:2147–50.

47. Kim KH, Lee JY, Kang DH, Lee H, Seo JT, Cho KS. Impact of surgical varicocele repair on pregnancy rate in subfertile men with clinical varicocele and impaired semen quality: a meta-analysis of randomized clinical trials. Korean J Urol. 2013;54:703–9.

48. Evers J, Collins J, Clarke J. Surgery or embolisation for varicoceles in subfertile men. Cochrane Database Syst Rev. 2008;3:CD000479.

49. de Campos FG. Surgery or embolization for varicoceles in subfertile men. Sao Paulo Med J. 2013;131:67.

50. Kroese AC, de Lange NM, Collins J, Evers JL. Surgery or embolization for varicoceles in subfertile men. Cochrane Database Syst Rev. 2013;131(1):67.

51. Ficarra V, Cerruto MA, Liguori G, Mazzoni G, Minucci S, Tracia A, et al. Treatment of varicocele in subfertile men: the cochrane review—A contrary opinion. Eur Urol. 2006;49:258–63.

52. Esteves SC, Roque M, Agarwal A. Outcome of assisted reproductive technology in men with treated and untreated varicocele: systematic review and meta-analysis. Asian J Androl. 2016;18:254–8. https://doi.org/10.4103/1008-682X.163269.

53. Chen SS, Huang WJ, Chang LS, et al. Attenuation of oxidative stress after varicocelectomy in subfertile patients with varicocele. J Urol. 2008;179(2):639–42.

54. Abdelbaki S, Sabry J, Al-Adl A, et al. The impact of coexisting sperm DNA fragmentation and seminal oxidative stress on the outcome of varicocelectomy in infertile patients: a prospective controlled study. Arab J Urol. 2017;15(2):131–9.

55. Ni K, Steger K, Yang H, et al. A comprehensive investigation of sperm DNA damage and oxidative stress injury in infertile patients with subclinical, normozoospermic, and astheno/oligozoospermic clinical varicocoele. Andrology. 2016;4(5):816–24.

56. Ozturk U, Ozdemir E, Buyukkagnici U, et al. Effect of spermatic vein ligation on seminal total antioxidant capacity in terms of varicocele grading. Andrologia. 2012;44(SUPPL.1):199–204.

57. Mancini A, Meucci E, Milardi D, et al. Seminal antioxidant capacity in pre- and postoperative varicocele. J Androl. 2004;25(1):44–9.

58. Baker K, McGill J, Sharma R, et al. Pregnancy after varicocelectomy: impact of postoperative motility and DFI. Urology. 2013;81(4):760–6.

59. Wang YJ, Zhang RQ, Lin YJ, Zhang RG, Zhang W. Relationship between varicocele and sperm DNA damage and the effect of varicocele repair: a meta-analysis. Reprod Biomed Online. 2012;25:307–14.

60. Qiu D, Shi Q, Pan L. Efficacy of varicocelectomy for sperm DNA integrity improvement: a meta-analysis. Andrologia. 2021;53:1–7. https://doi.org/10.1111/and.13885.

61. Lira Neto FT, Roque M, Esteves SC. Effect of varicocelectomy on sperm deoxyribonucleic acid fragmentation rates in infertile men with clinical varicocele: a systematic review and meta-analysis. Fertil Steril. 2021;116:696–712.

62. Pfeifer S, Butts S, Dumesic D, et al. Diagnostic evaluation of the infertile male: a committee opinion. Fertil Steril. 2015;103(3):e18–25.

63. Minhas S, Bettocchi C, Boeri L, Capogrosso P, Carvalho J, Cilesiz NC, Cocci A, Corona G, Dimitropoulos K, Gül M, Hatzichristodoulou G, Jones TH, Kadioglu A, Martínez Salamanca JI, Milenkovic U, Modgil V, Russo GI, Serefoglu EC, Tharakan T, Verze P, Salonia A, EAU Working Group on Male Sexual and Reproductive Health. European Association of Urology Guidelines on Male Sexual and Reproductive Health: 2021 Update on Male Infertility. Eur Urol. 2021;80(5):603–20. https://doi.org/10.1016/j.eururo.2021.08.014.

64. Moazzam A. Oxidative stress induced infertility in varicocele. Andrology. 2016;5(1):156.

65. Agarwal A, Finelli R, Panner Selvam MK, et al. A global survey of reproductive specialists to determine the clinical utility of oxidative stress testing and antioxidant use in male infertility. World J Mens Health. 2021;39:470–88.

66. Busetto GM, Agarwal A, Virmani A, Antonini G, Ragonesi G, Del Giudice F, Micic S, Gentile V, De Berardinis E. Effect of metabolic and antioxidant supplementation on sperm parameters in oligo-astheno-teratozoospermia, with and without varicocele: a double-blind placebo-controlled study. Andrologia. 2018;50(3) https://doi.org/10.1111/and.12927.

67. Oliva A, Dotta A, Multigner L. Pentoxifylline and antioxidants improve sperm quality in male patients with varicocele. Fertil Steril. 2009;91(4 SUPPL):1536–9.

68. Takihara H, Cosentino MJ, Cockett ATK. Zinc sulfate therapy for infertile male with or without varicocelectomy. Urology. 1987;29(6):638–41.

69. Gamidov SI, Ovchinnikov RI, Popova AV, et al. Current approach to therapy for male infertility in patients with varicocele. Ter Arkh. 2012;84(10):56–61.

70. Cyrus A, Kabir A, Goodarzi D, et al. The effect of adjuvant vitamin C after varicocele surgery on sperm quality and quantity in infertile men: a double blind placebo controlled clinical trial. Int Braz J Urol. 2015;41(2):230–8.

71. Barekat F, Tavalaee M, Deemeh MR, et al. A preliminary study: N-acetyl-L-cysteine improves semen quality following varicocelectomy. Int J Fertil Steril. 2016;10(1):120–6.

72. Nematollahi-Mahani SN, Azizollahi GH, Baneshi MR, et al. Effect of folic acid and zinc sulphate on endocrine parameters and seminal antioxidant level after varicocelectomy. Andrologia. 2014;46(3):240–5.

73. Kızılay F, Altay B. Evaluation of the effects of antioxidant treatment on sperm parameters and pregnancy rates in infertile patients after varicocelectomy: a randomized controlled trial. Int J Impot Res. 2019;31(6):424–31.

74. Pourmand G, Movahedin M, Dehghani S, et al. Does L-carnitine therapy add any extra benefit to standard inguinal varicocelectomy in terms of deoxyribonucleic acid damage or sperm quality factor indices: a randomized study. Urology. 2014;84(4):821–5.

75. Agarwal A, Leisegang K, Majzoub A, et al. Utility of antioxidants in the treatment of male infertility: clinical guidelines based on a systematic review and analysis of evidence. World J Mens Health. 2021;39(2):233–90.

76. Showell MG, Brown J, Yazdani A, et al. Antioxidants for male subfertility. Cochrane Database Syst Rev. 2011;3:CD007411.

77. Showell MG, Mackenzie-Proctor R, Brown J, et al. Antioxidants for male subfertility. Cochrane Database Syst Rev. 2014;12:CD007411.

78. Smits RM, Mackenzie-Proctor R, Yazdani A, et al. Antioxidants for male subfertility. Cochrane Database Syst Rev. 2019;2019(3):CD007411.

79. Ali M, Martinez M, Parekh N. Are antioxidants a viable treatment option for male infertility? Andrologia. 2020;53(1):e13644.

80. Virtanen HE, Toppari J. Epidemiology and pathogenesis of cryptorchidism. Hum Reprod Update. 2008;14:49–58.

81. Czeizel A, Erodi E, Toth J. Genetics of undescended testis. J Urol. 1981;126:528–9.

82. Savion M, Nissenkorn I, Servadio C, et al. Familial occurrence of undescended testes. Urology. 1984;23:355–8.

83. Foresta C, Zuccarello D, Garolla A, et al. Role of hormones, genes, and environment in human cryptorchidism. Endocr Rev. 2008;29:560–80.

84. Thorup J, Cortes D, Petersen BL. The incidence of bilateral cryptorchidism is increased and the fertility potential is reduced in sons born to mothers who have smoked during pregnancy. J Urol. 2006;176:734–7.

85. Jensen MS, Bonde JP, Olsen J. Prenatal alcohol exposure and cryptorchidism. Acta Paediatr. 2007;96:1681–5.

86. Jensen MS, Rebordosa C, Thulstrup AM, et al. Maternal use of acetaminophen, ibuprofen, and acetylsalicylic acid during pregnancy and risk of cryptorchidism. Epidemiology. 2010a;21:779–85.

87. Gill WB, Schumacher GF, Bibbo M, et al. Association of diethylstilbestrol exposure in utero with cryptorchidism, testicular hypoplasia and semen abnormalities. J Urol. 1979;122:36–9.

88. Josso N, Picard JY, Rey R, et al. Testicular anti-Müllerian hormone: history, genetics, regulation and clinical applications. Pediatr Endocrinol Rev. 2006;3:347–58.

89. Sasagawa I, Nakada T, Ishigooka M, et al. Chromosomal anomalies in cryptorchidism. Int Urol Nephrol. 1996;28:99–102.

90. Balsara ZR, Martin AE, Wiener JS, et al. Congenital spigelian hernia and ipsilateral cryptorchidism: raising awareness among urologists. Urology. 2014;83:457–9.

91. Main KM, Skakkebaek NE, Toppari J. Cryptorchidism as part of the testicular dysgenesis syndrome: the environmental connection. Endocr Dev. 2009;14:167–73. https://doi.org/10.1159/000207485.

92. Lewis JM, Kaplan WE. Anatomy and embryology of the male reproductive tract and gonadal development. In: Lipshultz LI, Howards SS, Niederberger CS, editors. Infertility in the male. 4th ed. New York: Cambridge University Press; 2009. p. 1–13.

93. Hughes IA, Acerini CL. Factors controlling testis descent. Eur J Endocrinol. 2008;159(Suppl. 1):S75–82.

94. Barthold JS, González R. The epidemiology of congenital cryptorchidism, testicular ascent and orchiopexy. J Urol. 2003;170:2396–401.

95. Lee PA. Fertility after cryptorchidism: epidemiology and other outcome studies. Urology. 2005;66:427–31.

96. Moretti E, Di Cairano G, Capitani S, et al. Cryptorchidism and semen quality: a TEM and molecular study. J Androl. 2007;28:194–9.

97. Snodgrass W, Bush N, Holzer M, et al. Current referral patterns and means to improve accuracy in diagnosis of undescended testis. Pediatrics. 2011;127:e382–8.

98. Hadziselimovic F. Examinations and clinical findings in cryptorchid boys. In: Cryptorchidism: management and implications. Berlin: Springer-Verlag; 1983. p. 93–8.

99. Cortes D, Thorup JM, Visfeldt J. Cryptorchidism: aspects of fertility and neoplasms. A study including data of 1,335 consecutive boys who underwent testicular biopsy simultaneously with surgery for cryptorchidism. Horm Res. 2001;55:21–7.

100. Docimo SG. The results of surgical therapy for cryptorchidism: a literature review and analysis. J Urol. 1995;154:1148–52.

101. Cendron M, Huff DS, Keating MA, et al. Anatomical, morphological and volumetric analysis:

a review of 759 cases of testicular maldescent. J Urol. 1993;149:570–3.

102. Kraft KH, Mucksavage P, Canning DA, et al. Histological findings in patients with cryptorchidism and testis-epididymis nonfusion. J Urol. 2011;186:2045–9.

103. Lee PA, Coughlin MT, Bellinger MF. Paternity and hormone levels after unilateral cryptorchidism: association with pretreatment testicular location. J Urol. 2000;164:1697–701.

104. Elder JS. Ultrasonography is unnecessary in evaluating boys with a nonpalpable testis. Pediatrics. 2002;110:748–51.

105. Kolon TF, Herndon CD, Baker LA, et al. Evaluation and treatment of cryptorchidism: AUA guideline. J Urol. 2014;192:337–45.

106. Tasian GE, Copp HL, Baskin LS. Diagnostic imaging in cryptorchidism: utility, indications, and effectiveness. J Pediatr Surg. 2011;46:2406–13.

107. Krishnaswami S, Fonnesbeck C, Penson D, et al. Magnetic resonance imaging for locating nonpalpable undescended testicles: a meta-analysis. Pediatrics. 2013;131:e1908–16.

108. Elder JS. Laparoscopy for impalpable testes: significance of the patent processus vaginalis. J Urol. 1994;152:776–8.

109. Moore RG, Peters CA, Bauer SB, et al. Laparoscopic evaluation of the nonpalpable tests: a prospective assessment of accuracy. J Urol. 1994;151:728–31.

110. Hutcheson JC, Cooper CS, Snyder HM 3rd. The anatomical approach to inguinal orchiopexy. J Urol. 2000a;164:1702–4.

111. Bianchi A, Squire BR. Transscrotal orchidopexy: orchidopexy revised. Pediatr Surg Int. 1989;4:189–92.

112. Rogers E, Teahan S, Gallagher H, et al. The role of orchiectomy in the management of postpubertal cryptorchidism. J Urol. 1998;159:851–4.

113. Wenzler DL, Bloom DA, Park JM. What is the rate of spontaneous testicular descent in infants with cryptorchidism? J Urol. 2004;171:849–51.

114. Kollin C, Karpe B, Hesser U, et al. Surgical treatment of unilaterally undescended testes: testicular growth after randomization to orchiopexy at age 9 months or 3 years. J Urol. 2007;178:1589–93; discussion 1593

115. Eijsbouts SW, de Muinck Keizer-Schrama SM, Hazebroek FW. Further evidence for spontaneous descent of acquired undescended testes. J Urol. 2007;178:1726–9.

116. van der Plas E, Meij-de Vries A, Goede J, et al. Testicular microlithiasis in acquired undescended testis after orchidopexy at diagnosis. Andrology. 2013;1:957–61.

117. Pyorala S, Huttunen NP, Uhari M. A review and meta-analysis of hormonal treatment of cryptorchidism. J Clin Endocrinol Metab. 1995;80:2795–9.

118. Henna MR, Del Nero RG, Sampaio CZ, et al. Hormonal cryptorchidism therapy: systematic review with meta-analysis of randomized clinical trials. Pediatr Surg Int. 2004;20:357–9.

119. Grasso M, Buonaguidi A, Lania C, et al. Postpubertal cryptorchidism: review and evaluation of the fertility. Eur Urol. 1991;20:126–8.

120. Negri L, Albani E, DiRocco M, et al. Testicular sperm extraction in azoospermic men submitted to bilateral orchidopexy. Hum Reprod. 2003;18:2534–9.

121. Wiser A, Raviv G, Weissenberg R, et al. Does age at orchidopexy impact on the results of testicular sperm extraction? Reprod Biomed Online. 2009;19:778–83.

122. Raman JD, Schlegel PN. Testicular sperm extraction with intracytoplasmic sperm injection is successful for the treatment of nonobstructive azoospermia associated with cryptorchidism. J Urol. 2003;170(4 Pt. 1):1287–90.

123. Valli-Pulaski H, Peters KA, Gassei K, Steimer SR, Sukhwani M, Hermann BP, Dwomor L, David S, Fayomi AP, Munyoki SK, Chu T, Chaudhry R, Cannon GM, Fox PJ, Jaffe TM, Sanfilippo JS, Menke MN, Lunenfeld E, Abofoul-Azab M, Sender LS, Messina J, Klimpel LM, Gosiengfiao Y, Rowell EE, Hsieh MH, Granberg CF, Reddy PP, Sandlow JI, Huleihel M, Orwig KE. Testicular tissue cryopreservation: 8 years of experience from a coordinated network of academic centers. Hum Reprod. 2019;34(6):966–77. https://doi.org/10.1093/humrep/dez043.

124. Hildorf S, Cortes D, Gül M, Dong L, Kristensen SG, Jensen CFS, Clasen-Linde E, Fedder J, Andersen CY, Hoffmann ER, Sønksen J, Fossum M, Thorup J. Parental acceptance rate of testicular tissue cryopreservation in Danish boys with cryptorchidism. Sex Dev. 2019;13(5–6):246–57. https://doi.org/10.1159/000511158.

125. Pellati D, Mylonakis I, Bertoloni G, Fiore C, Andrisani A, Ambrosini G, et al. Genital tract infections and infertility. Eur J Obstet Gynecol Reprod Biol. 2008;140:3–11.

126. Sandoval JS, Raburn D, Muasher S. Leukocytospermia: overview of diagnosis, implications, and management of a controversial finding. Middle East Fertil Soc J. 2013;18:129–34.

127. Azenabor A, Ekun AO, Akinloye O. Impact of inflammation on male reproductive tract. J Reprod Infertil. 2015;16:123–9.

128. Comhaire FH, Mahmoud AM, Depuydt CE, Zalata AA, Christophe AB. Mechanisms and effects of male genital tract infection on sperm quality and fertilizing potential: the andrologist's viewpoint. Hum Reprod Update. 1999;5:393–8.

129. Koak I, Yenisey C, Dündar M, Okyay P, Serter M. Relationship between seminal plasma interleukin-6 and tumor necrosis factor alpha levels with semen parameters in fertile and infertile men. Urol Res. 2002;30:263–7.

130. Haidl F, Haidl G, Oltermann I, Allam JP. Seminal parameters of chronic male genital inflammation

are associated with disturbed sperm DNA integrity. Andrologia. 2015;47:464–9.

131. Nickel JC, Downey J, Hunter D, Clark J. Prevalence of prostatitis-like symptoms in a population based study using the National Institutes of Health chronic prostatitis symptom index. J Urol. 2001;165:842–5.

132. Choi HI, Yang DM, Kim HC, Kim SW, Jeong HS, Moon SK, et al. Testicular atrophy after mumps orchitis: ultrasonographic findings. Ultrasonography. 2020;39:266–71.

133. Ness RB, Markovic N, Carlson CL, Coughlin MT. Do men become infertile after having sexually transmitted urethritis? An epidemiologic examination. Fertil Steril. 1997;68:205–13.

134. Brill JR. Diagnosis and treatment of urethritis in men. Am Fam Physician. 2010;81:873–8.

135. Köhn FM, Erdmann I, Oeda T, el Mulla KF, Schiefer HG, Schill WB. Influence of urogenital infections on sperm functions. Andrologia. 1998;30(Suppl 1):73–80.

136. Mazzoli S, Cai T, Addonisio P, Bechi A, Mondaini N, Bartoletti R. Chlamydia trachomatis infection is related to poor semen quality in young prostatitis patients. Eur Urol. 2010;57:708–14.

137. Liu J, Wang Q, Ji X, Guo S, Dai Y, Zhang Z, et al. Prevalence of Ureaplasma urealyticum, mycoplasma hominis, chlamydia trachomatis infections, and semen quality in infertile and fertile men in China. Urology. 2014;83:795–9.

138. Ouzounova-Raykova V, Ouzounova I, Mitov I. Chlamydia trachomatis infection as a problem among male partners of infertile couples. Andrologia. 2009;41:14–9.

139. Alexander RB, et al. Elevated levels of proinflammatory cytokines in the semen of patients with chronic prostatitis/chronic pelvic pain syndrome. Urology. 1998;52:744.

140. Alexander RB, et al. Chronic prostatitis: results of an internet survey. Urology. 1996;48:568.

141. Skerk V, et al. The role of unusual pathogens in prostatitis syndrome. Int J Antimicrob Agents. 2004;24(Suppl 1):S53.

142. Zegarra Montes LZ, et al. Semen and urine culture in the diagnosis of chronic bacterial prostatitis. Int Braz J Urol. 2008;34:30.

143. Budia A, et al. Value of semen culture in the diagnosis of chronic bacterial prostatitis: a simplified method. Scand J Urol Nephrol. 2006;40:326.

144. Perletti G, et al. Antimicrobial therapy for chronic bacterial prostatitis. Cochrane Database Syst Rev. 2013;8:CD009071.

145. Cai T, et al. Serenoa repens associated with Urtica dioica (ProstaMEV) and curcumin and quercitin (FlogMEV) extracts are able to improve the efficacy of prulifloxacin in bacterial prostatitis patients: results from a prospective randomised study. Int J Antimicrob Agents. 2009;33:549.

146. Aliaev IG, Vinarov AZ, Akhvlediani ND. Wardenafil in combined treatment of patients with chronic bacterial prostatitis. Urologiia. 2008;6:52–5.

147. Harnisch JP, et al. Aetiology of acute epididymitis. Lancet. 1977;1:819.

148. Street E, et al. The 2016 European guideline on the management of epididymo-orchitis. Int J STD AIDS. 2017;28(8):744–9.

149. Street E, Joyce A, Wilson J. BASHH UK guideline for the management of epididymo-orchitis, 2010. Int J STD AIDS. 2011;22(7):361–5.

150. Workowski KA, Bolan GA, Centers for Disease Control and Prevention. Sexually transmitted diseases treatment guidelines, 2015. MMWR Recomm Rep. 2015;64(RR-03):1–137.

151. Horner PJ, et al. 2016 European guideline on the management of non-gonococcal urethritis. Int J STD AIDS. 2016;27:928.

152. Workowski KA, et al. Sexually transmitted diseases treatment guidelines, 2015. MMWR Recomm Rep. 2015;64:1.

153. Jensen JS, et al. 2016 European guideline on mycoplasma genitalium infections. J Eur Acad Dermatol Venereol. 2016;30:1650.

154. Lanjouw E, et al. 2015 European guideline on the management of chlamydia trachomatis infections. Int J STD AIDS. 2016;27:333.

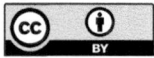

Giorgio Franco, Antonio Franco, and Flavia Proietti

15.1 Introduction

Azoospermia is defined as the absence of sperm in the ejaculate. This diagnosis is confirmed by centrifugation of a semen specimen for 15 min and at least two semen samples obtained more than two weeks apart should be examined [1].

Azoospermia should be distinguished from cryptozoospermia, when rare nemasperms (<500,000) are present after centrifugation of the seminal fluid, and aspermia, defined as the complete absence of seminal fluid emission during orgasm.

Supplementary Information The online version contains supplementary material available at [https://doi.org/10.1007/978-3-031-11701-5_15].

G. Franco (✉) · F. Proietti
Department of Urology, Policlinico Umberto I, Rome, Italy
e-mail: GIORGIO.FRANCO@UNIROMA1.IT;
flavia.proietti@uniroma1.it

A. Franco
Department of Urology, S. Andrea Hospital, Rome, Italy
e-mail: antonio.franco@uniroma1.it

15.2 Classification

Although many causes of azoospermia have been described, all etiologies can be categorized in pre-testicular, testicular, and post-testicular conditions:

- **Pre-testicular** causes include hypothalamic-pituitary-gonadal axis abnormalities.
- **Testicular** causes include intrinsic disorders of spermatogenesis inside the testes.
- **Post-testicular** etiologies include obstruction at any location of the male seminal tract and ejaculatory disfunctions.

In most cases, the assessment of both clinical and laboratory findings, including semen volume, testicular volume, palpable vas deferens and serum FSH, LH, and inhibin B levels, will facilitate the differentiation between the three categories.

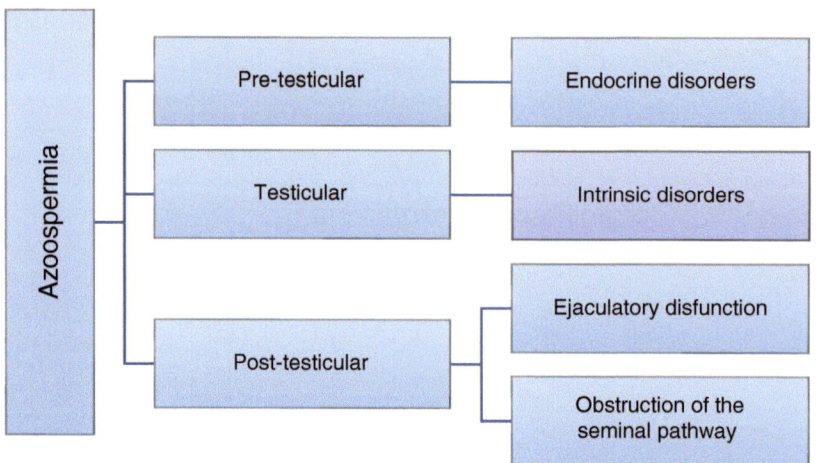

However, azoospermia is more commonly classified into two large groups:

- **Nonobstructive azoospermia (NOA)** or **secretory azoospermia** due to a sperm production impairment (pre-testicular and testicular etiologies).
- **Obstructive azoospermia (OA)** due to an obstruction of the passage of sperm along the seminal tract, leading to a complete absence of sperm in the ejaculate (post-testicular etiologies).

15.3 Epidemiology

The prevalence of azoospermia is approximately 1% among the general male population and ranges between 10% and 15% among infertile men [2]. The prevalence of OA and NOA is variable and depends on geographic areas and authors. However, NOA represents the main cause of azoospermia (60–75%). When considering fertility prognosis, OA showed more favorable outcomes.

15.4 Etiology

15.4.1 Pre-Testicular Etiology

15.4.1.1 Hypogonadotropic Hypogonadism (HH)

It is a very rare cause of NOA (<1%). The condition is characterized by decreased secretion of gonadotropins due to dysfunction of the hypothalamus or the pituitary gland.

HH recognizes both congenital and acquired causes. Congenital HH can be idiopathic (1/3 of the cases) or due to genetic syndromes (Kallmann syndrome, Prader-Willi syndrome). Acquired HH may be caused by pituitary lesions (tumor, granuloma, abscess) or injuries (irradiation, trauma, surgery), illicit drugs intake (anabolic steroids, opiates), alcohol abuse, hyperprolactinemia, and iron overload.

This condition is treatable with medical therapy that consists of gonadotropins (hCG, FSH), androgens, or GnRH administration. Therapeutic management depends on patient's desire for future fertility. Androgen replacement alone (testosterone) is indicated for men who already have children or have no desire for children. Conversely, in men willing to reach fatherhood, treatment with human chorionic gonadotropin (hCG) alone or in combination with follicle-stimulating hormone (FSH) is mandatory to stimulate spermatogenesis.

15.4.2 Testicular Etiology

In almost all cases of NOA, the defect is at gonadal level. Intrinsic disorders of spermatogenesis are derived from genetic mutations, gonadotoxic effects from drugs, undescended testes, varicocele-induced testicular damage, testicular torsion, orchitis, and idiopathic causes.

Despite definition of the exact etiology being desirable, subsequent conventional medical or surgical treatments are ineffective and sperm retrieval represents the only option.

15.4.2.1   Genetic Mutations

Chromosome alterations represent the most frequent genetic cause of azoospermia (15%) [3]. Several conditions have been identified:

Klinefelter syndrome is the most common numerical chromosome anomaly observed in infertile men occurring in 1:500 males [4]. It is characterized by X chromosome polysomy (47, XXY), even if a mosaicism has been also described (10% of cases). Affected men show small and hard testicles, azoospermia, and high levels of gonadotropins with low testosterone levels; the classical phenotype is characterized by tall eunuchoid body proportions.

47, XYY syndrome is caused by paternal non-disjunction during meiosis and occurs in 1:1000 men [5]. Patients present tall stature, azoospermia with normal serum testosterone level.

Y-chromosome microdeletion is caused by mutations of the gene localized in the AZF region (Yq). Three different forms have been identified due to mutation in AZFa, AZFb, and AZFc locus [6]; complete deletion of the AZFa and AZFb loci is always associated with the absence of spermatogenesis, with subsequent worse fertility prognosis [7].

15.4.2.2   Gonadotoxins

Medications (chemotherapy agents, irradiation, androgens, or antiandrogens) or environmental toxins (pesticides, solvents) can directly damage germ cells in the testis or cause disfunction of the Sertoli-cells [8]: in any case spermatogenesis is compromised. Many patients recover a normal sperm production months or years afterwards; however, in some cases, azoospermia is permanent.

15.4.2.3   Undescended Testis

Also defined cryptorchidism, it is a condition characterized by undescended testes/testis into the scrotum during embryonic development. Usually, the testicle remains in the inguinal canal (70%) or in the pre-scrotal region (20%); in these cases, germ cells count is compromised in 20–40% of patients. Conversely, if intra-abdominal retention occurs (8%), spermatogenetic dysfunction is recorded in 90% of cases. The probability of infertility is correlated with bilaterality and degree of retention.

15.4.2.4   Varicocele

The role of varicocele in determining azoospermia is still debated. In most cases, the two conditions are concomitant and not directly correlated. However, some authors have reported a beneficial effect of varicocele treatment in azoospermic patients, with the appearance of sperm in the ejaculate after correction. In particular, this improvement seems to be more likely when a histological diagnosis of hypospermatogenesis is present [9].

Current practice in azoospermic patients with clinically significant varicocele and no other clear causes of azoospermia is to schedule a bilateral TESE for sperm search, freezing, and histological evaluation, with simultaneous or delayed varicocele correction in selected cases [10].

15.4.2.5   Idiopathic Cause

Unfortunately, in almost 50% of NOA, it is not possible to determine the etiology of azoospermia. It is likely that in many of these conditions, an unknown genetical or congenital defect or a previous exposition to toxins is present.

15.4.3 Post-testicular Etiology

Obstruction of sperm transit and ejaculatory dysfunction represent post-testicular causes of azoospermia.

15.4.3.1   Obstruction of the Seminal Pathway

Obstructive conditions may affect:

- Proximal seminal ducts.
  - Efferent ductules (testis).
  - Epididymis.
  - Vas deferens.
- Distal seminal ducts.
  - Deferential ampullas.
  - Ejaculatory ducts.

Testicular Obstruction

Total absence of spermatozoa in the epididymis with preserved spermatogenesis is an extremely rare condition in the isolated form, and it is usually due to congenital malformation. Most commonly, it is associated with epididymal obstruction because of inflammation or infection.

Epididymal Obstruction

This condition is frequently diagnosed in patients with azoospermia (30–67%). Congenital obstruction could be secondary to bilateral agenesis of vas deferens (frequently associated with cystic fibrosis gene mutation) or Young's syndrome. Acquired forms are mostly due to sexually transmitted infections (*N. gonorrhoeae, Chlamydia*) or iatrogenic (blow-out of the epididymal tubules in vasectomized patients, fibrosis after epididymal aspiration, hydrocele repair, or orchiopexy).

Vas Deferens Absence

Congenital bilateral absence of the vas deferens (CBAVD) is found in 1% of infertile men and in up to 6% of those with obstructive azoospermia [11]. There are two possible mechanisms responsible for this condition:

- Mutation of the cystic fibrosis transmembrane conductance regulator (CFTR) gene. More than 800 different mutations have been described, but deletion in exon 10 (delta F508) is the most common mutation found in Caucasian population [12]. CFTR gene mutations have been detected in 80% of patients with congenital bilateral absence of the vas deferens and in 43% of men with unilateral absence [13].
- Abnormalities in the differentiation of the mesonephric duct [14]. Any insult to the Wolffian duct before week seven of gestation may impair urinary and reproductive tract formation including partial epididymal aplasia, seminal vesicle aplasia, or hypospadias, which may lead to a low ejaculate volume. Secondary findings include ipsilateral renal agenesis and imaging confirmation is imperative in patients with unilateral or bilateral absence of the vas deferens, without CFTR gene mutations.

The clinical features of CBAVD include normal testicular volume with normal spermatogenesis and normal levels of FSH. The caput epididymis is always present, but corpus and cauda are found only occasionally. Seminal vesicles are often absent or atrophic, but may also be enlarged or cystic. Spermatozoa can be easily retrieved from the testis or the caput epididymis.

Vas Deferens Obstruction

Vasal obstruction etiologies include vasectomy, inguinal or scrotal surgery such as hernioplasty or hydrocelectomy, infection, or trauma. Inadvertent injury of vas deferens during surgical hernia repair is a common cause of the obstruction. Entrapment for fibrosis induced by contact with the mesh can be also possible. However, the most common cause of obstruction is vasectomy performed for selective sterilization [15]. The diagnosis is suspected when examination reveals normal testicular volume and epididymis full and firm.

Ejaculatory Duct Obstruction

Ejaculatory duct obstruction (EDO) is an uncommon cause of male infertility (1–5%) [16] and represents almost 10% of the obstructive forms of OA. It is characterized by the obstruction of one or both ejaculatory ducts and may be congenital or acquired [17].

Congenital causes of EDO include congenital atresia or stenosis of ED and prostatic cysts (utricular, Mullerian duct, and wolffian duct cysts). Acquired causes include iatrogenic trauma secondary to prolonged catheterization, pelvic or bladder outlet surgeries or pelvic trauma, infectious etiologies, stones, and prostatic abscesses which all may lead to calculi, inflammation, and scarring [17].

Bilateral complete EDO is characterized by low volume (<1.5 mL), low pH, and azoospermia without fructose in the ejaculate in the setting of normal hormonal values. In cases of partial obstruction, the patient may have oligoasthenospermia (OAT) with low-normal volume and low-normal pH. In addition to infertility, other symptoms may include pelvic or scrotal pain exacerbated by ejaculation and rarely hematospermia. Seminal vesicles study usually show dilation.

In absence of anatomic obstruction, there may be dysfunctional voiding of the ejaculatory apparatus without a physical obstruction [18].

Ejaculatory Dysfunctions

Although these represent a relatively unusual cause of male infertility, disorders of ejaculation include a variety of conditions with individualized treatment. Ejaculatory dysfunction should be suspected in any patient with low volume or absent ejaculate. Retrograde ejaculation can be defined as the abnormal backward flow of semen into the bladder with ejaculation; the etiology may be iatrogenic postsurgical, anatomic, neurogenic, pharmacologic, or idiopathic. The diagnosis is made by finding sperm in the post-ejaculate urinalysis.

15.5   Diagnosis

Accurate andrological evaluation is crucial to understanding the etiology of azoospermia.

15.5.1 Medical History

The first step for azoospermia assessment includes a detailed personal history: childhood illness (cryptorchidism, orchitis, testicular tor-

sion), previous testicular trauma or surgery, history of irradiation, or medications.

15.5.2 Physical Examination

General examination can reveal typical phenotypes (Klinefelter syndrome, Kallmann syndrome) and allows sexual development evaluation. Testicular consistency and volume and presence of epididymis, vas deferens, and varicocele should be assessed.

15.5.3 Lab Tests

An endocrine evaluation based on serum testosterone and FSH levels helps to diagnose the majority of clinically significant endocrinopathies. If the testosterone level is low, complete evaluation including free and total testosterone, luteinizing hormone (LH), prolactin (PRL), inhibin B, and estradiol levels should be performed.

Semen analysis can reveal the nature of azoospermia via the evaluation of volume, pH, and fructose. The ejaculate volume is an essential tool in the evaluation of an azoospermic patient, differentiating distal seminal tract obstructions from proximal ones, considering that seminal fluid is mainly due to seminal vesicle production.

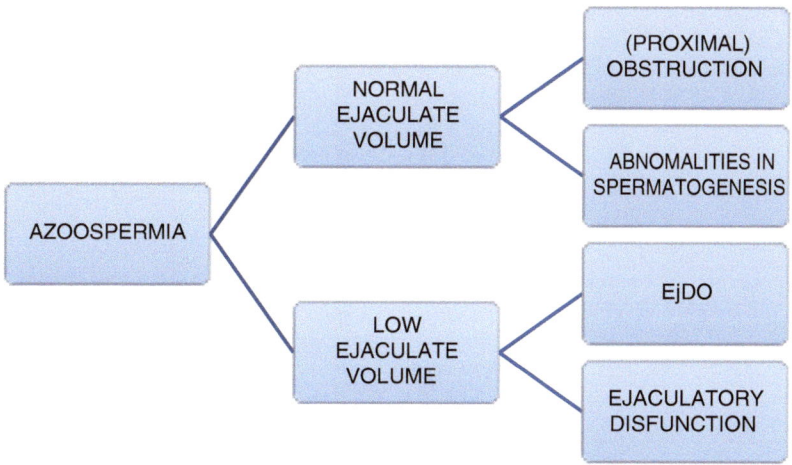

15.5.4 Genetic Screening

Karyotype, chromosome Y microdeletions, and CFTR gene mutations evaluations are advised for patients with azoospermia. Particularly, karyotype and chromosome Y microdeletion assessment must be done when NOA is suspected and in any case before assisted reproductive technique. Conversely, CFTR gene mutation screening is suggested in patients with obstruction. When assisted reproduction techniques (ART) are scheduled, screening should be extended to the partner, to define the risk of development of cystic fibrosis in the newborn.

15.5.5 Radiological Assessment

Testicular ultrasound adds information regarding structure of testicular tissue, testicular volume, epididymal aspect, and presence of varicocele or unpalpable tumor.

Transrectal ultrasound (TRUS) could be useful when ejaculate volume ≤1.5 mL and EjDO is suspected: obstruction should be suspected when seminal vesicle (SV) width is >1.5 cm and ejaculatory duct diameter is >2.3 mm or when cyst or duct calcification is observed [19]. However, TRUS did not show high specificity for EjDO

diagnosis: only 50% of men need surgery based on TRUS findings.

Magnetic resonance imaging (MRI) is showed to be beneficial for soft-tissue and cystic lesions; however, it is expensive, time consuming, and accuracy is not greater than TRUS [20].

15.5.6 Invasive Diagnostic Tools

Seminovesciculography, vasography, testicular fine needle aspiration, open testicular biopsy, and transurethral cyst aspiration can be used to confirm the diagnosis. Today, they are hardly used for pure diagnostic purposes.

15.6 Surgical Treatment

Clinical management depends on etiology of azoospermia. Two main different options are available to procreate:

- Surgical correction, with the goal to restore natural fertility and allow the couple to conceive naturally. It is a valid, and often preferred, option in selected cases of OA.
- Sperm retrieval for assisted reproductive techniques (ART) purposes. It is the only option in case of NOA and in many cases of OA.

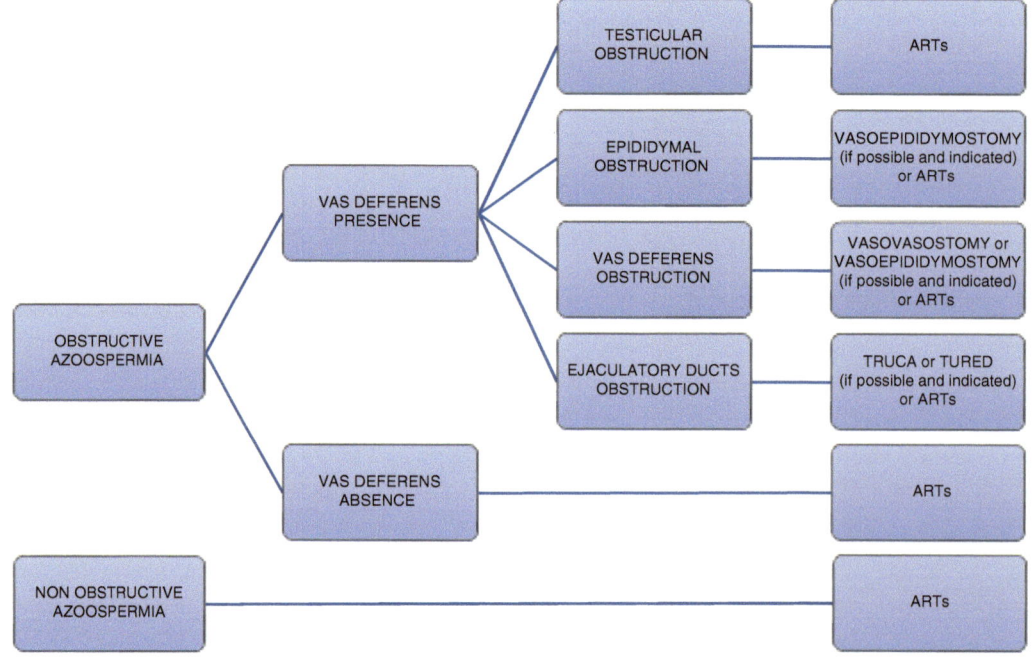

15.6.1 Recanalization of the Proximal Seminal Pathways

15.6.1.1 Vasoepididymostomy

This approach should be considered as first option when epididymal or vasal obstruction is present. The distal cauda epididymis represents the best site to perform the anastomosis due to presence of more robust tubules at this level and a long tract of epididymal tubule left for sperm maturation and motility acquirement. However, multifocal epididymal obstructions require that the anastomosis is performed proximally to all sites of obstruction. Proof of proximal patency is given by finding whole sperm in the open epididymal tubule. A standard microscope for sperm identification in the aspirated fluid is therefore necessary in the operating theatre.

Surgical technique consists in 3–4 cm vertical incision in the anterior aspect of the scrotum, preferably in the median raphe to expose the testis. The vas deferens is identified and transected close to the epididymal cauda. Several techniques have been described for microsurgical vasoepididymostomy, including end-to-side tubulovasostomy, triangulation, and tubular intussusception techniques [21]. However, the end-to-side anastomosis, firstly described by Thomas, is currently the most commonly used technique. It consists of a 1–2 mm incision of the epididymal tubule followed by a two-layer microsurgical anastomosis: a mucosal edge of 4–5 interrupted 10–0 nylon sutures and an additional 10–12 interrupted 9–0 nylon sutures for the outer muscular layer (Fig. 15.1).

Despite the operating microscope representing the gold standard to perform the procedure, robot-assisted surgery has been proposed, but its use is not widespread at present [22].

15.6.1.2 Vasovasostomy

It consists of an end-to-end anastomosis of the vasal stumps, after resection of the obstructed segment. Scrotal, inguinal, or infrapubic incision can be performed [23]. Adequate mobilization of the vas, without compromising vascularization, should be performed to ensure a tension-free anastomosis. However, in case of multifocal obstruction along the vas, recanalization is not indicated.

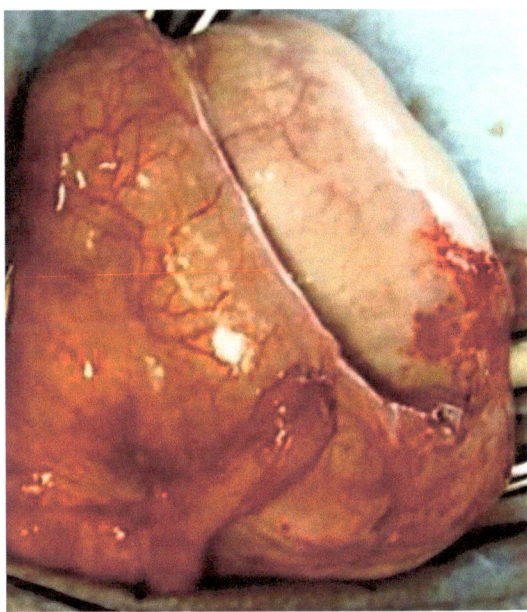

Fig. 15.1 End to side vasoepididymostomy

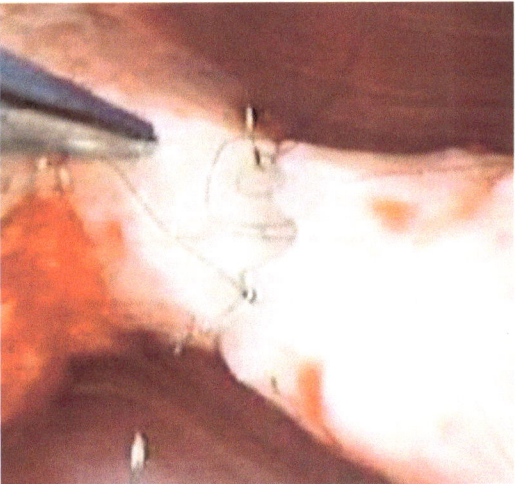

Fig. 15.2 Microsurgical two-layer vasovasostomy

Most surgeons perform vasovasostomy using two-layer microsurgical anastomosis, described by Silber. Like the vasoepididymostomy technique, the procedure consists of 5–6 interrupted 10–0 nylon sutures in the inner mucosal edges of the vas deferens, followed by 10–12 additional interrupted 9–0 nylon sutures in the outer muscular layer (Fig. 15.2) [24]. A modified one-layer anastomosis using interrupted 9–0 nylon suture through the mucosal and muscular layers of the vas has also been described [25]. Again, a robotic vasovasostomy has also been proposed with apparently good results and very high costs (Video 15.6).

The quality of the semen retrieved in the testicular stump represents the most important predictor of outcome and should be considered to assess the best surgical approach. Testicular vasal fluid has been graded according to the quality of the seminal fluid, as follow:

- Grade 1: Prevalence of normal motile sperm.
- Grade 2: Prevalence of normal nonmotile sperm.
- Grade 3: Prevalence of sperm heads.
- Grade 4: Only sperm heads.
- Grade 5: Absence of sperm.

Vasovasostomy should be performed for grades 1–4 [26]. For grade 5 vasal fluid, vasovasostomy should be performed if the fluid is watery and copious. If the fluid is thick and creamy, successful rate of vasovasostomy is low and vasoepididymostomy should be considered, particularly when magnification reveals discolored or indurated area in the epididymis (tubule rupture due to back pressure) or demarcation between collapsed and dilated tubules.

Other variables to consider are obstructive interval, length of the testicular vasal stump, presence of sperm granuloma, prior vasectomy reversal, and surgeon skills [21].

Robot-assisted approach for scrotal or intra-abdominal vasovasostomy as an alternative to microsurgery has been applied to obviate the need for an operating microscope [27].

15.6.2 Recanalization of the Distal Seminal Pathways

Preoperative assessment is crucial to determine appropriate surgical approach. When prostatic cyst is diagnosed, the communication with the ejaculatory ducts should be evaluated.

15.6.2.1 Trans Rectal Ultrasound-Guided Cyst Aspiration (TRUCA)

It is the treatment of choice when a noncommunicating prostatic cyst determines an ab-extrinsic compression and obstruction of the ejaculatory ducts. Both transrectal and transperineal access have been described. The procedure is performed using a sterile disposable needle guidance device mounted over the ultrasound probe puncture; a fine needle (20–22-gauge, 200 mm-long) is inserted into the cyst under real-time ultrasound guidance (Fig. 15.3). Cyst fluid is aspirated and analyzed to evaluate the presence of sperm (400× magnification). Contrast agent is injected to determine the relation with ejaculatory ducts. If the diagnosis of noncommunicating cyst is confirmed (Fig. 15.4) by absence of sperm and radiologic imaging, cyst sclerotization using ethanol 90% is performed.

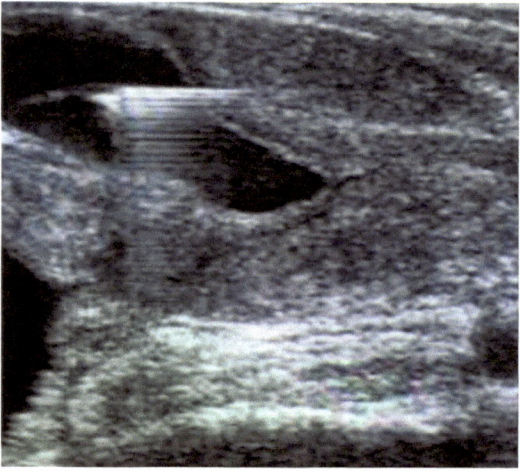

Fig. 15.3 TRUCA: Ultrasonographic guidance of needle into the cyst

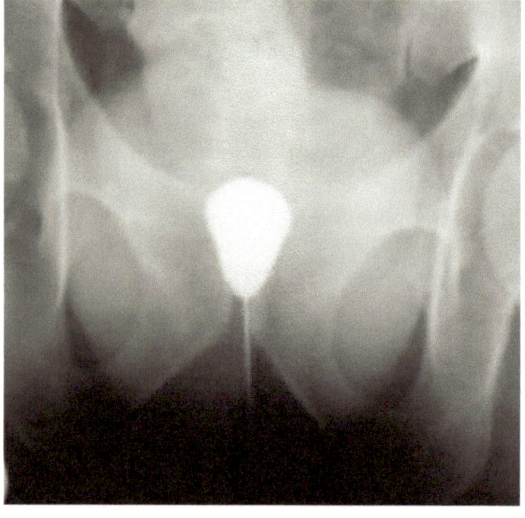

Fig. 15.4 TRUCA: Noncommunicating prostatic cyst

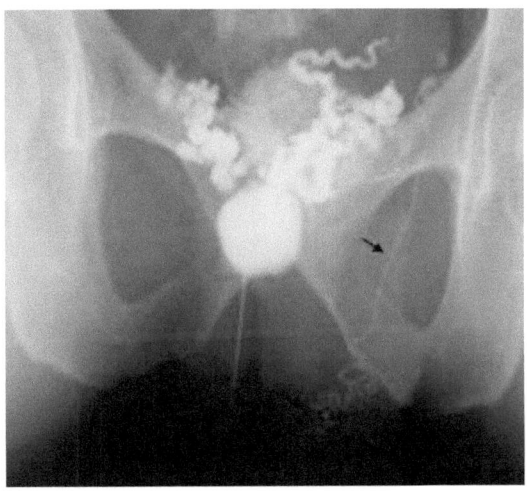

Fig. 15.5 TRUCA: Prostatic communicating cyst. Injection of contrast through transperineal fine needle shows median prostatic cyst communicating with both seminal vesicles and vas deferens (arrows)

15.6.2.2 Transurethral Resection of Ejaculatory Duct (TURED)

In 1973, Farley and Barnes first described stenosis of the ejaculatory duct (ED) and management with transurethral resection [27]. The rationale is to restore the continuity of the seminal ducts, through the resection of the intraprostatic tract of the ejaculatory ducts or the incision of an obstructing prostatic cyst. Surgical technique depends on obstruction etiology. When communicating cyst is diagnosed (Fig. 15.5), its anterior wall is incised using a Collings loop, allowing voiding of the cyst into the prostatic urethra (Video 15.4). Conversely, a "true" resection in performed in case of intrinsic obstruction/stenosis of the ejaculatory ducts, using a U loop. Prior injection of methylene blue into the seminal vesicles can help in identifying the ejaculatory ducts during resection. Simultaneous transrectal ultrasound control could be useful to perform the procedure in a safe manner (Video 15.5). In presence of extraprostatic stenosis or extended atresia of ejaculatory ducts, recanalization is not possible and indicated [28].

15.6.3 Sperm Retrieval Techniques

Sperm retrieval techniques for intracytoplasmic sperm injection (ICSI) represent the only thera-

peutic option in patients with nonobstructive azoospermia (NOA), in those with untreatable obstructive azoospermia (OA), and in cases where female factors are present and require the use of ART. In case of OA, any sperm retrieval technique might be used, either percutaneous or open surgical (MESA; TESA; TESE; PESA), with high probability of obtaining the material needed for ICSI; on the contrary, in case of NOA, it is necessary to use open surgical techniques, TESE or Micro-TESE, with lower chances of success [29].

Obstructive Azoospermia	
MESA	MICROsurgical Epididymal Sperm Aspiration
TESA/ TEFNA	TEsticular sperm aspiration/fine needle
TESE	TEsticular sperm extraction
PESA	Percutaneous epididymal sperm aspiration
Nonobstructive azoospermia	
TESE	TEsticular sperm extraction
Micro-TESE	MICROsurgical testicular sperm extraction

It should be noted that clinical situations might be complex and are best handled by an expert in the field, particularly on surgery of the male reproductive tract, no matter whether specialist in Andrology or Gynaecology. Techniques available today include:

15.6.3.1 MESA

MESA has been considered in the past the gold standard for spermatozoa collection in any cases of OA, as it allowed to obtain more than 1 million/mL sperm counts [30]. The original technique is rarely adopted today due to longer surgical times and higher costs. We developed a simplification of the original technique, named Mini-MESA, which combines the advantages of percutaneous and microsurgical surgery (x). It is performed through a window scrotal incision, allowing exposure of the epididymis head; at this level, the puncture is performed with an insulin needle under direct vision. This procedure allows to recover larger number of gametes, providing plenty of material for cryopreservation. Many studies have compared ICSI results using freshly retrieved or frozen-thawed sperm and the majority of these have concluded that there is no difference in terms of fertilization, implantation, and pregnancy rates [31].

15.6.3.2 TESA/TEFNA

This is the simplest percutaneous technique indicated in case of OA. It permits collection of spermatozoa for immediate ICSI and sometimes for one or more subsequent cycles.

This procedure consists in puncturing the testicle with a butterfly 21 G needle, followed by aspiration of the testicular fluid, which is then analyzed by biologist for retrieving spermatozoa. By maintaining aspiration during the extraction, it is often possible to remove a seminiferous tubule (Fig. 15.6), which is fragmented in a Petri plate for sperm extraction (Video 15.2).

15.6.3.3 PESA

This procedure is similar to TESA, differing only for sampling site, which in this case is represented by the head of the epididymis (Fig. 15.7). The number of gametes that can be obtained is generally higher than TEFNA technique and it is almost always possible to freeze the sample for subsequent cycles. PESA is particularly indicated in case of vas deferens agenesis and in all the other situations where a surgical restoration of the seminal tract is not possible.

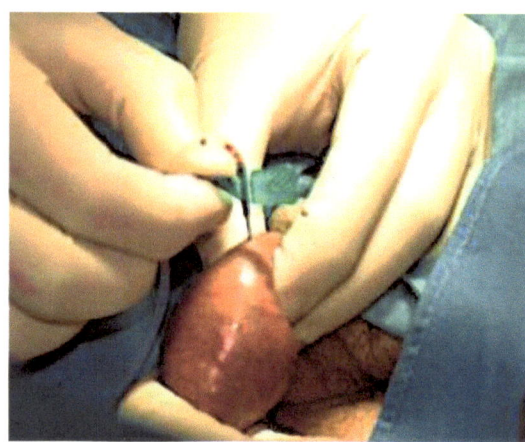

Fig. 15.7 Butterfly 21G needle inserted in the head of epididymis during PESA

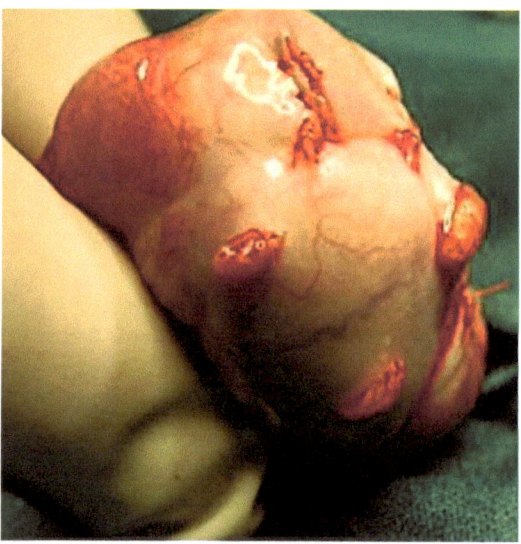

Fig. 15.8 Multiple conventional TESE

15.6.3.4 TESE

This technique is the gold standard in case of NOA. In this case, a surgical biopsy is performed, single or multiple (Fig. 15.8), monolateral or bilateral, with window technique (Fig. 15.9) or with delivery of the testicle. This procedure is more invasive, but allows a good amount of material to be obtained. It is therefore indicated when there is the possibility of cryopreservation, after failure of percutaneous techniques or when differential diagnosis between OA and NOA is not yet discovered. If no spermatozoa are found at first biopsy, multi-

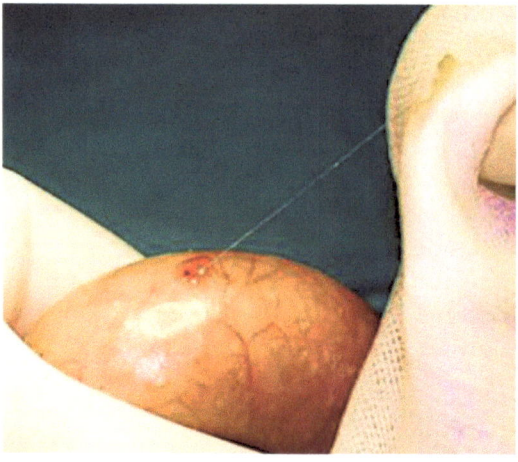

Fig. 15.6 Seminiferous tubule obtained by aspiration during TESA

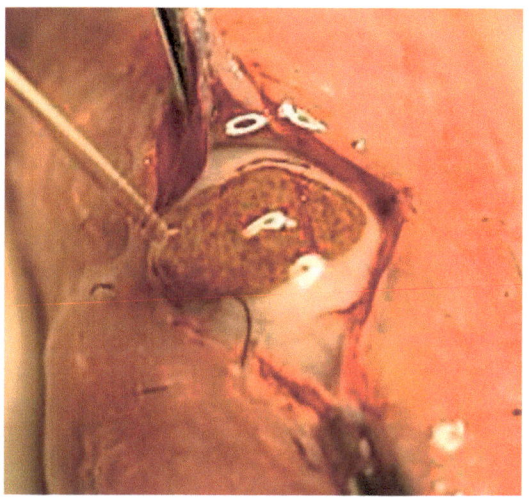

Fig. 15.9 TESE: Window technique

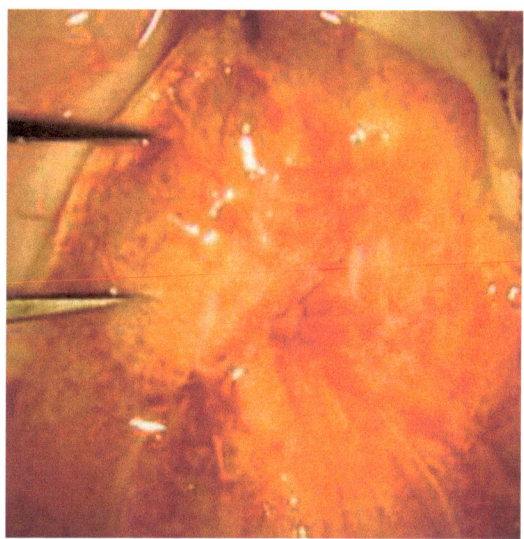

Fig. 15.10 Micro-TESE in a Klinefelter patient. Area of dilated tubules is visible between the forceps tips

ple biopsies are taken at different testicular sites [32]. Sperm recovery rate in NOA is around 50–60% [33], in contrast to OA cases where gametes can be recovered in all patients [34]. The appropriate number of biopsies to be performed is variable, but studies have shown that if gametes are present, they are often found within the first 4 biopsies [35]. Approximately half of the cases with positive results occur on the first sample [36] (Video 15.3).

15.6.3.5 MICRO-TESE

This approach, also known as Microdissection TESE, proposed by Schlegel in 1999, presents, as important innovation, the use of an operating microscope for gamete retrieval, resulting in higher success rate and fewer complications compared to TESE with multiple biopsies [37]. It consists in a single equatorial incision of the tunica albuginea and opening of the testicle; then, single seminiferous tubules are sampled from different areas of the testicular parenchyma by using microsurgical forceps and an operating microscope, and then sent to the laboratory for spermatozoa extraction. Optical magnification of the microscope enables to recognize and collect seminiferous tubules of larger diameter (Fig. 15.10), more likely containing spermatozoa [38]. This scenario of focally dilated tubules, typical of some patients with incomplete Sertoli Cells Only Syndrome (SCOS), is unfortu-

nately detectable in only 30% cases of NOA. At the end, the incision is closed with a running suture with minimal scarring (Video 15.1).

The advantages of Micro-TESE over multiple TESE are: less vascular damage, minor tissue loss, less postoperative pain due to reduced retraction of the albuginea, and less compression of the testicular parenchyma [37]. According to literature, this technique is often chosen in case of failure of conventional TESE or in severe conditions of azoospermia (SCOS, Klinefelter's syndrome) [32, 33]. Considering that in approximately 50% of naïve NOA cases, spermatozoa are recovered at the first biopsy, a 'gradual' Micro-TESE technique has been proposed by our group [39]. Under general or local anaesthesia (cord block and skin infiltration), an initial scrotal window incision is performed, similarly to traditional TESE, and a single testicular biopsy is extracted from mid-portion of the testis. The sample is immediately sent to the biological laboratory together with a specimen for histology and, if spermatozoa are found, the procedure is ended. If no spermatozoa are found, however, the incision is extended equatorially until the testis is fully opened and Micro-TESE is performed. In this way, a considerable saving of Micro-TESE procedures and consequent surgical invasiveness on testis may be achieved, with significant reduction in operating time and costs. This makes sense, if we consider that a significant hormonal impairment has been described after one or more Micro-TESE procedures [39, 40]. Histological examination is also highly desirable during TESE and Micro-TESE (at least one sample per testicle). This will provide useful prognostic information for possible re-interventions and may exclude intratubular germ cell neoplasia presence, a well-known possibility in azoospermic subjects, in consideration of the links between male infertility and germ cell neoplasia.

15.6.3.6 New Horizons

One of the major challenges in sperm retrieval surgery is represented by the preoperative prediction of successful sperm retrieval. Many predictive markers or models have been proposed such as histology, FSH, or other hormones levels and testicular volume, with debated values of efficacy. For the future, the presence of some omics in seminal plasma, particularly microRNA, appears particularly promising in detecting testes which contain areas of spermatogenesis [41].

Although micro-TESE has become first-line in sperm retrieval in men with NOA, there are some challenges with the procedure. For this reason, new interesting methods have been proposed: some of the latest advances on the horizon, such as multiphoton microscopy (MPM), Raman spectroscopy (RS), and full-field optical coherence tomography (FFOCT), have demonstrated the potential to better identify areas of spermatogenesis and improve sperm extraction success. Furthermore, ORBEYE (a novel 4 K three-dimensional [3D] surgical exoscope), Contrast Enhanced Ultrasonography (CEUS), and artificial intelligence have been mentioned, nowadays, as new strategies to enhance sperm retrieval for ART [42].

Although these new procedures seem to appear very sophisticated, showing higher magnification of the surgical field, faster operating time and, in some cases, less invasiveness, their reproducibility and higher costs and the absence of strong and solid human clinical trial indicate that their role in sperm retrieval surgery is still to be established.

References

1. WHO. World Health Organization: WHO Laboratory manual for the examination and processing of human semen—5th ed. Geneva: WHO Press, 2010.
2. Jarow JP, Espeland MA, Lipshultz LI. Evaluation of the azoospermic patient. J Urol. 1989;142(1):62–5. https://doi.org/10.1016/s0022-5347(17)38662-7.
3. Pandiyan N, Jequier AM. Mitotic chromosomal anomalies among 1210 infertile men. Hum Reprod. 1996;11(12):2604–8. https://doi.org/10.1093/oxfordjournals.humrep.a019178.
4. Van Assche E, Bonduelle M, Tournaye H, Joris H, Verheyen G, Devroey P, Van Steirteghem A, Liebaers I. Cytogenetics of infertile men. Hum Reprod. 1996;11(Suppl 4):1–24.; discussion 25-6. https://doi.org/10.1093/humrep/11.suppl_4.1.
5. Turek PJ, Pera RA. Current and future genetic screening for male infertility. Urol Clin North Am. 2002;29(4):767–92. https://doi.org/10.1016/s0094-0143(02)00090-3.
6. Vogt P, Chandley AC, Hargreave TB, Keil R, Ma K, Sharkey A. Microdeletions in interval 6 of the Y chromosome of males with idiopathic sterility point to disruption of AZF, a human spermatogenesis gene. Hum Genet. 1992;89(5):491–6. https://doi.org/10.1007/BF00219172.
7. European Association of Urology. Guidelines on male infertility. Eur Urol. 2012;62:324–32.
8. Nudell DM, Monoski MM, Lipshultz LI. Common medications and drugs: how they affect male fertility. Urol Clin North Am. 2002;29(4):965–73. https://doi.org/10.1016/s0094-0143(02)00079-4.
9. Cocuzza M, Cocuzza MA, Bragais FM, Agarwal A. The role of varicocele repair in the new era of assisted reproductive technology. Clinics (Sao Paulo). 2008;63(3):395–404. https://doi.org/10.1590/s1807-59322008000300018.
10. Esteves SC, Oliveira FV, Bertolla RP. Clinical outcome of intracytoplasmic sperm injection in infertile men with treated and untreated clinical varicocele. J Urol. 2010;184(4):1442–6. https://doi.org/10.1016/j.juro.2010.06.004.
11. Ferlin A, Raicu F, Gatta V, Zuccarello D, Palka G, Foresta C. Male infertility: role of genetic background. Reprod Biomed Online. 2007;14(6):734–45. https://doi.org/10.1016/s1472-6483(10)60677-3.
12. Uzun S, Gökçe S, Wagner K. Cystic fibrosis transmembrane conductance regulator gene mutations in infertile males with congenital bilateral absence of the vas deferens. Tohoku J Exp Med. 2005;207(4):279–85. https://doi.org/10.1620/tjem.207.279.
13. Claustres M. Molecular pathology of the CFTR locus in male infertility. Reprod Biomed Online. 2005;10(1):14–41. https://doi.org/10.1016/s1472-6483(10)60801-2.
14. McCallum T, Milunsky J, Munarriz R, Carson R, Sadeghi-Nejad H, Oates R. Unilateral renal agenesis associated with congenital bilateral absence of the vas

deferens: phenotypic findings and genetic considerations. Hum Reprod. 2001;16(2):282–8. https://doi.org/10.1093/humrep/16.2.282.

15. Costabile RA, Spevak M. Characterization of patients presenting with male factor infertility in an equal access, no cost medical system. Urology. 2001;58(6):1021–4. https://doi.org/10.1016/s0090-4295(01)01400-5.

16. Modgil V, Rai S, Ralph DJ, Muneer A. An update on the diagnosis and management of ejaculatory duct obstruction. Nat Rev Urol. 2016;13(1):13–20. https://doi.org/10.1038/nrurol.2015.276.

17. Pryor JP, Hendry WF. Ejaculatory duct obstruction in subfertile males: analysis of 87 patients. Fertil Steril. 1991;56(4):725–30. https://doi.org/10.1016/s0015-0282(16)54606-8.

18. Font MD, Pastuszak AW, Case JR, Lipshultz LI. An infertile male with dilated seminal vesicles due to functional obstruction. Asian J Androl. 2017;19(2):256–7. https://doi.org/10.4103/1008-682X.179858.

19. Avellino GJ, Lipshultz LI, Sigman M, Hwang K. Transurethral resection of the ejaculatory ducts: etiology of obstruction and surgical treatment options. Fertil Steril. 2019;111(3):427–43. https://doi.org/10.1016/j.fertnstert.2019.01.001.

20. Engin G, Kadioğlu A, Orhan I, Akdöl S, Rozanes I. Transrectal US and endorectal MR imaging in partial and complete obstruction of the seminal duct system. A comparative study. Acta Radiol. 2000;41(3):288–95. https://doi.org/10.1080/028418500127345271.

21. Practice Committee of the American Society for Reproductive Medicine in collaboration with the Society for Male Reproduction and Urology. Electronic address: asrm@asrm.org. The management of obstructive azoospermia: a committee opinion. Fertil Steril. 2019;111(5):873–80. https://doi.org/10.1016/j.fertnstert.2019.02.013.

22. Parekattil SJ, Gudeloglu A, Brahmbhatt J, Wharton J, Priola KB. Robotic assisted versus pure microsurgical vasectomy reversal: technique and prospective database control trial. J Reconstr Microsurg. 2012;28(7):435–44. https://doi.org/10.1055/s-0032-1315788.

23. Belker AM. Infrapubic incision for specific vasectomy reversal situations. Urology. 1988;32(5):413–5. https://doi.org/10.1016/0090-4295(88)90412-8.

24. Silber SJ. Perfect anatomical reconstruction of vas deferens with a new microscopic surgical technique. Fertil Steril. 1977;28(1):72–7.

25. Herrel LA, Goodman M, Goldstein M, Hsiao W. Outcomes of microsurgical vasovasostomy for vasectomy reversal: a meta-analysis and systematic review. Urology. 2015;85(4):819–25. https://doi.org/10.1016/j.urology.2014.12.023.

26. Sigman M. The relationship between intravasal sperm quality and patency rates after vasovasostomy. J Urol. 2004;171(1):307–9. https://doi.org/10.1097/01.ju.0000102322.90257.8b.

27. Barazani Y, Kaouk J, Sabanegh ES Jr. Robotic intra-abdominal vasectomy reversal: a new approach to a difficult problem. Can Urol Assoc J. 2014;8(5–6):E439–41. https://doi.org/10.5489/cuaj.1947.

28. Farley S, Barnes R. Stenosis of ejaculatory ducts treated by endoscopic resection. J Urol. 1973;109(4):664–6. https://doi.org/10.1016/s0022-5347(17)60510-x.

29. Lee R, Li PS, Goldstein M, Schattman G, Schlegel PN. A decision analysis of treatments for nonobstructive azoospermia associated with varicocele. Fertil Steril. 2009;92(1):188–96. https://doi.org/10.1016/j.fertnstert.2008.05.053.

30. Bernie AM, Ramasamy R, Stember DS, Stahl PJ. Microsurgical epididymal sperm aspiration: indications, techniques and outcomes. Asian J Androl. 2013;15(1):40–3. https://doi.org/10.1038/aja.2012.114.

31. Oates RD, Lobel SM, Harris DH, Pang S, Burgess CM, Carson RS. Efficacy of intracytoplasmic sperm injection using intentionally cryopreserved epididymal spermatozoa. Hum Reprod. 1996;11(1):133–8. https://doi.org/10.1093/oxfordjournals.humrep.a019006.

32. Turunc T, Gul U, Haydardedeoglu B, Bal N, Kuzgunbay B, Peskircioglu L, Ozkardes H. Conventional testicular sperm extraction combined with the microdissection technique in nonobstructive azoospermic patients: a prospective comparative study. Fertil Steril. 2010;94(6):2157–60. https://doi.org/10.1016/j.fertnstert.2010.01.008.

33. Marconi M, Keudel A, Diemer T, Bergmann M, Steger K, Schuppe HC, Weidner W. Combined trifocal and microsurgical testicular sperm extraction is the best technique for testicular sperm retrieval in "low-chance" nonobstructive azoospermia. Eur Urol. 2012;62(4):713–9. https://doi.org/10.1016/j.eururo.2012.03.004.

34. Greco E, Scarselli F, Iacobelli M, Rienzi L, Ubaldi F, Ferrero S, Franco G, Anniballo N, Mendoza C, Tesarik J. Efficient treatment of infertility due to sperm DNA damage by ICSI with testicular spermatozoa. Hum Reprod. 2005;20(1):226–30. https://doi.org/10.1093/humrep/deh590.

35. Shah R. Surgical sperm retrieval: techniques and their indications. Indian J Urol. 2011;27(1):102–9. https://doi.org/10.4103/0970-1591.78439.

36. Ostad M, Liotta D, Ye Z, Schlegel PN. Testicular sperm extraction for nonobstructive azoospermia: results of a multibiopsy approach with optimized tissue dispersion. Urology. 1998;52(4):692–6. https://doi.org/10.1016/s0090-4295(98)00322-7.

37. Ramasamy R, Ricci JA, Leung RA, Schlegel PN. Successful repeat microdissection testicular sperm extraction in men with nonobstructive azoospermia. J Urol. 2011;185(3):1027–31. https://doi.org/10.1016/j.juro.2010.10.066.

38. Caroppo E, Colpi EM, Gazzano G, Vaccalluzzo L, Piatti E, D'Amato G, Colpi GM. The seminiferous tubule caliber pattern as evaluated at high magnification during microdissection testicular sperm extraction predicts sperm retrieval in patients with non-obstructive azoospermia. Andrology. 2019;7(1):8–14. https://doi.org/10.1111/andr.12548.

39. Franco G, Scarselli F, Casciani V, De Nunzio C, Dente D, Leonardo C, Greco PF, Greco A, Minasi MG, Greco E. A novel stepwise micro-TESE approach in non obstructive azoospermia. BMC Urol. 2016;16(1):20. https://doi.org/10.1186/s12894-016-0138-6.

40. Takada S, Tsujimura A, Ueda T, Matsuoka Y, Takao T, Miyagawa Y, Koga M, Takeyama M, Okamoto Y, Matsumiya K, Fujioka H, Nonomura N, Okuyama A. Androgen decline in patients with nonobstructive azoospemia after microdissection testicular sperm extraction. Urology. 2008;72(1):114–8. https://doi.org/10.1016/j.urology.2008.02.022.

41. Zarezadeh R, Nikanfar S, Oghbaei H, et al. Omics in seminal plasma: an effective strategy for predicting sperm retrieval outcome in non-obstructive azoospermia. Mol Diagn Ther. 2021;25:315–25. https://doi.org/10.1007/s40291-021-00524-8.

42. Kresch E, Efimenko I, Gonzalez D, Rizk PJ, Ramasamy R. Novel methods to enhance surgical sperm retrieval: a systematic review. Arab J Urol. 2021;19(3):227–37. https://doi.org/10.1080/2090598X.2021.1926752.

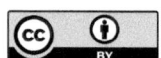

Pathophysiology of Female Reproduction and Clinical Management

16

Luigi Nappi, Felice Sorrentino, Francesca Greco,
Laura Vona, Francesco Maria Zullo,
and Stefano Bettocchi

Fecundability is the ability to conceive. Successful pregnancy requires a complex sequence that includes ovulation, ovum pick-up by a fallopian tube, fertilization, transport of a fertilized ovum into the uterus, and implantation into a receptive uterine cavity. Various studies show a monthly probability of conceiving up to 20–25%.

The female genital system is made up of dynamic organs that change during the woman's life cycle.

Schematically, during the period between two menses, it can be divided into:

- **Ovarian Cycle**: It consists of the growth and development of the ovarian follicle, its bursting, and transformation into the corpus luteum with relative production of estrogens and progesterone.
- **Menstrual Cycle**: It consists of the modifications of the endometrium, affected by ovarian hormones, that has to be prepared to accommodate the fertilized egg.

The normal menstrual cycle is the result of the integration of the primary neuroendocrine complex (the hypothalamus–pituitary–ovarian axis) into a control system regulated by a series of peripheral mechanisms of feedback and nerve signals that result in the release of a **single mature oocyte** from a pool of hundreds of thousands of primordial oocytes [1, 2].

16.1 Hypothalamic–Pituitary Axis [3–5]

The hypothalamus is made up of a series of nuclei located at the base of the brain, whose neurons contract synapses throughout the central nervous system. It is linked with the anterior pituitary gland by the portal system of blood supply. The posterior pituitary gland or neurohypophysis is like a "repository" for the hypothalamic hormones ADH and oxytocin. In fact, it contains the axonal terminals of neurons arising in the supraoptic (SO) nucleus that produces ADH and paraventricular nucleus (PVN) that produces oxytocin of the hypothalamus.

The hypothalamus produces GnRh, a decapeptide which stimulates gonadotropins biosynthesis and secretion: follicle-stimulating hormone (FSH) and luteinizing hormone (LH). Pulsatile GnRh input is required for activation and maintenance of GnRh receptors; changes in GnRh pulse frequency affect the absolute levels and the ratio of LH and FSH release.

L. Nappi (✉) · F. Sorrentino · F. Greco · L. Vona
F. M. Zullo · S. Bettocchi
Department of Medical and Surgical Sciences,
Institute of Obstetrics and Gynecology, University of
Foggia, Foggia, Italy
e-mail: l.nappi@unifg.it; stefano.bettocchi@unifg.it

© The Author(s) 2023
C. Bettocchi et al. (eds.), *Practical Clinical Andrology*,
https://doi.org/10.1007/978-3-031-11701-5_16

The anterior pituitary gland contains five hormone-producing cell types: gonadotrophs (LH and FSH), lactotrophs (PRL), somatotrophs (GH), thyrotrophs (TSH), and adrenocortico-trophs (ACTH). All the pituitary hormones are stimulated by hypothalamic neuroendocrine secretion, while PRL is under tonic inhibition and its expression is primarily under inhibitory regulation by dopamine. In fact, the gonadotro-pins (LH and FSH) are regulated by GnRH. The biosynthesis of ACTH is stimulated by the corticotropin-releasing hormone. The secretion of TSH is induced by the Thyrotropin-releasing hormone.

By convention, the first day of menses repre-sents the first day of the cycle (day 1). The cycle is then divided into two phases: follicular and luteal.

- The follicular phase begins with the onset of menses and ends on the day before the LH surge.
- The luteal phase begins on the day of the LH surge and ends at the onset of the next menses.

An average menstrual cycle lasts from 28 to 35 days, with approximately 14 to 21 days in the follicular phase and 14 days in the luteal phase [1, 2]. Changes in the intermenstrual interval are primarily due to changes in the follicular phase; in comparison, the luteal phase remains relatively constant.

16.2   Early Follicular Phase

In the early follicular phase, the ovary is least hor-monally active, resulting in low serum estradiol and progesterone concentrations. Influenced from the negative feedback effects of estradiol, proges-terone and probably inhibin, there is an increase in gonadotropin-releasing hormone (GnRH) pulse frequency and a subsequent increase in serum fol-licle-stimulating hormone (FSH) concentrations of approximately 30% [6]. This small increase in FSH secretion appears to be required for the recruitment of the next cohort of developing folli-cles, one of which will become the dominant and then ovulatory follicle during that cycle [7–9]. There is also a rapid increase in LH pulse fre-quency at this time, from one pulse every four hours in the late luteal phase to one pulse every 90 min in the early follicular phase [10]. Serum anti-Müllerian hormone (AMH) has been used as a potential marker of ovarian health and aging. It is secreted by small antral follicles and correlates with the total number of ovarian antral follicles. The variability of serum AMH across the men-strual cycle appears to be minimal [11].

16.2.1   Ovaries and Endometrium

The ovary is quiescent in the early follicular phase, except for the occasionally visible resolv-ing corpus luteum from the previous cycle. It is possible to see small follicles of 3 to 8 mm in diameter at this time. The endometrium is rela-tively indistinct during menses becoming a thin line once menses are completed.

16.3   Mid-Follicular Phase

The moderate rise in follicle-stimulating hor-mone (FSH) secretion progressively stimulates folliculogenesis and estradiol production, leading to progressive growth of the cohort of follicles selected. When several follicles initially grow to the antral stage, their granulosa cells increase in the size and divide, producing increasing serum concentrations of estradiol via FSH stimulation of aromatase and then inhibin A from the granu-losa cells in the ovaries. The increase in estradiol production negatively affects the hypothalamus–pituitary axis, suppressing the FSH and LH con-centrations as well as the LH pulse amplitude. At the same time, the gonadotropin-releasing hor-mone (GnRH) pulse generator accelerates slightly to a mean LH pulse frequency of approx-imately one per hour (versus one per 90 min in the early follicular phase). This GnRH stimula-tion is probably due to the negative feedback effects of progesterone from the previous luteal phase.

16.3.1 Ovarian and Endometrial Changes

Several antral follicles of 9–10 mm are visible on ovarian ultrasonography. There is a proliferation of the uterine endometrium that becomes thicker with an increase in the number of glands and the typical aspect of a "triple stripe" due to the increased concentrations of estradiol [12].

16.4 Late Follicular Phase

During the week before ovulation, the growing follicle induces the increase of estradiol and inhibin A. This increase of the estradiol is responsible for reducing the concentrations of FSH and luteinizing hormone LH due to negative feedback effects. Once the dominant follicle has been selected, FSH induces LH receptors in the ovary and increases ovarian secretion of intrauterine growth factors.

16.4.1 Ovarian, Endometrial, and Cervical Mucus Changes

A single dominant follicle has been selected. It increases in size 2 mm per day until a mature size of 20 to 26 mm is reached. The rest of the growing cohort of follicles gradually stop developing and undergo atresia. There is a gradual thickening of the uterine endometrium due to the rising of estradiol concentrations and changes of the cervical mucus; in particular, there is an increase in the amount and "stringiness".

16.5 Midcycle Surge and Ovulation

One day before the ovulation, an important neuroendocrine phenomenon occurs: the midcycle surge [10, 13]. It consists of a switch from negative feedback control of LH secretion by ovarian hormones (such as estradiol and progesterone) to a sudden positive feedback effect, resulting in an increase in serum LH concentrations and a smaller rise in FSH concentrations. This is probably due to an increase in the number of pituitary gonadotropin-releasing hormone (GnRH) receptors, but there is probably no change in GnRH input to the pituitary gland [14]. At this time, the amplitude of the LH pulses increases drastically even if the frequency of LH pulses continues to be approximately one per hour [15].

16.5.1 Ovarian Changes

The LH surge is responsible for important changes in the ovary. The oocyte in the dominant follicle completes its first meiotic division, then it is released from the follicle at the surface of the ovary approximately 36 h after the LH surge. It then travels down the fallopian tube to the uterine cavity. At the same time, there is an increase of secretion of plasminogen activator and other cytokines required for the process of ovulation [16, 17]. Before the oocyte is released, the granulosa cells begin to luteinize and produce progesterone. Progesterone is responsible for reducing LH pulse that becomes less frequent by the termination of the surge. There is a close relation of follicular rupture and oocyte release to the LH surge; as a result, measurements of serum or urine LH can be used to estimate the time of ovulation in women.

16.5.2 Endometrium

The endometrium becomes more uniformly bright, the "triple stripe" image is lost. This is due to the impact of progesterone increase that it is responsible for cessation of mitoses and "organization" of the glands [12, 18].

16.6 Luteal Phase

The corpus luteum induces the rising of progesterone concentrations in the middle and late luteal phase [19]. This increase causes the progressive slowing of LH pulses down to one pulse every four hours. A decrease in LH secretions results in a gradual fall in progesterone and estradiol production by the corpus luteum in the absence of a fertilized oocyte [20]. However, if the oocyte becomes fertilized, several days after ovulation starts its implantation in endometrium. The early embryo begins to make chorionic gonadotropin, which maintains the corpus luteum and progesterone production. Inhibin A is also produced by the corpus luteum, and serum concentrations of inhibin A reach peak in the mid-luteal phase. Inhibin B secretion is virtually absent during the luteal phase.

16.6.1 Endometrial Changes

In response to estradiol and progesterone decline due to the resolving of corpus luteum, the endometrium lose the blood supply. Menstruation is the cyclic, orderly sloughing of the uterine lining approximately 14 days after the LH surge [6]. Simultaneously, the hypothalamic–pituitary axis induces the LH rise and a new cycle starts.

16.7 Puberty

After birth, the gonads are quiescent until they are activated by gonadotropins from the pituitary gland to bring about the final maturation of the reproductive system (gonadarche). This period of transition to final sexual maturation is known as puberty. The age at the time of puberty is variable, generally occurring between the ages of 8 and 13 in girls depending on race/ethnic background and weight status. Between 5 and 12% of girls have menarche younger than 11 years of age [21]. The main physiological events in puberty are:

- **Gonadarche**: the activation of the gonads by gonadotropins from the pituitary gland. In details, the follicle-stimulating hormone (FSH) stimulates the growth of ovarian follicles and LH stimulates production of estradiol by the ovaries. At the onset of puberty, estradiol induces breast development and growth of the skeleton, leading to pubertal growth acceleration. Later in puberty, the interaction between pituitary secretions of gonadotropins and the secretion of estradiol by ovarian follicles leads to ovulation and menstrual cycles [22].

- **Adrenarche**: An increase in the secretion of adrenal androgens by the adrenal cortex. Typically happens in females before the onset of puberty occurring at age of 8–10 years. It is probably due to a rise in a 17α-hydroxylase activity. There is a gradual decline in this activity as plasma adrenal androgen secretion declines to low levels in old age.

Most adolescents have a predictable path for pubertal maturation, although there is some variability between individuals in terms of timing and sequence.

The first event of puberty is **thelarche**, the development of breasts. The breasts develop under the influence of the ovarian hormones, estradiol and progesterone, with estradiol primarily responsible for the growth of ducts and progesterone primarily responsible for the growth of lobules and alveoli.

Thelarche is then followed by **pubarche**, the development of axillary and pubic hair. The adrenal androgens significantly contribute to the growth of axillary and pubic hair.

Finally, there is **menarche**, the first menstrual period. The initial periods are generally anovulatory and occurs up to 2–2.5 years after the onset of puberty. A physiologic leukorrhea which is a thin, white, non-foul-smelling vaginal discharge occurs up 6 to 12 months before menarche for the estrogen stimulation of the vaginal mucosa [23–26].

The initial manifestation and the earlier onset of puberty has a lot of clinical implications. Earlier menarche (before 12 years of age) is associated with higher BMI during adulthood as compared with later menarche [27]. The earlier onset of puberty has important implications for the diagnosis of precocious puberty that has been defined as breast development prior to eight years of age in girls. Earlier puberty is associated with increased risk of adult pathological conditions. Multiple studies have reported the association of earlier age at menarche with breast cancer, with a 7% decreased risk for premenopausal breast cancer and 3% decreased risk for postmenopausal breast cancer for every year menarche is delayed [28]. Earlier puberty is also associated with increased risk for other reproductive cancers: endometrial and ovarian cancer in women and prostate cancer in men [29]. The relationship of pubertal timing and cardiovascular disease is more complex; in women, both earlier and later age at menarche are associated with increased risk of coronary heart and cerebrovascular diseases [30]. Additionally, earlier age at menarche is associated with increased risk for type 2 diabetes and impaired glucose tolerance; part of this association is mediated by increased adiposity and part is independent from adiposity [31]. Later puberty onset includes lower bone mineral density, increased fracture risk, and in men, increased risk for depression and anxiety. The pathophysiological processes for these associations are not known [32, 33].

16.8 Menopause

Natural menopause is the permanent cessation of menstrual periods, determined retrospectively after a woman has experienced 12 months of amenorrhea without any other obvious pathologic or physiologic cause. It is a reflection of complete, or near complete, ovarian follicular depletion, with resulting hypoestrogenemia and high FSH concentrations. Perimenopause is characterized by irregular menstrual cycles, endocrinological changes, and many symptoms. Early menopause begins between the ages of 40 and 45 years and late menopause after age of 55 years.

16.8.1 Clinic

Perimenopause starts about several years before the final menstrual cycle and results in various physiological changes that may affect woman's quality of life. It is characterized by irregular menstrual cycles and hormonal fluctuations.

Some of the symptoms are:

- Neurovegetative symptoms (the most frequent clinical manifestation of menopause are hot flushes (80%)) [34]. Palpitations and insomnia also occur.
- Sleep disorders.
- Atrophy of the urogenital system.
- Mood fluctuations.
- Emotional instability, nervousness, decreased libido, concentration difficulties, memory loss.
- Atrophy, dryness, and itching of skin and mucous membranes.
- Higher cardiovascular risk [35].
- Osteoporosis [36].
- Body composition (in the early postmenopausal years women usually gain fat mass and lose lean mass with a central fat distribution) [37].

16.8.2 Menopausal Endocrinology

During menopause, there is a gradual decrease in estradiol and inhibin and an increase in gonadotropins (more FSH than LH) as there is no negative feedback of ovarian steroid hormones [38]. The main source of estrogens will be the peripheral conversion of adrenal androgens to estrogens; estrone is the most important estrogen in menopause.

Other endocrine changes through the menopausal transition include a progressive decrease in serum inhibin B and AMH. Also, ovarian antral follicle count (AFC) declines steadily across the reproductive years until postmenopause.

16.8.3 Diagnosis

Generally, it is clinical: amenorrhea for 1 year accompanied by climacteric symptoms. Hormonal determinations also can be carried out: FSH >40 mU/mL, estradiol <20 pg/mL, and AMH < 10 pg/mL [39]. However, hormonal concentrations are less predictive of menopausal stage than clinical criteria, so they should not be used alone [40].

16.8.4   Treatment

Postmenopausal women experience vulvovaginal symptoms including dyspareunia and atrophy, which can be treated by local administration of estrogen. Osteoporosis is treated with calcium-rich diets, moderate exercise, calcitonin, and/or bisphosphonates. Coffee, tobacco, and alcohol should be avoided. Hormone replacement therapy is indicated for the management of menopausal symptoms, but not to prevent chronic disease such as cardiovascular disease, osteoporosis, or dementia [41, 42]. Indications are: symptomatic menopause (systemic estrogens are the most effective treatment available for relief of hot flashes) and early menopause (surgical or nonsurgical). Absolute contraindications are:

- Hormone-dependent gynecological carcinomas (breast, endometrial).
- Thrombophilia.
- History of coronary or cerebrovascular disease.
- Ongoing severe hepatopathy or liver tumors.
- Abnormal uterine bleeding of unknown cause.

There are two categories of menopausal hormone therapy: combined estrogen-progestin therapy and estrogen-alone therapy. The protective and side effects of both therapies have been investigated [41].

16.9   Amenorrhea

Approximately 2.5% of the population is affected by primary amenorrhea, defined as the absence of menses by age of 13 years in the absence of normal growth or secondary sexual development, or the absence of menses by age of 15 years in the setting of normal growth and secondary sexual development.

Secondary amenorrhea is defined as the absence of menses, in a previously menstruating woman, for more than three cycle intervals, or six consecutive months.

Regular and spontaneous menstruation requires:

- Functional hypothalamic–pituitary–ovarian endocrine axis.
- An endometrium able to respond to steroid hormone stimulation.
- An intact outflow tract from internal to external genitalia.

16.9.1   Causes of Amenorrhea

Frequent:

- Pregnancy.
- Hypothalamic amenorrhea.
- Galactorrhea-amenorrhea syndrome.
- Polycystic ovarian syndrome.
- Pituitary amenorrhea.

Less frequent:

- Premature ovarian failure (POF).
- Asherman's syndrome.
- Sheehan's syndrome.
- Drug-induced amenorrhea.

Rare:

- Diabetes.
- Hyperthyroidism or hypothyroidism.
- Cushing's syndrome.
- Addison's disease.
- Cirrhosis.
- Infection (tuberculosis, syphilis, encephalitis/meningitis, sarcoidosis).
- Chronic renal failure.
- Malnutrition.
- Irradiation or chemotherapy.
- Hemosiderosis.
- Surgery.

16.9.2   Causes of Primary Amenorrhea

Primary amenorrhea is mainly due to genetic and anatomical disorders. The most common etiologies are Gonadal dysgenesis, Mullerian agenesis,

Polycystic ovary syndrome (PCOS), and isolated GnRH deficiency.

Ovarian dysgenesis is caused primary by chromosomal abnormalities of the X. Most of the patients have Turner syndrome (45, XO or 45, XO/XX mosaics) and present with primary amenorrhea. Women with Turner syndrome are missing an X chromosome. The oocytes and follicles go into apoptosis even before the fetus is born. The ovaries are replaced by steak gonads, and in the absence of follicles, there is no secretion of ovarian estrogen, resulting in primary amenorrhea. However, the external female genitalia, uterus, and fallopian tubes develop normally until puberty, when estrogen-induced development does not occur. However, some patients with mosaic abnormalities may experiment secondary amenorrhea [43].

Müllerian dysgenesis: It results from agenesis or hypoplasia of the Müllerian duct system, with different degrees of severity according to the absent anatomical components. All or part of the vagina will be absent while the other female sexual characteristics are normal.

Other anatomic defects include **imperforate hymen**, **transverse vaginal septum**, and isolated absence of the vagina or cervix. These conditions present with cyclic pain and an accumulation of blood behind the obstruction, which can lead to endometriosis and pelvic adhesions [44].

Polycystic ovary syndrome: It is the most common reproductive disorder in women, accounts for approximately 20% of cases of secondary amenorrhea, but may account for approximately 50% of cases of oligomenorrhea [48]. It is a rare cause of primary amenorrhea. After exclusion of other etiologies, the diagnosis is based on the presence of at least two of the following criteria: (1) oligo- or anovulation, (2) clinical and/ or biochemical signs of hyperandrogenism, and (3) polycystic ovaries on ultrasound [45]. Even if the exact mechanics are not clear, it appears that insulin resistance and hyperinsulinemia are involved [46].

Isolated GnRH deficiency is rare and is called idiopathic hypogonadotropic hypogonadism or Kallmann syndrome if it is associated with anosmia [47].

Steroid Enzyme Defects alter ovary steroidogenesis in the different steps leading to testosterone and estradiol synthesis. The resulting clinical picture is different depending on the involved enzyme. They are a rare cause of primary amenorrhea.

16.9.3 Causes of Secondary Amenorrhea

The most common causes of secondary amenorrhea are, in order of frequency, pregnancy, functional hypothalamic amenorrhea, pituitary defects, polycystic ovary syndrome, premature ovarian insufficiency, and intrauterine adhesions.

Functional hypothalamic amenorrhea (FHA) is one of the most common causes of secondary amenorrhea and excludes pathologic disease. Several factors can lead to this condition, including a significant weight loss or restricted diet, intense exercise, and stress.

Pituitary Defects: acquired pituitary dysfunction can follow local radiation or surgery or Sheehan's syndrome, characterized by postpartum amenorrhea, in women with significant postpartum blood loss. This may result in ischemic necrosis of the pituitary gland and hypopituitarism [48]. Hyperprolactinemia is the most common pituitary cause of secondary amenorrhea. Prolactin-secreting adenomas are the most common subtype of secretory pituitary adenoma. These tumors are usually benign, and prolactin levels typically correlate with tumor size. Elevated prolactin levels lead to amenorrhea, but the mechanisms underlying are unclear [47]. Isolated hyperprolactinemia is an infrequent cause of primary amenorrhea. The diagnosis is suggested by a history of galactorrhea and elevated serum prolactin level. Medications such as antipsychotic, antidepressant, and prokinetics can increase serum prolactin levels and lead to amenorrhea. TRH also induces prolactin secretion, so primary hypothyroidism will result in elevated TRH, hyperprolactinemia, and galactorrhea-amenorrhea syndrome [49].

Premature Ovarian Failure (POF): If menopause occurs before age 40 year, it is marked by amenorrhea, increased gonadotropin levels, and estrogen deficiency. Causes of premature ovarian failure may be different: Turner syndrome, fragile X premutation, autoimmune ovarian destruction, radiation therapy, or chemotherapy with alkylating agents or unknown [50].

Intrauterine synechiae are often caused by a complicated dilatation and curettage (Asherman's syndrome).

16.9.4 Differential Diagnosis

16.9.4.1 Diagnosis of Primary Amenorrhea

A pelvic examination and an ultrasound scan can be used to define the presence of uterus, vagina, and no outflow obstruction that may cause the absence of menses.

Moreover, FSH serum level should be measured too. If hypergonadotropic hypogonadism is present, the probable diagnosis is gonadal dysgenesis, and a karyotype should be done.

In case of Mullerian agenesis, serum gonadotropins are in the range and the uterus is absent.

In case of obstructed outflow, FSH is normal, uterus is present, but instrumental examination reveals accumulation of blood in the uterus or vagina. A story of pelvic pain will be attended.

If the FSH is low, the uterus is present and there's no evidence of breast development, most likely the patient has a hypothalamic-pituitary disorder. Distinction of hypothalamic from pituitary disorders can be obtained by the injection of GnRH, but pituitary causes are rare and can often be diagnosed by history alone.

16.9.4.2 Diagnosis of Secondary Amenorrhea

The first cause of secondary amenorrhea is pregnancy, so measurement of beta-hCG is recommended.

History of weight loss, extreme exercise, diet, or illness should be indagated to discover a functional hypothalamic amenorrhea. If there are clinical evidences of hyperandrogenism, an ultrasound should be done to study the ovaries and serum total testosterone should be measured. If a

patient has no history of dilatation and curettage, we can almost certainly exclude Asherman's syndrome. Karyotype genetic test is indicated for all women who present with primary ovarian failure. Serum PRL, FSH, and TSH should be tested. If PRL is initially higher than 50–200 ng/mL, the patient must be studied to discover a prolactinoma. If prolactin level is in the range of 20–50 ng/mL, TSH levels should be measured. If TSH levels are high, hypothyroidism must be corrected and prolactin must be measured again. Estrogen status can be assessed with a progestin challenge. Withdrawal bleeding after progestin discontinuation indirectly determines that endometrium has been prepared with ovarian estrogen. Absence of bleeding can be due to hypoestrogenism or an outflow obstruction.

16.9.5 Amenorrhea Complications

Many are the complications of amenorrhea, including infertility and psychosocial disorders. Hypoestrogenism can lead to the development of severe osteoporosis [36]. In patients responding to progesterone challenge, hyperestrogenism not counterbalanced by progestin is a risk factor for endometrial hyperplasia and cancer.

16.9.6 Treatment

16.9.6.1 Ovulation Induction in Patient Desiring Pregnancy

Dopamine agonist drugs remain the first-line therapy in patients with both micro and macroadenomas. These drugs can decrease prolactin secretion and tumor size. Thyroid replacement therapy should be used in patient with hypothyroidism. In patients with a negative progestin-challenge, estrogen levels are low, and the pituitary does not produce high quantities of LH and FSH, so exogenous gonadotropins are the first-line therapy. Patients with a positive progestin challenge would probably respond to clomiphene citrate, which has important antiestrogenic activity on the hypothalamus and pituitary, preventing negative feedback on GnRH release and leading an increase in endogenous FSH.

Most of the premature ovarian failures are idiopathic and cannot be treated.

16.9.6.2 Patient Not Desiring Pregnancy Can Be Divided into Two Categories

Hypoestrogenic patients must be treated with both estrogen and progestin to prevent complications due to the absence of these two hormones. Oral contraceptives can be used. Patients who respond to the progestin challenge require sporadic progestin delivery to prevent endometrial hyperplasia and carcinoma. In patients with hyperprolactinemia, prolactin should be measured periodically, and they must be studied for the development of macroadenomas.

16.10 Infertility

16.10.1 Definition

- Infertility is defined as the inability of a couple to conceive within 1 year of regular, unprotected sexual intercourse.
- Primary infertility applies to those who have never conceived.
- Secondary infertility designates those who have conceived in the past.
- Sterility implies an intrinsic inability to achieve pregnancy.
- Fecundability is the probability of being pregnant in a single menstrual cycle.
- Fecundity is the probability of achieving a live birth within a single cycle.

The prevalence of women diagnosed with infertility is approximately 13%, with a range from 7 to 28%, depending on the age of the woman [51]. The incidence of primary infertility has increased, with a concurrent decrease in secondary infertility, most likely because of social changes such as delayed childbearing. In normal fertile couples having frequent intercourse, the fecundability is estimated to be approximately 20–25%. Approximately 85–90% of couples with unprotected intercourse will conceive within 1 year.

16.10.2 Timing of Infertility Evaluation

Infertility evaluation should be undertaken for couples who have not been able to conceive after 12 months of unprotected and frequent intercourse, but earlier evaluation should be undertaken based on medical history and physical findings, and in women over 35 years of age [52].

An inverse relationship exists between fecundity and the age of the woman. This decline in fertility is multifactorial. Females are born with a fixed number of oocytes, which decreases with age. The quality of oocytes also falls with age because meiotic errors occur more frequently with increasing age [53]. During the menstrual cycle, the process to select a dominant follicle for ovulation does not exclude genetically abnormal oocytes. In addition to the endogenous accumulation of genetic errors in the oocyte pool, other factors such as smoking, other environmental exposures, and certain medical and surgical treatments can compromise oocyte quality, ovarian reserve, and chance for a healthy outcome for pregnancy [54].

16.10.3 Most Common Female Factors of Infertility

Female factor infertility was reported in 37% of infertile couples in developed countries. The most common identifiable female factors, which accounted for 81% of female infertility, were:

- Ovulatory disorders (25%).
- Tubal abnormalities (20%).
- Endometriosis (15%).
- Pelvic adhesions (12%).
- Hyperprolactinemia (7%).

16.10.3.1 Ovulatory Disorders
An **ovulatory dysfunction** is responsible for approximately 20–25% of infertility cases. The

history, including the onset of menarche, menstrual cycle length, and presence or absence of premenstrual symptoms, should be investigated. Signs and symptoms of systemic disease, especially of hypothyroidism, and physical signs of endocrine disease (i.e., hirsutism, galactorrhea, and obesity) should be focused on. The degree and intensity of exercise and a history of weight loss and of hot flushes are clinical clues of possible endocrine or ovulatory dysfunction. Progesterone serum levels of 3 ng/mL or greater in the mid-luteal phase are coherent with ovulation, which can be supported by pelvic ultrasonography. In the follicular phase, the developing follicle can be monitored until maturation and subsequent rupture. The disappearance of the follicle and appearance of free fluid can document ovulation. A secretory endometrium confirms ovulation. To detect the LH surge, the patient can use urinary LH kits or serum LH assay. Ovulation occurs 24–36 hours after the onset of the LH surge and 10–12 hours after the peak of the LH.

Ovarian reserve is the functional capacity of the ovary and it is determined by the number and the quality of oocytes at a certain time. It depends on age, exposure to toxic factors (i.e., smoking, surgery, gonadotropic therapies), and individual follicular wealth.

Initially, the basal FSH level in the early follicular phase was used as a test of ovarian reserve. However, FSH has considerable intra- and intercycle variability, and this greatly limits its reliability [55].

The most appropriate quantitative tests are the AMH assay [54] and the transvaginal ultrasound count of pre-antral follicles (AFC), which are used as predictors of the potential success of fertility treatments.

AMH is secreted exclusively by the granulosa cells of the pre-antral pool and small FSH-independent antral follicles, so it can be assayed at any stage of the cycle.

The antral follicle count (AFC) is calculated by adding up the number of follicles between 2 and 10 mm in size in both ovaries. Ninety nine percent of the follicles in the ovary are primordial follicles, plus a proportion of follicles in the early growth phase that are too small to be seen by ultrasound. However, a proportion of these follicles mature into antral follicles with a diameter of more than 2 mm, forming the recruitable pool responsive to FSH. These follicles can be detected by transvaginal ultrasound.

16.10.3.2 Pelvic Factor

The pelvic factor includes abnormalities of the uterus, fallopian tubes, ovaries, and adjacent pelvic structures. A history of pelvic infection, the use of intrauterine devices, endometritis, and septic abortion are suggestive for diagnosis.

Endometriosis may be suggested by worsening dysmenorrhea, dyspareunia, or previous surgical reports. Endometriosis decreases fertility due to anatomic distortion from pelvic adhesions, damage to ovarian tissue by endometrioma formation and surgical resection, and the production of substances such as cytokines and growth factors which impair the normal processes of ovulation, fertilization, and implantation [56].

Uterus: An impaired implantation, due to mechanical factors or reduced endometrial receptivity, is the uterine cause of infertility.

Uterine fibroids are common benign smooth muscle monoclonal tumors. Apparently, fibroids with a submucosal or intracavitary component can reduce implantation rates [57].

Uterine abnormalities, like Müllerian anomalies, are a significant cause of recurrent pregnancy loss. The septate uterus is associated with the poorest reproductive outcome [58, 59].

Any history of ectopic pregnancy, adnexal surgery, leiomyomas, or exposure to diethylstilbestrol (DES) in utero should be noted as possibly contributory to the diagnosis of a pelvic factor.

A pelvic examination can give many information (a fixed uterus is suggestive of adhesions, leiomyomas, or adnexal masses).

A transvaginal ultrasound examination can add information (hydrosalpinx, leiomyoma, ovarian cysts, including endometriomas, can often be observed).

16.10.3.3 Tubal Disease

The main cause of tubal factor infertility is pelvic inflammatory disease caused by pathogens such as Gonorrhea, Chlamydia trachomatis, or Mycoplasma genitalium [60]. Other conditions that may interfere with tubal transport include severe endometriosis, adhesions from previous surgery or non-tubal infection (i.e., appendicitis, inflammatory bowel disease), pelvic tuberculosis, and salpingitis isthmica nodosa (i.e., diverticulosis of the fallopian tube).

16.10.3.4 Cervical Factors

Congenital malformations and trauma to the cervix may result in stenosis and inability of the cervix to produce normal mucus, which usually facilitates the transport of sperm.

Cervix abnormalities may be indicated by a history of abnormal Pap-test, postcoital bleeding, or surgery. The best evaluation of the cervix is performed with speculum examination, which can reveal evidence of cervicitis or cervical stenosis, especially in a patient with prior history of surgery (i.e., conization or cryotherapy).

16.10.3.5 Genetic Causes

Infertile couples have a higher prevalence of karyotype abnormalities than the general population. The most common aneuploidies associated with infertility are 45, X (Turner syndrome) in women and 47, XXY (Klinefelter syndrome) in men [61].

16.10.3.6 Unexplained Infertility

Diagnosis of unexplained infertility generally implies normal uterine cavity, bilateral patent tubes, normal semen analysis, and evidence of ovulation.

16.10.4 Essentials of Infertility Diagnosis

- History

In presence of oligomenorrhea, amenorrhea, short or very irregular menstrual cycles, or when ovulation is not confirmed, evaluation of the hypothalamic–pituitary–ovarian axis is advised. A usual initial assessment includes the serum concentrations of FSH, estradiol, prolactin, and TSH.

- **Ovarian Factor.**
  - Ovarian reserve.
  - Day 3 serum follicle-stimulating hormone and estradiol levels.
  - AMH.
  - Antral follicle count.
- **Confirmation of Ovulation.**
  - History.
  - Serum progesterone assay.
  - Pelvic ultrasonography.
  - Changes in cervical mucus.
  - Luteal phase defect.
- **Pelvic Factor.**
  - Physical exam.
  - Ultrasound examination.
  - Hysterosalpingogram to evaluate uterine cavity and fallopian tubes.
  - Possible saline sonogram to evaluate uterine cavity.
  - Laparoscopy to assess endometriosis when indicated.
- **Cervical Factor.**
  - History.
  - PAP test.
  - Speculum examination.
- **Metabolic Disease.**
  - Thyroid assessment.

References

1. Treloar AE, Boynton RE, Behn BG, Brown BW. Variation of the human menstrual cycle through reproductive life. Int J Fertil. 1967;12:77.
2. Sherman BM, Korenman SG. Hormonal characteristics of the human menstrual cycle throughout reproductive life. J Clin Invest. 1975;55:699.
3. Mahendro MS, Cunningham FG. Parturition. In: Cunningham FG, Leveno KJ, Bloom SL, et al., editors. Williams obstetrics. 23th ed. New York: McGraw-Hill; 2010a. p. 159.
4. Mahendro MS, Cunningham FG. Implantation and placental development. In: Cunningham FG, Leveno KJ, Bloom SL, et al., editors. Williams obstetrics. 25th ed. New York: McGraw-Hill; 2018a. p. 81.
5. Mahendro MS, Cunningham FG. Parturition. In: Cunningham FG, Leveno KJ, Bloom SL, et al., editors. Williams obstetrics. 25th ed. New York: McGraw-Hill; 2018b. p. 406.
6. Hall JE, Schoenfeld DA, Martin KA, Crowley WF Jr. Hypothalamic gonadotropin-releasing hormone secretion and follicle-stimulating hormone dynamics during the luteal-follicular transition. J Clin Endocrinol Metab. 1992;74:600.

7. Gougeon A. Dynamics of follicular growth in the human: a model from preliminary results. Hum Reprod. 1986;1:81.

8. Welt CK, Martin KA, Taylor AE, et al. Frequency modulation of follicle-stimulating hormone (FSH) during the luteal-follicular transition: evidence for FSH control of inhibin B in normal women. J Clin Endocrinol Metab. 1997;82:2645.

9. Welt CK, McNicholl DJ, Taylor AE, Hall JE. Female reproductive aging is marked by decreased secretion of dimeric inhibin. J Clin Endocrinol Metab. 1999;84:105.

10. Filicori M, Santoro N, Merriam GR, Crowley WF Jr. Characterization of the physiological pattern of episodic gonadotropin secretion throughout the human menstrual cycle. J Clin Endocrinol Metab. 1986;62:1136.

11. Kissell KA, Danaher MR, Schisterman EF, et al. Biological variability in serum anti- Müllerian hormone throughout the menstrual cycle in ovulatory and sporadic anovulatory cycles in eumenorrheic women. Hum Reprod. 2014;29:1764.

12. Fleischer AC, Kalemeris GC, Entman SS. Sonographic depiction of the endometrium during normal cycles. Ultrasound Med Biol. 1986;12:271.

13. Adams JM, Taylor AE, Schoenfeld DA, et al. The midcycle gonadotropin surge in normal women occurs in the face of an unchanging gonadotropin-releasing hormone pulse frequency. J Clin Endocrinol Metab. 1994;79:858.

14. Taylor AE, Whitney H, Hall JE, et al. Midcycle levels of sex steroids are sufficient to recreate the follicle-stimulating hormone but not the luteinizing hormone midcycle surge: evidence for the contribution of other ovarian factors to the surge in normal women. J Clin Endocrinol Metab. 1995;80:1541.

15. Martin KA, Welt CK, Taylor AE, et al. Is GnRH reduced at the midcycle surge in the human? Evidence from a GnRH-deficient model. Neuroendocrinology. 1998;67:363.

16. Richards JS. Hormonal control of gene expression in the ovary. Endocr Rev. 1994;15:725.

17. Tsafriri A, Chun SY, Reich R. Follicular rupture and ovulation. In: The ovary, Adashi EY, Leu ng PCK (Eds), Raven Press, New York 1993. 227.

18. Noyes RW, Hertig AT, Rock J. Dating the endometrial biopsy. Fertil Steril. 1950;1:3.

19. Stocco C, Telleria C, Gibori G. The molecular control of corpus luteum formation, function, and regression. Endocr Rev. 2007;28:117.

20. Filicori M, Butler JP, Crowley WF Jr. Neuroendocrine regulation of the corpus luteum in the human. Evidence for pulsatile progesterone secretion. J Clin Invest. 1984;73:1638.

21. Dunger DB, Ahmed ML, Ong KK. Early and late weight gain and the timing of puberty. Mol Cell Endocrinol. 2006;254–255:140.

22. Wu FC, Butler GE, Kelnar CJ, Sellar RE. Patterns of pulsatile luteinizing hormone secretion before and during the onset of puberty in boys: a study using an immunoradiometric assay. J Clin Endocrinol Metab. 1990;70:629.

23. Marshall WA, Tanner JM. Variations in pattern of pubertal changes in girls. Arch Dis Child. 1969;44:291.

24. Biro FM, Huang B, Crawford PB, et al. Pubertal correlates in black and white girls. J Pediatr. 2006;148:234.

25. Taranger J, Engström I, Lichtenstein H, Svennberg-RI. VI. Somatic pubertal development. Acta Paediatr Scand Suppl. 1976;258:121–35.

26. Susman EJ, Houts RM, Steinberg L, et al. Longitudinal development of secondary sexual characteristics in girls and boys between ages 91/2 and 151/2 years. Arch Pediatr Adolesc Med. 2010;164:166.

27. Yang L, Li L, Millwood IY, et al. Adiposity in relation to age at menarche and other reproductive factors among 300 000 Chinese women: findings from China Kadoorie biobank study. Int J Epidemiol. 2017;46:502.

28. Clavel-Chapelon F, E3N-EPIC Group. Differential effects of reproductive factors on the risk of pre- and postmenopausal breast cancer. Results from a large cohort of French women. Br J Cancer. 2002;86:723–7.

29. Day FR, Thompson DJ, Helgason H, et al. Genomic analyses identify hundreds of variants associated with age at menarche and support a role for puberty timing in cancer risk. Nat Genet. 2017;49:834.

30. Canoy D, Beral V, Balkwill A, et al. Age at menarche and risks of coronary heart and other vascular diseases in a large UK cohort. Circulation. 2015;131:237.

31. Cheng TS, Day FR, Lakshman R, Ong KK. Association of puberty timing with type 2 diabetes: a systematic review and meta-analysis. PLoS Med. 2020;17:e1003017.

32. Day FR, Elks CE, Murray A, et al. Puberty timing associated with diabetes, cardiovascular disease and also diverse health outcomes in men and women: the UK biobank study. Sci Rep. 2015;5:11208.

33. Chan YM, Feld A, Jonsdottir-Lewis E. Effects of the timing of sex-steroid exposure in adolescence on adult health outcomes. J Clin Endocrinol Metab. 2019;104:4578.

34. Woods NF, Mitchell ES. Symptoms during the perimenopause: prevalence, severity, trajectory, and significance in women's lives. Am J Med. 2005;118:14–24.

35. Derby CA, Crawford SL, Pasternak RC, Sowers M, Sternfeld B, Matthews KA. Lipid changes during the menopause transition in relation to age and weight: the Study of Women's Health Across the Nation. Am J Epidemiol. 2009;169(11):1352–61.

36. Cosman F, de Beur SJ, LeBoff MS, Lewiecki EM, Tanner B, Randall S, et al. Clinician's guide to prevention and treatment of osteoporosis. Osteoporos Int. 2014;25(10):2359–81.

37. Sternfeld B, Wang H, Quesenberry CP, Abrams B, Everson-Rose SA, Greendale GA, et al. Physical activity and changes in weight and waist circumference in midlife women: findings from the Study of

Women's Health Across the Nation. Am J Epidemiol. 2004;160(9):912–22.

38. Hall JE. Neuroendocrine physiology of the early and late menopause. Endocrinol Metab Clin North Am. 2004;33(4):637–59.

39. Finkelstein JS, Lee H, Karlamangla A, Neer RM, Sluss PM, Burnett-Bowie S-AM, et al. Antimullerian Hormone and Impending Menopause in Late Reproductive Age: The Study of Women's Health Across the Nation. J Clin Endocrinol Metab. 2020;105(4):e1862–71.

40. Randolph JF, Crawford S, Dennerstein L, Cain K, Harlow SD, Little R, et al. The value of follicle-stimulating hormone concentration and clinical findings as markers of the late menopausal transition. J Clin Endocrinol Metab. 2006;91(8):3034–40.

41. Manson JE, Chlebowski RT, Stefanick ML, Aragaki AK, Rossouw JE, Prentice RL, et al. Menopausal hormone therapy and health outcomes during the intervention and extended poststopping phases of the Women's Health Initiative randomized trials. JAMA. 2013;310(13):1353–68.

42. ACOG Practice Bulletin No. 141: management of menopausal symptoms. Obstet Gynecol. 2014;123(1):202–16.

43. Fourman LT, Fazeli PK. Neuroendocrine causes of amenorrhea—an update. J Clin Endocrinol Metab. 2015;100(3):812–24.

44. Practice Committee of the American Society for reproductive medicine. Current evaluation of amenorrhea. Fertil Steril. 2006;86(5 Suppl 1):S148–55.

45. The Rotterdam ESHRE/ASRM-sponsored PCOS consensus workshop group. Revised 2003 consensus on diagnostic criteria and long-term health risks related to polycystic ovary syndrome (PCOS). Hum Reprod. 2004;19(1):41–7.

46. Diamanti-Kandarakis E. Polycystic ovarian syndrome: pathophysiology, molecular aspects and clinical implications. Expert Rev Mol Med. 2008;10:e3.

47. Turner's syndrome. West J Med. 1982;137(1):32–44.

48. Zargar AH, Singh B, Laway BA, Masoodi SR, Wani AI, Bashir MI. Epidemiologic aspects of postpartum pituitary hypofunction (Sheehan's syndrome). Fertil Steril. 2005;84(2):523–8.

49. Kakuno Y, Amino N, Kanoh M, Kawai M, Fujiwara M, Kimura M, et al. Menstrual disturbances in various thyroid diseases. Endocr J. 2010;57(12):1017–22.

50. Rebar RW. Premature Ovarian Failure. Obstet Gynecol. 2009;113(6):1355–63.

51. Chandra A, Copen CE, Stephen EH. Infertility and impaired fecundity in the United States, 1982–2010: data from the National Survey of Family Growth. Natl Health Stat Report. 2013;67:1–18.

52. Practice Committee of the American Society for Reproductive Medicine. Optimal evaluation of the infertile female. Fertil Steril. 2006;86(5):S264–7.

53. Jones KT. Meiosis in oocytes: predisposition to aneuploidy and its increased incidence with age. Hum Reprod Update. 2008;14(2):143–58.

54. Nappi L, Angioni S, Sorrentino F, Cinnella G, Lombardi M, Greco P. Anti-Mullerian hormone trend evaluation after laparoscopic surgery of monolateral endometrioma using a new dual wavelengths laser system (DWLS) for hemostasis. Gynecol Endocrinol. 2016;32(1):34–7. https://doi.org/10.3109/09513590.2015.1068754.

55. Parry JP, Koch CA. Ovarian reserve testing. In: Feingold KR, Anawalt B, Boyce A, Chrousos G, de Herder WW, Dhatariya K, Dungan K, Hershman JM, Hofland J, Kalra S, Kaltsas G, Koch C, Kopp P, Korbonits M, Kovacs CS, Kuohung W, Laferrère B, Levy M, McGee EA, McLachlan R, Morley JE, New M, Purnell J, Sahay R, Singer F, Sperling MA, Stratakis CA, Trence DL, Wilson DP, editors. Endotext. South Dartmouth (MA), MDText.com, Inc.; 2019.

56. Giudice LC, Kao LC. Endometriosis. Lancet. 2004;364(9447):1789–99.

57. Practice Committee of the American Society for reproductive medicine. Electronic address: ASRM@asrm.org, practice Committee of the American Society for reproductive medicine. Removal of myomas in asymptomatic patients to improve fertility and/or reduce miscarriage rate: a guideline. Fertil Steril. 2017;108(3):416–25.

58. Nappi L, Pontis A, Sorrentino F, Greco P, Angioni S. Hysteroscopic metroplasty for the septate uterus with diode laser: a pilot study. Eur J Obstet Gynecol Reprod Biol. 2016;206:32–5. https://doi.org/10.1016/j.ejogrb.2016.08.035.

59. Nappi L, Falagario M, Angioni S, et al. The use of hysteroscopic metroplasty with diode laser to increase endometrial volume in women with septate uterus: preliminary results. Gynecol Surg. 2021;18:11. https://doi.org/10.1186/s10397-021-01093-8.

60. Soper DE. Pelvic inflammatory disease. Obstet Gynecol. 2010;116(2 Pt 1):419–28.

61. Clementini E, Palka C, Iezzi I, Stuppia L, Guanciali-Franchi P, Tiboni GM. Prevalence of chromosomal abnormalities in 2078 infertile couples referred for assisted reproductive techniques. Hum Reprod. 2005;20(2):437–42.

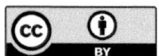

Stefano Bettocchi, Ferdinando Murgia,
Francesca Greco, Maria Grazia Morena, Tea Palieri,
Ambra Pisante, Fabiana Divina Fascilla,
and Luigi Nappi

17.1 Introduction

Infertility is a disease of the male or female reproductive system defined by the failure to achieve a pregnancy after 12 months or more of regular unprotected sexual intercourse [1].

This condition affects millions of people worldwide with subsequent impact on their families and communities. Estimates suggest that between 48 million couples and 186 million individuals live with infertility globally [2].

Management of infertility is a difficult challenge, and the couple should be aware that delaying pregnancy increases the rates of infertility and complicated pregnancies. In the era of artificial intelligence, different functional in vitro fertilization prediction models for tailoring personalized treatment of infertile couples have been proposed. [3].

Practically, evaluation of the couple should begin after 12 months in a woman under 35 years, and after 6 in a woman over 35 and should be initiated even earlier in a woman older than 40 years, as age seems to play a role in the quality of oocytes, which appears to be a central point not only for infertility, but also in order to reach a viable pregnancy.

The assessment of infertility should be carried out by experienced physicians trained in the field of both diagnostics and surgery in a context of a multidisciplinary team.

The first step is a complete personal and familiar interview, in order to customize the following steps. In particular, it is essentially a complete obstetric, sexual, and menstrual history.

Moreover, it is important to assess any previous pelvic surgery or any possible symptom of endometriosis (dysmenorrhea, dyspareunia, dischezia), previous chemotherapy or irradiation, and also lifestyle habits that can interfere with conception such as alcohol or tobacco abuse.

BMI should be assessed at first visit as both obesity and underweight can reduce fertility.

Also, a complete physical examination should be performed looking for signs of discrinia, congenital Mullerian anomalies, and secondary sexual characteristics.

S. Bettocchi (✉) · F. Greco · M. G. Morena ·
T. Palieri · A. Pisante · L. Nappi
Department of Medical and Surgical Sciences,
Institute of Obstetrics and Gynecology,
University of Foggia, Foggia, Italy
e-mail: info@stefanobettocchi.com

F. Murgia
Gynecologic Oncology Unit, Department of
Obstetrics and Gynecology, "F. Miulli" General
Regional Hospital, Bari, Italy

F. D. Fascilla
Obstetrics and Gynecologic Unit, Department of
Obstetrics and Gynecology, "Di Venere" General
Hospital, Bari, Italy

17.2 Laboratory Tests in Infertility

Some couples deserve laboratory tests in order to assess causes of infertility. Among others:

1. Semen analysis to exclude male factor.
2. Assessment of ovarian reserve: it can be either performed with ultrasound or biochemical tests. All women with infertility should perform:
   (a) a dosage of Anti Mullerian hormone (AMH). AMH is produced by the granulosa cells of early follicles and it is a good marker of ovarian reserve. It is also gonadotropin-independent, so it can be measured in all phases of the menstrual cycle. Moreover, AMH is a good predictor of success in IVF (in vitro fertilization);
   (b) an early-follicular-phase dosage of inhibin b, produced by preantral follicles. In advanced age, both AMH and early-follicular phase inhibin b tend to decline, reducing negative feedback on pituitary gland, and therefore on FSH secretion;
   (c) Follicle-stimulating hormone (FSH) is therefore an indirect marker of ovarian reserve. It should be dosed like inhibin b on the third day of the menstrual cycle. FSH stimulates the selection of a new pool of oocytes and therefore is higher in women with low ovarian reserve;
   (d) Clomiphene Citrate Challenge Test (CCCT): it is performed with measurements of FSH on the third day of the menstrual cycle and on day 10, after treatment with clomiphene citrate (100 mg from day 5 to 9). Women with a high level of FSH after CCCT have a lower ovarian reserve.

      However, CCCT is not superior as a marker of ovarian reserve than basal FSH combined with antral follicle count.
3. Assessment of ovulation: women who refer regular menses are likely to ovulate. In order to confirm it, a dosage of progesterone during mid-luteal phase can be useful (around day 21): a value >3 ng/mL confirms ovulation.

It is also possible to confirm ovulation with serial ultrasound transvaginal scans from the appearance of follicles to the selection of the dominant one till it disappears at ovulation.

Irregularity in menses should be checked for the most common causes of anovulation, such as thyroid dysfunction, PCOS, and PRL function. All these tests are not mandatory in evaluation of infertile women, but become necessary in case of suspicion of anovulation.

17.3 Imaging in Infertility

First of all, we must ask ourselves: is this enough to assess tubal patency and at the same time neglecting functional aspects of the tubal epithelium?

17.3.1 Hysterosalpingography

Even if hysterosalpingography (HSG) is still widely considered as the second step in the diagnostic approach to infertile women, it grants very low sensitivity in diagnosis of proximal (51%) and distal (42%) tubal occlusion [4].

Hysterosalpingography is performed with no analgesia as an outpatient procedure even if it is proven to be quite painful; van Welie et al. (2022) [5] showed that the mean pain score for HSG on the 1–10 Visual Analogue Scale (VAS) was 5.4 (SD 2.5), significantly high especially when compared to less expensive or less invasive techniques without leading to substantial differences in pregnancy rates. On the other hand, sonohysterography (HyFoSy) is associated with significantly less pain [6].

HSG only assesses tubal and cavity patency; the injection of contrast allows the evaluation of various genital tract anomalies using X-rays, but it needs further instrumental examinations to confirm diagnosis in several situations:

(a) Filling defects, such as polyps, myomas, and synechiae, are indistinguishable in hysterosalpingograms and always require further evaluations;

(b) Uterine contour anomalies, such as adenomyosis, and Mullerian anomalies, (single horn uterus, arcuate uterus, didelphys uterus, or uterine septa). However, for differential diagnosis, it is often mandatory to evaluate the diagnosis with magnetic resonance, 3D ultrasound, hysteroscopy, and/or laparoscopy.

So we may conclude that HSG is an obsolete technique with very poor performance.

Given those evidences since 2013, the National Institute for Care and Health Excellence (NICE) proposes sonohysterography (HyFoSy) as an effective alternative to HSG [7].

This imaging does not require contrast media, reducing the risk for allergic reactions, or adverse events such as Wolff-Chaikoff effect or thyrotoxicosis.

HyFoSy should be scheduled, like HSG, during mid-luteal phase, when the endometrium is very thin in order to avoid false positives. Using a small catheter, saline water-based infusion media is injected in utero. Uterine cavity is then studied both in longitudinal axis and coronal planes. If fluid passes in the Douglas, at least one of the two tubes is patent.

Maheux-Lacroix et al. in 2014 demonstrated that HyFoSy, performed alternatively to HSG in the evaluation of tubal patency, grants best performances for the evaluation of uterine cavity and gives the benefit of simultaneous evaluation of both ovaries and myometrium [8].

17.3.2 Ultrasounds

Together with HyFoSy, a Three-Dimensional ultrasound (3D) scan is nowadays an essential tool to optimize the infertility treatment outcomes [9]. It allows to see several renderings that wouldn't be possible with a 2D technique.

An ultrasound assessment is an essential searching for infertility causes in several conditions:

1. Congenital uterine anomalies: Since Congenital Uterine anomalies are mostly asymptomatic, it is difficult to determine the exact prevalence.

(a) Arcuate uterus, a milder abnormality, consists in a midline indentation, sometimes associated with a fundal cavity indentation. It is not associated with pregnancy adverse outcomes in literature. Ultrasound scan shows a <1 cm depth from the interstitial line to the apex of the fundal indentation and an indentation angle greater than 90°;

(b) Septate or subseptate uterus, the most common Mullerian anomaly. A 3D US coronal view allows diagnosing a septate uterus using the following criteria: the depth from the interstitial line to the apex of the indentation is >1 cm, and the angle of indentation is less than 90°. MRI could be an option, especially if expertise in 3D-US is not available. Septate uterus is strongly associated with preterm birth, breech presentation, and abruption and has been associated with several pregnancy adverse outcomes;

(c) Bicornuate uterus: A 3D-US scan will show two separate endometrial cavities and an indentured uterine contour. Pregnancy adverse outcomes are quite common;

(d) Didelphys uterus comes from the failure of Mullerian ducts fusion. US shows two separate horns with a wide fundal indentation. In this case, MRI is the gold standard for definitive diagnosis. High rates of abortion and premature delivery have been reported, 32% and 28%, respectively. Surgical treatment (metroplasty) must be considered in case of RPL or pelvic pain.

(e) Unicornuate uterus, only one Mullerian duct evolves correctly, so one normal emicavity is associated with a rudimentary horn which can communicate with the uterus or may not. A noncommunicant horn exposes the patient to higher risk of ectopic pregnancies, chronic pelvic pain, first and second-trimester abortion, preterm birth.

In 2013, the CONUTA scientific committee proposed a new classification system for Mullerian abnormalities (the ESGE/ESHRE

2013 CONUTA classification System). The main classes are designed to focus on the embryological origin of the uterine malformation, while each subclass is designed focusing on the different degree of uterine deformity and its clinical significance [10].

2. Fibroids and Polyps: A recent meta-analysis conducted by Somigliana et al. showed insufficient evidence to confirm a cause-effect relationship between fibroids and infertility. Nevertheless, fibroids affect up to 27% of women looking for pregnancy. Fibroids distort the cavity with subsequent alteration of endometrial receptivity, and sometimes sexual discomfort. Ultrasonography is the preferred initial imaging modality for diagnosis of fibroids. Based on the position in the myometrium, fibroids are defined as intramural, subserous, and submucosal.

   In 1993, Wamsteker suggested the following fibroid classification based on myometrial penetration assessed by ultrasound and hysteroscopic findings; this classification is still recommended by the European Society of Gynecological Endoscopy (ESGE).
   (a) G0 Myoma's development is completely inside the uterine cavity.
   (b) G1 The myoma is inside the uterine cavity for more than 50%.
   (c) G2 The myoma is inside myometrial thickness for more than 50%.

   Moreover, in 2011, FIGO classification system (PALM COEIN), for causes of abnormal uterine bleeding in women of reproductive age, added 6 more classes [11]:
   (a) Type 3, entirely submucosal myoma.
   (b) Type 4, entirely intramural myoma.
   (c) Type 5 subserosal, at least 50% intramural.
   (d) Type 6 subserosal, less than 50% intramural.
   (e) Type 7 subserosal, attached to the serosal by a stalk.

3. Pelvic inflammatory disease: Pelvic inflammatory disease is a polymicrobial infection-induced inflammation that involves upper female genital tract, sometimes including endometrium, fallopian tubes, ovaries, and peritoneum. It primarily affects sexually active young women.

   Organisms most commonly isolated are Neisseria Gonorrhoeae and Chlamydia Trachomatis.

   Sonographic markers of acute salpingitis are [12]:
   (a) Tubal wall thickness >5 mm.
   (b) Sausage-like structure.
   (c) "Cogwheel" sign
   (d) Incomplete septa.
   (e) Fluid in the Pouch of Douglas.
   (f) Tubo-ovarian complex.

17.3.3 Laparoscopy

Unluckily, both HSG and ultrasound can evaluate less more than patency and cannot assess tubal mucosa nor permit direct vision of the pelvis.

On the other hand, laparoscopy (LPS) offers a direct vision of the entire abdomen and allows diagnosis and eventually treatment of other pathologies such as endometriosis, pelvic adhesions, and some Mullerian anomalies.

Laparoscopy with chromo-pertubation allows direct vision of the tubes and it is possible to inject a dye through a catheter directly in utero and then it flows through fallopian tubes [13].

However, laparoscopy requires general anesthesia and it is an invasive procedure and consequently it is not usually performed in the beginning of the workup of an infertile woman; as a matter of fact, the National Institute for Care and Health Excellence (NICE) recommends laparoscopy only in women suspected for comorbidities such as endometriosis which can be cured at the same time [14].

Laparoscopy with cromo-salpingoscopy provides direct vision of the external surface of fallopian tubes and its patency as HSG and HyFoSy, respectively.

In the early 80s, in order to overcome these limits, salpingoscopy was proposed as a new endoscopic technique, useful for direct vision of tubal mucosa other than the presence or absence of anatomical distortions [15].

Salpingoscopy was done in infertile women who underwent diagnostic laparoscopy and showed at least one patent tube on chromopertubation test, during postmenstrual phase (day 5–day 9) under general anesthesia.

Laparoscopy was done through a standard 3-trocar access (5-mm ports for ancillary instruments) and salpingoscope. Laparoscopic external tubal morphology can be assessed, but at the same time for salpingoscopy, a 2-mm, 30 rigid salpingoscope (Karl Storz, Germany Hopkins II) with an outer sheath of 2.8 mm diameter is used.

Salpingoscopic mucosal appearance can also be graded according to Brosens and Puttemans classification (1989) as follows:

– Grade I: normal mucosal folds (both major and minor).
– Grade II: the major folds are separated and flattened, but otherwise normal/dye staining of mucosa/minimal flattening.
– Grade III: focal adhesions between mucosal folds and variable flattening.
– Grade IV: extensive adhesions between mucosal folds and disseminated flat areas.
– Grade V: complete loss of mucosal fold pattern.

Other classifications have been proposed by Kerin et al. [16] and Hershlag et al. [17].

With salpingoscopy, lesions of the infundibulum and ampullary region can also be detected in patients for whom HSG has shown apparently normal tubes [18].

According to previous studies, laparoscopy and salpingoscopy probably complement; unfortunately, this technique is no longer performed and disappeared maybe for complexity of instrumentation and consequent lack of investments.

17.3.4 Hysteroscopy

In infertile women, a complete assessment of the uterine cavity is essential, and among several modalities, hysteroscopy is considered the gold standard.

Since the early 90s, our group advisedly decided to abandon previous dogmas and look at the uterine cavity from a completely different perspective.

Methodically implementing some great intuitions time after time, we first put aside the traditional and outdated approach to hysteroscopy and nowadays clinicians performing office hysteroscopy worldwide use the vaginoscopic approach: quicker and less painful [19].

By not using the speculum and the tenaculum before hysteroscopic examination, we eliminated discomfort not related to the technique itself and reduced the number of instruments necessary. It is ideal for office hysteroscopy and in patients who otherwise might require general anesthesia.

Two recent randomized studies with several critical biases failed to demonstrate a real advantage of hysteroscopy before IVF in increasing live birth rates.

The inSIGHT study is a multicenter, randomized, comparative study. InSIGHT concerned women scheduled for IVF (in vitro fertilization) and a normal transvaginal ultrasound. Women were randomized for proceeding directly for IVF or performing an hysteroscopy before IVF. Routine hysteroscopy did not increase live birth rate, therefore is not recommended in case of normal US scan [20].

In 2016, a similar study (the TROPHY study) involved women with at least two failed IVF and a normal US scan, randomized for performing routine hysteroscopy or directly another IVF cycle. Hysteroscopy did not increase the live birth rate [21].

Otherwise, we must be aware that the real innovation constituted by hysteroscopy is the so-called see & treat' approach, which introduced the concept of a single procedure in which the operative part is perfectly integrated in the diagnostic workup.

Despite the great advantages and cost savings of such philosophy, the number of gynecologists who prefer to perform operative procedures in an outpatient setting rather than in the operative theatre continues to be low.

Apart from this new perspective, our group proposed a contemporary approach to almost every concept in the field of hysteroscopy such as myomas and cervical stenosis, and on the other hand, we helped to develop increasingly less invasive and effective devices.

Absolute indications for hysteroscopy in infertile women include intracavitary abnormalities such as endometrial polyps, submucous fibroids, uterine septum, endometritis, and adhesions (Figs. 17.1, 17.2, 17.3, and 17.4).

Several intracavitary pathologies that may cause infertility can be diagnosed and at the same time treated with an outpatient hysteroscopy:

– Endometrial Polyps can cause infertility with different mechanisms, including irregular endometrial bleeding, inflammatory response, interference in the interaction between embryo and endometrium, and interference with normal patterns of endo-

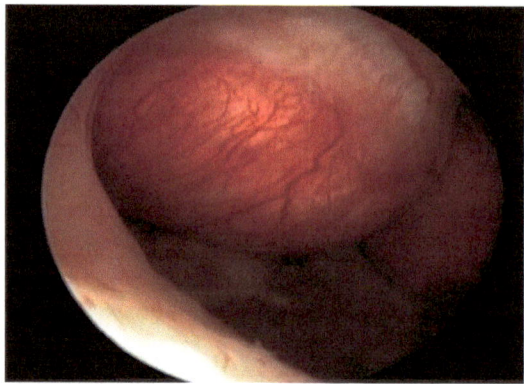

Fig. 17.3 Sub-mucous myomas. (Reproduced from Bettocchi et al. 2021)

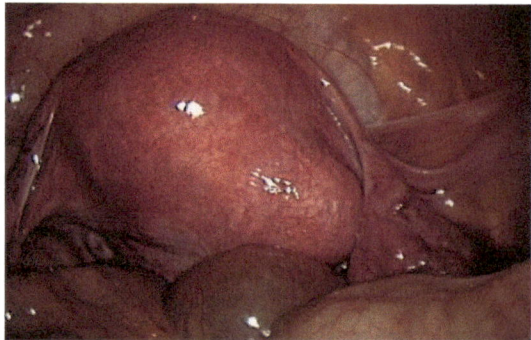

Fig. 17.4 Uterus with fibroids, Laparoscopy. (Reproduced from Bettocchi et al. 2021)

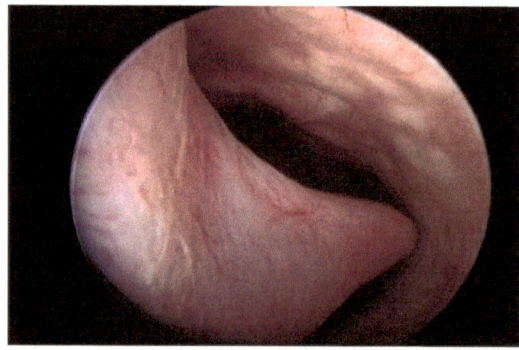

Fig. 17.1 Endometrial polyp. (Reproduced from Bettocchi et al. 2021)

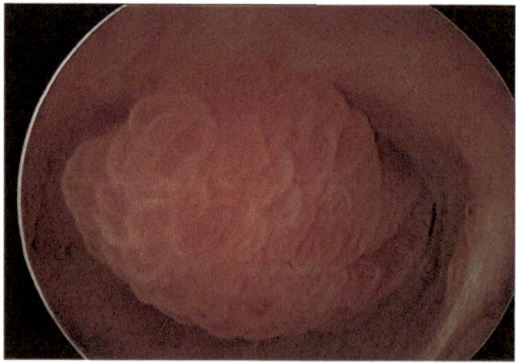

Fig. 17.2 Cervical polyp. (Reproduced from Bettocchi et al. 2021)

crine function. Moreover, polyps were commonly associated with chronic endometritis and the majority are positive for CD-138 staining, suggesting a link between chronic inflammation, a debated cause of infertility, and Eps [22]. Hysteroscopic polypectomy can be performed with cold instruments, such as miniaturized forceps or scissors, with bipolar instruments or with laser devices mostly in an outpatient modality;

– Submucosal Fibroids: as polyps do, fibroids can cause infertility in different ways: distortion of the cavity, abnormal uterine contractility, obstruction of tubal ostia, abnormalities in uterine vascularization, impaired endometrial receptivity, and subsequent implantation failure. Only hysteroscopy allows a complete mapping of the localization of the myoma and depth of myometrial invasion. Vaginal approach for submucosal myomectomy is feasible, secure, and with low discomfort for the patient.

Nowadays, hysteroscopic myomectomy is the gold standard in order to improve cumulative pregnancy rate as well as live birth rate in selected women with submucosal myomas and history of reproductive failure.

The rate of live birth increases and the rate of abortion decreases after hysteroscopic myomectomy. Pregnancy rate is higher in women who underwent a hysteroscopic myomectomy compared with those with fibroids left in situ even if the evidence is still widely debated [23].

Myomectomy could be performed with several techniques apart from the classical slicing technique [24]. Sometimes this technique upfront could be somehow challenging, especially when facing some large G1 or G2 submucosal fibroids. OPPIuM technique has been proposed and seems to achieve the downgrading of these types of leiomyomas in approximately 93% of cases, without any significant surgical complications or the need of hormonal agents' administration. In this way, the safer and quicker subsequent complete myomectomy is facilitated [25].

This technique developed by our group more than a decade ago consisted of an incision of the endometrial mucosa covering the myoma by means of cold scissors or bipolar Versapoint Twizzle electrode, along its reflection line on the uterine wall, up to the precise identification of the cleavage surface between the myoma and its pseudo-capsule. Such procedure was aimed at triggering the protrusion of the intramural portion of the myoma into the uterine cavity during the following menstrual cycles, thus facilitating the subsequent total removal of the lesion via resectoscopic surgery [26].

In the last few years, new other minimally invasive techniques have been developed for the treatment of uterine fibroids. There are some incisionless procedures that use various forms of energy to heat and ablate uterine fibroids like radiofrequency, focused ultrasound, and microwaves (Figs. 17.5 and 17.6).

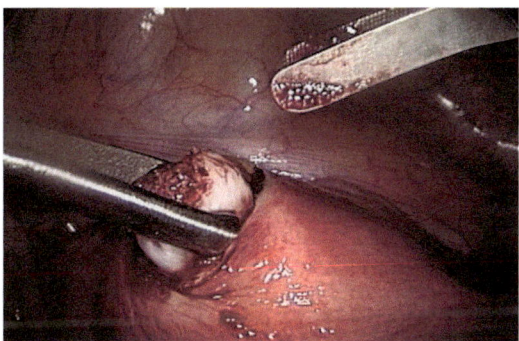

Fig. 17.5 Laparoscopic myomectomy. (Reproduced from Bettocchi et al. 2021)

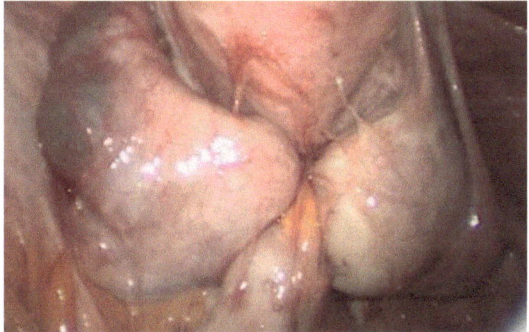

Fig. 17.6 Endometriosis—kissing ovaries. (Reproduced from Bettocchi et al. 2021)

Recently, MR-guided focused ultrasound (MRgFUS), another modality of hyperthermic ablation, has been approved by the US Food and Drug Administration as a validated treatment for fibroids in women seeking pregnancy.

Radiofrequency myolysis (RFM) is the latest uterine-conserving technique, generates thermal effects inside the myoma (60–80 °C), and it results in distinct histological changes: necrosis of tissue cells from coagulation, vascular thrombosis, and inactivation of hormonal receptors within the myoma that prevents tumor tissue from growing [27].

Other incisionless techniques include the use of surgical lasers (Argon, CO_2, Yag, KTP, and others). Diode lasers have been used in hysteroscopic surgery with many advantages.

The main disadvantages for the clinical application of this technology might be the cost because laser equipment currently tend to be expensive and an adequate learning curve to better understand the instrumentation technical characteristics [28].

Recent literature strongly supports hysteroscopic approach even in the treatment of uterine septum, as it has proven to be simple, with minimal postoperative sequelae, improving reproductive outcomes.

These findings have been strong enough to lead to a more liberalized approach, which includes the treatment not only of patients with recurrent pregnancy loss or premature labor, but also the ones with infertility or with IVF plans [29, 30].

We usually perform each metroplasty during the early proliferative phase (day 4 to 9) under general anesthesia using a bipolar 15 Fr. Mini-Resectoscope (Karl Storz Co., Tuttlingen, Germany is connected to an advanced bipolar generator (Autocon III 400, Karl Storz Co., Tuttlingen, Germany). Intrauterine pressure is carefully kept stable (around 45 mmHg) using a dedicated pump (Endomat, Karl Storz Co, Tuttlingen, Germany).

Usually the septum is initially incised "in a classic fashion," adopting an "L-shape" bipolar electrode (Karl Storz Co., Tuttlingen, Germany) up to the fundal area. The septum is then longitudinally transected into two parts, forming an anterior and a posterior triangle on each uterine wall, with the base on the fundus.

Thanks to a careful analysis, we are nowadays able to describe the fine anatomy of the muscle bundles taking part to the septum: this entity should no longer be considered as a fibrous notch in the middle of the cavity, but as a real three-dimensional structure with a "myoma-like" component.

Once we got rid of previous misconceptions, we developed and proposed a new surgical approach based on fine anatomy of the septum: first of all, we completely incise/resect those symmetric fibrous bundles at the base of the septum and then we resect the apex of the septum until the central muscular core is reached.

During this step and given the parallel arrangement of muscular fibers in this area, the fundal area spontaneously flattens and the central muscular core is finally resected [31].

Apart from adequate anatomical knowledge which is essential for successful clinical practice [30], our proposal in resectoscopic surgery should also persuade from a technical point of view as relies on the implementation in our clinical practice of the 15 Fr.

Mini-Resectoscope itself grants at least two more great advantages. First of all, it's a native bipolar system and carries itself all the clear advantages of bipolar energy: the plasma effect of bipolar current allows better cut and coagulation. Moreover, it has minor risk of interference on other electronic equipment (electrocardiogram, pace makers, and others) simultaneously connected to the patient.

Incidence of overflow syndrome in gynecology and TUR syndrome in urology varies considerably in the literature, ranging from 0.18% to 10.9%.

The use of saline solution for distension media of the uterine cavity is the principal advantage of this technology avoiding hypotonic nonelectrolyte solution that can cause fluid overload during the surgical procedure.

Everything said up to now represents a new frontier in the modern hysteroscopic surgical approach to intrauterine pathology in order to increase fertility [32]; the relevance of this technique has been emphasized over during the recent pandemic [33]. Otherwise, large multicentric trials are needed in order to evaluate and reevaluate the endometrial function after surgery and its impact on fertility, of which we know relatively little or nothing.

References

1. WHO. International classification of diseases, 11th Revision (ICD-11). Geneva: WHO; 2018.
2. Mascarenhas MN, Flaxman SR, Boerma T, et al. National, regional, and global trends in infertility prevalence since 1990: a systematic analysis of 277 health surveys. PLoS Med. 2012;9(12):e1001356.
3. Siristatidis C, Vogiatzi P, Pouliakis A, Trivella M, Papantoniou N, Bettocchi S. Predicting IVF outcome: a proposed web-based system using artificial intelligence. In Vivo. 2016;30(4):507–12.
4. Ngowa JD, Kasia JM, Georges NT, Nkongo V, Sone C, Fongang E. Comparison of hysterosalpingograms

with laparoscopy in the diagnostic of tubal factor of female infertility at the Yaoundé general hospital, Cameroon. Pan Afr Med J. 2015;22:264.

5. Van Welie N, van Rijswijk J, et al. Can hysterosalpingo-foam sonography replace hysterosalpingography as first-choice tubal patency test? A randomized non-inferiority trial. Hum Reprod. 2022;37(5):969–79.

6. Ahmad G, Duffy J, Watson AJ. Pain relief in hysterosalpingography. Cochrane Database Syst Rev. 2007;2:CD006106.

7. Assessment and Treatment for People with Fertility Problems. NICE clinical guideline 156; 2013.

8. Maheux-Lacroix S, Boutin A, Moore L, Bergeron ME, Bujold E, Laberge P, Lemyre M, Dodin S. Hysterosalpingosonography for diagnosing tubal occlusion in subfertile women: a systematic review with meta-analysis. Hum Reprod. 2014;29(5):953–63.

9. Di Spiezio SA, Zizolfi B, Bettocchi S, Exacoustos C, Nocera C, Nazzaro G, da Cunha VM, Nappi C. Accuracy of hysteroscopic metroplasty with the combination of presurgical 3-dimensional ultrasonography and a novel graduated intrauterine palpator: a randomized controlled trial. J Minim Invasive Gynecol. 2016;23(4):557–66.

10. Grimbizis GF, Gordts S, Di Spiezio SA, Brucker S, De Angelis C, Gergolet M, Li TC, Tanos V, Brölmann H, Gianaroli L, Campo R. The ESHRE-ESGE consensus on the classification of female genital tract congenital anomalies. Gynecol Surg. 2013;10(3):199–212.

11. Munro MG, Critchley HO, Broder MS, Fraser IS. FIGO working group on menstrual disorders. FIGO classification system (PALM-COEIN) for causes of abnormal uterine bleeding in nongravid women of reproductive age. Int J Gynaecol Obstet. 2011;113(1):3–13.

12. Timor-Tritsch IE, Lerner JP, Monteagudo A, Murphy KE, Heller DS. Transvaginal sonographic markers of tubal inflammatory disease. Ultrasound Obstet Gynecol. 1998;12(1):56–66.

13. Dun EC, Nezhat CH. Tubal factor infertility: diagnosis and management in the era of assisted reproductive technology. Obstet Gynecol Clin North Am. 2012;39(4):551–66.

14. NHS (National Institute for Clinical Excellence), Full Guideline. Fertility: assessment and treatment for people with fertility problems. London: RCOG Press; 2004.

15. Puttemans PJ, De Bruyne F, Heylen SM. A decade of salpingoscopy. Eur J Obstet Gynecol Reprod Biol. 1998;81(2):197–206.

16. Kerin JF, Surrey ES, William DB, et al. Falloscopic observations of endotubal mucus plugs as a cause of reversible obstruction and their histological characterization. J Laparoendosc Surg. 1991;1:103–10.

17. Hershlag A, Seifer DB, Carcangiu ML, et al. Salpingoscopy: light microscope and electron microscopic correlations. Obstet Gynaecol. 1991;77:399–405.

18. Nakagawa K, Inoue M, Nishi Y, et al. A new evaluation score that uses salpingoscopy to reflect fallopian tube function in infertile women. Fertil Steril. 2010;94(7):2753–7.

19. Bettocchi S, Selvaggi L. A vaginoscopic approach to reduce the pain of office hysteroscopy. J Am Assoc Gynecol Laparosc. 1997;4(2):255–8.

20. Smit JG, Kasius JC, Eijkemans MJC, Koks CAM, van Golde R, Nap AW, Scheffer GJ, Manger PAP, Hoek A, Schoot BC, van Heusden AM, Kuchenbecker WKH, Perquin DAM, Fleischer K, Kaaijk EM, Sluijmer A, Friederich J, Dykgraaf RHM, van Hooff M, Louwe LA, Kwee J, de Koning CH, Janssen ICAH, Mol F, Mol BWJ, Broekmans FJM, Torrance HL. Hysteroscopy before in-vitro fertilisation (inSIGHT): a multicentre, randomised controlled trial. Lancet. 2016;387(10038):2622–9.

21. El-Toukhy T, Campo R, Khalaf Y, Tabanelli C, Gianaroli L, Gordts SS, Gordts S, Mestdagh G, Mardesic T, Voboril J, Marchino GL, Benedetto C, Al-Shawaf T, Sabatini L, Seed PT, Gergolet M, Grimbizis G, Harb H, Coomarasamy A. Hysteroscopy in recurrent in-vitro fertilisation failure (TROPHY): a multicentre, randomised controlled trial. Lancet. 2016;387(10038):2614–21.

22. Cicinelli E, Bettocchi S, de Ziegler D, Loizzi V, Cormio G, Marinaccio M, Trojano G, Crupano FM, Francescato R, Vitagliano A, Resta L. Chronic endometritis, a common disease hidden behind endometrial polyps in premenopausal women: first evidence from a case-control study. J Minim Invasive Gynecol. 2019;26(7):1346–50.

23. Metwally M, Raybould G, Cheong YC, Horne AW. Surgical treatment of fibroids for subfertility. Cochrane Database Syst Rev. 2020;1(1):CD003857.

24. Zhang W, Liu J, Wu Q, Liu Y, Wang C, Ma C. A modified technique of bipolar loop resectoscopic slicing for treating submucous fibroids with enucleation makes the operation safer. Front Surg. 2021;8:746936.

25. Cicinelli E, Mitsopoulos V, Fascilla FD, Sioutis D, Bettocchi S. The OPPIuM technique: office hysteroscopic technique for the preparation of partially intramural leiomyomas. Minerva Ginecol. 2016;68(3):328–33.

26. Bettocchi S, Di Spiezio SA, Ceci O, Nappi L, Guida M, Greco E, Pinto L, Camporiale AL, Nappi C. A new hysteroscopic technique for the preparation of partially intramural myomas in office setting (OPPIuM technique): a pilot study. J Minim Invasive Gynecol. 2009;16(6):748–54.

27. Fasciani A, Turtulici G, Siri G, Ferrero S, Sirito R. A prospective intervention trial on tailored radiofrequency ablation of uterine myomas. Medicina (Kaunas). 2020;56(3):122.

28. Nappi L, Sorrentino F, Angioni S, Pontis A, Greco P. The use of laser in hysteroscopic surgery. Minerva Ginecol. 2016;68(6):722–6.

29. Homer HA, Li TC, Cooke ID. The septate uterus: a review of management and reproductive outcome. Fertil Steril. 2000;73(1):1–14.

30. McShane PM, Reilly RJ, Schiff I. Pregnancy outcomes following tompkins metroplasty. Fertil Steril. 1983;40(2):190–4.
31. Fascilla FD, Resta L, Cannone R, De Palma D, Ceci OR, Loizzi V, Di Spiezio SA, Campo R, Cicinelli E, Bettocchi S. Resectoscopic metroplasty with uterine septum excision: a histologic analysis of the uterine septum. J Minim Invasive Gynecol. 2020;27(6):1287–94.
32. Bettocchi S, Achilarre MT, Ceci O, Luigi S. Fertility-enhancing hysteroscopic surgery. Semin Reprod Med. 2011;29(2):75–82.
33. Carugno J, Di Spiezio SA, Alonso L, Haimovich S, Campo R, De Angelis C, Bradley L, Bettocchi S, Arias A, Isaacson K, Okohue J, Farrugia M, Kumar A, Xue X, Cavalcanti L, Laganà AS, Grimbizis G. COVID-19 pandemic. impact on hysteroscopic procedures: a consensus statement from the global congress of hysteroscopy scientific committee. J Minim Invasive Gynecol. 2020;27(5):988–92.

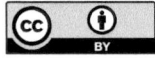

Maria Matteo

18.1 Introduction

The human species is biologically distinguished by low fertility.

In fact, with each menstrual cycle, a couple at the peak of their reproductive capacity has only about a 30% chance of conceiving. This percentage, already quite modest, is significantly reduced in the presence of factors that can reduce reproductive capacity. The World Health Organization (WHO) states that it is the decision of each individual and couple, according to their conscience, to determine whether they intend to have a pregnancy and if so, when they wish to have a child, as well as determining the size of the family unit. However, fertility problems may affect the possibility of pregnancy. The WHO states infertility as "*a disease of the reproductive system defined by the failure to achieve a clinical pregnancy after 12 months or more of regular unprotected intercourse*" [1] It is reported that one in four couples in developing countries has been affected by infertility. In 2012, infertility in women remained within a similar range over 20 years, from 1990 to 2010. However, in 2019, infertility increased worldwide, as it was found that the age-standardized infertility preva-lence rate increased by 0.37% per year for women and by 0.29% per year for men. Since a significant percentage of couples manage to have a child after at least 2 years of trying, many prefer to talk about infertility after 24 months. The term "sub fecundity", on the other hand, indicates a fertility index three or four times lower: this means that some couples will have to wait longer to conceive. Although it is difficult to assess the impact of the various factors on the causes of infertility, the data regarding the incidence and the main causes of infertility are similar worldwide. About 20–30% of infertility cases are due to male infertility, 20–35% are due to female infertility, and 25–40% are due to combined problems in both parts. In 10–20% cases, no cause is found.

Common contributory factors-causes of *female infertility,* include:

- Ovarian disorders and hormonal imbalances (e.g., polycystic ovarian syndrome-PCOS), premature ovarian failure (POF), hypothalamic dysfunction, hyperprolactinemia.
- Fallopian tubal damage (including previous tubal ligation).
- Pelvic inflammatory disease (PID) caused by infections like tuberculosis.
- Age-related factors.
- Uterine problems (benign polyps fibroids).
- Cervical disorders (benign polyps or tumors and cervical stenosis).
- Endometriosis.
- Advanced maternal age.

M. Matteo (✉)
Department of Medical and Surgical Sciences, University of Foggia, Foggia, Italy

Phisiopathology and Assisted Reproductive Unit, University Hospital of Foggia, Foggia, Italy
e-mail: maria.matteo@unifg.it

C. Bettocchi et al. (eds.), *Practical Clinical Andrology*,
https://doi.org/10.1007/978-3-031-11701-5_18

The main cause of *male infertility* is low semen quality. In men who have the necessary reproductive organs to procreate, infertility can be caused by low sperm count due to endocrine problems, drugs, radiation, or infection. There may be testicular malformation, hormone imbalance, or blockage of man's duct system.

Male and female infertility: in some cases, both the man and woman may be infertile or subfertile, and couple's infertility arises from the combination of these conditions. In other cases, the cause is suspected to be.

Infertility due to unknown cause (idiopathic): In the US, up to 20% of infertile couples have unknown (unexplained) infertility. In these cases, abnormalities are likely to be present but not detected by current methods.

18.2 Assisted Reproductive Technology

Assisted reproductive technology (ART) consists of all treatments or procedures that include the in vitro handling of both human oocytes and sperm or of embryos, for the purpose of establishing a pregnancy. Increasingly, couples are turning to ART for help with conceiving and ultimately giving birth to a healthy live baby of their own. In July 1978, Louise Brown was the first child successfully born after her mother received IVF treatment. Brown was born as a result of natural-cycle IVF, where no stimulation was made. The procedure took place at Dr. Kershaw's Cottage Hospital (now Dr. Kershaw's Hospice) in Ryton, Oldham, England. Robert G. Edwards was awarded the Nobel Prize in Physiology or Medicine in 2010. The physiologist codeveloped the treatment together with Patrick Steptoe and embryologist Jean Purdy, but the latter two were not eligible for consideration as they had died and the Nobel Prize is not awarded posthumously. Since the first baby was born after in vitro fertilization (IVF) in the United Kingdom in 1978, assisted reproductive technology (ART), including IVF and embryo transfers (ETs), has been widely used for infertility treatment worldwide. The International Committee for Monitoring

Assisted Reproductive Technologies reported that more than one million babies were born after ART between 2008 and 2010.

18.3 Art Techniques and Indications

The techniques are usually divided into three broad categories:

- *First level techniques:* the simpler and less invasive ones, such as intrauterine insemination (IUI) with or without ovarian stimulation.
- *Second level techniques* the more complex and more invasive ones that can be performed under local anesthesia or deep sedation, which differ from the basic techniques as they involve manipulation of female and male gametes and because they require in vitro fertilization. Among these techniques, the IVF (In Vitro Fertilization and Embryo Transfer), ICSI (Intracytoplasmic Sperm Injection), and the possible cryopreservation of male and female gametes and embryos.
- *Third level techniques* procedures that require general anesthesia with intubation, including:
  - laparoscopic egg retrieval, intra-tubal transfer of male and female gametes (GIFT), zygotes (ZIFT) and /or embryos (TET) laparoscopically;
  - microsurgical sampling of gametes from the testicle: Testicular Sperm Extraction (TESE), Microsurgical Testicular Sperm Extraction (microTESE), Testicular Sperm Aspiration (TESA);
  - microsurgical sampling of gametes from the epididymides: Percutaneous Epididymal Sperm Aspiration (PESA) and Microsurgical Epididymal Sperm Aspiration (MESA).

In all assisted reproduction techniques, the seminal fluid receives a treatment able to induce capacitation "in vitro" so that the activated spermatozoa, at the threshold of the acrosomal reaction, can interact with the mature oocytes.

The goal of the preparation is twofold:

1. Separate sperm from seminal plasma which contains decapacitating factors, bacteria, leukocytes, and cell debris.
2. Concentrate as many spermatozoa as possible with good progressive motility in a small volume.

18.3.1 First Level Technique: Intrauterine and Intracervical Insemination IUI/ICI

Intrauterine insemination is used most often in couples who have:

- Donor sperm treatment.
- Unexplained infertility.
- Endometriosis stage I –II-related infertility.
- Mild male factor infertility (subfertility).
- Cervical factor infertility.
- Ovulatory factor infertility.

In an IUI cycle, the male partner's sperm is prepared and placed directly in the womb around the time of ovulation. The sperm can be inseminated in natural cycles or in cycles with ovarian stimulation.

In natural cycles, the timing of insemination may be determined by measuring urinary luteinizing hormone (LH). Detection of a rise in the LH level can also be done in the clinic, with daily blood samples. Finally, transvaginal ultrasound, in combination with the administration of human chorionic gonadotropin (hCG), may be used to time the insemination [2]. In cycles with OH, women receive clomiphene citrate, an antiestrogen, or gonadotrophins to induce the growth of up to three follicles. The timing of insemination is determined by transvaginal ultrasound, combined with hCG-triggered ovulation.

When the follicle reaches an estimated size of 15–20 mm, human chorionic gonadotrophin (hCG) is administered intramuscularly and final maturation of the oocyte is thereby induced [3]. Many sperm preparation procedures are available, but there are three main methods (Fig. 18.1) used to select the best spermatozoa from native sperm (Fig. 18.1a).

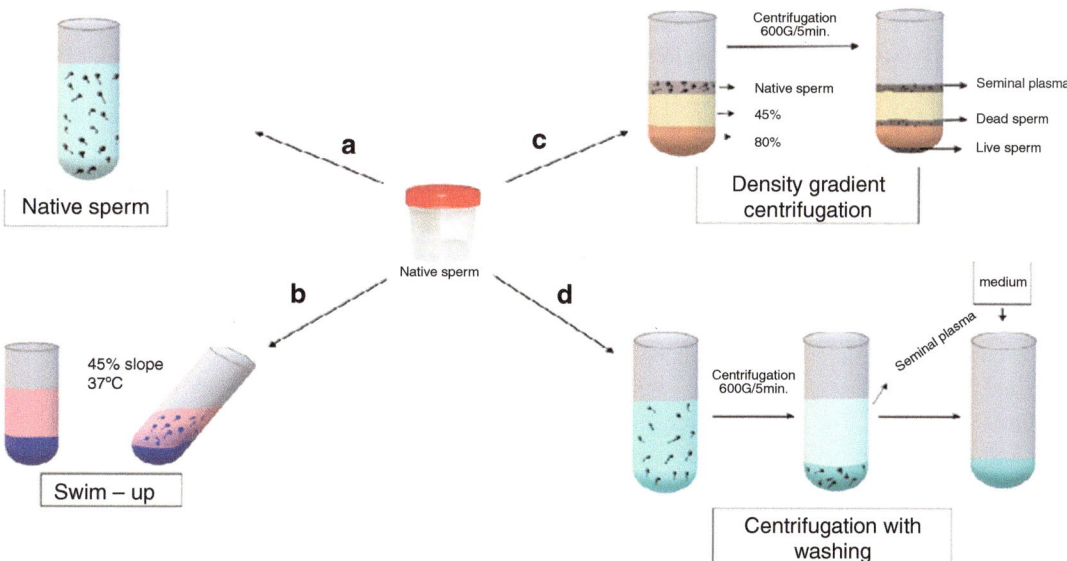

Fig. 18.1 Description of the compared sperm preparation procedures (**a**) Native sperm; (**b**) Swim-up; (**c**) Density Gradient Centrifugation, and (**d**) Centrifugation with washing

18.3.1.1 Sperm Preparation Techniques

- *Swim-up*: The spermatozoa may be selected on their ability to swim, known as the *"swim-up technique"* (Fig. 18.1b). This technique is performed by layering culture medium over the liquefied semen. Motile spermatozoa then swim into the culture. The upper part of the supernatant is then carefully removed for further use.
- *Density gradients* The second method of selecting spermatozoa is by the use of *density gradients* (Fig. 18.1c). The semen sample is pipetted on top of the density column and then centrifuged. Density gradient centrifugation separates spermatozoa according to their density. This way you can select the motile, morphologically spermatozoa in the solution with the highest concentration of gradient, which is aspirated for further use [4].
- The third method is the *conventional wash method in combination with centrifugation* (Fig. 18.1d). The semen sample is diluted with a medium and centrifuged. Subsequently, the pellet is resuspended in a bit of medium and incubated until the time of insemination.

Concerning IUI outcomes, recent evidences suggest that treatment with IUI with ovarian stimulation probably results in a higher live birth rate, compared to expectant management without ovarian stimulation, in couples with a low prediction score of natural conception. Similarly, treatment with IUI in a natural cycle probably results in a higher cumulative live birth rate compared to treatment with expectant management in a stimulated cycle [5]. At present, the most important indication for IUI is in donor sperm treatment. In these cases, the sperm can be introduced by intrauterine insemination (IUI) or by intracervical insemination (ICI). The main difference between IUI and ICI is the processing of the sperm [6].

18.3.2 Second Level Techniques: In Vitro Fertilization (IVF)

Fertility treatments are complex, and each cycle consists of several steps. If one of these steps is incorrectly applied, conception may not occur.

18.3.2.1 Indications

In vitro fertilization is indicated in couples who are unable to conceive for:

- Tubal-peritoneal factor (acquired or congenital tubal disease).
- Moderate male infertility when medical-surgical treatment or previous intrauterine inseminations have failed or have been judged inappropriate.
- Severe male factor infertility.
- Grade III or IV endometriosis.
- Immunological factor.
- Idiopathic infertility if the previous intrauterine insemination treatment did not give results or was not judged appropriate for that couple.
- Cryopreserved semen, in relation to semen quality after thawing.
- Repeated abortion.
- Genetic Diseases/Preimplantation Genetic Screening or Diagnosis (PGT-A or PGT-M).

The following steps make up an IVF cycle:

- Drugs are initiated to stimulate growth of multiple ovarian follicles, while at the same time other medications are given to suppress the natural menstrual cycle and downregulate the pituitary gland.
- After ovarian stimulatory drugs are initiated, monitoring is undertaken at intervals to assess the growth of follicles. When the follicles have reached an appropriate size (19–20 mm), a drug is administered to bring about final maturation of the eggs (known as ovulation triggering). The next step involves egg collection (usually with a transvaginal ultrasound probe to guide the pickup) and, in some cases of male infertility, sperm retrieval.
- Next is the fertilization process, which usually is completed by in vitro fertilization (IVF) or intracytoplasmic sperm injection (ICSI).
- Embryos are then placed into the uterus. Issues of importance here include endometrial preparation, the best timing for embryo transfer, how many embryos to transfer, what type

of catheter to use, the use of ultrasound guidance, need for bed rest, etc.

Then comes luteal phase support, for which several options are available, including administration of progesterone, estrogen (E_2), and human chorionic gonadotrophin (hCG).

Finally, adverse effects, such as ovarian hyperstimulation syndrome, can be associated with the assisted reproduction process.

18.3.2.2 Controlled Ovarian Stimulation in IVF

Controlled ovarian stimulation comprises three basic elements.

1. Exogenous gonadotrophins to stimulate multi-follicular development.
2. Cotreatment with either gonadotropin-releasing hormone (GnRH) agonist or antagonists to suppress pituitary function and prevent premature ovulation.
3. Triggering of final oocyte maturation 36–38 h prior to oocyte retrieval.

Gonadotrophin preparations available for use include human menopausal gonadotrophin (hMG), a urinary product with follicle-stimulating hormone (FSH) and luteinizing hormone (LH) activity, purified FSH (p-FSH) and highly purified FSH (hp-FSH), and various recombinant FSH (rFSH) and LH (rFSH/rLH) preparations. In addition, IVF in an unstimulated cycle with the anticipation of only collecting a mature single egg is offered by some clinics, but this practice is not widely established [7].

GnRH agonists or antagonists have been used in a number of different protocols. In the so-called 'long protocol', the GnRH agonist is started at least 2 weeks before stimulation and continued up until oocyte maturation is achieved. Alternatively, a 'short protocol' is used in which the GnRH agonist is commenced simultaneously with stimulation and continued up until the day of oocyte maturation trigger. Yet another option is the use of GnRH antagonists. These involve a shorter duration of use compared with the agonist 'long protocol' and are started a few days after initiation of

stimulation, continuing up until administration of a drug to trigger oocyte maturation.

18.3.2.3 Controlled Ovarian Stimulation and Ovarian Response

On the basis of ovarian response patients are classified into normoresponders, poor responders, and hyperresponders. Although no unequivocal definition of the *poor responders* has been universally accepted, the Bologna classification [8] defines poor responders by two of the following characteristics:

– Maternal age 40 years or older, or other risk factors for poor ovarian response (such as excision of bilateral ovarian endometriomas)
– Poor ovarian response in previous IVF cycle(s) (defined as retrieval of three or fewer oocytes in a conventional stimulation IVF protocol).
– Low antral follicle count (AFC) (less than 5–7 follicles), or low anti-Müllerian hormone (AMH) below 0.5–1.1 ng/mL (3.5–8 pmol/L).

Hyperresponders patients, with a prior risk for development of hyperstimulation (OHSS), are those with polycystic ovaries (PCOs), low body mass index (BMI), high antral follicle count (AFC), increased anti-Muller hormone (AMH) levels, and elevated serum estradiol (E2) concentrations [7]. Ovarian stimulation protocols are chosen on the basis of the expected response of patients. Duiring controlled ovarian stimulation, the number and size of follicles, visualized at transvaginal ultrasound sonography, provide an estimate of ovarian response and hCG is used to trigger ovulation when a certain number of follicles reach a certain size. Estradiol, which is produced by developing follicles, provides additional information which is believed to further improve the decision making process; follicle maturity is supported by adequate estradiol levels while there is an increased risk of OHSS in the presence of very high levels. At the end of the stimulation phase of an IVF cycle, a drug is used to trigger the final oocyte maturation, which is used to mimic the natural endogenous LH surge and initiate the process of ovulation before the mature eggs are collected from the woman and fertilized with sperm in the laboratory. Two drugs are currently used: human chorionic gonadotropin (HCG), which is the most common drug, or GnRH agonist in an antagonist protocol.

18.3.3 IVF—ICSI: Laboratory Phase

In Vitro Fertilization (IVF) and Intracitoplasmatic Sperm Injection (ICSI) are laboratory techniques that both involve the aspiration of oocytes from the follicles. Therefore, the therapy to be carried out by the patient and the egg retrieval are absolutely the same in the two techniques. Which technique to adopt is a decision that is made "in the laboratory" after the egg retrieval.

18.3.3.1 In Vitro Fertilization
IVF consists of placing the spermatozoa close to the oocyte and letting one of these fertilize it nat-

urally (Fig. 18.2). This technique can be used when sperm has the adequate number of spermatozoa with sufficient motility to fertilize the egg.

18.3.3.2 Intracitoplasmatic Sperm Injection (ICSI)
In vitro fertilization with ICSI is an assisted reproduction technique that allows to inseminate an oocyte (female reproductive cell) by microinjection into it of a single sperm. The ICSI requires a sperm to be selected and injected into the oocyte, forcing its fertilization (Fig. 18.3).

Once fertilized, the oocyte becomes a preembryo and is transferred inside the uterus so that it continues its development (Fig. 18.4).

ICSI is a complementary tool to conventional in vitro fertilization. The previous and subsequent stages are the same as those of insemination (stimulation of the ovaries, follicular puncture, and embryo transfer); only the insemination technique changes. This technique is used

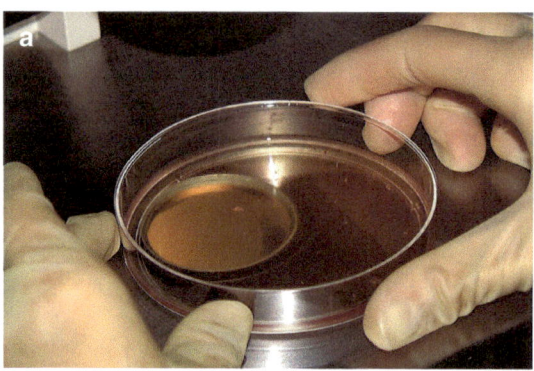
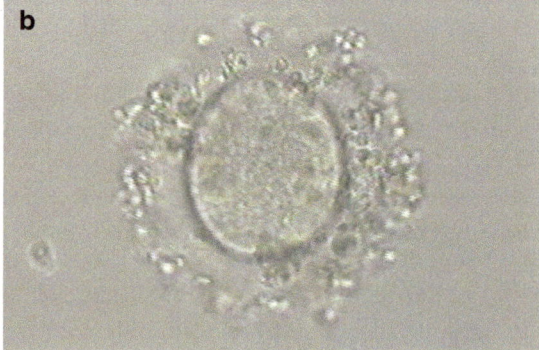

Fig. 18.2 (**a**) IVF: Sperms are placed along with eggs and leave them to their natural process of fertilization. (**b**) Microscopic sperm cells around human egg

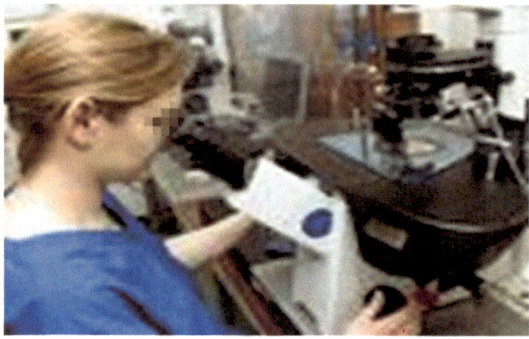
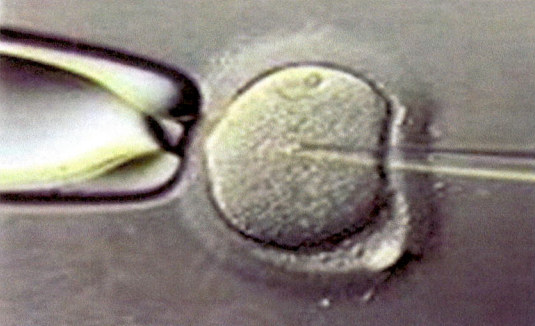

Fig. 18.3 ICSI procedure: a single spermatozoa is injected directly into an egg to achieve fertilization

Day 1   Day 2

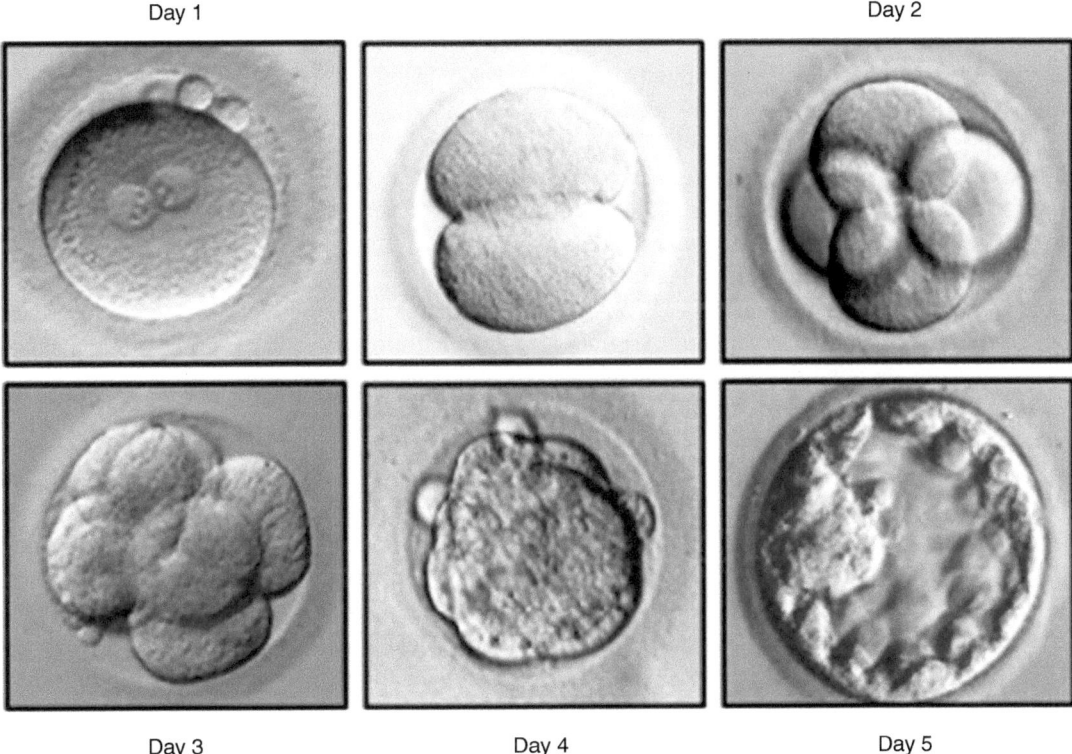

Day 3   Day 4   Day 5

Fig. 18.4 Stages of embryo development from zygote (day 1) to blastocyst (day 5)

when the spermatozoa are in very small numbers and their motility is very low. With this technique, there is an evident saving of sperm: only one sperm is needed for each oocyte, while in conventional IVF, between 50,000 and 100,000 sperm are needed. IVF technique reproduces more faithfully than ICSI what probably occurs in nature; allowing the sperm to enter in a very natural way, without having to create a microtrauma on the oocyte wall (the microinjection of ICSI). Let the sperm that fertilizes the egg be "selected by nature". However, we do not yet know for sure whether this selection process is better than the one performed in the laboratory with ICSI. Since sperm and oocytes remain in contact for a long time, the slightly immature oocytes develop and be fertilized even many hours after pick-up. On the other hand, ICSI technique is the only technique through which it is possible to obtain pregnancy when the seminal damage is severe or when the spermatozoa must be retrieved directly from the testicle and not from the ejaculate. It ensures that if there is a

problem where the sperm is unable to "pass" the egg wall, it is overcome by microinjecting the sperm beyond the wall. It is the only technique that fertilizes oocytes if the frosted oocytes are used. It is therefore clear that in some cases the choice of ICSI is an opportune and obligatory choice which has revolutionized the world of assisted procreation, allowing fertilization with very badly damaged seminal fluids. It is also true that in cases where it is applicable, IVF remains an effective and highly successful technique. Therefore, the use of routine ICSI is not indicated but only in specific cases. The most appropriate technique will therefore be chosen according to the clinical situation of the couple.

18.3.4 Third Level Techniques: IVF in Azoospermic Patients

The absence of sperm in semen does not necessarily mean that they are not produced at all. In the case of azoospermia, crypto-azoospermia, necrozoospermia, and anejaculation, the spermatozoa can be identified in other sites—testis or epididymis—and even if in small numbers they can be collected using various techniques. Testicular Sperm Extraction (TESE) and Microsurgical Testicular Sperm Extraction (microTESE) or Testicular Sperm Aspiration (TESA) allow the recovery of spermatozoa from the testicles; other techniques as Percutaneous Epididymal Sperm Aspiration (PESA)and Microsurgical Epididymal Sperm Aspiration (MESA) from the epididymides. What are the main withdrawal techniques in details:

- PESA, MESA, and TESA are procedures performed by needle aspiration: the sampling is carried out with different techniques in the epididymis.
- TESE and micro TESE are surgical procedures: the collection takes place through the skin of the testicle.

TESE: is a biopsy of testicular tissue, a procedure that allows the recovery of spermatozoa from a small fragment of surgically removed testicle tissue. TESE can be performed under local, locoregional anesthesia, or deep sedation. The surgeon cuts into the tissue covering the testicle (tunica albuginea) and takes a section of the seminiferous tubules the size of an orange seed. The removed fragment is delivered inside a sterile test tube to the biologists for the extraction of spermatozoa. The sampling can be single or multiple in the same testicle. A histological examination is also routinely performed which allows for a precise diagnosis of azoospermia and to intercept occult tumor forms, frequent in nonobstructive azoospermia. *Sperm recovery success rates:* In obstructive azoospermias (OA), in obstructive crypto-azoospermias, in necrozoospermia, and in anejaculation, the recovery rate of "useful" spermatozoa for ICSI is close to 100%. In nonobstructive azoospermias (NOAs) and secretory crypto-azoospermias, the recovery rate of "useful" spermatozoa is 50%. Generally, it is performed before carrying out the ovarian stimulation in the female partner, cryopreserving the sperma-

tozoa, to optimize the time and avoid hormonal treatments to the woman in case of absence of spermatozoa.

18.3.5 Genetic Diseases/ Preimplantation Genetic Testing

One additional indication for IVF is to provide genetic testing on embryos prior to implantation. Preimplantation Genetic Screening (PGS) and Preimplantation Genetic Diagnosis (PGD) are highly specialized procedures which involve removing three to four cells from a 5–6 days old blastocyst and testing it for chromosomal abnormalities prior to transferring the embryo into a woman's uterus. Following a revision of definitions used in infertility care, the previous terms of preimplantation genetic diagnosis (PGD) and preimplantation genetic screening (PGS) have been replaced by the term PGT, including PGT for aneuploidies (PGT-A), PGT for monogenic/single gene defects (PGT-M), and PGT for chromosomal structural rearrangements (PGT-SR) [9]. PGT was first clinically applied in the early 90s, and was initially utilized in sexing cases for couples who were at risk of transmitting an X-linked recessive disorder [10]. Since that time, the number of diseases diagnosed has increased dramatically, as have the different patient groups who use PGT to achieve a healthy pregnancy. At present, PGT is considered as an alternative to prenatal diagnosis [11], while the related method known as preimplantation genetic screening (PGS) is employed to increase success rates of ART. PGD is indicated in the following categories of patients: (1) Carriers of single gene disorders, dominant and recessive, autosomal or X-linked. (2) Carriers of structural chromosome abnormalities, reciprocal and Robertsonian translocations, inversions, deletions, insertions, etc. In most cases, these can lead to chromosomal rearrangements not compatible with life or result in repeated miscarriages (3) Women of advanced maternal age, to avoid having chromosomally abnormal offspring. (4) Couples with repeated

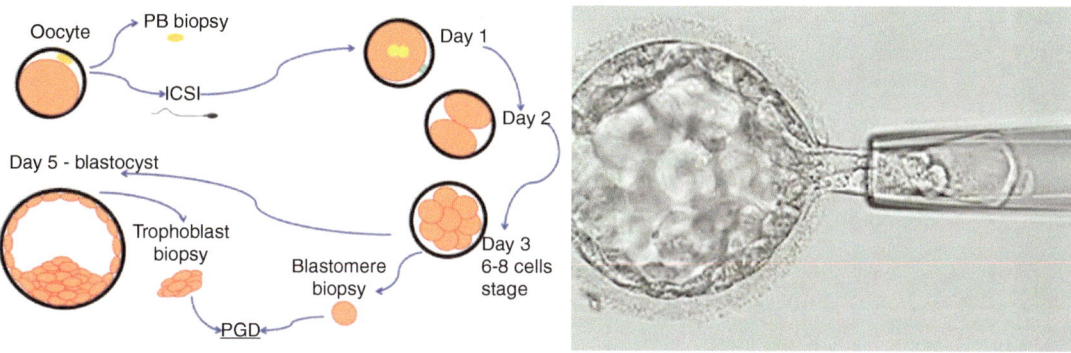

Fig. 18.5 Blastocyst trophectoderm biopsy

implantation failure following assisted reproduction treatments (ART). (5) Couples with repeated unexplained miscarriage. PGT-A and PGT-M techniques permit the selection and subsequent transfer of embryos which are less likely to have chromosomal abnormalities or free of a known single gene disorder, hence increasing the chances for a successful pregnancy, decreased risk of miscarriage, and healthy baby.

Patients who need PGT-A or PGT-M undergo a typical IVF cycle. After the patient's eggs are retrieved, they are fertilized with the husband's or donor sperm in the laboratory. The lab waits for fertilization to occur and lets the embryos develop for 5–6 days into the 80–100 cell blastocyst stage. Trophectoderm biopsy (Fig. 18.5) has replaced cleavage-stage biopsy as the preferential method for biopsy for PGT-A and for concurrent PGT-M. This shift in the biopsy method is linked to the implementation of comprehensive genetic testing.

At the blastocyst stage, embryologists remove three to four cells from each embryo after creating a precise microscopic hole in the outer shell with a laser (embryo biopsy) and then these cells undergo the chromosomal analysis. Once chromosomally normal embryos are confirmed, patients receive a frozen embryo transfer after appropriate ovarian suppression and uterine preparation using hormonal stimulation. The frozen embryo transfer can occur as soon as 5–6 weeks after initial egg retrieval, but this is dependent on several factors. In most cases, it will subsequently only transfer at the most two blastocysts, and in most cases, recommend transfer of one chromosomally tested normal blastocyst in order to avoid the increased risk of higher order multiples. According to the last data report of the ESHRE PGT Consortium, the top five of PGT-M indications are: cystic fibrosis, Huntington's disease, and myotonic dystrophy type 1 that remain frequent indications, while testing for hereditary breast cancer syndromes and neurofibromatosis has become more frequent than analyses for hereditary haemoglobinopathies and fragile X [12]. The efficiency of diagnostic testing is high (over 94%) for PGT-SR, PGT-A, and concurrent PGT-M/SR and PGT-A, whereas a slightly poorer efficiency (88%) is obtained for PGT-M. It remains to be seen whether in the coming years efficiency can be improved with new comprehensive techniques.

18.3.6 IVF Outcomes in European Countries

According to data reported from the European IVF-Monitoring Consortium (EIM) for the European Society of Human Reproduction and Embryology (ESHRE), the clinical pregnancy rates (PR) per aspiration and per transfer are 28.0% and 34.8%, respectively. After ICSI, the corresponding rates are 24% and 33.5% (Table 18.1) [13]. The pregnancy and delivery rates are higher for frozen embryo replacement (FER) cycles than for both fresh IVF and ICSI cycles. When considering the stage of replaced embryos, data showed PR for blastocyst transfers

Table 18.1 Pregnancy and delivery rates (DR) after IVF or ICSI and after FER (after both IVF and ICSI) reported in European countries in 2017

Country	IVF				ICSI			FER			ART infants	ART infants per national births (%)
	Initiated Cycles IVF + ICSI	Aspirations	Pregnancies per aspiration (%)	Deliveries per aspiration (%)	Aspirations	Pregnancies per aspiration (%)	Deliveries per aspiration (%)	Thawings FER	Pregnancies per thawing (%)	Deliveries per thawing (%)		
Albania	105	0			105	37.1	29.5	82	28.0	20.7	65	
Armenia	1155	492	42.3	40.9	636	38.2	36.8	675	36.7	33.0	884	2.2
Austria	10 216	1702	31.6	28.0	5298	28.5	24.4	2801	32.9	28.4	2824	3.2
Belarus	2741	1117	36.5	27.6	1511	35.3	25.8	663	39.1	24.7	1066	1.0
Belgium	18 681	2819	24.1	18.0	13 133	22.2	15.8	12 881	27.1	18.8	5711	4.8
Bosnia-Herzegovina, Federation part	82				72	25.0	23.6	80	38.7	20.0	172	
Bulgaria	4955	311	30.9	21.9	4644	20.3	14.9	1365	28.4	21.1		
Croatia	4334											
Czech Republic	15 557				15 122	22.4	14.0	13 907	29.7	17.7	6191	5.4
Denmark	13 656	6525	22.6	13.1	5659	23.5	16.9				3411	5.6
Estonia	1840	620	28.1	21.6	1199	29.6	21.9	890	27.9	18.8	725	5.3
Finland	4261	2341	22.9	17.5	1679	21.0	16.6					
France	67 703	20 768	21.0	17.7	41 412	21.2	18.3	37 469	22.9	19.2	20 966	2.7
Germany	71 969	17 771	25.1	17.8	50 863	26.6	19.0	27 234	26.5	17.7	21 292	
Greece	15 754	2166	24.9	18.1	13 588	18.4	12.7	5192	43.4	24.2	6276	
Hungary	5408	1326			4003							
Iceland		259	28.2	25.5	221	26.7	21.7	267	41.9	32.2	229	5.6
Italy	53 014	7201	21.8	14.8	40 710	19.0	12.2	17 281	29.3	20.2	12 638	2.8
Kazakhstan	5161	1285	24.3	14.1	3497	23.7	13.1	2416	49.1	26.5	1700	5.7
Latvia	846	265	28.7	20.8	581	25.3	18.2	549	43.0	29.5	401	
Lithuania	395							187	36.4	3.2	125	0.4
Luxembourg	717	234	28.6	20.5	419	27.9	21.2	429	29.1	17.2	243	3.9
Malta	231	17			204						48	1.1
Moldova	960				891	33.8	24.7	346	38.7	21.4		
Montenegro	582				575	24.3	19.0	84	26.2	23.8	170	2.3
North-Macedonia	2521	385	34.0	10.4	1885	32.9	27.5	277	41.9	31.0	747	4.7
Norway	6960	3759	24.6	20.8	2856	23.7	20.5	4476	22.0	17.8		
Poland	14 565	465	27.7	22.2	13 923	26.6	16.3	10 390	35.8	22.0	5680	1.4
Portugal	6327	2521	27.4	20.5	3490	21.7	16.1	2317	33.7	24.8	2436	2.8
Romania	2900	1138	26.9	20.3	1631	25.6	20.4	1452	33.5	26.4	1105	0.6
Russia	87 613	37 275	29.2	21.2	47 500	25.1	17.4	35 979	40.2	27.7	34 173	2.0
Serbia	222	146	31.5	26.0	74	29.7	24.3	34	41.2		74	

Results generated from European registries by ESHRE

to be higher: 41.7% vs. 29.4% for cleavage stage embryos, for fresh IVF and ICSI cycles, respectively. Regarding treatment modalities, while ICSI remains the most applied with a trend to stabilization of its use during recent years, frozen embryo replacement is the second most used technique and there is a progressive increase in the proportion of transfer of frozen embryo relative to fresh IVF and ICSI cycles .

18.4　Art Complications

ART can alleviate the burden of infertility on individuals and families, but it can also present challenges to public health as evidenced by the high rates of multiple delivery, preterm delivery, and low birth-weight delivery experienced with ART. Monitoring the outcomes of technologies that affect ART has become an important public health activity. The potential health risks for both mothers and infants are described as follows.

18.4.1　Ovarian Hyperstimulation Syndrome (OHSS)

Ovarian hyperstimulation syndrome (OHSS) is an iatrogenic complication of assisted reproduction technology. The syndrome is characterized by cystic enlargement of the ovaries and a fluid shift from the intravascular to the third space due to increased capillary permeability and ovarian neoangiogenesis. Its occurrence is dependent on the administration of human chorionic gonadotrophin (hCG). To understand OHSS and its management, one must first be aware of its classifications of severity [14].

Grades of OHSS are described as follows:

- Mild OHSS
  - Grade 1—Abdominal distention and discomfort
  - Grade 2—Grade 1 disease plus nausea, vomiting, and/ or diarrhea plus ovarian enlargement from 5 to 12 cm.
- Moderate OHSS
  - Grade 3—Features of mild OHSS plus ultrasonographic evidence of ascites.
- Severe OHSS
  - Grade 4—Features of moderate OHSS plus clinical evidence of ascites and/or hydrothorax and breathing difficulties.
  - Grade 5—All of the above plus a change in the blood volume, increased blood viscosity due to hemoconcentration, coagulation abnormalities, and diminished renal perfusion and function.

18.4.1.1 Prevention of OHSS: Effective Interventions

Dopamine agonist is effective for prevention of moderate or severe OHSS in women at high risk of OHSS. However, dopamine agonists might increase the risk of adverse events, such as gastrointestinal symptoms [15]. Moreover, the use of gonadotrophin-releasing hormone antagonists (GnRHa) compared with long GnRHa protocols is associated with a large reduction in OHSS, and no evidence suggested a difference in live birth rates [16]. OHSS rates are reduced with GnRHa triggering. However, a lower live birth rate, a reduced ongoing pregnancy rate, and a higher miscarriage rate are registered among women who received GnRHa versus hCG [17].

18.4.2 Multiple Pregnancies and Preterm Birth

Because multiple embryos are transferred in most ART procedures, ART often results in multiple-gestation pregnancies and multiple births. In Europe, according to data of the last report of the European IVF-monitoring Consortium (EIM) [13], as a result of decreasing numbers of embryos replaced per transfer, the proportion of both twin and triplet deliveries continued to decrease. In 2017, twin and triplet rates for fresh IVF and ICSI cycles together were 14.2% and 0.3%, respectively. Corresponding results for frozen embryo replacement were 11.2% and 0.2%. Risks to the mother from a multiple-birth pregnancy include higher rates of caesarean delivery, maternal hemorrhage, pregnancy-related hypertension, and gestational diabetes. Risks to the infant include preterm birth, low birth weight, death, and greater risk for birth defects and developmental disability. Further, also singleton infants conceived with ART might have higher risk for low birthweight and prematurity than singletons not conceived with ART [18]. According to data reported from CDC ART surveillance [19], in the United States, although rates of ART-conceived preterm and low birthweight infants have been declining steadily, the percentage of infants born with low birthweight and preterm is higher among ART-conceived infants than among all infants. The percentage of preterm births is higher among infants conceived with ART (29.9%) than among all infants born in the total birth population (9.9%). ART-conceived infants contribute to 5.3% of all preterm (gestational age <37 weeks) infants.

18.4.3 Long-Term Effects of ART on Women

Hormonal and reproductive factors are involved in the etiology of breast cancer and cancers of the female genital tract. Many studies have not been able to reach solid conclusions. In a large-scale cohort study in The Netherlands, after a follow-up of 5 ± 8 years, no increased risk of breast and ovarian cancer was found in women who had undergone IVF, as compared with subfertile women who had received no IVF [20]. For endometrial cancer, an increased risk was observed in those exposed to IVF as well as in the unexposed group, suggesting a subfertility-related effect which needs further evaluation.

18.4.4 Long-Term Effects of ART on Offspring

Much concern has been expressed about the health of children born after ART. In particular, the risk of boys born to couples with male factor subfertility has drawn attention, since in a substantial number of male factor subfertility cases, a genetic cause can be suspected. These include Y-chromosomal microdeletions, X-chromosomal and autosomal aberrations (i.e., Robertsonian translocations), syndromal disorders featuring infertility (i.e., Kallmann's syndrome), and ultrastructural sperm defects with a genetic basis (Meschede et al., 2000). Theoretically, with ICSI these defects may be transmitted to the following male generation. Moreover, according to recent statements, [21] the use of ART is associated with increased risks of a major nonchromosomal birth defect, cardiovascular defect and any defect in singleton children, and chromosomal defects in twins. The use of ICSI further increases this risk, the most with male factor infertility. These findings support the correct use of ICSI only when medically indicated. The relative contribution of ART treatment parameters versus the biology of the subfertile couple to this increased risk remains unclear and warrants further study [21].

18.5 Art Legislation and Regulation in European Countries

Thirty-nine European countries reported specific legislation on ART; Accessibility is legally restricted to heterosexual couples in 11 countries: Albania, Bosnia and Herzegovina, Czech Republic, France, Italy, Lithuania, Poland, Slovakia, Slovenia, Switzerland, and Turkey. A total of 30 countries offer treatments to single women and 18 to female couples. In five countries, ART and IUI are permitted for treatment of all patient groups, being infertile couples, single women, and same sex couples, male and female. Use of donated sperm is allowed in 41 countries, egg donation in 38, the simultaneous donation of sperm and egg in 32, and embryo donation in 29. Embryo donation is not allowed in 14 countries (Austria, Armenia, Belarus, Bosnia and Herzegovina, Bulgaria, Denmark, Iceland, Italy, Kazakhstan, Norway, Slovenia, Sweden, Switzerland, and Turkey). Information on individual principal countries is shown in Table 18.2. Preimplantation genetic testing (PGT) for monogenic disorders or structural rearrangements is not allowed in two countries, and PGT for aneuploidy is not allowed in 11; surrogacy is accepted in 16 countries. With the exception of marital/sexual situation, female age is the most frequently reported limiting criteria for legal access to ART, minimal age is usually set at 18 years, and maximum ranging from 45 to 51 years with some countries not using numeric definition. Male maximum age is set in very few countries. Where permitted, age is frequently a limiting criterion for third-party donors (male maximum age 35–55 years; female maximum age 34–38 years). Other legal constraints in third-party donation are the number of children born from the same donor (in some countries, number of families with children from the same donor) and, in 10 countries, a maximum number of egg donations. The legislations of 6 principal european countries are reported in Table 18.2.

Table 18.2 Principal countries in Europe and their ART regulations

Art regulations

Country	Current legislation/regulations	Year	Specifications
Spain	*Human Assisted Reproduction Technique Law 14/2006* *Biomedical Law 14/2007*	2006 2007	It prohibits reproductive cloning, transfer of more than three embryos per reproductive cycle, germline modification, non-medical sex selection and the use of PGT for non-medical purposes Surrogacy is not recognized
United Kingdom	*Surrogacy Arrangement Act* *The Human Embryology and Fertilization Act* *Human Reproductive Cloning Act* *Human Fertilization and Embryology (Mitochondrial Donation) Regulations 2015, Nº 572*	1985 1990 1990 2005	Prohibit reproductive cloning, germline modification, non-medical sex selection, commercial egg and sperm donation, and commercial surrogacy. Regulates the use of donor gametes, assisted fertilization, PGT, gamete and reproductive tissue banking, and human embryo research
Italy	*Law No. 40. Medically Assisted Procreation Law*	2004	2009: the Constitutional Court declared as unconstitutional the maximum limit of embryos to be produced and transferred for each cycle (three, according to the original version) 2014: the Constitutional Court allowed heterologous assisted reproduction 2015: the Constitutional Court granted the right to access ART to couples who are fertile but carriers of genetic diseases
France	*Law on the Donation and Use of Elements and Products of the Human Body, Medically Assisted Procreation, and Prenatal Diagnosis, No. 94–654* *Bioethics Law No. 2004–800*	1994 2004	The Bioethics Law prohibits reproductive and research cloning, germline modification, non-medical sex selection and surrogacy PGT is only allowed when a parent or close relative has a serious genetic disease
Germany	*Federal Embryo Protection Law* *Adoption Brokerage Law* *Guideline of the German Federal Medical Chamber*	1990 2006 2006	Reproductive and research cloning, gamete donation, creation of hybrid embryos, cryopreservation of fertilized eggs, sex selection (except sperm selection for the prevention of certain sex-related genetic disorders), PGT and all forms of surrogacy are prohibited
Switzerland	*Federal Law on Medically Assisted Reproduction* *Federal Act on Research Involving Embryonic Stem Cells* *Federal Law on Medically Assisted Reproduction*	1998 2003 2004	Reproductive and research cloning, egg and embryo donation, creation of an embryo for research purposes, creation of a hybrid embryo, germline modification, PGT, non-medical sex selection and surrogacy are prohibited. The destruction of cryopreserved gametes and embryos is mandated after 5 years

References

1. Zegers-Hochschild F, Adamson GD, de Mouzon J, Ishihara O, Mansour R, Nygren K, Sullivan E, Vanderpoel S. for ICMART and WHO. International Committee for Monitoring Assisted Reproductive Technology (ICMART) and the World Health Organization (WHO) revised glossary of ART terminology, 2009. Fertil Steril. 2009;92:1520–4.
2. Allersma T, Farquhar C, Cantineau AEP. Natural cycle in vitro fertilisation (IVF) for subfertile couples Cochrane Gynaecology and Fertility Group. Cochrane Database Syst Rev. 2013;2013(8):CD010550.
3. Nargund G, Waterstone J, Bland J, Philips Z, Parsons J, Campbell S. Cumulative conception and live birth rates in natural (unstimulated) IVF cycles. Hum Reprod. 2001;16(2):259–62.
4. WHO. 1999 Laboratory manual for the examination of human sperm and sperm-cervical mucus interaction. 4th ed. Cambridge: Cambridge University Press; 1999.
5. Ayeleke RO, Asseler JD, Cohlen BJ, Veltman-Verhulst SM. Intra-uterine insemination for unexplained subfertility. Cochrane Database Syst Rev. 2020;3:CD001838.
6. Kop PAL, Mochtar MH, O'Brien PA, Van der Veen F, van Wely M. Intrauterine insemination versus intracervical insemination in donor sperm treatment. Cochrane Database Syst Rev. 2018;2018:CD000317.
7. Gallos ID, Eapen A, Price MJ, Sunkara SK, Macklon NS, Bhattacharya S, Khalaf Y, Tobias A, Deeks JJ, Rajkhowa M, Coomarasamy A. Controlled ovarian stimulation protocols for assisted reproduction: a network meta-analysis. Cochrane Database Syst Rev. 2017;2017(3):CD012586.
8. Ferraretti AP, La Marca A, Fauser BC, Tarlatzis B, Nargund G, Gianaroli L. ESHRE consensus on the definition of 'poor response' to ovarian stimulation for in vitro fertilization: the Bologna criteria. Hum Reprod. 2011;26:1616–24.
9. Zegers-Hochschild F, Adamson GD, Dyer S, Racowsky C, de Mouzon J, Sokol R, Rienzi L, Sunde A, Schmidt L, Cooke ID, et al. The international glossary on infertility and fertility care, 2017. Hum

Reprod. 2017;32:1786–801.

10. Handyside AH, Kontogianni EH, Hardy K, Winston RM. Pregnancies from biopsied human preimplantation embryos sexed by Y-specific DNA amplification. Nature. 1990;344:768–70.

11. Delhanty JD, Harper JC. Pre-implantation genetic diagnosis. Baillieres Best Pract Res Clin Obstet Gynaecol. 2000;14:691–708.

12. Van Montfoort A, Carvalho F, Coonen E, Kokkali G, Moutou C, Rubio C, Goossens V, De Rycke M. ESHRE PGT Consortium data collection XIX-XX. Hum Reprod Open. 2021;2021(3):hoab024.

13. Wyns C, De Geyter C, Calhaz-Jorge C, Kupka MS, Motrenko T, Smeenk J, Bergh C, Tandler-Schneider A, Rugescu IA, Vidakovic S, Goossens V. ART in Europe, 2017: Results generated from European registries by ESHRE. Hum Reprod Open. 2021;3:1–17.

14. Golan A, Ron-el R, Herman A, Soffer Y, Weinraub Z, Caspi E. Ovarian hyperstimulation syndrome: an update review. Obstet Gynecol Surv. 1989;44:430–40.

15. Tang H, Mourad S, Zhai S-D, Hart RJ. Dopamine agonists for preventing ovarian hyperstimulation syndrome. Cochrane Database Syst Rev. 2016;11:CD008605.

16. Al-Inany HG, Youssef MA, Ayeleke RO, Brown J, Lam WS, Broekmans FJ. Gonadotrophin-releasing hormone antagonists for assisted reproductive technology. Cochrane Database Syst Rev. 2016;4:CD001750.

17. Youssef M, Mourad S. Volume expanders for the prevention of ovarian hyperstimulation syndrome. Cochrane Database Syst Rev. 2016;8:CD001302.

18. Pandey S, Shetty A, Hamilton M, Bhattacharya S, Maheshwari A. Obstetric and perinatal outcomes in singleton pregnancies resulting from IVF/ICSI: a systematic review and meta-analysis. Hum Reprod Update. 2012;18:485–503.

19. Sunderam S, et al. Assisted Reproductive Technology Surveillance—US. MMWR. 2019;64(6):1–29.

20. Klip H, Burger CW, Kenemans P, Van Leeuwen FE. Cancer risk associated with subfertility and ovulation induction: a review. Cancer Causes Control. 2000;11:319–44.

21. Luke B, Brown MB, Wantman E, Forestieri NE, Browne ML, Fisher SC, Yazdy MM, et al. The risk of birth defects with conception by ART. Hum Reprod. 2021;36(1):116–29.

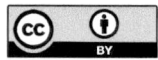

Nicola Bianchi, Olga Prontera, Mauro Dicuio,
Sergio Concetti, Alessandra Sforza,
and Giovanni Corona

19.1 Introduction

Male sexual function is the result of the communication among organic relational and intrapsychic components, which mutually interact supporting and maintaining a satisfying sexual relationship [1–9]. Endocrine and nervous systems represent the key messengers connecting and regulating all the involved phases. Both systems detect all the environmental changes affecting the body and work together to provide the best appropriate response to such events. The nervous system is based on electrical stimulations to communicate, whereas hormones a heterogeneous group of steroid or peptide-derived molecules, produce a messenger system regulating distant target organs.

Sexual sensations collected through the sense organs such as sight, hearing, smell, and touch are detected by peripheral nerves and the codified information reaches the most important centers within the central nervous system, including the septal nuclei, the amygdala, and the hippocampus [5, 10, 11]. The latter are brain areas widely interconnected with each other and with other regulatory centers of endocrine activity, such as the hypothalamus. At the appropriate time, the symphonic activity of hormones and neurotransmitters determines the readiness towards sexuality, which eventually results in intense vascularization of the corpora cavernosa and, eventually in penile erection.

Several hormonal pathways are involved in the latter process. Testosterone (T) represents the most important hormonal regulator of male sexuality acting either at central or peripheral level [11, 12]. Thyroid system seems to be more involved in the regulation of the ejaculatory reflex, although a possible contribution in sexual desire as well as in penile erection has also been supposed [12–15]. Prolactin (PRL) is mainly involved in the modulation of sexual desire, whereas its contribution in the pathogenesis of erectile dysfunction (ED) is more conflicting [12, 16]. Similarly, the role of other hormonal pathways in the regulation of male sexual response appears negligible [12].

In the following sections, the available evidence supporting the role endocrine system in the regulation of male sexual response will be summarized and critically discussed. In particular, the specific contribution on sexual desire erectile function and ejaculation will be analyzed in details.

N. Bianchi · O. Prontera · A. Sforza · G. Corona (✉)
Endocrinology Unit, Medical Department,
Azienda Usl, Bologna Maggiore-Bellaria Hospital,
Bologna, Italy

M. Dicuio
Urology Unit, Surgical Department, Azienda Usl,
Bologna Maggiore-Bellaria Hospital, Bologna, Italy

Department of Urology, Sahlgrenska University
Hospital, Goteborg, Sweden

S. Concetti
Urology Unit, Surgical Department, Azienda Usl,
Bologna Maggiore-Bellaria Hospital, Bologna, Italy

© The Author(s) 2023
C. Bettocchi et al. (eds.), *Practical Clinical Andrology*,
https://doi.org/10.1007/978-3-031-11701-5_19

19.2 Steroids

Testosterone (T) is the main circulating sex steroid in males, essentially derived from testis production (daily production 5–10 mg) with a negligible contribution of the adrenal glands [17–19].

About 6–8% of daily T production is reduced into the more potent androgen, dihydrotestosterone (DHT), through the action of two distinct 5 α reductase (5αR) isoforms, 5αR type 1 and 2 [19]. In addition, T and its precursor, Δ4 androstenedione, can be actively transformed, through P450 aromatase, to other bioactive metabolites, such as estrone and 17-β-estradiol (E2) (daily production about 45 μg), which activate estrogen receptors (ERs).

During fetal life, androgens play a crucial role in regulating the differentiation of internal (mainly T) and external (mainly DHT) genitalia. During puberty, the new T rise contributes to the development of secondary sexual characteristics, growth acceleration, and body composition as well as to psychological modifications, which eventually allow reaching the adulthood male appearance. During adulthood, androgens, and T in particular, are mainly involved in maintaining and sustaining the psycho-biological modifications occurred during puberty [19–21]. The regulation of male sexual response is probably one of the most important functions modulated by T during adulthood and aging [18, 22–24]. According to the results derived from the European Male Aging Study (EMAS), a survey performed on more than 3400 community-dwelling men recruited from eight European centers, sexual symptoms—particularly ED, reduced frequency of morning erections, and reduced libido—are the most sensitive and specific symptoms in identifying patients with reduced T levels [25]. Similar results were thereafter reported by our group investigating a large sample ($n = 4890$) of subjects seeking medical care for ED [26]. Conversely, the role of other sex steroids including DHT and estrogens in regulating male sexual functioning is more conflicting. In the following section, the specific role of sex steroids on the regulation of sexual desire, erectile function, and ejaculation will be analyzed more in details.

19.2.1 Sexual Desire

T represents the fuel of sex drive and it is the most important determinant of the motivation to seek sexual contact (Table 19.1). Data derived from the general population [25, 27] as well as those detected from subjects consulting for ED [28, 29] have clearly documented an inverse relationship between circulating T levels and sexual desire. Similar data were observed in subjects undergoing androgen deprivation therapy for prostate cancer [30–32] or in those with hypogonadism related to androgenetic steroid abuse [33]. Accordingly, several clinical trials have documented that T replacement therapy (TRT) significantly improves sexual desire, spontaneous sexual thoughts, and attractiveness to erotic stimuli in hypogonadal (total T below 12 nmol/L; 3.5 ng/mL) subjects [34–39]. Data derived from animal studies and using functional magnetic resonance imaging (fMRI) have clearly documented that androgen receptors (AR) are widely expressed in specific brain areas, including temporal, preoptic, hypothalamus, amygdala, midbrain, frontal and prefrontal cortex areas, and cingulate gyrus which play an essential role in regulating male sexual drive [40]. Accordingly, the acute T administration activates most of them, as derived from fMRI [41]. Similarly, erotic visual stimulation, in healthy volunteers, leads to

Table 19.1 Role of several hormonal pathways in the control of male sexual response

	Sexual desire	Erection	Ejaculation
Steroids			
Testosterone	+++	+++	++
DHT	++ −	+++	− − −
Estrogens	+ − −	− − −	+ − −
DHEA/DHEAS	− − −	− − −	− − −
Glucocorticoids	+ − −	− − −	− − −
Aldosterone	− − −	+ − −	− − −
Other hormones			
Thyroid hormones	+ − −	+ − −	++ −
Prolactin	+++	+ − −	+ − −
Oxitocyn	− − −	+ − −	+ − −
Melacortin	− − −	− − −	− − −

DHT dihydrotestosterone, *DHEA* dehydroepiandrosterone, *DHEAS* dehydroepiandrosterone sulfate a significant activation of the inferior frontal lobe, cingulate gyrus, insula gyrus, corpus callosum, thalamus, caudate nucleus, globus pallidus, and inferior temporal lobe [42]. Interestingly, the same results were not confirmed when hypogonadal men were considered [42]. Finally, in line with previous results, Stoleru et al. [43] using positron emission tomography (PET) documented that sexually explicit visual stimulation is able to produce T plasma level increase and to activate several paralimbic areas. Hence, taking together the aforementioned results support a strong role of T through AR activation in regulating male sexual desire [40]. However, given the possibility that other sex steroids, besides T, can support its role within the brain, acting on AR or through T, conversion to estrogens on ERs cannot be ruled out.

The role of DHT is quite conflicting (Table 19.1). Data derived from a clinical model of congenital 5αR type 2 deficiency, characterized by the impairment of T into DHT, showed that affected subjects often report normal sexual desire [44]. Similarly, data derived from population-based studies showed no relationship between mass-derived DHT and sexual desire [45]. In apparent contrast with the previous results, data derived from studies using 5αR inhibitors (5ARIs) for androgenetic alopecia [46] or prostate hyperplasia (BPH; [47]) showed an association with an increased risk of ED and reduced sexual desire. An intriguing working hypothesis supports the concept that 5ARIs can impair the formation of other 5α-reduced steroid metabolites, acting as neurosteroids in modulating sexual desire [48].

Limited evidence supports a possible role of estrogens (Table 19.1). In a double-blind placebo-controlled randomized controlled trial (RCT), Finkelstein et al., [49] by experimentally inducing a clinical condition of secondary hypogonadism through the administration of GnRH-analogue in 400 healthy men, aged from 20 to 50 years, reported that either E2 or T contributed to the observed decline of sexual desire. In line with the latter evidence, data derived from men with aromatase deficiency showed that transdermal E2 administration was able to improve sexual desire

[50]. Conversely, adrenal hormones including dehydroepiandrosterone (DHEA) and its sulfate (DHEAS) [51], as well as cortisol and aldosterone, seem to not be involved in the regulation of male sexual desire [12] (Table 19.1).

19.2.2   Erectile Function

Data derived from animal models and in vitro studies have documented that T controls most of the signaling pathways involved in the control of penile erection, including nitric oxide (NO) production and degradation, adenosine signaling, calcium sensitization through the RhoA-ROCK pathway, and even penile smooth muscle differentiation [52] (Table 19.1). Despite this evidence, data derived from clinical studies showed only a milder association between self-reported severe ED and circulating T levels [11, 53, 54]. Conversely, more solid data support the association between sleep-related erections and T levels [55–57]. These observations deserve a better discussion. Penile erection is essentially a neurovascular phenomenon characterized by the increase in blood flow within the lacunar spaces of the penis. Increasing age and associated morbidities can largely reduce the influence of T on erectile function by impairing penile vascular flow. Accordingly, we recently reported that age and comorbidities were the best predictors of the relationship between prostaglandin E1 (PGE1)-stimulated penile blood flow and T levels in a cohort of more than 2500 men complaining of sexual dysfunction [11]. Similar data were previously reported by us [58] and other groups [59, 60]. Hence, the main physiological action of T is to timely adjust the erectile process as a function of sexual desire, therefore finalizing erections with sex. However, it should be important to recognize that we recently reported that the combination of low T and associated morbidities could often result in more severe sexual problems [58].

In line to what derived from clinical evidence, all the available meta-analyses have shown that TRT is able to significantly improve erectile function in hypogonadal (total T < 12 nmol/L, 3.5 ng/mL) subjects [36, 37, 39, 61]. Interestingly, however, TRT induced a modest 8% increase in International Index of erectile function domain score [11, 39], which should be considered clinically meaningful only in patients with milder forms of ED according to Rosen et al. [62]. Accordingly, the effects of TRT are more limited in more complicated patients such as those with obesity and diabetes mellitus [11, 35, 39]. The combination between phosphodiesterase type 5 inhibitors (PDE5i) and TRT has been suggested a possible strategy to overcome the limited effects of TRT in more severe ED. However, the present data are still conflicting and final conclusions cannot be drawn [11, 63].

Data derived from animal models seem not to support any difference when T is compared to DHT in the regulation of the main androgen-dependent pathway involved in penile erection and detumescence [18, 52] (Table 19.1). Accordingly, the possible association between the use of 5ARIs and ED seems more related to a drug effect rather than to reduction of DHT circulating levels. In line with the latter hypothesis, experimental studies showed that 5ARIs induce a structural and functional alteration in penile tissue, resulting in penile fibrosis through a modulation of cholinergic and adrenergic sensitivity, with no apparent changes in PDE5 expression and activity [64].

Estrogens and adrenal androgens (DHEAS and DHEA) play a negligible role in regulating erectile function, whereas limited evidence supports a possible role of glucocorticoids and mineralocorticoids [12] (Table 19.1).

19.2.3 Ejaculation

As previously reported for erectile function and sexual desire, T is deeply involved also in the modulation of ejaculatory reflex acting either at central or peripheral level [15, 65] (Table 19.1). Several central brain areas, including medial preoptic area, the bed nucleus of the stria terminalis, the median amygdala, and the posterior thalamus, are crucial for the supraspinal control of ejaculation express AR [15, 65]. In addition, bulbo-cavernosus muscle as well as other mus-

cles of the pelvic floor involved in the ejection of the seminal bolus are under T control [15, 65]. Furthermore, T positively modulates also the emission phase by regulating the integrated system NO-PDE5, which represents one of the most important factor involved in the contractility of the male genital tract [65, 66]. In line with this evidence, we originally reported that low T levels and the presence of hypogonadal symptoms are associated with an overall lower propensity to ejaculate [66–68].

Accordingly, TRT is able to improve ejaculatory domain and orgasm when hypogonadal (total T < 12 nmol/L, 3.5 ng/mL) patients are considered [11, 69].

ERs have been identified in the epididymis of several animal species including humans [15]. At this level, estrogens are involved in the regulation of luminal fluid reabsorption and sperm concentration [15]. In addition, a possible role in the modulation of epididymal contractility has been also suggested [15]. In particular, estrogens might positively regulate endothelin-1 (ET-1) and oxytocin (OT)-mediated contractility either by increasing the expression of OT receptors or by activating a common downstream effector of the contractile mechanisms: the calcium-sensitizing RhoA/Rho-kinase system (see below; [70]) (Table 19.1).

No evidence supports a role of adrenal androgens (DHEAS and DHEA) as well as glucocorticoids and mineralocorticoids in the control of ejaculatory reflex [12, 15]. Similarly, no specific effect of DHT has been supposed [15] (Table 19.1).

19.3 Prolactin

PRL is a polypeptide secreted by the anterior pituitary and mainly regulated through tonic hypothalamic inhibition, by dopamine (DA) secretion [71, 72]. Hence, disruptions of the latter pathway or portal circulation perturbation, as well as sellar or parasellar tumors, are all associated with the development of marked hyperprolactinemia. The same condition can be associated with a primary hypothyroidism, since thyroid-stimulating hormone (TRH) exerts positive effects on PRL secretion, or with the use of drugs blocking dopaminergic or increasing serotoninergic transmission such as antipsychotics or antidepressants [16]. The prevalence of milder forms of hyperprolactinemia (MHPRL, PRL >420 mU/L or 20 ng/mL) in male subjects with sexual dysfunction ranges from more than 13% [73] to less than 2% [74]. Conversely, more severe forms (SHPRL, PRL > 735 mU/L or 35 ng/mL) are less frequently observed (less than 1%; [74, 75]). In the presence of MHPRL, repeat blood sampling, in adequate conditions, results in normal PRL values in about 50% of cases, most probably due to venipuncture stress [74]. False positive cases can be derived from the presence of macroprolactin (around 10%), in the presence of SHPRL [74]. The latter is a biologically inactive complex of PRL and IgG which can be easily ruled out by reproducible polyethylene glycol (PEG) test [76]. Finally, it is also important to recognize that SHPRL is frequently (around 60%) supported by an organic problem in the hypothalamic-pituitary region, whereas a drug-induced condition can be found in almost 1/3 of cases [74].

Despite the well-known role of PRL in promoting breast-feeding in females, the specific role of this hormone in males is still not completely clarified. However, much evidence documented that elevated PRL levels in males are associated with a negative perturbation of sexual function [12, 16, 18, 29]. In the following sections, the specific contribution of PRL perturbation on male sexual function will be analyzed in details.

19.3.1 Sexual Desire

PRL receptors (PRLR) are expressed in brain, testis, accessory glands, and even at penis level [16]. A large body of evidence has clearly documented that SHPRL is tightly associated with reduced sexual desire in males [28, 29, 74, 77], whereas milder forms of hyperprolactinemia are less frequently associated with reduced libido [28, 77, 78] (Table 19.1). The specific molecular mechanisms through which PRL can impair sex-

ual desire are not completely clarified. PRL can interfere with gonadotropin releasing hormone (GnRH) inducing a development of secondary hypogonadism. However, the latter can explain, only partially, the association between SHPRL and reduced libido [72]. Accordingly, TRT is not effective in restoring sexual desire in patients with SHPRL [79]. Hence, possible direct mechanisms of PRL have been advocated. Accordingly, PRL can modulate the turnover of DA in several brain areas partially involved in the regulation of sexual behavior such as the nigrostriatal and the mesolimbic tracts [72] Furthermore, experimental data have documented that PRL is involved in decreasing DA pathway in the diencephalic incertohypothalamic dopaminergic system, which represents the most important area for the control of motivational and consummatory aspects of sexual behavior [16, 80]. In line to what reported above, DA agonists such as bromocriptine and cabergoline are considered the first line treatments for SHPRL, particularly in patients with PRL-secreting adenomas [81]. Conversely, when possible, the modification or the withdrawn of interfering drugs should be advocated [81]. DA can normalize sexual desire and T levels in up to 90% of patients [16]. If hypogonadism persists, even after PRL normalization, TRT can be added resulting in better outcomes [16].

19.3.2 Erectile Dysfunction

The role of PRL in the regulation of erectile process is more conflicting (Table 19.1). Some studies have reported worse erectile function in subjects with SHPRL [73, 75]. However, we were unable to detect any association between SHPRL and severe ED after adjustment for T levels [74]. The latter observation suggests that PRL plays a major indirect effect (SHPRL-induced hypogonadism) on ED. Interestingly, we more recently reported that low PRL (<10 ng/mL or 210 mU/L) rather than high PRL was associated with arteriogenic ED in a large sample of patients seeking medical care for sexual dysfunction [82]. These results were confirmed in the general population [78, 83]. The latter observations support a positive effect of PRL on initiating or maintaining sexual behavior. The specific mechanisms underlying these findings are still unclear. However, an intriguing hypothesis supports the view that low PRL, in the peripheral circulation, could mirror, within the hypothalamus, both an increase of dopaminergic and a decreased serotoninergic signaling [16].

19.3.3 Ejaculation

Several observational studies have reported a PRL increase following male orgasm [84–86], supporting a possible role of PRL in the regulation of the postorgasmic refractory period [16]. However, it should be important to recognize that the observed postorgasmic rise in PRL is similar in men and women, which are less inclined to experience postorgasmic refractoriness. Hence, it is conceivable support that the observed PRL increases during orgasm reflect the emotional and stressful situation related to the sexual stimulation [16].

Similar to what was reported for ED, we originally documented that relatively low PRL levels were associated with a higher risk of premature ejaculation (PE) even after adjustment for confounders [82] (Table 19.1). In the same study, we did not observe any difference in the risk of PE when lifelong or acquired forms were considered [82]. Hence, by supporting PE-related *Waldinger's neurobiological hypothesis*, dealing with a disturbance in the central serotonin pathway, our data support the view that even secondary causes of PE would act mainly influencing the brain serotonergic system [16].

19.4 Thyroid Hormones

Free fractions (FT3 and FT4) represent the biological active fraction of the thyroid hormones (TH) produced by thyroid glands under thyroid-stimulating hormone (TSH) control [15]. TH are involved in regulating protein, fat, and carbohydrate metabolism so that no organs or tissues can

be unaffected by thyroid diseases [87]. Accordingly, thyroid receptors are widely expressed within male genitalia tract, although the specific role of TH on male sexual function is still conflicting.

19.4.1 Sexual Desire

In a first open-label observational pilot study, Carani et al. [13] reported that hypothyroidism was associated with low sexual desire, which was improved after normalizing TH levels. Similar results were reported by other authors [88]. Although the raised PRL levels due to hypothyroidism status have been advocated as a possible supporting mechanism mediating the negative effects of low TH on sexual desire, a direct action of TH on the serotoninergic system has been also suggested [12, 18]. However, it should be important to recognize that no association between low TH and sexual desire has been reported in a larger series of subjects either from the general population or from patients seeking medical care for sexual dysfunction [14]. Hence, more studies are advisable to better clarify the role of TH on sexual desire (Table 19.1).

19.4.2 Erectile Dysfunction

Similar to what was reported for sexual desire, the role of TH in regulating male erectile function is still conflicting (Table 19.1). Limited evidence has documented a possible association between either hypo or hyperthyroidism and ED [13, 88–90]. In addition, some authors also reported that the restoration of normal TH was associated with an amelioration of erectile function [13, 88, 89]. The largest study published so far including 3203 subjects seeking medical care for sexual dysfunction and more than 3400 patients enrolled in the EMAS study showed that hyperthyroidism but not hypothyroidism was associated with an increased risk of severe ED, after adjusting for confounding factors [14]. The latter results were confirmed by Keller et al. [91] in a retrospective analysis of a Health Insurance Database representative of Taiwan's general population. Data derived from animal models have shown that hyperthyroidism is associated with an impairment of NO-dependent relaxation of corpora cavernosa (CC; [92, 93]). In addition, in the same experimental model either acetylcholine- or electrical field stimulation-induced relaxation of CC was impaired, whereas sensitivity to the NO donor, sodium nitroprusside, was unchanged [93]. However, it is important to recognize that the prevalence of thyroid disorders in patients seeking medical care for ED is rather low (<1%) and not different from that observed in the general population [94]. The latter observations limit the specific direct role of TH on erectile function.

19.4.3 Ejaculation

More robust data have supported a possible role of TH in the regulation of the ejaculatory reflex (Table 19.1). In 2004, we originally reported, for the first time, a significant association between hyperthyroidism, even in the subclinical form, and PE in a consecutive series of 755 men presenting with sexual dysfunction [95]. In line with this observation, Carani et al. [13] thereafter confirmed an association between PE and hyperthyroidism and that the opposite condition, hypothyroidism, resulted in a twofold increase in ejaculatory latency. Similar results were confirmed by other authors [66, 96]. Data from animal models showed that experimentally induced hyperthyroidism in rats caused an increased frequency of seminal vesicle contraction and bulbospongiosus muscle contractile activity, supporting the role of TH in regulating either the emission or the expulsion phases of the ejaculation process [97]. To further support the possible contribution of TH in the modulation of ejaculation, the aforemtioned studies also documented that achieving euthyroidism at follow-up was associated with an improvement of PE [13, 96] or reduction in ejaculatory time [13], respectively. Finally, more recently a meta-analysis of the available data confirmed that hyperthyroidism was associated with twofold increased risk of PE and that delayed ejaculation was related to hypo-

thyroid [98]. The same study also confirmed that treatment of underlining thyroid disorders improved the mean intravaginal ejaculatory latency time measures of the subjects [98].

19.5 Other Hormones

Oxytocin (OT): is a short peptide synthesized in the supraoptic (SON) and paraventricular nuclei (PVN) of the hypothalamus and released by posterior pituitary. OT in men is released during sexual activity and orgasm and it can activate the secretion of ET-1 and OT itself in the epididymis, creating a reciprocal and synergic cross-activation of contractile factors involved in the regulation of male genitalia tract contractility favoring sperm progression [15]. Despite this evidence, the role of OT in regulating penile erection is limited and still conflicting [12] (Table 19.1).

Other hormones Limited evidence has documented a possible contribution of other hormones in the regulation of male sexual functioning, including growth hormone [99] and melanocortin [100]; however, available data are too preliminary and not supported by robust evidence-based data [12] (Table 19.1).

19.6 Conclusions

A large body of evidence supports the crucial role of T in the regulation of male sexual response. PRL is mainly involved in modulating sexual desire, whereas TH plays a major role in regulating ejaculatory reflex. All available guidelines strongly encourage investigating T levels in all subjects complaining of sexual dysfunction [18, 22–24]. TRT can improve all aspects of sexual function and should be considered the first treatment, especially in hypogonadal patients with milder forms of ED. Dopaminergic drugs are highly effective in restoring male sexual desire in subjects with severe hyperprolactinemia, whereas the treatment of underlying thyroid diseases can improve ejaculatory problems. Further studies are advisable to better characterize the role of other hormones.

References

1. Boddi V, Corona G, Fisher AD, Mannucci E, Ricca V, Sforza A, et al. "It takes two to tango": the relational domain in a cohort of subjects with erectile dysfunction (ED). J Sex Med. 2012;9(12):3126–36.
2. Corona G, Ricca V, Bandini E, Mannucci E, Petrone L, Fisher AD, et al. Association between psychiatric symptoms and erectile dysfunction. J Sex Med. 2008;5(2):458–68.
3. Corona G, Ricca V, Bandini E, Rastrelli G, Casale H, Jannini EA, et al. SIEDY scale 3, a new instrument to detect psychological component in subjects with erectile dysfunction. J Sex Med. 2012;9(8):2017–26.
4. Jannini EA, Nappi RE. Couplepause: a new paradigm in treating sexual dysfunction during menopause and Andropause. Sex Med Rev. 2018;6(3):384–95.
5. Rastrelli G, Corona G, Maggi M. Testosterone and sexual function in men. Maturitas. 2018;112:46–52.
6. Rastrelli G, Corona G, Lotti F, Aversa A, Bartolini M, Mancini M, et al. Flaccid penile acceleration as a marker of cardiovascular risk in men without classical risk factors. J Sex Med. 2014;11(1):173–86.
7. Boddi V, Corona G, Monami M, Fisher AD, Bandini E, Melani C, et al. Priapus is happier with Venus than with Bacchus. J Sex Med. 2010;7(8):2831–41.
8. Dewitte M, Bettocchi C, Carvalho J, Corona G, Flink I, Limoncin E, et al. A psychosocial approach to erectile dysfunction: position statements from the European Society of Sexual Medicine (ESSM). Sex Med. 2021;9(6):100434.
9. Marieke D, Joana C, Giovanni C, Erika L, Patricia P, Yacov R, et al. Sexual desire discrepancy: a position statement of the European Society for Sexual Medicine. Sex Med. 2020;8(2):121–31.
10. Rastrelli G, Guaraldi F, Reismann Y, Sforza A, Isidori AM, Maggi M, et al. Testosterone replacement therapy for sexual symptoms. Sex Med Rev. 2019;7(3):464–75.
11. Corona G, Rastrelli G, Vignozzi L, Maggi M. Androgens and male sexual function. Best Pract Res Clin Endocrinol Metab. 2022;101615. https://doi.org/10.1016/j.beem.2022.101615.
12. Corona G, Isidori AM, Aversa A, Burnett AL, Maggi M. Endocrinologic control of men's sexual desire and arousal/erection. J Sex Med. 2016;13(3):317–37.
13. Carani C, Isidori AM, Granata A, Carosa E, Maggi M, Lenzi A, et al. Multicenter study on the prevalence of sexual symptoms in male hypo- and hyperthyroid patients. J Clin Endocrinol Metab. 2005;90(12):6472–9.
14. Corona G, Wu FC, Forti G, Lee DM, O'Connor DB, O'Neill TW, et al. Thyroid hormones and male sexual function. Int J Androl. 2012;35(5):668–79.
15. Corona G, Jannini EA, Vignozzi L, Rastrelli G, Maggi M. The hormonal control of ejaculation. Nat Rev Urol. 2012;9(9):508–19.

16. Rastrelli G, Corona G, Maggi M. The role of prolactin in andrology: what is new? Rev Endocr Metab Disord. 2015;16(3):233–48.
17. Mason KA, Schoelwer MJ, Rogol AD. Androgens during infancy, childhood, and adolescence: physiology and use in clinical practice. Endocr Rev. 2020;41(3):bnaa003.
18. Salonia A, Bettocchi C, Boeri L, Capogrosso P, Carvalho J, Cilesiz NC, et al. European association of urology guidelines on sexual and reproductive health-2021 update: male sexual dysfunction. Eur Urol. 2021;80(3):333–57.
19. Salonia A, Rastrelli G, Hackett G, Seminara SB, Huhtaniemi IT, Rey RA, et al. Paediatric and adult-onset male hypogonadism. Nat Rev Dis Primers. 2019;5(1):38.
20. Corona G, Vena W, Pizzocaro A, Giagulli VA, Francomano D, Rastrelli G, et al. Testosterone supplementation and bone parameters: a systematic review and meta-analysis study. J Endocrinol Invest. 2022;45(5):911–26.
21. Corona G, Guaraldi F, Rastrelli G, Sforza A, Maggi M. Testosterone deficiency and risk of cognitive disorders in aging males. World J Mens Health. 2021;39(1):9–18.
22. Bhasin S, Brito JP, Cunningham GR, Hayes FJ, Hodis HN, Matsumoto AM, et al. Testosterone therapy in men with hypogonadism: an Endocrine Society clinical practice guideline. J Clin Endocrinol Metab. 2018;103(5):1715–44.
23. Lunenfeld B, Mskhalaya G, Zitzmann M, Corona G, Arver S, Kalinchenko S, et al. Recommendations on the diagnosis, treatment and monitoring of testosterone deficiency in men. Aging Male. 2021;24(1):119–38.
24. Corona G, Goulis DG, Huhtaniemi I, Zitzmann M, Toppari J, Forti G, et al. European academy of andrology (EAA) guidelines on investigation, treatment and monitoring of functional hypogonadism in males: endorsing organization: European society of endocrinology. Andrology. 2020;8(5):970–87.
25. Wu FC, Tajar A, Beynon JM, Pye SR, Silman AJ, Finn JD, et al. Identification of late-onset hypogonadism in middle-aged and elderly men. N Engl J Med. 2010;363(2):123–35.
26. Rastrelli G, Corona G, Tarocchi M, Mannucci E, Maggi M. How to define hypogonadism? Results from a population of men consulting for sexual dysfunction. J Endocrinol Invest. 2016;39(4):473–84.
27. Travison TG, Morley JE, Araujo AB, O'Donnell AB, McKinlay JB. The relationship between libido and testosterone levels in aging men. J Clin Endocrinol Metab. 2006;91(7):2509–13.
28. Corona G, Petrone L, Mannucci E, Ricca V, Balercia G, Giommi R, et al. The impotent couple: low desire. Int J Androl. 2005;28(Suppl 2):46–52.
29. Corona G, Rastrelli G, Ricca V, Jannini EA, Vignozzi L, Monami M, et al. Risk factors associated with primary and secondary reduced libido in

male patients with sexual dysfunction. J Sex Med. 2013;10(4):1074–89.

30. Corona G, Baldi E, Maggi M. Androgen regulation of prostate cancer: where are we now? J Endocrinol Invest. 2011;34(3):232–43.

31. Corona G, Filippi S, Comelio P, Bianchi N, Frizza F, Dicuio M, et al. Sexual function in men undergoing androgen deprivation therapy. Int J Impot Res. 2021;33(4):439–47.

32. Corona G, Gacci M, Baldi E, Mancina R, Forti G, Maggi M. Androgen deprivation therapy in prostate cancer: focusing on sexual side effects. J Sex Med. 2012;9(3):887–902.

33. Corona G, Rastrelli G, Marchiani S, Filippi S, Morelli A, Sarchielli E, et al. Consequences of anabolic-androgenic steroid abuse in males; sexual and reproductive perspective. World J Mens Health. 2021;40(2):165–78.

34. Pizzocaro A, Vena W, Condorelli R, Radicioni A, Rastrelli G, Pasquali D, et al. Testosterone treatment in male patients with Klinefelter syndrome: a systematic review and meta-analysis. J Endocrinol Invest. 2020;43(12):1675–87.

35. Corona G, Torres LO, Maggi M. Testosterone therapy: what we have learned from trials. J Sex Med. 2020;17(3):447–60.

36. Boloña ER, Uraga MV, Haddad RM, Tracz MJ, Sideras K, Kennedy CC, et al. Testosterone use in men with sexual dysfunction: a systematic review and meta-analysis of randomized placebo-controlled trials. Mayo Clin Proc. 2007;82(1):20–8.

37. Elliott J, Kelly SE, Millar AC, Peterson J, Chen L, Johnston A, et al. Testosterone therapy in hypogonadal men: a systematic review and network meta-analysis. BMJ Open. 2017;7(11):e015284.

38. Isidori AM, Giannetta E, Gianfrilli D, Greco EA, Bonifacio V, Aversa A, et al. Effects of testosterone on sexual function in men: results of a meta-analysis. Clin Endocrinol (Oxf). 2005;63(4):381–94.

39. Corona G, Rastrelli G, Morgentaler A, Sforza A, Mannucci E, Maggi M. Meta-analysis of results of testosterone therapy on sexual function based on international index of erectile function scores. Eur Urol. 2017;72(6):1000–11.

40. Pfaus JG. Pathways of sexual desire. J Sex Med. 2009;6(6):1506–33.

41. Heany SJ, van Honk J, Stein DJ, Brooks SJ. A quantitative and qualitative review of the effects of testosterone on the function and structure of the human social-emotional brain. Metab Brain Dis. 2016;31(1):157–67.

42. Park K, Seo JJ, Kang HK, Ryu SB, Kim HJ, Jeong GW. A new potential of blood oxygenation level dependent (BOLD) functional MRI for evaluating cerebral centers of penile erection. Int J Impot Res. 2001;13(2):73–81.

43. Stoléru S, Grégoire MC, Gérard D, Decety J, Lafarge E, Cinotti L, et al. Neuroanatomical correlates of visually evoked sexual arousal in human males. Arch Sex Behav. 1999;28(1):1–21.

44. Brinkmann L, Schuetzmann K, Richter-Appelt H. Gender assignment and medical history of individuals with different forms of intersexuality: evaluation of medical records and the patients' perspective. J Sex Med. 2007;4(4 Pt 1):964–80.

45. Hsu B, Cumming RG, Blyth FM, Naganathan V, Le Couteur DG, Seibel MJ, et al. The longitudinal relationship of sexual function and androgen status in older men: the Concord health and ageing in men project. J Clin Endocrinol Metab. 2015;100(4):1350–8.

46. Lee S, Lee YB, Choe SJ, Lee WS. Adverse sexual effects of treatment with finasteride or dutasteride for male androgenetic alopecia: a systematic review and meta-analysis. Acta Derm Venereol. 2019;99(1):12–7.

47. Corona G, Tirabassi G, Santi D, Maseroli E, Gacci M, Dicuio M, et al. Sexual dysfunction in subjects treated with inhibitors of 5α-reductase for benign prostatic hyperplasia: a comprehensive review and meta-analysis. Andrology. 2017;5(4):671–8.

48. Diviccaro S, Melcangi RC, Giatti S. Post-finasteride syndrome: an emerging clinical problem. Neurobiol Stress. 2020;12:100209.

49. Finkelstein JS, Lee H, Burnett-Bowie SA, Pallais JC, Yu EW, Borges LF, et al. Gonadal steroids and body composition, strength, and sexual function in men. N Engl J Med. 2013;369(11):1011–22.

50. Rochira V, Carani C. Aromatase deficiency in men: a clinical perspective. Nat Rev Endocrinol. 2009;5(10):559–68.

51. Corona G, Rastrelli G, Giagulli VA, Sila A, Sforza A, Forti G, et al. Dehydroepiandrosterone supplementation in elderly men: a meta-analysis study of placebo-controlled trials. J Clin Endocrinol Metab. 2013;98(9):3615–26.

52. Podlasek CA, Mulhall J, Davies K, Wingard CJ, Hannan JL, Bivalacqua TJ, et al. Translational perspective on the role of testosterone in sexual function and dysfunction. J Sex Med. 2016;13(8):1183–98.

53. Yafi FA, Jenkins L, Albersen M, Corona G, Isidori AM, Goldfarb S, et al. Erectile dysfunction. Nat Rev Dis Primers. 2016;2:16003.

54. Yassin AA, Saad F. Testosterone and erectile dysfunction. J Androl. 2008;29(6):593–604.

55. Corona G, Rastrelli G, Balercia G, Sforza A, Forti G, Mannucci E, et al. Perceived reduced sleep-related erections in subjects with erectile dysfunction: psychobiological correlates. J Sex Med. 2011;8(6):1780–8.

56. Granata AR, Rochira V, Lerchl A, Marrama P, Carani C. Relationship between sleep-related erections and testosterone levels in men. J Androl. 1997;18(5):522–7.

57. Schiavi RC, White D, Mandeli J, Schreiner-Engel P. Hormones and nocturnal penile tumescence in healthy aging men. Arch Sex Behav. 1993;22(3):207–15.

58. Rastrelli G, Corona G, Maggi M. Both comorbidity burden and low testosterone can explain symp-

toms and signs of testosterone deficiency in men consulting for sexual dysfunction. Asian J Androl. 2020;22(3):265–73.

59. Rhoden EL, Telöken C, Sogari PR, Souto CA. The relationship of serum testosterone to erectile function in normal aging men. J Urol. 2002;167(4):1745–8.

60. Kang J 2nd, Ham BK, Oh MM, Kim JJ, Moon du G. Correlation between serum total testosterone and the AMS and IIEF questionnaires in patients with erectile dysfunction with testosterone deficiency syndrome. Korean J Urol. 2011;52(6):416–20.

61. Corona G, Isidori AM, Buvat J, Aversa A, Rastrelli G, Hackett G, et al. Testosterone supplementation and sexual function: a meta-analysis study. J Sex Med. 2014;11(6):1577–92.

62. Rosen RC, Allen KR, Ni X, Araujo AB. Minimal clinically important differences in the erectile function domain of the international index of erectile function scale. Eur Urol. 2011;60(5):1010–6.

63. Zhu J, Zhang W, Ou N, Song Y, Kang J, Liang Z, et al. Do testosterone supplements enhance response to phosphodiesterase 5 inhibitors in men with erectile dysfunction and hypogonadism: a systematic review and meta-analysis. Transl Androl Urol. 2020;9(2):591–600.

64. Pinsky MR, Gur S, Tracey AJ, Harbin A, Hellstrom WJ. The effects of chronic 5-alpha-reductase inhibitor (dutasteride) treatment on rat erectile function. J Sex Med. 2011;8(11):3066–74.

65. Alwaal A, Breyer BN, Lue TF. Normal male sexual function: emphasis on orgasm and ejaculation. Fertil Steril. 2015;104(5):1051–60.

66. Corona G, Jannini EA, Lotti F, Boddi V, De Vita G, Forti G, et al. Premature and delayed ejaculation: two ends of a single continuum influenced by hormonal milieu. Int J Androl. 2011;34(1):41–8.

67. Corona G, Mannucci E, Petrone L, Fisher AD, Balercia G, De Scisciolo G, et al. Psychobiological correlates of delayed ejaculation in male patients with sexual dysfunctions. J Androl. 2006;27(3):453–8.

68. Corona G, Jannini EA, Mannucci E, Fisher AD, Lotti F, Petrone L, et al. Different testosterone levels are associated with ejaculatory dysfunction. J Sex Med. 2008;5(8):1991–8.

69. Corona G, Vignozzi L, Sforza A, Maggi M. Risks and benefits of late onset hypogonadism treatment: an expert opinion. World J Mens Health. 2013;31(2):103–25.

70. Fibbi B, Filippi S, Morelli A, Vignozzi L, Silvestrini E, Chavalmane A, et al. Estrogens regulate humans and rabbit epididymal contractility through the RhoA/rho-kinase pathway. J Sex Med. 2009;6(8):2173–86.

71. Bachelot A, Binart N. Reproductive role of prolactin. Reproduction. 2007;133(2):361–9.

72. Freeman ME, Kanyicska B, Lerant A, Nagy G. Prolactin: structure, function, and regulation of secretion. Physiol Rev. 2000;80(4):1523–631.

73. Buvat J, Lemaire A. Endocrine screening in 1,022 men with erectile dysfunction: clinical significance and cost-effective strategy. J Urol. 1997;158(5):1764–7.

74. Corona G, Mannucci E, Fisher AD, Lotti F, Ricca V, Balercia G, et al. Effect of hyperprolactinemia in male patients consulting for sexual dysfunction. J Sex Med. 2007;4(5):1485–93.

75. Buvat J. Hyperprolactinemia and sexual function in men: a short review. Int J Impot Res. 2003;15(5):373–7.

76. Fahie-Wilson MN, John R, Ellis AR. Macroprolactin; high molecular mass forms of circulating prolactin. Ann Clin Biochem. 2005;42(Pt 3):175–92.

77. Corona G, Mannucci E, Petrone L, Giommi R, Mansani R, Fei L, et al. Psycho-biological correlates of hypoactive sexual desire in patients with erectile dysfunction. Int J Impot Res. 2004;16(3):275–81.

78. Corona G, Wu FC, Rastrelli G, Lee DM, Forti G, O'Connor DB, et al. Low prolactin is associated with sexual dysfunction and psychological or metabolic disturbances in middle-aged and elderly men: the European Male Aging Study (EMAS). J Sex Med. 2014;11(1):240–53.

79. Carter JN, Tyson JE, Tolis G, Van Vliet S, Faiman C, Friesen HG. Prolactin-screening tumors and hypogonadism in 22 men. N Engl J Med. 1978;299(16):847–52.

80. Sachs BD. Contextual approaches to the physiology and classification of erectile function, erectile dysfunction, and sexual arousal. Neurosci Biobehav Rev. 2000;24(5):541–60.

81. Melmed S, Casanueva FF, Hoffman AR, Kleinberg DL, Montori VM, Schlechte JA, et al. Diagnosis and treatment of hyperprolactinemia: an Endocrine Society clinical practice guideline. J Clin Endocrinol Metab. 2011;96(2):273–88.

82. Corona G, Mannucci E, Jannini EA, Lotti F, Ricca V, Monami M, et al. Hypoprolactinemia: a new clinical syndrome in patients with sexual dysfunction. J Sex Med. 2009;6(5):1457–66.

83. Gettler LT, McDade TW, Feranil AB, Kuzawa CW. Prolactin, fatherhood, and reproductive behavior in human males. Am J Phys Anthropol. 2012;148(3):362–70.

84. Krüger TH, Haake P, Chereath D, Knapp W, Janssen OE, Exton MS, et al. Specificity of the neuroendocrine response to orgasm during sexual arousal in men. J Endocrinol. 2003;177(1):57–64.

85. Krüger TH, Haake P, Hartmann U, Schedlowski M, Exton MS. Orgasm-induced prolactin secretion: feedback control of sexual drive? Neurosci Biobehav Rev. 2002;26(1):31–44.

86. Exton MS, Krüger TH, Koch M, Paulson E, Knapp W, Hartmann U, et al. Coitus-induced orgasm stimulates prolactin secretion in healthy subjects. Psychoneuroendocrinology. 2001;26(3):287–94.

87. Corona G, Croce L, Sparano C, Petrone L, Sforza A, Maggi M, et al. Thyroid and heart, a clinically relevant relationship. J Endocrinol Invest. 2021;44(12):2535–44.

88. Krysiak R, Szkróbka W, Okopień B. The effect of L-thyroxine treatment on sexual function and depressive symptoms in men with autoimmune hypothyroidism. Pharmacol Rep. 2017;69(3):432–7.

89. Krassas GE, Tziomalos K, Papadopoulou F, Pontikides N, Perros P. Erectile dysfunction in patients with hyper- and hypothyroidism: how common and should we treat? J Clin Endocrinol Metab. 2008;93(5):1815–9.

90. Veronelli A, Masu A, Ranieri R, Rognoni C, Laneri M, Pontiroli AE. Prevalence of erectile dysfunction in thyroid disorders: comparison with control subjects and with obese and diabetic patients. Int J Impot Res. 2006;18(1):111–4.

91. Keller J, Chen YK, Lin HC. Hyperthyroidism and erectile dysfunction: a population-based case-control study. Int J Impot Res. 2012;24(6):242–6.

92. Bates JN, Kohn TP, Pastuszak AW. Effect of thyroid hormone derangements on sexual function in men and women. Sex Med Rev. 2020;8(2):217–30.

93. Krassas GE, Poppe K, Glinoer D. Thyroid function and human reproductive health. Endocr Rev. 2010;31(5):702–55.

94. Maseroli E, Corona G, Rastrelli G, Lotti F, Cipriani S, Forti G, et al. Prevalence of endocrine and metabolic disorders in subjects with erectile dysfunction: a comparative study. J Sex Med. 2015;12(4):956–65.

95. Corona G, Petrone L, Mannucci E, Jannini EA, Mansani R, Magini A, et al. Psycho-biological correlates of rapid ejaculation in patients attending an andrologic unit for sexual dysfunctions. Eur Urol. 2004;46(5):615–22.

96. Cihan A, Demir O, Demir T, Aslan G, Comlekci A, Esen A. The relationship between premature ejaculation and hyperthyroidism. J Urol. 2009;181(3):1273–80.

97. Oztürk M, Koca O, Tüken M, Keleş MO, Ilktaç A, Karaman MI. Hormonal evaluation in premature ejaculation. Urol Int. 2012;88(4):454–8.

98. Cihan A, Esen AA. Systematic review and meta-analysis for the value of thyroid disorder screening in men with ejaculatory dysfunction. Int J Clin Pract. 2021;75(10):e14419.

99. Lotti F, Rochira V, Pivonello R, Santi D, Galdiero M, Maseroli E, et al. Erectile dysfunction is common among men with acromegaly and is associated with morbidities related to the disease. J Sex Med. 2015;12(5):1184–93.

100. Ückert S, Bannowsky A, Albrecht K, Kuczyk MA. Melanocortin receptor agonists in the treatment of male and female sexual dysfunctions: results from basic research and clinical studies. Expert Opin Investig Drugs. 2014;23(11):1477–83.

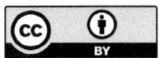

Elisabetta Lavorato, Antonio Rampino,
and Valentina Giorgelli

20.1 Introduction

The nosography of Gender Dysphoria (GD) has recently been object of an important change. In the Statistical and Diagnostic Manual of Mental Disorders, DSM V [1], this diagnosis was separated from paraphilias and sexual disorders, becoming an independent category. The most important innovative aspect introduced by the DSM V concerns the condition known as "Gender Identity Disorder", which is now referred to as "Gender Dysphoria". The new nomenclature emphasizes the salient aspect of distress overcoming the stigmatizing definition of "disorder", previously used.

Literature reports that Gender Dysphoria (GD)—defined as marked incongruence between one's expressed gender and her/his assigned gender [2] (APA 2014)—is associated with psychological suffering characterized by anxiety, depression, impaired relationships, and suicidal ideation. The difference between one's expressed gender and her/his physical sexual characteristics is expressed by the desire to get rid of them and/or to have the primary and secondary sexual characteristics of the opposite gender. The peculiarity of this disorder is the coexistence of medical aspects (biological sex) and psychological aspects (subjective experience). Previous studies highlight that psychological risk does not derive from the gender inconsistency, but from childhood traumatic experiences in different contexts, such as family, school, and because of non-recognition of psychological and sexual identity [3]. The community non-acceptance persists in adulthood, magnified by cultural stereotypes.

Therefore, Gender Dysphoria (GD) represents the condition of partial or complete discordance between assigned sex, based on external genitalia, and the gender recognized by the brain. So, it is characterized by suffering, malaise, and stress. This existential state has an intrinsic complexity that deserves as much attention and management as the medical issues related. Therefore, in a service dedicated to GD, it is necessary to create a multidisciplinary team dealing with all aspects of the transition process. Accordingly, an elective modality of "cure" has been proposed: on the one hand, the person carrying GD is supported from a psychological point of view; on the other hand, s/he is allowed to choose how to transform his/her morphological characteristics according to his/her subjective experience of identity, through endocrinological and surgical treatments. Of

E. Lavorato (✉)
"Azienda Ospedaliera Universitaria Policlinico di Bari"—Psychiatry Unit, Bari, Italy

A. Rampino · V. Giorgelli
Group of Psychiatric Neuroscience, Department of Basic Medical Sciences, Neuroscience and Sense Organs, University of Bari Aldo Moro, Bari, Italy

note, Law number 164 on 14th April 1982 (*"Rules on the rectification of gender attribution"*) establishes the possibility of carrying out a Surgical Sex Reassignment (SSR) and/or a change of sex at registry office even without SSR. In any case, it is permitted only after a clear diagnosis of GD has been formulated by a psychiatrist.

In Italy, the Observatory on Gender Identity (ONIG) has identified the centres able to take care of these cases throughout the national territory. Such centres must meet the criteria of Standards of Care (SOC) of the World Professional Association for Transgender Health [4], as defined by the Harry Benjamin International Gender Dysphoria Association. In fact, in all countries of the world, this Association reunited and supported people who, despite different skills, desire to develop the best possible practices and the most useful support to improve the quality of life of this population.

As a general expectation, people born with male sex identify themselves as men, while those born with female sex as women. Nonetheless, this is not what real experience teaches us and can be prejudicial if not detached from reality. In fact, a person, who experiences a so-called "Gender Variance", does not recognize him/herself in this binary system occurring at birth. He/she does not perceive the gender identity as corresponding to birth assigned sex.

In fact, while there is biological sex depending on differences in chromosome numbers and genital conformation, gender identity is a more intimate feeling of belonging to the male or female gender, or to some combination of them. Therefore, Gender Identity allows people to say: "I am a man", "I am a woman", "I am a genderqueer", regardless of the birth assigned sex.

The term *Transgender* refers to identities or gender expressions that differ from social expectations typically based on the birth assigned sex. Transgender people can have a binary gender identity (identifying themselves as women if at birth they were men or as men if at birth they were women) or non-binary (identifying themselves with subjective combination of genres). Not all people living "Gender Variance" express psychological or physical

discomfort. Most of them find balance between the perception of oneself and the subjective model of relationships. On the other hand, if there is a psychological or physical distress, the so-called *Gender Dysphoria,* the person could feel the need to adapt the external reality (anatomical and personal data) to his or her emotional inner world. This is possible thanks to different interventions, including intake of feminizing or masculinizing hormones, surgical interventions, and/or modification of personal data. There are currently no data indicating a prevalence of people with gender variance. Nevertheless, there are data on the prevalence of Gender Dysphoria based on people entering specialized centres. Specifically, the World Professional Association for Transgender Health Standards of Care reported a prevalence of 1 in 11,900–45,000 for people assigned at birth to the male gender and 1 in 30,400–200,000 for people assigned at birth to the female gender.

The personal gender identity develops influenced by emotionally significant relationships and by social-educational environment, based on predisposing biological characteristics. Most of clinical and psycho-social studies agree on multifactorial nature of this process, focusing on the combined action of biological, psychological, social, and cultural factors.

20.2 Basic Concepts: Sexual and Gender Identity

To understand the experiences of Transgender people, we refer to behavioural and phenomenological markers of psychosexual development. Most of scholars refer to a tripartite model based on *gender identity, gender role,* and *sexual orientation.* Some authors also consider a further construct: *gender expression.* These components drive and guide the development of *sexual identity.* There are different definitions of *gender identity*; first, it is not a stable construct because it is acquired step by step in the entire existence and it is influenced by different experiences. The *sexual identity* consists of biological sex (male or female according to certain biological parameters), gender identity (feeling male or female), gender role (adherence to the expectations of social context related to both biological sex and one's own gender identity experience), and then sexual orientation (the gender towards which the individual feels sexual attraction).

The *biological sex* is the set of all biological characteristics of being female or male (biological sex): the sex chromosomes (XY for males and XX for females), the gonads (testes for males and ovaries for females), external genitalia, and secondary sexual characteristics (development of breasts, presence of face hair, tone of the voice, etc.) which appear during the sexual development (puberty).

Gender is a more complex construct and refers to characteristics depending on cultural, social, and psychological factors that define typical behaviours for men and women. For most people, biological sex and gender identity match. The term *transgender* identifies people with gender identity other than biological sex: for example, a person born as male, but feeling female (or vice versa). The condition that gender identity differs from biological sex is known as gender incongruence. *The gender incongruence is not a disorder.* In the last edition of International statistical classification of diseases and related health problems (ICD-11), gender incongruence was declassified from the chapter of mental health and included in the chapter of *sexual health*. If psychological discomfort of gender incongruence is structured in persistent and specific symptoms with an associated alteration of the global functioning, that is Gender Dysphoria.

Epidemiological data: as previously reported, prevalence data of *Gender Dysphoria* in adults (>18 years) are collected by specialized centres. Such data are most probably underestimated because not all people with gender incongruence develop Gender Dysphoria, then not all people affected by Gender Dysphoria come to a specialized centre. The estimated prevalence of GD is 0.005–0.014% of people with biological male sex and 0.002–0.003% of people with biological female sex [5]. Therefore, gender dysphoria is more common in the MtF form with a male/female ratio of approximately 3:1. In children

under 12, the male/female ratio ranges from 3:1 to 2:1; while in teenagers, over 12 years, the male/female ratio is about 1:1.7 [5]. We highlight Gender Dysphoria is independent from sexual preference, which indicates sexual and emotional attraction for a person of the same sex (homosexuality), of opposite sex (heterosexuality), or of both genders (bisexuality). Transgender people can have any sexual and sentimental orientation, for example, they can be heterosexual or lesbian, gay or bisexual.

20.3   Symptoms

Gender Dysphoria appears as malaise and discomfort towards one's body, felt as a stranger; the same sense of strangeness is experienced towards behaviours and attitudes that are typical of one's sex, within which the person does not recognize her/himself.

The first symptoms of gender dysphoria may appear from the very early years of life, 2–3 years. In studies on childhood, it was seen gender dysphoria remains until adulthood for 6–23% among males and 12–27% among females. In other words, less than a third of children, in whom gender dysphoria has been diagnosed, will maintain this condition even during adolescence. However, when gender dysphoria persists in the early stage of sexual development (puberty), it rarely disappears over time, and nearly all adolescents with gender dysphoria maintain this condition well into adulthood.

20.3.1   Children

Characteristic behaviours of gender dysphoria among children may include:

- Desire to wear clothes, use toys or take part to games typically associated to the other gender, preferring to play with children of opposite biological sex.
- Refusal to urinate as other children of the same biological sex do (standing for boys or sitting for girls).

- Desire to get rid of their genitals and want to have genitals of the opposite biological sex (for example a boy may say he wants to get rid of his penis and a girl may wish to have a penis).
- Extreme discomfort with the changes in the body that occur during puberty.

These behaviours in gender dysphoria are associated with deep suffering and distress at school and in relationships. Rather consistently, in children with gender dysphoria, anxiety and depression are common.

20.3.2 Teenagers and Adults

In teenagers and adults, symptoms may include:

- Certainty that one's true gender is not aligned with one's body.
- Disgust towards one's own genitals.
- Strong desire to get rid of one's genitals and other characteristics of one's biological sex.

It is very difficult to have or suppress these feelings, and as a result, people with gender dysphoria may present with anxiety, depression, engage in self-harm, and have suicidal thoughts.

In the Diagnostic and Statistical Manual of Mental disorders, fifth edition (DSM-5—American Psychiatric Association) details about the diagnostic criteria for gender dysphoria according to age (children, adolescents, and adults) are reported.

20.3.3 DSM 5

20.3.3.1 Gender Dysphoria Criteria in Adults

A. A marked incongruence between one's experienced/expressed gender and their assigned gender, lasting at least 6 months, as manifested by at least two of the following:
1. A marked incongruence between one's experienced/expressed gender and primary and/or secondary sex characteristics (or in young adolescents, the anticipated secondary sex characteristics).
2. A strong desire to get rid of one's primary and/or secondary sex characteristics because of a marked incongruence with one's experienced/expressed gender (or in young adolescents, a desire to prevent the development of the anticipated secondary sex characteristics).
3. A strong desire for the primary and/or secondary sex characteristics of the other gender.
4. A strong desire to be of the other gender (or some alternative gender different from one's assigned gender).
5. A strong desire to be treated as the other gender (or some alternative gender different from one's assigned gender).
6. A strong conviction that one has the typical feelings and reactions of the other gender (or some alternative gender different from one's assigned gender).
B. The condition must also be associated with clinically significant distress or impairment in social, occupational, or other important areas of functioning.

20.3.3.2 Gender Dysphoria Criteria in Children

A. A marked incongruence between one's experienced/expressed gender and their assigned gender, lasting at least 6 months, as manifested by at least two of the following (one of which must be the first criterion):
1. A strong desire to be of the other gender or an insistence that one is the other gender (or some alternative gender different from one's assigned gender).
2. In boys (assigned gender), a strong preference for cross-dressing or simulating female attire; or in girls (assigned gender), a strong preference for wearing only typical masculine clothing and a strong resistance to the wearing of typical feminine clothing.
3. A strong preference for cross-gender roles in make-believe play or fantasy play.

4. A strong preference for the toys, games, or activities stereotypically used or engaged in by the other gender.
5. A strong preference for playmates of the other gender.
6. In boys (assigned gender), a strong rejection of typically masculine toys, games, and activities and a strong avoidance of rough-and-tumble play; or in girls (assigned gender), a strong rejection of typically feminine toys, games, and activities.
7. A strong dislike of one's sexual anatomy.
8. A strong desire for the physical sex characteristics that match one's experienced gender.

B. The condition must be associated with clinically significant distress or impairment in social, occupational, or other important areas of functioning.

Specify whether a Sexual Development Disorder is present.

20.3.3.3 Gender Dysphoria Criteria in Adolescents

A. A marked incongruence between one's experienced/expressed gender and their assigned gender, lasting at least 6 months, as manifested by at least two of the following:
   1. A marked incongruence between one's experienced/expressed gender and primary and/or secondary sex characteristics (or in young adolescents, the anticipated secondary sex characteristics).
   2. A strong desire to get rid of one's primary and/or secondary sex characteristics because of a marked incongruence with one's experienced/expressed gender (or in young adolescents, a desire to prevent the development of the anticipated secondary sex characteristics).
   3. A strong desire for the primary and/or secondary sex characteristics of the other gender.
   4. A strong desire to be of the other gender (or some alternative gender different from one's assigned gender).
   5. A strong desire to be treated as the other gender (or some alternative gender different from one's assigned gender).
   6. A strong conviction that one has the typical feelings and reactions of the other gender (or some alternative gender different from one's assigned gender).

B. The condition must also be associated with clinically significant distress <u>or impairment in social, occupational, or other important areas of functioning</u>.

Specify whether a Sexual Development Disorder is present.

After confirming the diagnosis, the person affected by Gender Dysphoria must be informed about all strategies of treatments, as well as about the associated risks and the irreversibility of some of them. The symptoms described above explain the need to provide adequate responses to specific needs, bearing in mind, as we are about to clarify, the multifactorial nature of the condition of gender incongruence and of Gender Dysphoria.

20.4 Causes: Etiological Theories

The causes of Gender Dysphoria are still unclear and both psychosocial and biological factors have been implicated. Currently, the most accepted hypothesis is that both factors contribute to its development [6, 7]. Even if social factors, such as education, environment, and events of life, are of great importance in emergence of gender dysphoria, there is still no experimental evidence to support this theory.

Studies carried out on twin populations have shown that in monozygotic twins (i.e. generated by the same egg-cell and, therefore, with the same genetic makeup) the possibility of gender dysphoria occurring in both twins is higher than in heterozygous twins (generated by two distinct egg cells and therefore with 50% of the same genetic makeup). This suggests genetic factors are important in gender dysphoria. There are also numerous theories that consider the influence of sex hormones on the onset of gender dysphoria.

As established by animal model experiments, the process of sexual differentiation is not limited to the development of the genitals, but it involves the structures of the central nervous system that regulate sexual behaviours. Since the differentiation of the genitals occurs in the first 2 months of intrauterine life, while that of the central nervous system begins in the second half of pregnancy and becomes manifest in adult life, it has been hypothesized that in subjects with gender dysphoria these two processes occur in a disharmonic way. In this regard, the importance of prenatal male sex hormones, particularly testosterones, in development of male sexual identity was suggested. Indeed, some studies highlighted that low levels of testosterone in male foetuses can be associated with an increased incidence of Gender Dysphoria. Furthermore, a reduced sensitivity to testosterone and, therefore, a defective functioning of this hormone has been evidenced in MtF people.

Other studies focused on brain area differences between male and female population and suggested that cerebral architecture of individuals with Gender Dysphoria resembles the one of individuals with the same gender identity rather than those with the same biological sex, thus suggesting that non-biological factors may play a predominant role in GD genesis. The diagnosis of Gender Dysphoria requires evaluation by a mental health expert (psychologist or psychiatrist). In general, a psychologist or a psychiatrist assesses whether Gender Dysphoria criteria are satisfied, with a focus on the way feelings and behaviours develop over time, and on the family and social context (if it is present and supportive). The team also assesses all condition for differential diagnosis, i.e. a non-compliance to stereotyped gender role behaviours, or a strong desire to belong to another gender than the one assigned and the degree and pervasiveness of activities and interests that vary with respect to gender for reasons inherent to the gender role rather than identity. GD must be distinguished from Transvestic Disorder, a cross-dressing behaviour that generates sexual arousal and causes suffering and/or impairment without questioning one's primary gender. GD differs

from Body Dysmorphism; the focus is on the alteration or removal of a specific part of the body as it is perceived as abnormal and not because it is representative of an assigned gender that is repudiated. It should also be distinguished from psychotic mental disorders, in which gender inconsistency can be underlying a delusional construct.

20.5 Treatment

Treatment of Gender Dysphoria aims to reduce, or remove, suffering based on teamwork of psychologists, psychiatrists, endocrinologists, and surgeons. There are standards of care proposed by the World Professional Association of Transgender Health (WPATH, [8]) and international guidelines [9] which health workers refer to. Some people with Gender Dysphoria decide to modify their body to make it more alike to how they feel, through a *"path of affirmation of gender"* that proceeds in successive phases and can include hormonal and/or surgical treatment. Treatments are not always necessary and the treatment process is not the same for all people. Indeed, the procedure is different according to real needs of the individual.

20.5.1 Treatment for Children and Adolescents

First line treatment of GD in children and adolescents is psychological intervention that must be provided by mental health experts (child psychologists and neuropsychiatrists), especially if specialized in issues related to developmental age. Psychological support allows to face current problems and provides help to reduce emotional suffering sometimes allowing for more drastic treatment avoidance.

Non-medical intervention is planned. So far, there is no consensus about the best intervention with *children* with GD, because the studies on the effectiveness of the different psychological approaches are poor and inconclusive. However, there is expert convergence on the opinion that the aim of a clinical intervention in children with GD must be to reduce discomfort and—if present—the associated emotional difficulties. The goal is the psychological well-being of the child. The better described approach is the so-called *watchful waiting*, which has the aim to encourage people with GD to explore their gender identity for it to develop in a natural and spontaneous way, while the individual maintains a neutral attitude towards any development outcome. The aim of the clinician (psychologist and/or psychotherapist) is to inform and to train the family about GD and to support it in making decisions following a careful evaluation of costs and benefits. Major associations dealing with developmental age or transgender health, such as the World Professional Association for Transgender Health (WPATH) and the American Academy of Child and Adolescent Psychiatry, condemned all interventions aimed at identity gender modification as unethical or attempts at prevention of a future non-heterosexual orientation.

The approach to Gender Dysphoria in *adolescence* requires careful evaluation, with particular care in making differential diagnoses with other conditions in order to define individualized paths. For example, it is important to distinguish Gender Dysphoria from internalized homophobia that occurs in some adolescents who, failing to accept their homosexual orientation, may require a medical gender reassignment (GR). Depending on the cultural context, their belief system, or even stereotyped views of social arrangements, some homosexual adolescents may mistake their sexual orientation for gender identity, due to a history of borderline behaviours and cross-gender interests in childhood. First, differential diagnosis needs to exclude the "Transvestic Disorder". Transvestism mostly characterizes male adolescents who occasionally wear female clothes without a connected sexual motivation; in fact, in adolescence this behavioural manifestation can represent a phase of experimentation. Transvestic Disorder in DSM-5 is among the Paraphilic Disorders and generally occurs in males of hetero- or bisexual orientation who experience sexual arousal in wearing women's clothing associated with emotional distress. Transvestism

disorder is distinguished from Gender Dysphoria because in the first case, gender identity is not in question. Gender Dysphoria must also be distinguished from "Body Dysmorphic Disorder" characterized by pervasive concern for presumed physical defects or imperfections, which are associated with repetitive behaviours in response to worries about such defects. In these cases, the modification or removal of a specific part of the body is required because it is perceived as abnormal or deformed, and not because it is attributable to the gender assigned at birth.

It is important to point out that Gender Dysphoria in adolescence is often accompanied by concomitant psychopathologies. Adolescents with Gender Dysphoria report higher levels of suicidal risk, depression, anxiety, social isolation, and bodily dissatisfaction.

The persistence of Gender Dysphoria in adolescence and the frequency of other associated psychopathologies—reactively to the condition of Gender Dysphoria—supports the importance of early intervention, including medical intervention. The guidelines of the Endocrine Society and the WPATH Standards of Care, together with the recommendations of the main national scientific societies, suggest to interrupt pubertal development with GnRH analogues (GnRHa) in adolescents with GD who meet specific criteria, i.e. an early onset of DG whose symptoms intensified during the early stages of puberty; the absence of psychosocial issues that may have interfered with diagnosis or treatment; a good understanding for the consequences of GR (Gender Reassignment) in one's existence. In addition to psychological support, the administration of GnRHa is indicated to postpone puberty when Tanner stage 2 has been reached. GnRH analogues, which are prescribed by the endocrinologist, work by suppressing the production of sex hormones, therefore they block the physical changes induced by puberty. Therefore, they allow adolescents for a longer exploration of their gender identity and the mental health experts to observe adolescents' gender identity while relieving the suffering that can come from contact with a body that develops in an unwanted direction. The effects of therapy with GnRH analogues are completely reversible:

if the treatment is interrupted, pubertal development immediately begins in the direction of biological sex. If GD persists and if specific eligibility criteria are met, it is possible to start a first hormonal GR, from 16 years onwards with the intake of cross-sex hormones (CHT). Surgery is also allowed as an extreme strategy, but better after age of 18.

20.5.2   Treatment for Adults

1. Psychological support if necessary.
2. Feminizing or masculinizing hormone treatment (cross-sex therapy).
3. Sex reassignment surgery.

In this section, we will deal with the *psychological support* provided to people with Gender Dysphoria, mentioning hormone therapy only in relation to the involvement of mental health professionals. The prerequisite for any psychotherapeutic approach can be summarized in some fundamental requirements that health professionals must apply always and in every area such as: the respect due to users with Gender Dysphoria without pathologizing the differences related to gender identities and expressions; the ability to provide adequate information about the services that transsexual, transgender and gender nonconforming people can benefit from the National Health System and, in particular, on the benefits and risks of the treatment; to guarantee personalized psychotherapeutic approaches, which are shaped on the individual needs; to facilitate the access to the most appropriate cures based on the condition of the individual. Taking charge of user with Gender Dysphoria provides for multiple paths and possibilities that the psychologist and/or psychotherapist are required to know. Indeed, some people do not feel the need to modify the somatic characteristics of their body—through medical-surgical paths of virilization or feminization—especially if capable of integrating their trans- or cross-gender experience in the gender assigned at birth. Alternatively, people may consider only a few changes in gender role or gender expression or wish to make a transition even

physical in line with the change in their gender role, requiring hormonal therapies but not surgery. Finally, people may wish surgery to complete the transition process and thus alleviate dysphoria but not other non-surgical strategies. It is therefore essential for health professionals, and especially for psychologists and psychotherapists, to make an effort to deeply understand the individual's life history and support him/her in an individualized way.

In fact, treatment of gender dysphoria should always explore the different possibilities of expression of identity. Psychotherapy (individual, couple, family, or group) therefore aims: to explore gender identity, role, and expression; to alleviate the stressful impact of Gender Dysphoria and social stigma on mental health; to reduce internalized transphobia; to provide tools for the user to enhance their social network and peers; to improve their body image; and ultimately to promote resilience.

Hormone therapy can be prescribed to all people with persistent and well-documented Gender Dysphoria; who are of age (if minors it is necessary to refer to guidelines for adolescents with gender dysphoria); they must be able to make a fully informed decision and to agree with the treatment and, finally, that they do not present medical or psychological problems.

In order to start hormone therapy, no minimum time for evaluation, psychological support, or social transition is required. However, the physician prescribing sex hormones (usually an endocrinologist) has the responsibility of making sure that hormone therapy is the best way to meet the user's needs and reduce their suffering, without inducing health problems. Therefore, it is considered appropriate to provide multidisciplinary care, so that different professional skills are continuously integrated. An accurate assessment of the psychological and existential status of the person, as well as their psychosocial context of reference, is necessary.

It is good to proceed to:

1. Analysis and evaluation of the psychological motivations that led the subject to undertake his/her treatment path;

2. Analysis of awareness of achievable goals and hypothesized emotional reactions related to the realistic change of the body according to the desired identity, to any sex reassignment surgery procedures, to the functionality of the genital system;

3. Assessment of the users' ability to share with their family and social context with respect to their transition process and assessment of the resources of the family and social context to welcome and support the user.

Such a general assessment is necessary in order to have a snapshot of the personal and relational situation of the user with Gender Dysphoria and make psychotherapeutic management personalized.

However, it is important to underline WPATH recognizes that health does not depend only on clinical care, but also on a social and political climate that guarantees social tolerance, equality, respect, and the full right of citizenship. Health is guaranteed with public policies and legal reforms that promote tolerance and fairness towards all gender differences and aimed to eliminate prejudice, discrimination, and stigmatization.

A significant part of transgender people's suffering originates precisely from the stigmatization deriving from a stereotyped vision of the concept of gender along with all additional stressors, connected to the stigma of gender nonconformity, and that may negatively affect the psycho-physical health of the individual. This phenomenon, known as *Minority Stress,* affects people belonging to social categories stigmatized and subjected to excessively high levels of stress, such as those derived from violence, discrimination, and stigmatization. Stigma can certainly be defined as a social process that negatively connotes a member or a community based on its characteristics to which inferior qualities are arbitrarily attributed. Stigma can be experienced on at least three levels: structural, interpersonal, and individual. Structural stigma refers to the level of social institutions and it constitutes a barrier to access to fundamentals, such as work or care; the interpersonal stigma is a particular behavioural structure which mani-fests itself through verbal abuse, physical or sexual violence, or threats; the individual stigma instead refers to the feelings and emotions that the stigmatized person feels or what he believes that others think of himself. All three types of stigma are widely represented among transgender people and connected with the adverse psycho-physical health outcomes. It is evident that psychotherapy work must focus on the individual's resources to promote resilience, while being aware that structural and interpersonal aspects of the stigma cannot be eradicated with psychotherapeutic work alone.

20.6 Conclusions

The formation and definition of transgender and transsexual identity have a high specific complexity, to which environmental and cultural stigmatizations add further complexity. However, it is essential to recognize that the transgender and transsexual evolutionary path preserves the typical dynamics of any identity construction process. Therefore, in clinical work with these people, it is important to consider both the identity structure of the person and the universal evolutionary processes. Approaching transsexual people with the prejudice of an absolute diversity in the formation of the self and identity can compromise the understanding of psychological processes behind while preventing from a fully empathic relationship, that is needed in order to establish a good therapeutic alliance.

References

1. American Psychiatric Association (APA). Diagnostic and statistical manual of mental disorders: fifth edition (DSM-5). Washington DC: American Psychiatric Association; 2013.
2. American Psychiatric Association (APA). Diagnostic and statistical manual of mental disorders: 5fth edition (DSM-5). Washington DC: American Psychiatric Association. 2013.
3. Lingiardi V, Giovanardi G, Fortunato A, Nassisi V, Speranza AM. Personality and Attachment in Transsexual Adults. Arch Sex Behav. 2017 Jul;46(5):1313-1323. https://doi.org/10.1007/s10508-017-0946-0. Epub 2017 Feb 16. PMID: 28210932.

4. WPATH 2012" World Professional Association for Transgender Health. Standards of Care for the Health of Transsexual, Transgender, and Gender Nonconforming People [7th Version]. (2012). https://www.wpath.org/publications/soc.
5. Zucker KJ. Epidemiology of gender dysphoria and transgender identity [Sintesi]. Sex Health. 2017;14(5):404–11.
6. Chipkin SR, Kim F. Ten Most important things to know about caring for transgender patients. Am J Med. 2017;130:1238–45.
7. Winter S, et al. Transgender people: health at the margins of society [Sintesi]. Lancet. 2016;388:390–400.
8. Coleman E, et al. Standards of Care for the Health of transsexual, transgender, and gender-nonconforming people, version 7 [Sintesi]. Int J Transgend. 2012;13(4):165–232.
9. Hembree WC, et al. Endocrine treatment of gender-dysphoric/gender-incongruent persons: an Endocrine Society clinical practice guideline. J Clin Endocrinol Metab. 2017;102:3869–903.

Link to Further Information

ICD-11. Gender incongruence of adolescence or adulthood: https://www.who.int/standards/classifications/frequently-asked-questions/gender-incongruence-and-transgender-health-in-the-icd.
Infotrans: https://www.infotrans.it/.
Mayo Clinic. Gender Dysphoria: https://www.mayoclinic.org/diseases-conditions/gender-dysphoria/symptoms-causes/syc-20475255.
NHS Choices. Gender Dysphoria: https://www.nhs.uk/conditions/gender-dysphoria/.
ONIG: https://www.onig.it/drupal8/.
World Professional Association for Transgender Health. Standards of care: https://www.wpath.org/soc8.

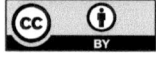

The Transgender: Endocrinological Assessment

21

Carlotta Cocchetti, Mario Maggi,
and Alessandra Daphne Fisher

21.1 Introduction

In the past, gender identity has always been conceived through a binary perspective, including only two possible choices: male or female. This conceptualization—named gender binarism—has been extended also to the transgender experience. Transgender represents an umbrella term used to describe those people who transiently or permanently identify with a gender different from the assigned one (AMAB for those assigned male at birth and AFAB for those assigned female at birth) [1, 2]. Contrastingly, the term cisgender refers to individuals whose gender identity matches with the assigned gender at birth. Since gender identity can be described as a spectrum with many possibilities, a complete identification with the opposite gender should not be considered as the only available option for transgender people. In line with that, recent studies highlighted a relevant prevalence of non-binary gender identity among transgender individuals [3, 4]. Thus, professionals dealing with transgender health should explore gender identity and desired body changes of each person, in order to guarantee an individualized approach during gender-affirming path [5]. This applies also to gender-affirming hormonal treatment, which should be tailored to the individual needs.

21.2 Initial Evaluation in Trans AFAB and AMAB People

Prior to start hormonal treatment, the endocrinologist should collect a detailed family and personal medical history, in order to assess pre-existing health risks and evaluate the presence of criteria for prescribing hormonal treatment (reported in Table 21.1) [6]. In particular, hormonal treatment in trans AMAB people is contraindicated in case of history of oestrogen-sensitive cancers, cholelithiasis, macroprolactinoma, cardiovascular/cerebrovascular disease, severe hypertriglyceridemia, if not recovered [6]. History of venous thromboembolism (VTE) should undergo evaluation and treatment before the start of hormonal treatment. Current guidelines do not routinely recommend screening for hereditary thrombophilia in all trans AMAB people [6]. In trans AFAB people, absolute contraindications for testosterone (T) treatment include pregnancy, whereas relative contraindications include erythrocytosis, sleep apnoea, and congestive heart failure [6, 7].

C. Cocchetti · A. D. Fisher (✉)
Andrology, Women's Endocrinology and Gender Incongruence Unit, Careggi University Hospital, Florence, Italy
e-mail: fishera@aou-careggi.toscana.it

M. Maggi
Endocrinology Unit, Department of Experimental and Clinical Biomedical Sciences "Mario Serio", Careggi Hospital, University of Florence, Florence, Italy

© The Author(s) 2023
C. Bettocchi et al. (eds.), *Practical Clinical Andrology*,
https://doi.org/10.1007/978-3-031-11701-5_21

Table 21.1 Eligibility criteria for gender-affirming hormonal treatment in adult transgender people

Criteria for gender-affirming hormonal treatment
1. Persistent gender dysphoria/gender incongruence
2. Capacity to make a fully informed decision and to give consent for treatment
3. The age of majority in a given country
4. Mental health concerns, if present, must be reasonably well-controlled

Considering the partial lack of data regarding long-term cardiovascular safety of hormonal treatment, all the modifiable risk factors (i.e. hypertension, dyslipidemia, obesity, tobacco use, sedentary lifestyle) should be managed before the start of hormonal treatment.

Furthermore, transgender people should be adequately informed by clinicians regarding the expected body changes during hormonal treatment and their timing, in order to avoid potential anxiety due to high expectations.

Since fertility may be affected, clinicians must inform all transgender people about the potential impact of medical treatment and discuss at that time the available fertility preservation options.

21.3　Full Masculinization in Trans AFAB People

21.3.1　Hormonal Treatment Strategies

Virilizing hormonal treatment in trans AFAB people is based on T administration. To date, clinicians can opt for several available T formulations, including parental injections (T esters or undecanoate), transdermal or oral T (as detailed in Table 21.2). At the present moment, relevant differences regarding short-term safety and satisfaction have not been observed among different preparations. However, injectable short-term T esters are associated with significant fluctuations of T levels, which may be associated with mood swings and higher risk of haematocrit increase [8, 9]. On the contrast, transdermal and long-acting intramuscular T allow to maintain more stable T levels simulating male production rate

Table 21.2 Hormonal treatment regimens in transgender people requesting full virilization or full de-virilization and feminization

Requested effect	Hormonal compounds	Administration route and recommended dosage
Full virilization	Mixed T esters preparations	Intramuscularly, 250 mg every 3 weeks
	T enanthate	Intramuscularly, 250 mg every 2–4 weeks
	T undecanoate[a]	Intramuscularly, 1000 mg every 12 weeks
	T gel 1–2%	Transdermal, 50 mg/day (available in dispenser pump or as single-dose sachets)
Full de-virilization	Cyproterone acetate	Oral, 10–50 mg/day
	Spironolactone	Oral, 100–200 mg/day
	GnRH agonist (leuprolide, triptorelin)	Intramuscularly or subcutaneously, 3.75 mg monthly or 11.25 mg every 3 months
Full feminization	Estradiol valerate	Oral, 2–6 mg/day
	Estradiol	Transdermal, patch 25–100 μg/24 h twice or once weekly
	Estradiol hemihydrate	Transdermal, gel 1.5–3 mg/day

[a]One thousand milligrams initially followed by an injection at 6 weeks then at 12 weeks

and rhythm. Oral T is usually not recommended because of the gastrointestinal absorption variability leading to multiple daily administrations need.

If a full virilization is required, T treatment should follow the principles of hormonal replacement treatment in hypogonadal cisgender men, achieving T levels within the adult cisgender men range (depending on the specific assay, but typically from 320 to 1000 ng/dL, or 11.1 to 34.7 nmol/L) [6].

In trans AFAB people undergoing oophorectomy, T treatment should be continued in order to avoid consequences of premature loss of hormonal support, such as osteoporosis, cardiovascular events, and cognitive impairment.

21.3.2 Virilizing Effects

Masculinizing effects include increase in facial and body hair, body composition and fat distribution changes, and voice deepening, which usually occur in the first 6 months of treatment [10–12]. Among dermatological effects, also increased skin oiliness, acne and—in genetically predisposed individuals—androgenetic alopecia have been reported [13]. T treatment results in clitoromegaly and amenorrhea. All T formulations lead to amenorrhea in the first 12–18 months of treatment, but transdermal T resulted associated with higher rates of persistent vaginal bleeding in the first months of treatment compared to T undecanoate [14]. If vaginal bleeding persists, clinicians may consider the addition of progestins or gonadotropin-releasing hormone analogues (GnRHa) [6]. Regarding sexual well-being, a transient increase in sexual desire has been reported in literature, probably due to the initial increase of T levels, as well as an improvement of sexual well-being in the midterm [15, 16].

21.3.3 Safety Concerns

If full virilization is requested, clinicians should maintain T levels in the physiologic normal male range avoiding adverse effects resulting from T excess [6]. Regarding safety profile, T treatment leads to a more atherogenic lipid profile with increased triglycerides and low-density lipoprotein cholesterol (LDL-c) levels and decreased high-density lipoprotein cholesterol levels (HDL-c) [17–20]. This may lead to increased cardiovascular risk [20], even if a recent systematic review of the literature stated that definitive conclusions on rates of cardiovascular/cerebrovascular events cannot be drawn due to very low-quality evidence [21]. Furthermore, data on cardiovascular outcomes in older trans AFAB people are mostly lacking. For this reason, long-term data on car-

diovascular safety of T treatment are needed. A recent study showed an increase in haemoglobin and haematocrit levels during T treatment within the range for cisgender AMAB people, reaching a plateau after the first year [9]. However, clinically significant erythrocytosis appears really uncommon [9].

With respect to bone health, T treatment may exert a protective effect on bone mediated by the peripheral conversion to oestradiol. Baseline bone mineral (BMD) levels in trans AFAB people are usually in the expected range for their birth-assigned gender [22]. No relevant changes of BMD seem to occur during T treatment unless adequate dosages and compliance are guaranteed [23]. Limited data on osteoporotic fracture risk of are available in trans AFAB people.

Long-term T treatment may be associated with some concerns around cancer incidence and mortality, although not supported by literature. The available data showed very few cancer events in trans AFAB people with cancer mortality rates similar to those of the general population [24–28]. Nevertheless, breast and cervical cancer screening protocols are advised in trans AFAB people not undergoing gender-affirming surgeries [6].

21.3.4 Monitoring During Hormonal Treatment

Periodical monitoring is advised in trans AFAB people after the start of T treatment, with a frequency of 3–4 monthly in the first year and 1 or 2 per year thereafter [6]. The monitoring aims both to identify possible side effects of T treatment and to monitor the development of desired body changes. Haematocrit and haemoglobin represent the most important biochemical parameters, due to the risk of erythrocytosis associated with T treatment. Furthermore, lipid profile, weight, waist, and blood pressure should be checked at regular intervals. Clinical and instrumental-suggested monitoring is summarized in Table 21.3. Dual-energy X-ray absorptiometry (DXA) should be performed at baseline only in case of anamnestic relevant risk of osteoporosis

Table 21.3 Periodical monitoring in trans AMAB and AFAB people before and after the start of hormonal treatment

	Baseline	First year of hormonal treatment (every 3 months)	After the first year of hormonal treatment (every 6–12 months)
Trans AMAB people	Clinical evaluation LH, FSH, total testosterone, estradiol, prolactin levels, blood counts, renal and liver function, lipid, and glucose profile BMD in older than 60 years or in those who are not compliant with hormone therapy	Clinical evaluation Testosterone, estradiol levels, LH (every 3 months); prolactin levels (once a year). Liver function, lipid, and glucose profile (every 3 months) Serum electrolytes (every 3 months in case of spironolactone use)	Clinical evaluation Testosterone, estradiol (every 6–12 months) levels; prolactin levels (every 2 years), blood counts, liver function, lipid, and glucose profile (every 6–12 months) Serum electrolytes (every 12 months, in case of spironolactone use) BMD evaluation after 60 years or in case of discontinuation of therapy after gonadectomy
Trans AFAB people	Clinical evaluation LH, FSH, total testosterone, estradiol, prolactin levels, blood counts, renal and liver function, lipid, and glucose profile BMD in older than 60 years or in those who are not compliant with hormone therapy	Clinical evaluation Testosterone, estradiol levels, LH (every 3 months); haematocrit, lipid, and glucose profile (every 3 months)	Clinical evaluation Testosterone, estradiol (every 6–12 months) levels; hematocrit, lipid, and glucose profile (every 6–12 months) BMD evaluation after 60 years or in case of discontinuation of therapy after gonadectomy

(smoking, excessive alcohol use, family history of fractures/osteoporosis, glucocorticoids use, and anorexia nervosa) and after gonadectomy in case of low compliance to hormonal treatment [6]. As stated before, periodical oncological screening of all present tissues is recommended, even if the adequate timing has not been yet elucidated.

21.4 Full Feminization and De-Masculinization in Trans AMAB People

21.4.1 Hormonal Treatment Strategies

In trans AMAB people, oestrogens are necessary to induce female secondary sexual characteristics. Among them, in the past ethinyl oestradiol was widely used especially through self-prescription. Given safety concerns due to the increased thromboembolic and cardiovascular risk, current guidelines recommend the use of oestradiol [6, 29]. Among oestrogen options, patients and clinicians can opt for oral micron-ized esterified (valerate) oestradiol or transdermal 17β-oestradiol (treatment regimens reported in Table 21.2). Transdermal formulations (patches or gel) do not undergo first hepatic metabolism, which may reduce the risk of pro-thrombotic effect. For this reason, transdermal compounds should be preferred in cases of higher thromboembolic risk (i.e. age >40 years, smoking, obesity, liver disease, diabetes mellitus with complications). If full feminization is desired, oestrogen is prescribed at dosages two or three times higher than the recommended doses for hormonal replacement treatment in postmenopausal cisgender women. In this case, the goal is to reach and maintain serum oestradiol and T in the normal range for premenopausal cisgender women (100–200 pg/mL and 50 ng/dL, respectively) [6].

Trans AMAB people often require the addition of anti-androgen therapies to achieve desired body changes (Table 21.2). In many European countries, cyproterone acetate (CPA) represents the most commonly prescribed androgen lowering compound. CPA is an anti-androgenic progestational compound with both peripheral and central action. Recently, its use has been limited by evidences of hepatotoxicity, increased incidence of depression and hyperprolactinemia, and association with multifocal meningiomas, which is a hormone-sensitive tumour expressing progesterone receptors [30–34]. According to a recent multicentric study, a daily dose of 10 mg is effective (equally to 50 mg/daily) in lowering testosterone concentrations in trans women, while showing fewer side effects [35].

Among androgen-lowering therapies, GnRHa may be considered as a valuable alternative due to their efficacy and safety profile. GnRHa reduce T levels through the downregulation of pituitary GnRH receptor. GnRHa are considered extremely safe and in one recent comparative study they showed a better metabolic profile with respect to CPA [36]. The main limitation to their use is represented by the high cost.

Spironolactone (100–300 mg/daily) is an antagonist of mineralocorticoid receptor with anti-androgen properties, frequently used in the United States where CPA is not available. Spironolactone 200 mg daily proved effective in reducing T levels in trans AMAB people into the cisgender female range [37]. However, spironolactone use is limited by the risk of hyperkalaemia, hypotension, and gastrointestinal bleeding [38].

Peripheral androgen receptor blockers such as flutamide (50–75 mg/daily) or bicalutamide (25–50 mg/daily) are not recommended in trans AMAB people, due to the lack of data regarding their efficacy and safety and the risk of hepatotoxicity described in cisgender women [39].

21.4.2 Feminizing and De-Virilizing Effects

Body changes occurring in the first months include dermatological effects such as a significant reduction of terminal facial and body hair—although often not satisfying—and a decreased skin oiliness [12]. During the first year of treatment, body composition changes occur, with increased body fat mainly in the gynoid regions and decreased lean body mass, in line with a more feminine body composition [40]. Breast development becomes relevant after 6 months and reaches a maximum at 2 years after the start of feminizing treatment [41]. Increase in breast size is strictly associated with decrease in body uneasiness [12]; however, less than 20% of trans AMAB people reach Tanner breast stage 4–5 after 24 months of hormonal treatment [12], with most people seeking mammoplasty. To date, data supporting a beneficial effect of progestins on breast development are scarce and do not allow to recommend their use, also considering the potential increase of cardiovascular risk [42, 43]. Testicular volume decreased by approximately 60% after 24 months, along with a reduction of spontaneous erections [12]. Voice frequency does not modify in trans AMAB people under hormonal treatment [44].

Regarding sexuality, hormonal treatment in trans AMAB people is associated with a transient decrease in sexual desire in the first 3–6 months of hormonal treatment [16], whereas sexual well-being increases in the mid-term, probably because of the improvement of body image perception [15].

21.4.3 Safety Concerns

In relation to safety profile, hormonal treatment in trans AMAB people resulted associated with favourable changes in lipid profile, with increased HDL-c and decreased LDL-c concentrations [19, 20]. A recent meta-analysis found only changes in triglycerides, whose levels were higher in trans AMAB people after 24 months of hormonal treatment [21]. Concerns raised about long-term effects of feminizing hormonal treatment on cardiovascular outcomes. A study conducted in Belgium over 200 trans AMAB people reported higher rates of myocardial infarction, venous thrombosis, and cerebrovascular disease compared to cisgender men and women [25]. Other studies confirmed higher rates of ischemic stroke in trans AMAB people compared to cisgender one [45], whereas myocardial infarction rates resulted higher in trans AMAB people with respect to matched cisgender AFAB individuals and similar to those found in cisgender AMAB people [46]. Furthermore, oestrogens have a known pro-thrombotic action. The incidence rate of VTE in trans AMAB people under feminizing hormonal treatment appeared to be 2.3 per 1000 person-year [47]. However, the previous use of ethinyl oestradiol may lead to overestimation of the rate of VTE. Besides, hormonal treatment under medical supervision can be considered safer than self-prescribed therapy.

Trans AMAB people have a lower baseline BMD with respect to age-matched cisgender men, probably because of lower outdoor physical activity leading to reduced levels of vitamin D [22]. Estrogen treatment in trans AMAB people seems to be associated with improvement of BMD, especially at the lumbar spine [48–50]. However, fracture rate during long-term hormonal treatment in trans AMAB people is unknown.

Regarding oncological risk, oestrogens and progestogens can play a role in the pathogenesis of some brain tumours. Since oestrogens can stimulate the growth of pituitary lactotroph cells, an increased risk of prolactinoma has been demonstrated in trans AMAB people [51]. For this reason, guidelines recommend periodical monitoring of prolactin levels, although a moderate increase during feminizing hormonal treatment is expected [6]. Furthermore, higher risk of meningioma has been described in trans AMAB people compared to cisgender AFAB people [51], thus CPA discontinuation after gender-affirming surgery and lower dosages in case of long-term treatment are suggested [29, 35]. Rates of incidence of hormone-sensitive cancers, such as breast and prostate cancers, seemed to be low among trans AMAB people. A large study reported no increase in breast cancer incidence in trans AMAB people compared to cisgender women [52]. Another large study conducted in USA found no increased risk of any cancer in trans AMAB people compared to cisgender women, whereas an increased risk of breast cancer was reported with respect to cisgender men [53].

21.4.4 Monitoring During Hormonal Treatment

As stated before, periodical monitoring is recommended also in trans AMAB people after the start of feminizing/de-virilizing hormonal treatment, with a frequency of 3–4 monthly in the first year and 1 or 2 per year thereafter [6]. The aims are to monitor for appropriate signs of feminization and for development of adverse reactions. Serum T and oestradiol should be checked every 3 months, adjusting dosages if appropriate range for full feminization is not reached. In case of spironolactone administration, serum electrolytes should be monitored every 3 months in the first years and then annually [6, 29]. Table 21.3 shows the suggested clinical and biochemical monitoring. As for trans AFAB people, routine cancer screening of all present tissue should be performed. DXA should be performed at baseline only in individuals at high risk of osteoporosis, whereas in individuals at low risk screening for osteoporosis should be conducted after 60 years [6].

21.5 Partial De−/Masculinization and/or De-/Feminization

21.5.1 Partial Virilization and/or De-Feminization in Trans AFAB People

Some trans AFAB people may desire only partial masculinization. In this case, T dosages can be adjusted or other hormonal compounds could be added in order to shape androgens' effect on the body [5, 29]. Particularly, T could be prescribed at lower dosages, without achieving normal male T levels, although metabolic and bone safety of these treatment strategies are not elucidated. If the desired effect is represented by body composition changes and voice deepening without male body hair distribution, 5α-reductase inhibitors can be added to T [5]. In fact, by reducing 5α-dihydro-testosterone (DHT) levels through 5α-reductase type 2 inhibition, finasteride use

(1 mg/daily) resulted effective in the treatment of androgenetic alopecia and hirsutism [54, 55]. Other options besides 5α-reductase inhibitors can be proposed, such as definitive hair removal or eflornithine [54].

Conversely, in trans AFAB people requesting partial body shape changes with greater beard development, topical minoxidil application can be added to variable dosages of T [56].

Furthermore, low T dosages cannot be able to stop menses. For this purpose, when partial virilization and amenorrhea are both required, progestins, GnRHa, progesterone-releasing intrauterine devices, or endometrial ablation can be used to obtain amenorrhea [5, 57].

21.5.2 Partial Feminization and/or De-Virilization in Trans AMAB People

Some trans AMAB people may desire feminization and no/partial de-masculinization. For this purpose, the endocrinologist could prescribe only oestrogens or oestrogens plus lower dosages of CPA (such as 10 mg/daily or 10 mg on alternative days) [5].

On the contrast when de-virilization with little or no feminization is requested, only androgen lowering compounds can be proposed. Despite the absence of long-term safety data, the main criticality of this approach is represented by BMD loss due to androgen deprivation [58]. To prevent this, administration of low oestrogen dosages or selective oestrogen receptor modulators should be discussed with clients [5]. Other options to reduce male or induce female body characteristics can be discussed, such as permanent methods of hair reduction, breast augmentation, and lipofilling.

21.6 Conclusions

Transgender health—and therefore the endocrinological management—has become a topic of growing interest in the medical and scientific community in recent years. Research in this field moved away from case reports and small series, with an increased number of large longitudinal studies and systematic reviews/metanalysis. Increasing evidences regarding efficacy and safety of standardized hormonal treatment protocols are available in literature, even if there are still some open questions and long-term data remain sparse. The clinical approach also changed in recent years. In fact, endocrinologists dealing with transgender health care should explore gender identity and desired body changes in each person, actively involving the person in decisions regarding hormonal treatment and providing a real personalized clinical approach. The lack of information about non-standardized therapies for non-binary people should be kept in mind, thus benefits and risks should be extensively discussed with patients.

Acknowledgement None.

Conflict of Interest The authors have no conflict of interest.

References

1. Arcelus J, Bouman WP. Language and terminology. In: Bouman WP, Arcelus J, editors. The transgender handbook: a guide for transgender people, their families and professionals. New York, NY: Nova; 2017.
2. Coleman E, Bockting W, Botzer M, Cohen-Kettenis P, DeCuypere G, Feldman J, Fraser L, Green J, Knudson G, Meyer WJ, Monstrey S. Standards of care for the health of transsexual, transgender and gender-nonconforming people, version 7. Int J Transgend. 2012;13:165–232.
3. Koehler A, Eyssel J, Nieder TO. Genders and individual treatment progress in (non-)binary trans individuals. J Sex Med. 2018;15(1):102–13.
4. Romani A, Mazzoli F, Ristori J, Cocchetti C, Cassioli E, Castellini G, Mosconi M, Meriggiola MC, Gualdi S, Giovanardi G, Lingiardi V, Vignozzi L, Maggi M, Fisher AD. Psychological wellbeing and perceived social acceptance in gender diverse individuals. J Sex Med. 2021;18(11):1933–44.
5. Cocchetti C, Ristori J, Romani A, Maggi M, Fisher AD. Hormonal treatment strategies tailored to non-binary transgender individuals. J Clin Med. 2020;9(6):1609.

6. Hembree WC, Cohen-Kettenis PT, Gooren L, Hannema SE, Meyer WJ, Murad MH, Rosenthal SM, Safer JD, Tangpricha V, T'Sjoen GG. Endocrine treatment of gender-dysphoric/gender-incongruent persons: an Endocrine Society clinical practice guideline. J Clin Endocrinol Metab. 2017;102(11):3869–903.

7. T'Sjoen G, Arcelus J, Gooren L, Klink DT, Tangpricha V. Endocrinology of transgender medicine. Endocr Rev. 2019;40(1):97–117.

8. Pelusi C, Costantino A, Martelli V, et al. Effects of three different testosterone formulations in female-to-male transsexual persons. J Sex Med. 2014;11(12):3002–11.

9. Defreyne J, Vantomme B, Van Caenegem E, et al. Prospective evaluation of hematocrit in gender-affirming hormone treatment: results from European Network for the investigation of gender incongruence. Andrology. 2018;6(3):446–54.

10. Meriggiola MC, Armillotta F, Costantino A, et al. Effects of testosterone undecanoate administered alone or in combination with Letrozole or Dutasteride in female to male transsexuals. J Sex Med. 2008;5(10):2442–53.

11. Irwig MS, Childs K, Hancock AB. Effects of testosterone on the transgender male voice. Andrology. 2017;5(1):107–12.

12. Fisher AD, Castellini G, Ristori J, et al. Cross-sex hormone treatment and psychobiological changes in transsexual persons: two-year follow-up data. J Clin Endocrinol Metab. 2016;101(11):4260–9.

13. Wierckx K, Van de Peer F, Verhaeghe E, et al. Short- and long-term clinical skin effects of testosterone treatment in trans men. J Sex Med. 2014;11(1):222–9.

14. Defreyne J, Vanwonterghem Y, Collet S, et al. Vaginal bleeding and spotting in transgender men after initiation of testosterone therapy: a prospective cohort study (ENIGI). Int J Transgend Health. 2020;21(2):163–75.

15. Ristori J, Cocchetti C, Castellini G, et al. Hormonal treatment effect on sexual distress in transgender persons: 2-year follow-up data. J Sex Med. 2020;17(1):142–51.

16. Defreyne J, Elaut E, Kreukels B, et al. Sexual desire changes in transgender individuals upon initiation of hormone treatment: results from the investigation of gender incongruence. J Sex Med. 2020;17(4):812–25.

17. Elamin MB, Garcia MZ, Murad MH, et al. Effect of sex steroid use on cardiovascular risk in transsexual individuals: a systematic review and meta-analyses. Clin Endocrinol (Oxf). 2010;72(1):1–10.

18. Berra M, Armillotta L, D'Emidio F, et al. Testosterone decreases adiponectin levels in female to male transsexuals. Asian J Androl. 2006;8(6):725–9.

19. Van Velzen DM, Paldino A, Klaver M, et al. Cardiometabolic effects of testosterone in transmen and estrogen plus Cyproterone acetate in transwomen. J Clin Endocrinol Metab. 2019;104(6):1937–47.

20. Cocchetti C, Castellini G, Iacuaniello D, et al. Does gender-affirming hormonal treatment affect 30-year cardiovascular risk in transgender persons? A two-

year prospective European study (ENIGI). J Sex Med. 2021;18(4):821–9.

21. Maraka S, Singh Ospina N, Rodriguez-Gutierrez R, Davidge-Pitts CJ, Nippoldt TB, Prokop LJ, Murad MH. Sex steroids and cardiovascular outcomes in transgender individuals: a systematic review and meta-analysis. J Clin Endocrinol Metab. 2017;102(11):3914–23.

22. Van Caenegem E, Wierckx K, Taes Y, et al. Body composition, bone turnover, and bone mass in trans men during testosterone treatment: 1-year follow-up data from a prospective case controlled study (ENIGI). Eur J Endocrinol. 2015;172(2):163–71.

23. Van Kesteren P, Lips P, Gooren LJG, et al. Long-term follow-up of bone mineral density and bone metabolism in transsexuals treated with cross-sex hormones. Clin Endocrinol (Oxf). 1998;48(3):347–54.

24. Dhejne C, Lichtenstein P, Boman M, Johansson AL, Langstrom N, Landen M. Long-term follow-up of transsexual persons undergoing sex reassignment surgery: cohort study in Sweden. PLoS One. 2011;6:e16885.

25. Wierckx K, Elaut E, Declercq E, Heylens G, De Cuypere G, Taes Y, Kaufman JM, T'Sjoen G. Prevalence of cardiovascular disease and cancer during cross-sex hormone therapy in a large cohort of trans persons: a case-control study. Eur J Endocrinol. 2013;169:471–8.

26. Gooren LJ, van Trotsenburg MA, Giltay EJ, van Diest PJ. Breast cancer development in transsexual subjects receiving cross-sex hormone treatment. J Sex Med. 2013;10:3129–34.

27. Van Kesteren PJ, Asscheman H, Megens JA, Gooren LJ. Mortality and morbidity in transsexual subjects treated with cross-sex hormones. Clin Endocrinol (Oxf). 1997;47:337–42.

28. Asscheman H, Giltay EJ, Megens JA, de Ronde WP, van Trotsenburg MA, Gooren LJ. A long-term follow-up study of mortality in transsexuals receiving treatment with cross-sex hormones. Eur J Endocrinol. 2011;164:635–42.

29. Fisher AD, Senofonte G, Cocchetti C, Guercio G, Lingiardi V, Meriggiola MC, Mosconi M, Motta G, Ristori J, Speranza AM, Pierdominici M, Maggi M, Corona G, Lombardo F. SIGIS-SIAMS-SIE position statement of gender affirming hormonal treatment in transgender and non-binary people. J Endocrinol Invest. 2021;45(3):657–73. https://doi.org/10.1007/s40618-021-01694-2.

30. Kim JH, Yoo BW, Yang WJ. Hepatic failure induced by cyproterone acetate: a case report and literature review. Can Urol Assoc J. 2014;8(5–6):E458–61.

31. Millet N, Longworth J, Arcelus J. Prevalence of anxiety symptoms and disorders in the transgender population: a systematic review of the literature. Int J Transgend. 2016;18(1):27–38.

32. Defreyne J, Nota N, Pereira C, et al. Transient elevated serum prolactin in trans women is caused by cyproterone acetate treatment. LGBT Health. 2017;4(5):328–33.

33. Mancini I, Rotilio A, Coati I, et al. Presentation of a meningioma in a transwoman after nine years of cyproterone acetate and estradiol intake: case report and literature review. Gynecol Endocrinol. 2018;34(6):456–9.

34. Ter Wengel PV, Martin E, Gooren L, et al. Meningiomas in three male-to-female transgender subjects using oestrogens/progestogens and review of the literature. Andrologia. 2016;48:1130–7.

35. Kuijpers SME, Wiepjes CM, Conemans EB, Fisher AD, T'Sjoen G, den Heijer M. Toward a lowest effective dose of Cyproterone acetate in trans women: results from the ENIGI study. J Clin Endocrinol Metab. 2021;106(10):e3936–45.

36. Gava G, Mancini I, Alvisi S, et al. A comparison of 5-year administration of cyproterone acetate or leuprolide acetate in combination with estradiol in transwomen. Eur J Endocrinol. 2020;183(6):561–9.

37. Liang JJ, Jolly D, Chan KJ, Safer JD. Testosterone levels achieved by medically treated transgender women in a United States endocrinology clinic cohort. Endocr Pract. 2018;24:135–42.

38. Gulmez SE, Lassen AT, Aalykke C, Dall M, Andries A, Andersen BS, Hansen JM, Andersen M, Hallas J. Spironolactone use and the risk of upper gastrointestinal bleeding: a population-based case-control study. Br J Clin Pharmacol. 2008;66:294–9.

39. Giorgetti R, di Muzio M, Giorgetti A, Girolami D, Borgia L, Tagliabracci A. Flutamide-induced hepatotoxicity: ethical and scientific issues. Eur Rev Med Pharmacol Sci. 2017;21:69–77.

40. Klaver M, de Blok CJM, Wiepjes CM, et al. Changes in regional body fat, lean body mass and body shape in trans persons using cross-sex hormonal therapy: results from a multicenter prospective study. Eur J Endocrinol. 2018;178(2):163–71.

41. Meyer WJ 3rd, Webb A, Stuart CA, Finkelstein JW, Lawrence B, Walker PA. Physical and hormonal evaluation of transsexual patients: a longitudinal study. Arch Sex Behav. 1986;15:121–38.

42. Prior JC. Progesterone is important for transgender women's therapy—applying evidence for the benefits of progesterone in ciswomen. J Clin Endocrinol Metab. 2019;104(4):1181–6.

43. Jain J, Kwan D, Forcier M. Medroxyprogesterone acetate in gender-affirming therapy for transwomen: results from a retrospective study. J Clin Endocrinol Metab. 2019;104(11):5148–56.

44. Bultynck C, Pas C, Defreyne J, et al. Self-perception of voice in transgender persons during cross-sex hormone therapy. Laryngoscope. 2017;127(12):2796–804.

45. Getahun D, Nash R, Flanders WD, et al. Cross-sex hormones and acute cardiovascular events in transgender persons: a cohort study. Ann Intern Med. 2018;169(4):205–13.

46. Alzahrani T, Nguyen T, Ryan A, et al. Cardiovascular disease risk factors and myocardial infarction in the transgender population. Circ Cardiovasc Qual Outcomes. 2019;12(4):e005597.

47. Khan J, Schmidt RL, Spittal MJ, Goldstein Z, Smock KJ, Greene DN. Venous thrombotic risk in transgender women undergoing estrogen therapy: a systematic review and meta-analysis. Clin Chem. 2019;65(1):57–66.

48. Wiepjes CM, Vlot MC, Klaver M, et al. Bone mineral density increases in trans persons after 1 year of hormonal treatment: a multicenter prospective observational study. J Bone Miner Res. 2017;32:1252–60.

49. Singh-Ospina N, Maraka S, Rodriguez-Gutierrez R, et al. Effect of sex steroids on the bone health of transgender individuals: a systematic review and meta-analysis. J Clin Endocrinol Metab. 2017;102:3904–13.

50. Rothman MS, Iwamoto SJ. Bone health in the transgender population. Clin Rev Bone Miner Metab. 2019;17(2):77–85.

51. Nota NM, Wiepjes CM, de Blok CJM, et al. The occurrence of benign brain tumours in transgender individuals during cross-sex hormone treatment. Brain. 2017;141(7):2047–54.

52. Brown GR, Jones KT. Incidence of breast cancer in a cohort of 5,135 transgender veterans. Breast Cancer Res Treat. 2015;149:191–8.

53. Silverberg MJ, Nash R, Becerra-Culqui TA, Cromwell L, Getahun D, Hunkeler E, Lash TL, Millman A, Quinn VP, Robinson B, Roblin D, Slovis J, Tangpricha V, Goodman M. Cohort study of cancer risk among insured transgender people. Ann Epidemiol. 2017;27:499–501.

54. Martin KA, Anderson RR, Chang RJ, et al. Evaluation and treatment of hirsutism in premenopausal women: an endocrine society clinical practice guideline. J Clin Endocrinol Metab. 2018;103:1233–57.

55. Unluhizarci K, Ozel D, Tanriverdi F, et al. A comparison between finasteride, flutamide, and finasteride plus flutamide combination in the treatment of hirsutism. J Endocrinol Invest. 2009;32:37–40.

56. Ingprasert S, Tanglertsampan C, Tangphianphan N. Efficacy and safety of minoxidil 3% lotion for beard enhancement: a randomized, double-masked, placebo-controlled study. J Dermatol. 2016;43:968–9.

57. Dickersin K, Munro MG, Clark M. Hysterectomy compared with endometrial ablation for dysfunctional uterine bleeding: a randomized controlled trial. Obstet Gynecol. 2007;110:1279–89.

58. Rachner TD, Coleman R, Hadji P, et al. Bone health during endocrine therapy for cancer. Lancet Diabetes Endocrinol. 2018;6:901–10.

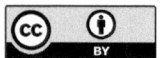

The Transgender: Legal Path to Surgery

Domenico Costantino

22.1 The Right to Gender Identity

The phenomenon of transsexualism has aroused a growing interest not only from a medical and sociological point of view, but also from a legal point of view, with particular regard to the human rights of trans and intersex people, also in order to avoid any discrimination based on gender identity and sexual characteristics.

Since medical science has made possible a realignment between the body and psyche of a person "affected" by gender dysphoria, there has been a need to legally regulate this process of "harmonization," providing for its conditions, limits, and effects.

Law no. 164 of 14 April 1982 filled the regulatory gaps in the matter, recognizing a real right to gender identity, as a specific declination, according to the now more consolidated private and public doctrine, of the rights to sexual identity and health, protected by Articles 2 and 32 of the Constitution.

It is not easy to define "gender identity," as the field of sex and gender has given rise to a proliferation of terms, whose meaning varies not only over time, but also within the same discipline and between one discipline and another.

Therefore, before proceeding to analyze the right to gender identity, it is appropriate to frame and define transsexualism, in order to fully grasp what have been the problems at the center of jurisprudential and doctrinal debates.

The WHO's International Statistical Classification of Diseases and Related Health Problems (ICD-10)[1] had included transsexualism within Gender Identity Disorders as *"the desire to live and be accepted as a member of the opposite sex, usually accompanied by a feeling of discomfort or inappropriateness related to one's anatomical sex and a desire to resort to hormonal treatments and surgeries to adapt your body as appropriate as possible to your favorite sex,"* and states that *"the transsexual identity must have been present persistently for at least two years."*

---

[1] Available on https://www.who.int/classifications/icd/ICD10Volume2_en_2010.pdf; for further analysis see F. Fontanarossa, *Il diritto all'identità di genere nel procedimento di rettificazione dell'attribuzione di sesso: cenni comparatistici*, in *Europa e Diritto Privato*, fasc. 2, 1 June 2018, pag. 709.

D. Costantino (✉)
Family Law at the Department of Law,
University of Bari, Bari, Italy
e-mail: domenico@studiolegalecostantino.it

© The Author(s) 2023
C. Bettocchi et al. (eds.), *Practical Clinical Andrology*,
https://doi.org/10.1007/978-3-031-11701-5_22

That definition, however, was reviewed in the context of ICD-11,[2] which, considering the evidence that trans-related and gender diverse identities are not conditions of mental ill health, and classifying them as such can cause enormous stigma, has replaced diagnostic categories like ICD-10's "transsexualism" and "gender identity disorder of children" with "gender incongruence of adolescence and adulthood" and "gender incongruence of childhood", respectively.

Similarly, the Diagnostic and Statistical Manual of Mental Disorders (DSM-5), following amendments aimed at *"reducing phenomena of social stigma,"* has also qualified transsexualism as gender dysphoria, understood as a *"general descriptive term"* that *"refers to affective/cognitive distress in relation to the assigned gender, but assumes a greater specificity only when it is used as a diagnostic category."* In the case of adults and adolescents, it must be possible to find for the purposes of diagnosis *"a marked inconsistency between the gender experienced/expressed by an individual and the assigned gender, lasting at least six months"*.[3]

With regard to the notion of gender, we read in the DSM-5 that *"the need to introduce the term* gender *arose from the observation that for individuals with contrasting or ambiguous sexual biological indicators (e.g.* intersex*) the role experienced by society and/or identification as male or female cannot be associated or predicted tout court by classical biological indicators and, moreover, some individuals develop an identity as male or female in contrast with their uniform set of traditional biological indicators"* and that therefore the term gender is used *"to indicate the public role lived (and generally recognized from the legal point of view) (...) but, contrary to some socio-constructionist theories, biological factors are considered a contribution, in interaction with social and psychological factors, to the development of gender"*.[4]

That said, the "right to gender identity" starts from the need to recognize, on the part of individuals, a right to self-determination that is considered, in the private and family field, absolute and insusceptible of conditions and limits to its exercise, in the sense that it pertains to that field of freedom that the legal system must protect from aggression, and that it itself cannot attack.

Already in 1985, the Constitutional Court, on the occasion of the judgment on the constitutional legitimacy of Article 1, paragraph 1, of Law no. 164 of 14 April 1982, had affirmed the need to recognize and respect gender identity, that is, the right of transsexual persons to live harmoniously their being in relation to others, also through the modification of personal data, as an expression of the right to personal identity, falling within the framework of the fundamental rights of the person, referred to Article 2 of the Constitution.[5] In fact, according to the Court, *"Law 164 of 1982 is therefore part of an evolving juridical civilization, ever more attentive to the values, freedom and dignity of the human person, who seeks and protects even in minority and anomalous situations. It is necessary, according to these incisive indications, that the interpretation of Law 164/82 takes into account the inclusion of the right to the recognition of gender identity in an evolving legal civilization as it is subject to changes in the scientific, cultural and ethical approach to issues inherent, in the present case, to questions of sex change and to the phenomenon of transsexualism and more generally to choices relating to gender and the sphere of sexual identity"*.[6]

It is important to understand if the concept of gender identity has been recalled by Italian jurisprudence, *primarily* the constitutional one, exclusively with a view to balancing the individual's interest in not undergoing health treatments (surgical or hormonal), extremely invasive and dangerous for health,[7] on the one hand, and the public

[2]The 11th edition of the International Statistical Classification of Diseases and Related Health Problems (ICD-11) is a document that provides standardized data and vocabulary to help diagnose and monitor health problems around the world.

[3]American Psychiatry Association, DSM-5, Italian edition, curated by M. Biondi, Milan, 2014, pp. 527–528.

[4]American Psychiatry Association, DSM-5, Italian edition, curated by M. Biondi, Milan, 2014, pp. 527–528.

[5]Constitutional Court, 23 May 1985, n. 161, https://www.giurcost.org/decisioni/1985/0161s-85.html.

[6]Constitutional Court, 23 May 1985, n. 161, https://www.giurcost.org/decisioni/1985/0161s-85.html.

[7]Article 13 Cost., which protects personal freedom, should also operate with respect to decisions concerning the body in its physical dimension, and therefore with respect to the desire to rectify one's own gender.

interest in the certainty of legal relationships, on the other.

With regard to the interests of the individual, the right to health and the right to personal identity are highlighted, in its component of sexual self-determination and gender identity.

The right to gender identity, often recurrent in Italian jurisprudential rulings without a precise identification of the "content", at international and supranational (community) level instead finds more references, although for the most part they are acts without normative value.[8]

It was with the judgment Christine Goodwin v United Kingdom of 11 July 2002[9] that the European Court of Human Rights began to look at the issue of transsexualism from the perspective of the protection of sexual identity, starting from the interpretation of Article 8 ECHR. The judges consider that this rule considers "personal freedom" as an important principle, which grants protection to the "personal sphere of each individual" and which includes "the right of each person to determine the particular characteristics of his identity as a human being." About the effects that the recognition of the possibility of rectification may have on civil society, the Court *"considers that it can reasonably be required of society that it accept certain inconveniences in order to allow persons to live in dignity and respect, in accordance with the sex-ual identity chosen by them at the price of great suffering."*

The scientific and cultural debate has profoundly changed the relationship between the right to gender identity and therefore to sexual self-determination,[10] and the right to health, two fundamental rights that, according to the originalist interpretation, had to be the object of choice by the individual in gender transition. The issue discussed concerned the need for surgery to adapt the primary sexual characteristics for transsexuals who want to obtain rectification.

On this point, the Supreme Court underlined how sexual identity lives on three elements: body *(soma)*, self-perception *(psyche)*, and social role *(polis)*[11], reflecting the concept of "health," which in the definition provided by the WHO develops on a trilateral form: *"a state of complete physical, mental and social well-being"*.[12]

We can therefore grasp a strong parallelism between the three elements of sexual identity and the three elements characterizing the concept of health, such that identity and health are not automatically in conflict, but are included, as the complete psycho-physical-social well-being can only be achieved if there is no suffering regarding the self-perception of one's gender, one's body, and one's social role. There is no doubt, therefore, that *"the interest in sexual identity, in so far as it involves the dignity of the human person, his fundamental right to the free development of the personality, the very right to health, understood, also and above all as mental health, is an essential interest of the person and, as such, destined to prevail over any other interest."*[13]

Therefore, in balancing the interests at stake, it is necessary to refer to a rigid principle of "proportionality," as underlined by the supranational

---

[8]For example, in 2009 the Commissioner for Human Rights published a thematic document of the European Council titled "Human rights and gender identity", which required member States to officially recognize the gender change of transgender persons, condemning the need for medical treatment to access sex and name change procedures, which were considered too long (T. HAMMABERGH, *I diritti umani e l'identità di genere*, http://transrespect. org/wp-content/uploads/2015/08/Hberg-Ital.pdf); always at the international level, worthy of mention are the "Princes of Yogyakarta", a set of principles laid down for the protection of the human rights of transgender persons, adopted at the International Congress held at the Gadjah Mada University, Yogyakarta, Indonesia in November 2006; these principles were considered in the document "Human rights and gender identity" whereas the European Council issued in July 2009 (The Yogyakarta Principles on the Application of International Human Rights Law in Relation to Sexual Orientation and Gender Identity, 2006, http://www.yogyakartaprinciples.org/principles-en/)

[9]ECHR, Christine Goodwin y. United Kingdom [GC], 11 July 2002, no. 28957, www.dejure.it

[10]ECHR, Van Kück c. Germany, 12 June 2003, No 35968/97, http://www.crisalide-azionetrans.it/CASE%20 OF%20VAN%20KUCK%20v.%20GERMANY.pdf.

[11]WHO, Ottawa Charter for Health Promotion, 1948.

[12]Court of Cassation, 20 July 2015, n. 15,138, www. dejure.it.

[13]On this point G. CARDACI, *Per un "giusto processo" di mutamento di sesso*, in *Diritto di Famiglia e delle Persone* (Il), fasc.4, 2015, p. 1459.

order,[14] also with specific regard to sexual reassignment.[15]

The European Court of Human Rights has clarified that gender identity is included in the non-exhaustive list of protected characteristics set out in Article 14 of the ECHR[16] and that States Parties to the European Convention on Human Rights have an obligation to legally recognize the preferred gender.[17]

22.2 The Procedure for Rectification of the Attribution of Sex

Before the entry into force of Law no. 164/1982, published in the Official Gazette no. 106 of 19 April 1982, it was not allowed to perform surgical interventions for the reassignment of sex other than that of birth. In fact, those who wished to access these treatments turned to foreign clinics to perform surgical interventions in the States that admitted this practice, and then returned to Italy and submitted an application for correction of gender data pursuant to articles 165 and 167 of Royal Decree 9 July 1939, n. 1238 (civil status system in force at the time) and art. 454 of the Italian Civil Code.

These provisions, however, were limited to cases of modification of material errors committed at the time of the birth certificate, as in the rare but still possible cases of ambiguity of the

external genitalia or of late natural development of the subject towards the opposite sex to that initially ascertained or even of the simultaneous presence in the same individual of the sexual characteristics of both sexes.

The Constitutional Court itself had been referred to the question of the legality of those provisions precisely because the living law did not consider them applicable to cases of voluntary change in the sexual characteristics of the individual, but the question had been rejected.[18]

---

[18]Constitutional Court, 26 July 1979 n. 98, www.giurcost. org: *"The question of constitutional legitimacy had been raised by the Court of Livorno, where the applicant had submitted an application for rectification of the birth certificate with attribution of the female sex, alleging that, although he was born with male sexual characteristics, he had always identified himself in the female gender, had undergone reconstructive demolition surgery in Casablanca and was socially integrated and accepted in his context of reference as a person of sex female. With a compliant result, the following year was also pronounced by the Court of Cassation, first section, judgment of 3/4/1980 n. 2161: The assessment and documentation of the sex of the person, carried out at the time of birth certificate, pursuant to Articles 67, 70 and 71 of the civil status system (R.D. 9 July 1939 n 1238), with exclusive regard to the external genital organs, are subject to subsequent rectification, pursuant to Articles. 165 et seq. of the aforementioned system, manifestly not in contrast with Articles 2 and 24 of the Constitution (judgment of the Constitutional Court no. 98 of 1979), only as a result of changes in sexual characteristics, for a natural and objective evolution of a situation originally not well defined or only apparently defined, although linked to the psychic orientation of the person himself, or assisted by surgical interventions aimed at highlighting already existing organs, and not also, therefore, for the mere finding of a psychosexuality contrasting with the clear characteristics of the sexual organs, or for manipulative or demolition surgical interventions, aimed at changing the natural anatomical reality"* (in terms 1236/75, mass. No. 374696; v 3948/74, mass No 372518). On the European scene, a very similar case was brought to the attention of the Commission of the European Court of Human Rights (decision of 9 May 1978, in the case of Daniel Oosterwijck v Belgian government). She was a Belgian citizen who, after undergoing hormone therapy and various surgeries, had assumed an outward appearance and male gender identity and had requested the correction of the personal data, denied at first instance and on appeal. The European Court of Human Rights (decision of 6 November 1980 in case no. 7654/76) which rejected it for failure to exhaust internal remedies).

---

[14]ECHR, Godelli c. Italy, 25 September 2012, n. 33,783/0, https://www.camera.it/application/xmanager/projects/leg17/attachments/sentenza/testo_ingleses/000/000/518/Godelli.pdf.

[15]Recommendation CM/Rec(2010) of the Committee of Ministers of the Council of Europe to the Member States on measures to combat discrimination based on sexual orientation or gender identity, 31 March 2010, sec. IV, § 20: *"The prerequisites, including physical modifications, necessary for the legal recognition of the once the sex change has taken place, they should be regularly reviewed in order to eliminate those that prove to be abusive"*.

[16]ECHR, Identoba and Others c. Georgia, 12 May 2015, no. 73235/2012, https://www.questionegiustizia.it/articolo/cedu_pillole-di-maggio_08-09-2015.php.

[17]ECHR, Christine Goodwin y. United Kingdom, 11 July 2002, no. 28957, www.dejure.it.

In Italy, it was time to await the entry into force of Law No 164 of 14 April 1982 laying down rules on the rectification of the attribution of sex, for a complete regulation of the procedural aspects of the relevant procedure. However, there were many critical issues encountered.

Article 1 of Law 164/1982 provides that *"rectification shall be made by virtue of a judgment of the Court of First Instance which has the force of res judicata attributing to a person sex other than that set out in the birth certificate following changes in his sexual characteristics."*

In interpreting the norm, a first problem that has been placed is that relating to the identification of what are the modifications of the "sexual characteristics" that legitimize the rectification of sex. It was taken, then, as a reference the third paragraph of the article 31 d.lgs. 150/2011, according to which *"where it is necessary to adapt the sexual characteristics to be carried out by means of medical and surgical treatment, the Court of First Instance authorizes it by a judgment which has the rule of res judicata,"* although it does not provide a clear definition of "sexual character" nor of "sex." Thus, in the jurisprudential and doctrinal debate, two different orientations have emerged.

The first orientation, linked to the need, of public policy, to preserve a degree of certainty with respect to the boundaries between the two genders, as well as to the idea of a necessary sterility of the transsexual person who obtains the rectification of sex, affirms the need, for the purposes of sex rectification, for a modification of the "primary" sexual characteristics identified in the genital and reproductive organs.[19] Therefore, also in accordance with the conclusions of the Court of Justice no. 161/1985, it was considered indispensable, for the transsexual who wanted to obtain the rectification of sex, the convergence "between soma and psyche" obtained with surgery to adapt the primary sexual characteristics.

Another orientation, now endorsed by the rulings of the Constitutional Court and the Court of Cassation but a minority in the 90s, evaluates as sufficient the modification of the "secondary aesthetic-somatic and hormonal sexual characteristics," considering that a surgical intervention that modifies the genital apparatus becomes necessary only when it ensures *"to the transsexual subject a stable psychophysical balance, that is to say when the discrepancy between anatomical sex and psychosexuality cause in the person concerned a conflictual attitude of rejection of his sexual organs"*[20] or, according to other jurisprudence, *"only in the case in which it is necessary to ensure the transsexual subject a stable psychophysical balance".*[21] According to this guideline, however, for the purposes of rectification, it seems that hormonal treatment that adapts "the phenotype to mental sex" seems to remain necessary, thus achieving "psychophysical stability and well-being".[22]

In the face of these different orientations of the jurisprudence of merit, the Court of Cassation, with judgment of 20 July 2015, no. 15138, interpreted Law no. 164/1982, as amended by Legislative Decree 150/2011, following the second orientation, and therefore considering it possible to rectify sex even in the absence of a surgical treatment modifying the primary sexual characteristics, considering, moreover, that the same judgment of the Constitutional Court of 1985[23] had defined the law in question as the result of a *"juridical civi-*

---

[19] In this sense Court Massa, 11 January 1989, in *Arch. Civ.*, 1989, II, 737; Court Vicenza, 2 August 2000, in *Dir. Fam.*, 2001, I, 220; Court Salerno, 15 June 2010, n. 1387, www.iusexplorer.it; Court Vercelli, 12 December 2014, n. 154, in *Dir. Fam.*, 2015, I, 1379; Court Rimini, 12 December 2014, www.studiolegaleleggiditalia.it.

[20] Court Rome, 18 October 1997, in *Dir. Fam.*, 1998, I, 1033, with note of M.C. LA BARBERA, *Transessualismo e mancata volontaria, seppur giustificata, attuazione dell'intervento chirurgico*; Court Rome, 14 April 2011, n. 5896, in *Fam. and Dir.*, 2012, 183, with note of M. TRIMARCHI, *L'attribuzione di una nuova identità sessuale in mancanza di intervento chirurgico.*

[21] Court Rovereto, 3 May 2013, in *Nuova Giur. Civ.*, 2013, I, 1116, with note of F. BILOTTA, *Identità di genere e diritti fondamentali della persona.*

[22] Court Messina, 4 November 2014, in *Nuova Giur. Civ.*, 2015, I, 543, with note of A. VESTO, *Fostering the emergence of sexual identity to protect human dignity in its uniqueness.*

[23] Constitutional Court, 5 February 1985, n. 161, http://www.giurcost.org/decisioni/1985/0161s-85.html.

lization in continuous evolution increasingly attentive to the values of freedom and dignity of the human person, which seeks and protects even in minority and anomalous situations" and as such cannot be subjected to a static reading, historically crystallized.[24] Ultimately, the relevance of the notion of "gender identity" emerges. According to the address expressed by the Supreme Court, the desire to realize *"a coincidence between soma and psyche"* is *"the result of an elaboration (...) of one's gender identity, realized with the support of necessary medical and psychological treatments"* and the path of *"adaptation"* is a *"process of self-determination"*. The construction of the "new gender identity" is conceived as the point of arrival of an individual process but, in any case, remains connected to a physical transformation that adapts the body to the "destination sex" according to objectively appreciated criteria. In fact, we read in the ruling that it remains *"unavoidable a rigorous assessment of the definitiveness of the choice based on the criteria deducible from the current landings and shared by medical and psychological science"*, and it becomes necessary *"a subjective path of recognition of this primary profile of personal identity neither short nor devoid of interventions amending the original somatic and hormonal characteristics."* The Court of Cassation seems to affirm the need for an intervention that modifies the body of the trans person; with regard to the adequacy of the amendments, the Judges of Legitimacy attach great importance to judicial control, which must consist in *"a rigorous assessment of the completion of this path,"* precisely in the face of the need, as anticipated, for a balance between the right to self-determine one's identity and the public interest in clarity in the identification of sexual genders and legal relationships.

The Constitutional Court, prompted by an order for the remission of the substantive juris-prudence aimed at declaring the unconstitutionality of Article 1, paragraph 1, of Law 14 April 1982 no. 164,[25] with judgment of 5 November 2015, no. 221, followed the interpretation of the Court of Cassation, and therefore excluded the need for surgical intervention for the purpose of rectification, as *"corollary of an approach that—in coherence with supreme constitutional values—it refers to the individual the choice of the methods through which to realize, with the assistance of the doctor and other specialists, his own transition path, which must in any case concern the psychological, behavioral and physical aspects that contribute to composing the gender identity."* The profound merit of this judgment is to understand that the right to identity and the right to health are never in opposition if the protection of the self-determination of the subject is put at the center and the protection of public interests is limited only to temperaments punctually enunciated, ensuring that the soma-psyche reunification is desirable only if it corresponds to the personal needs of the subject, but never as an exclusive safeguard of public interests (which are well protected through the irreversibility of the choice and the modification of secondary sexual characteristics). In this way, the doors of a complete transition are opened even to subjects who have not considered it appropriate to modify their primary characters, making the legal boundaries between transsexuals and transgenders fluid from now on.[26]

This approach was recently reconfirmed in two judgments concerning the constitutionality of Article 1 of Law no. 164/1982. In the proceedings in question, the Consulta had the opportunity to return to the subject of transsexualism, confirming the centrality, in the context of the sex change process, of the judicial verification phase and excluding, at the same time, that the pure and simple will be expressed by the subject who intends to change sex is sufficient to "overcome" the essential evaluation step

---

[24]On the need for an evolutionary interpretation when it comes to the rights of the person cf. in accordance with ECHR, Stafford v. United Kingdom [GC], 28 May 2002, no 46295/99, 2002, § 68; ECHR, Y.Y.c. Turkey, 10 March 2015, no. 14793/08, § 103.

[25]Court Trento, ord. 20 August 2014, no. 228, www. dejure.it.

[26]Constitutional Court, 5 November 2015, no. 221, www. dejure.it.

regarding the need for surgical intervention, the latter of exclusive judicial jurisdiction.[27]

Constitutional jurisprudence has therefore shown an "openness" towards the recognition of gender identity, with the consequent positions taken to simplify the individual's access to the sex change process.

In any case, it will be essential to appeal to the ordinary civil Court, and still following the ritual forms of the ordinary judgment of cognition, if the interested party intends to obtain the rectification of the civil status documents in the part relating to the indication of sex and forename, with an action, called, in fact, "rectification of sex attribution."

The Italian jurisprudence, first of all the constitutional one, intervened in the matter of rectification of the attribution of sex, has repeatedly reiterated that the aspiration of the individual to the correspondence of the sex resulting in the population registers with that subjectively perceived and lived constitutes an expression of the right to gender identity.

If it is true that public awareness is improving, it is equally true that people suffering from gender dysphoria continue to suffer from strong pressures social and the need for greater legal protection, through the adoption of necessary measures to guarantee the equality and non-discrimination based on gender identity, gender expression, and sexual characteristics, can no longer be overlooked.

---

[27]Constitutional Court, 13 July 2017, no. 185 and Constitutional Court, 13 July 2017, no. 180, www.dejure. it. The Constitutional Court no. 180/2017 clearly states that: "*in the light of the principles affirmed in Judgment no. 221 of 2015, it must be reiterated that the constitutionally adequate interpretation of the Law no. 164 of 1982 allows you to exclude the requirement of normoconformation surgery. And yet this does not exclude at all, but rather supports, the need for a rigorous assessment not only of the seriousness and univocality of the intent, but also of the objective transition of gender identity, which emerged in the path followed by the person concerned; path that corroborates and reinforces the intent thus manifested. Therefore, in line with the principles referred to in the judgment, it must be excluded that the only voluntarist element can be of priority or exclusive importance for the purpose of ascertaining the transition. In line with what was stated in the judgment referred to, it should once again be noted that the individual's aspiration to the correspondence of the sex attributed to him in the population registers, at the time of birth, with that subjectively perceived and lived undoubtedly constitutes an expression of the right to recognition of gender identity. In the system of Law No 164 of 1982, this is achieved through a judicial procedure that guarantees, at the same time, both the right of the individual and those requirements of certainty of legal relationships, on which the survey of the population registers is based. The reasonable balance between the multiple instances of guarantee was, in fact, identified by entrusting to the judge, in the assessment of the irrepressible peculiarities of each individual, the task of ascertaining the nature and extent of the changes in sexual characteristics, which contribute to determining personal and gender identity*".

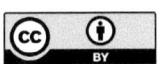

MtF Sex Reassignment Surgery: Trombetta Technique

Carlo Trombetta

23.1 Introduction

The challenging male-to-female sexual reassignment surgery requires good surgical technique and well-trained surgeons. My technique has been developed after 30 years of experience and after more than 400 patients treated. Herein are reported all preoperative, intraoperative, and postoperative steps [1–5].

23.2 Preoperative Procedures

At the time of their first surgical visit, patients are prompted to get perineal laser hair removal to avoid hair growth inside the neovagina [6]. One month before surgery, patients must stop oestrogen therapy due to well-known potential cardiovascular risks, whereas the antiandrogenic therapy can be continued [7, 8].

23.3 Position of the Surgeons

Since our initial experiences when we perform male-to-female surgery, we do so with two surgical teams who work in the same time and sometimes all together: with the patient in lithotomic position, two surgeons are placed on either side of the patient, and other two surgeons are positioned at the perineal side (Fig. 23.1) [9, 10].

All pictures are original, property of Dr. Migliozzi F.

C. Trombetta (✉)
Urology Clinic, Trieste, Italy
e-mail: trombcar@units.it

© The Author(s) 2023
C. Bettocchi et al. (eds.), *Practical Clinical Andrology*,
https://doi.org/10.1007/978-3-031-11701-5_23

Fig. 23.1 Surgical theatre setting: double equipe

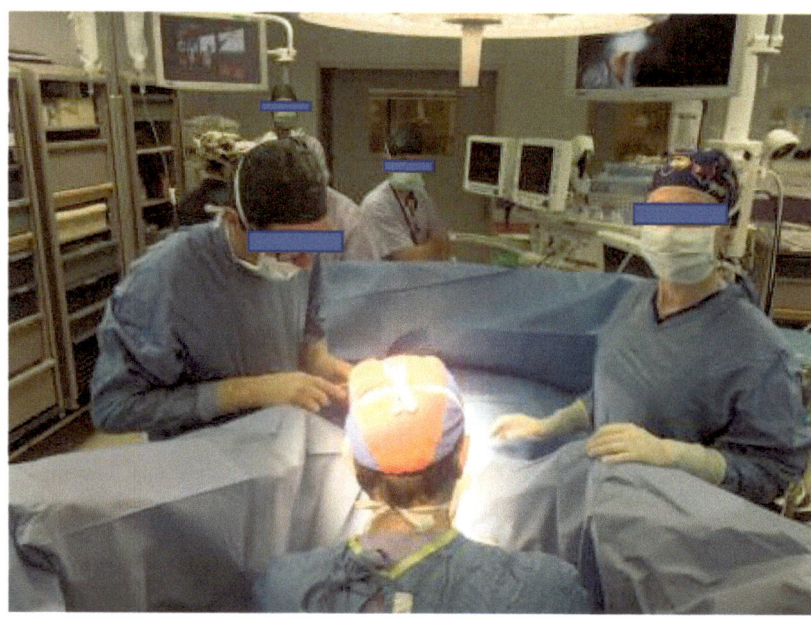

23.4 Markings

Before the beginning of the operation, we start by marking on the pubic-umbilical line, which is done for correctly locating all the structures. Another drawing is done at the scrotal level, *drop shaped* with the apex pointing towards the anus, which represents the scrotal flap. The correct distance between the anal verge and the apex of the drawing is 1–2 cm. The length of the scrotal flap varies between 12 and 15 cm. It is crucial that when measuring the length of the scrotal flap, there must not be tension at the apex of the skin flap after suturing. For the circumcision, another line is drawn in order to leave 1 cm of skin at the under the glans of penis.

The drawing is then continued for the length of the penis on ventral side (Figs. 23.2 and 23.3).

Fig. 23.2 Initial drawing of perineal and scrotal flap. Distance from anal rim should be 1,5-2cm

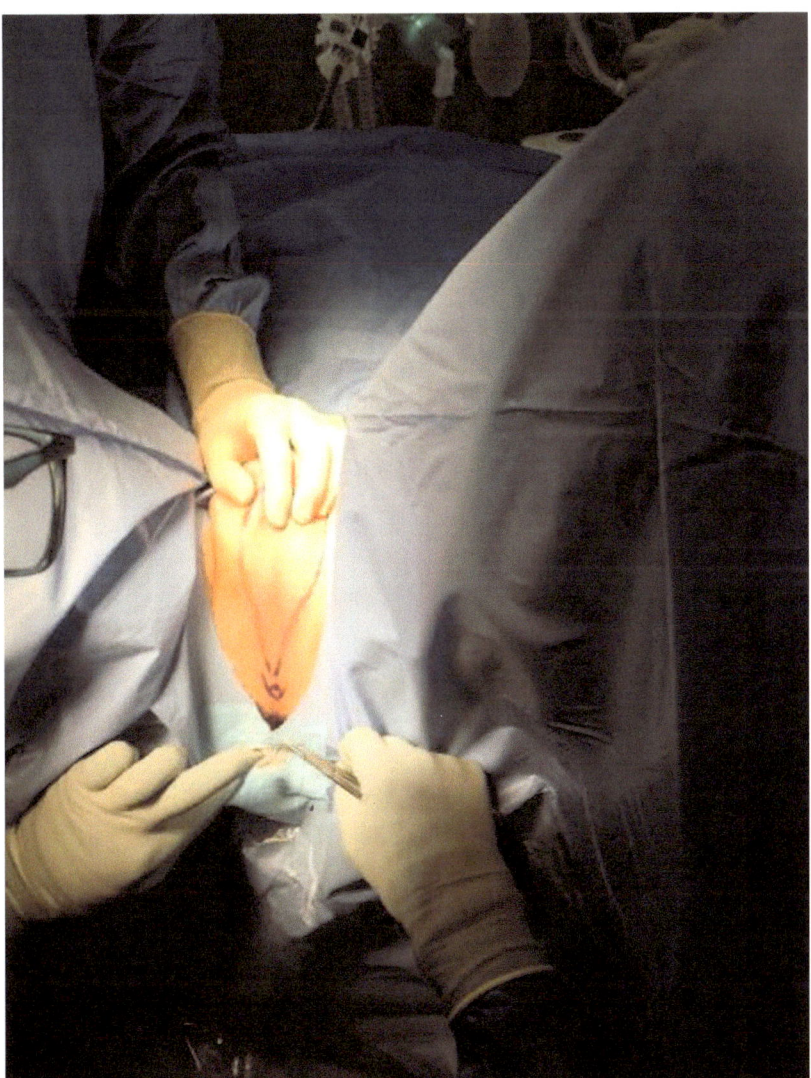

Fig. 23.3 Median line
supports symmetry

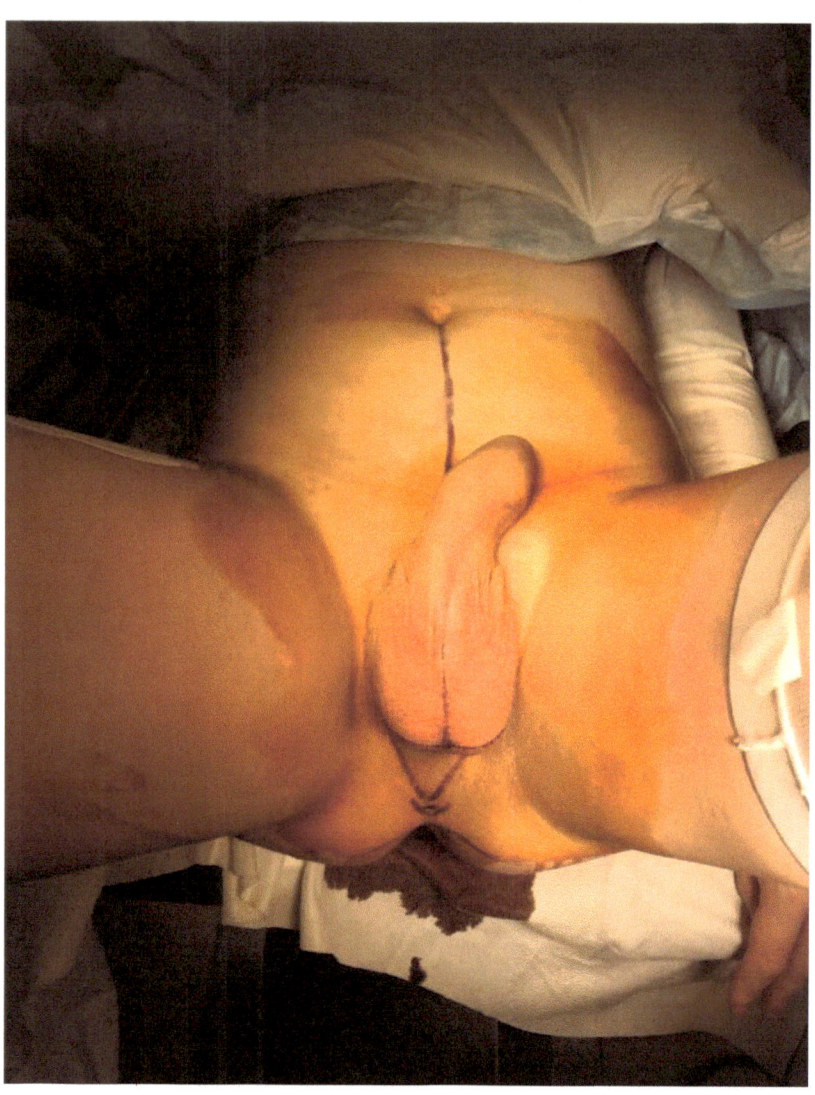

23.5   Devices

The sterile drape that we use for covering the
patient permits to access anal-rectal area (with
instruments or manually), without contaminating
the operatory field. This manoeuvre is determinant in avoiding rectal injuries during blunt dissection. It consists of a water-repellent drape
which can cover legs and has also a fluid collection pouch.

Power star bipolar scissors (Johnson &
Johnson Medical GmbH) are very useful especially to dissect urethra.

The surgical illuminator provides cool, shad-
owless, deep cavity lighting. Flexible or malleable, it may be attached to most retractors or
instruments, using two-side adhesives. Once
attached to the instrument, its thin profile takes
minimal space.

When connected to an ACMI cable and standard, 300 Watt xenon light source, it lights the
cavity as if a fluorescent light was switched on
inside the patient. The LightMat® brings bright,
cool light where it is needed—into the surgical
cavity, improving visualization, helping surgeons
save time and avoid complications.

The V-LocTM wound closure device (COVIDIEN) is a new technology that eliminates the need to tie knots, so you can close incisions up to 50% faster without compromising strength and security. The V-LocTM device offers secure, fast, and effective incision closure for our patients: in particular, the absence of knots into the neovagina avoids painful dilatation manoeuvres in the postoperative period. A small (9 cm × 4 cm → 100 mL of water) or medium (12 cm × 4 cm → 130 mL of water) vaginal stent is used. It is an inflatable cylinder made of biocompatible silicone with a clamp and a connector, specifically produced for trans women.

23.6 Perineal Surgery

The surgeon positioned at the perineal side, incises the skin along the line drawn on perineum.

The first step is the bilateral orchiectomy with dissection and suturing of both the spermatic cords at the level of the external inguinal rings. The peritesticular fat is preserved as support for the labia majora. The dissection is extended through the subcutaneous tissue until reaching the corpus spongiosum, which is then isolated from the corpora cavernosa. The urethra is severed at the pubic symphysis, and the terminal portion is spatulated and longitudinally split on the ventral midline so as to obtain a Y-shape. At this point, a urethral catheter is inserted (Fig. 23.4) [9].

The position of neo-urethral meatus is ensured by applying a knot at the apex of the incision. This becomes the reference point for positioning the neoclitoris, which will be surrounded by urethral mucosa (Figs. 23.5 and 23.6). The urethral bulb is carefully removed in order to prevent its bulging during sexual arousal and pain during penetration. Running absorbable suture of the two margins of the urethra decreases the risk of postoperative bleedings.

Surgery continues with the removal of the proximal corpora cavernosa, facilitated by the placement of a traction point at the apex of tissue, paying attention to the vascular bundle.

These manoeuvres allow the exposure of the perineal tendinous centre, which is then opened while monitoring the integrity of the rectal wall through the anal access provided by the sterile drop. At this point, the surgeon creates a neo-cavity in the rectoprostatic space which will accommodate the neovagina: we usually use a LigaSure device to sever the subcutaneous tissue, while sight is aided by an aspirator provided with a light source. The knowledge of the rectoprostatic space has been acquired, thanks to a large number of pelvic postoperative MRIs administered in order to have a precise anatomical visualization of all the structures involved in the surgery. These allow for measurements of inclination, length, and distance of the neovagina and its adjacent organs [11, 12].

When the catheter's balloon is palpated by the operator, it means that the neovagina is deep enough (Fig. 23.7). The fixation of the cul-de-sac in the rectoprostatic space is crucial to prevent the neovagina from prolapsing. Two Prolene double needle stitches are passed through the wall of the neo-cavity (anterior and posterior walls or the lateral walls), and both the ends of the sutures are passed through the penile-scrotal flap at the level of the cul-de-sac. In order to prevent prolapse, we also put another stitch through the scrotal flap and the subcutaneous tissue in proximity of the Denonvilliers' fascia incision.

Fig. 23.4 Positioning
of catheter before
proceeding with
spatulation of urethra

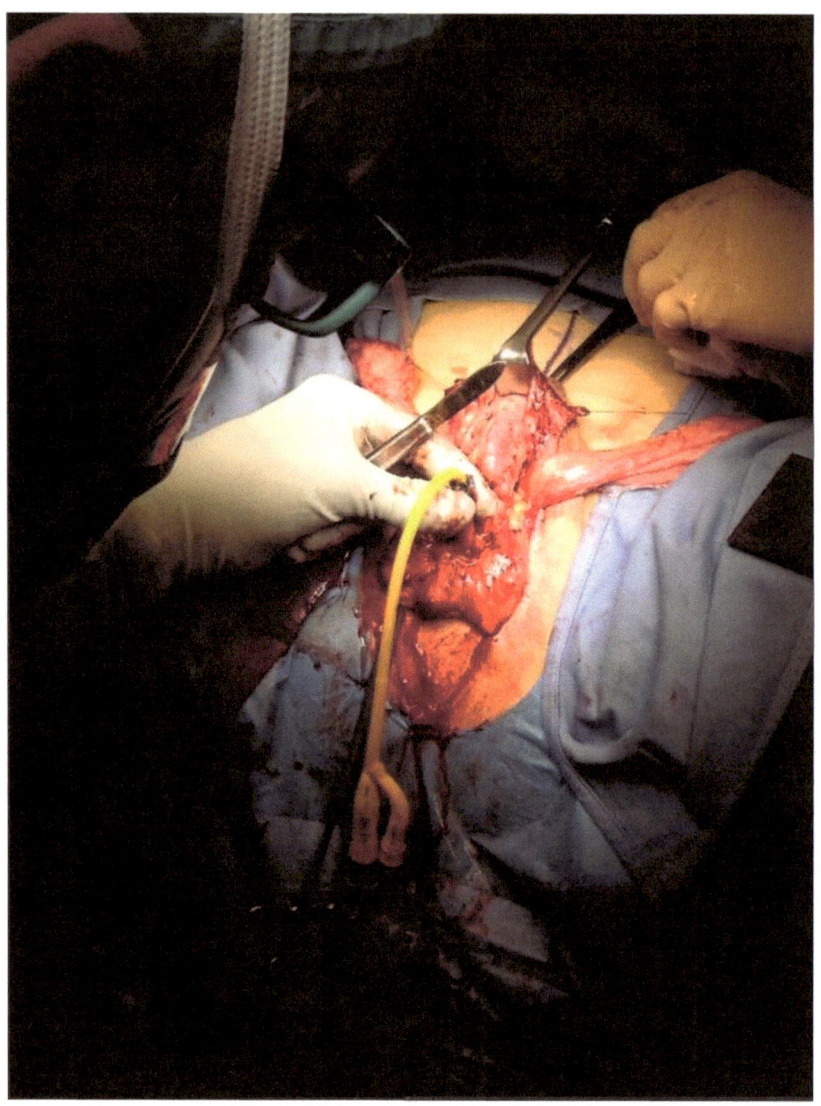

Fig. 23.5 Modeling of urethra to create neourethral-neoclitoral complex

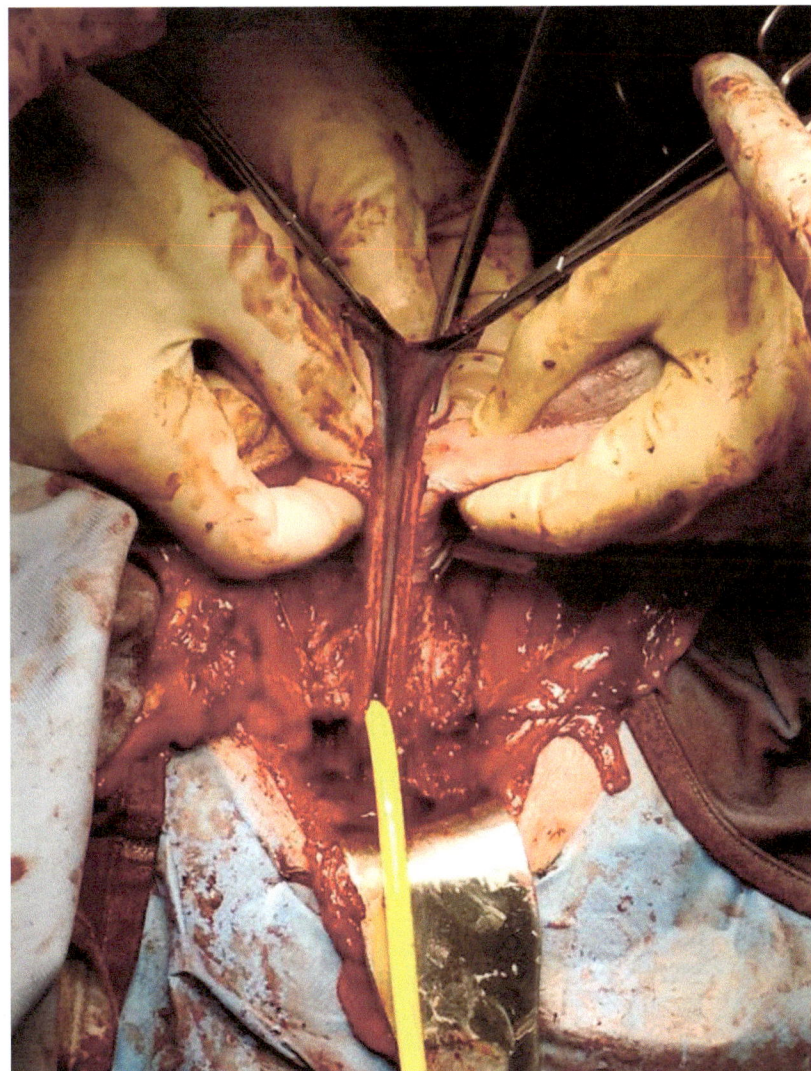

Fig. 23.6 Median incision of urethra to create the "Y" shape

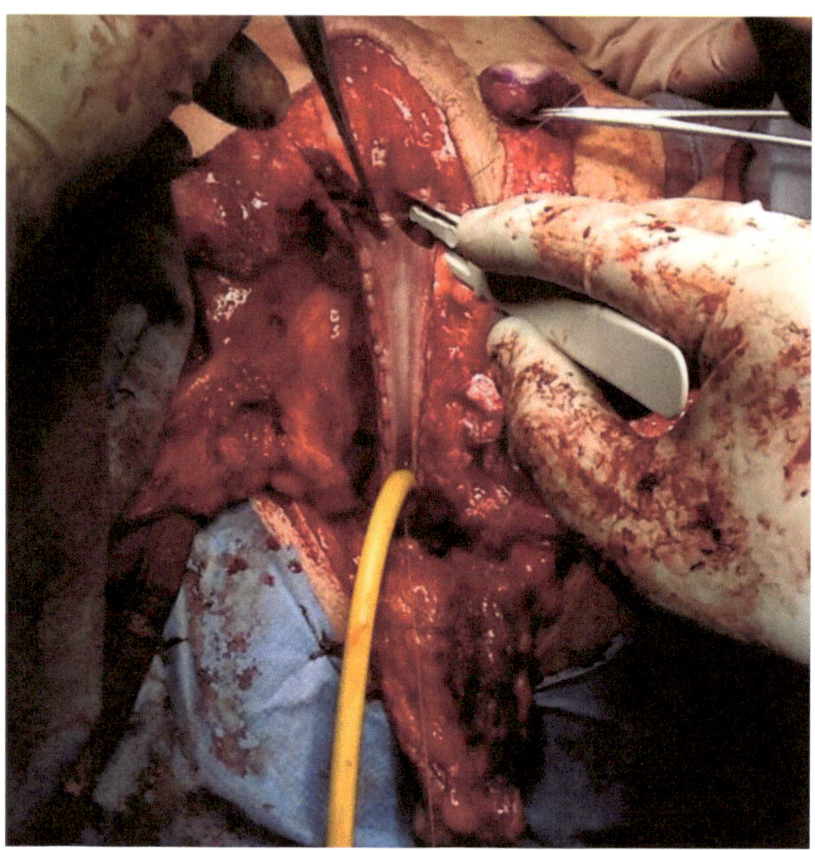

Fig. 23.7 Check of the depth of neovagina

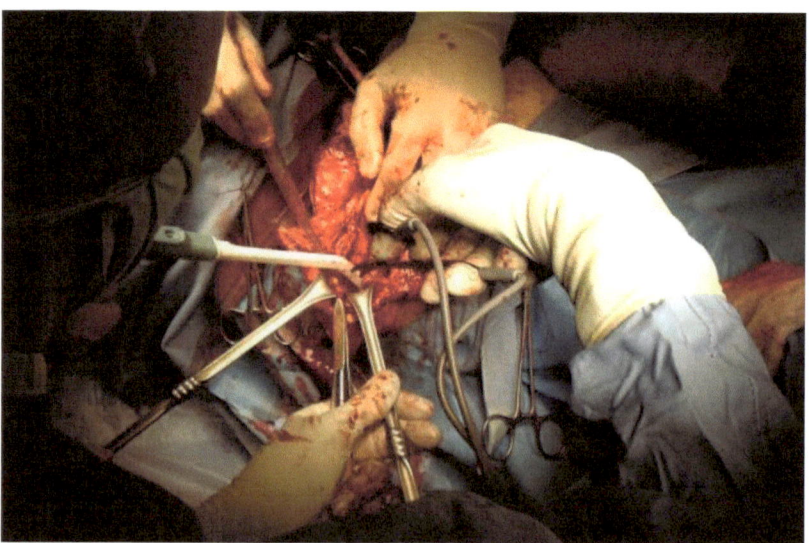

23.7 Penile Surgery

The two surgeons positioned on either side of the patient begin by performing incisions following the line previously drawn, and the penile flap is obtained by isolation from the corpora cavernosa, taking care to preserve vitality of the skin. Positioning a tourniquet around the corpora cavernosa and the urethra, it is possible to obtain a hydraulic erection using a butterfly needle and infusing saline solution into the corpora cavernosa. This is done to facilitate the blunt dissection of Buck's fascia from the tunica albuginea. Buck's fascia is identified and incised at a paraurethral level to avoid damage of the dorsal nerves of the penis. This procedure is done in order to permit the creation of a sensitive neoclitoris.

These structures need to be manipulated with delicate instruments, such as anatomical clamps, in order to reduce damage. For this same reason, bleeding is controlled with a bipolar coagulator.

After achieving the complete bilateral dissection of the neurovascular bundle, we insert two open tourniquets up to favourite glandulectomy. At the base of the penis, the dissection of the bundle is continued by positioning a Satinsky clamp at the level of the corpora cavernosa up to inhibit blood refilling so as to avoid wasting of blood. Removal of all corpora cavernosa avoids an eventual residual erection that can cause dyspareunia.

The glans is reduced and remodelled preserving a good amount of spongiosum tissue to create a well-vascularized neoclitoris: the dimensions of the resulting button are greater than that of the female clitoris. This is done so as to oppose eventual excessive hypotrophy of the tissues.

The bundle is folded on itself and fixed with a stitch: in this way, we create the mons pubis to better simulate the female form, and we also prevent the torsion of the flap avoiding neoclitoral ischemia. The neoclitoris is now joined to the urethral plate at the forking previously created. The suture is done in two layers, at the level of spongiosum tissue and the other at the level of urethral mucosa and neoclitoris epithelium. It is interesting to underline that the two layers have the same histological characteristics (Figs. 23.8 and 23.9) [13].

Creation of the urethra-clitoris complex is an innovative technique and presents two main advantages:

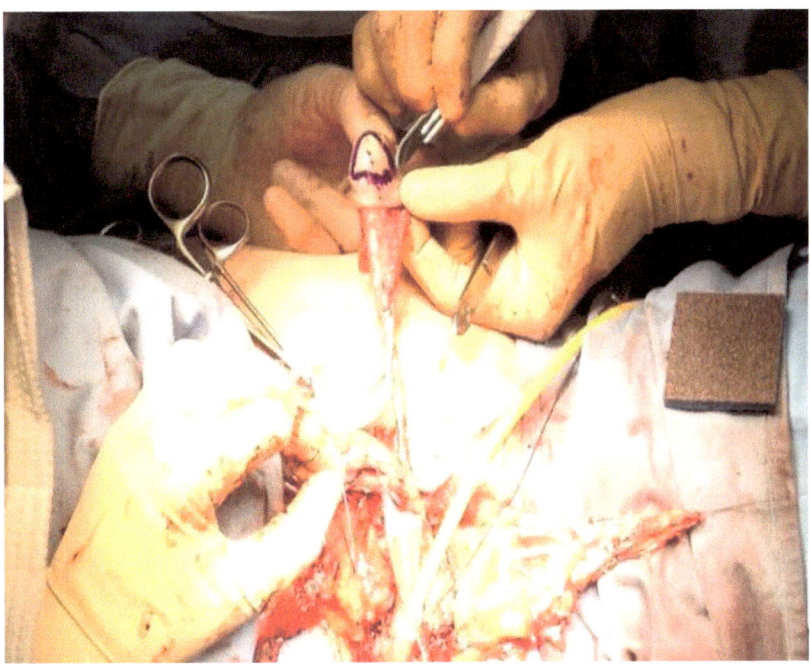

Fig. 23.8 Creation of neoclitoris from glans

Fig. 23.9 Arrangement of neoclitoris between the urethral flaps

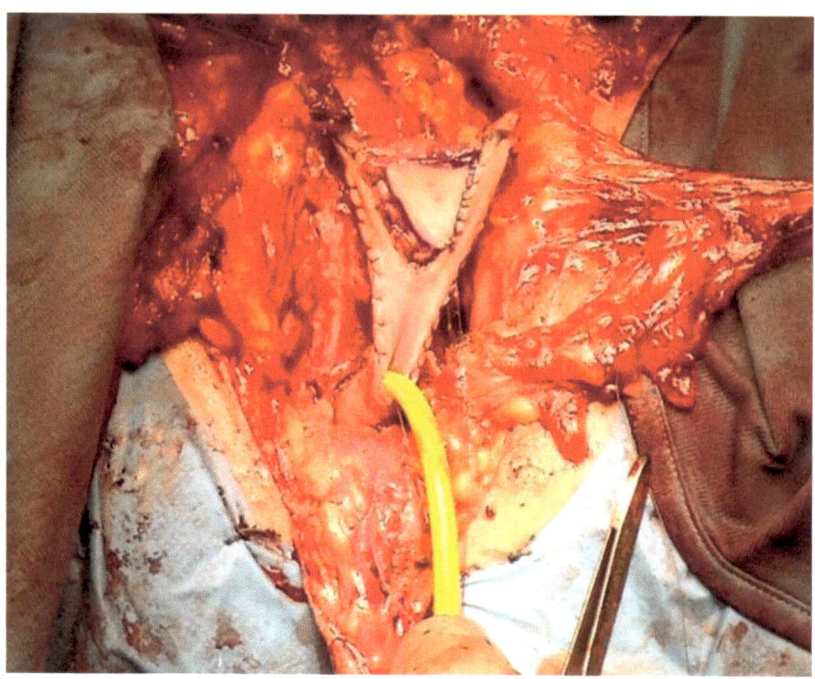

- It allows for the neoclitoris to be in a mucosal environment.
- The two-layer suture permits a reciprocal vascular support, useful in case of urethral or clitoral ischemia.

23.8 Tubularization of Penile-Scrotal Flap

At this point, the peritesticular fat is fixed at the perineal level. Scrotal and penile skin is sutured, using Vicryl 3/0, only bilaterally leaving an opening at the apex. We do this because no patient ever has enough skin to fully cover the entire length of the neocavity, and if we completely closed the neovaginal tube, there would be a possible loss of depth. Another option is to lengthen the penile-scrotal flap using redundant scrotal skin as a graft [14].

The two Prolene stitches we had put at prostatic and rectal level are now passed through the penile and scrotal flap. A frank demarcation between the labia minora and labia majora is obtained by placing four stitches between the outside of the penile-scrotal cylinder and the crura. Residual skin is excised. A longitudinal midline incision on the penile flap is performed in order to allow the exteriorization of the urethra-clitoris complex, catheter, and urethral meatus.

In order to avoid hypersensitivity of the neoclitoris, a cap is created from the residual preputial skin (Fig. 23.10). Now, the penile-scrotal cylinder of skin is introduced into the neo-cavity, now forming the neovagina, and the two Prolene stitches are safely knotted to hold it in place and avoid any eventual prolapse (Fig. 23.11) [15]. We have to remember the presence of ureters when we pass the two stitches into the deep part of the neocavity [16].

The surgical incision at the end of the procedure appears as a wide "U" and is closed with a V-loc running suture.

As the final step, a lubricated adjustable vaginal stent is inserted into the neovagina, making sure that it reaches the vault. The stent consists of a sealed silicone shell filled with polyurethane foam, fully adjustable by inflation (Fig. 23.12).

During insertion, the stent is deflated, only to be inflated once the position is satisfactory. After

Fig. 23.10 Labia majora and labia minora creation after fixation of neovagina

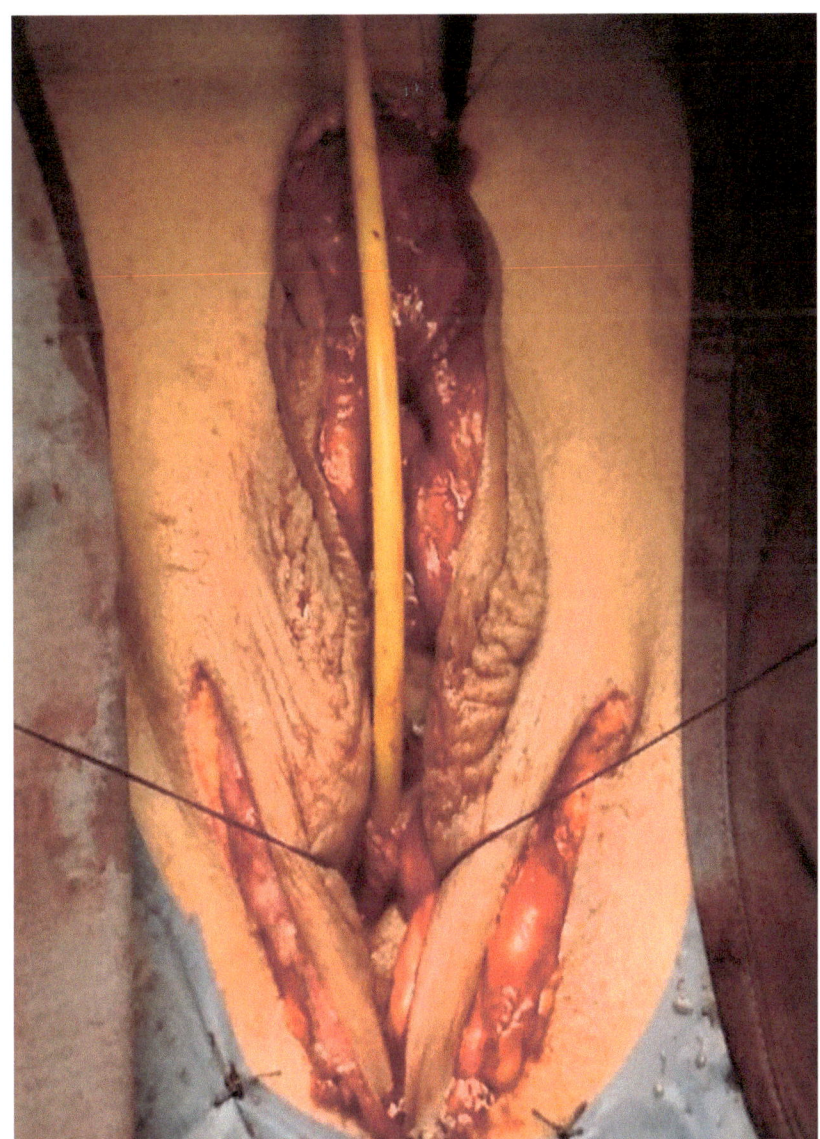

inflation, in order to avoid slipping due to the smooth surfaces of the stent, a cotton ball is always inserted in the vaginal introitus [17]. The usefulness of this vaginal stent is double: first, it prevents the vaginal walls from collapsing, and second, it is designed to permit the drainage of all secretions. A compressive packing is always done, in a crisscross fashion, using a wide adhesive gauze. A good compression avoids postoperative bleeding and swelling and helps maintain the stent in place.

Fig. 23.11 Modeling of penile flap to create labia minora

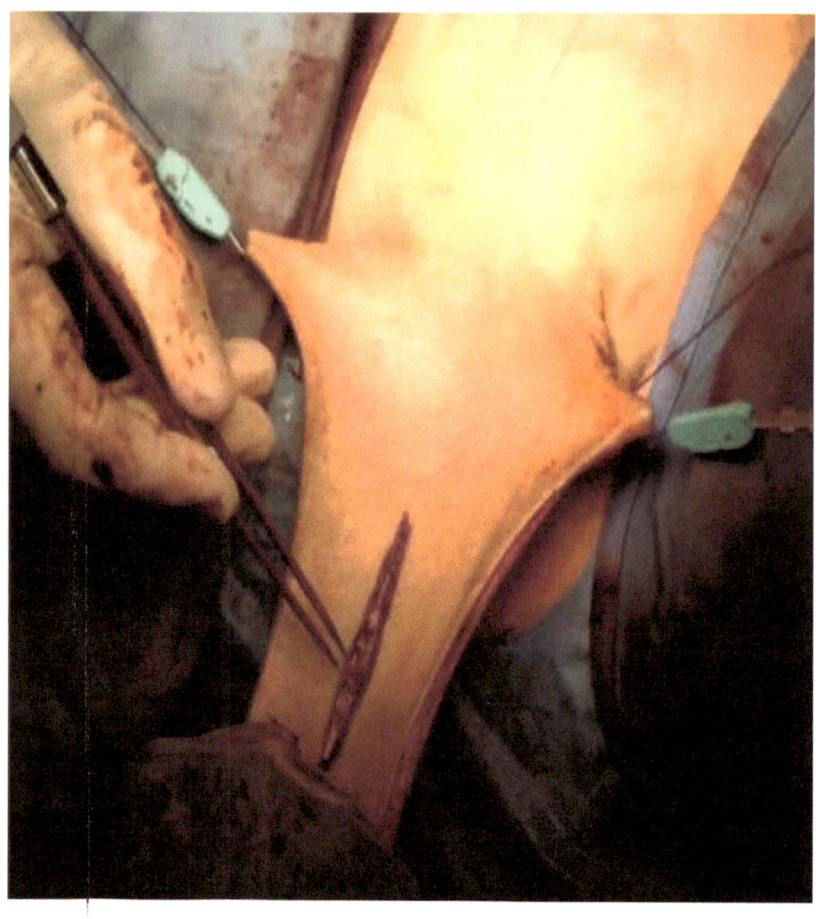

Fig. 23.12 Final result. Urethral catheter and neovaginal inflating dilator in place

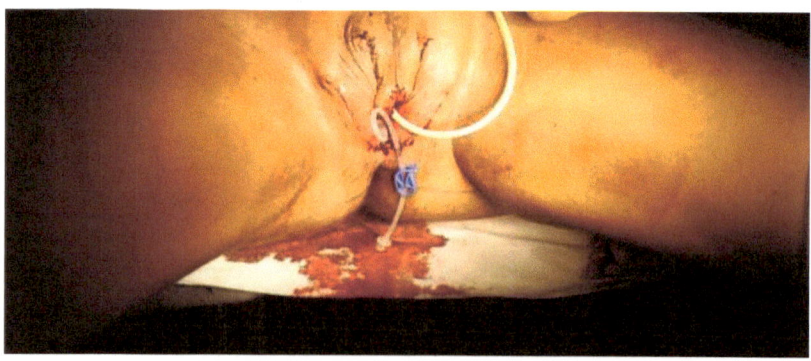

23.9   Postoperative Care

After surgery, the patient must stay in a supine position, for 2 days. During this period, it is crucial to conduct thrombo-embolic prophylaxis (heparin, antiembolic stockings, and mobilization of the feet and legs). Usually, the first day the patient is restricted to a liquid diet, and during the second day, she can begin a solid diet.

From the second day, washing of the neovagina is done by introducing a small amount of Iodine-saline solution through the stent.

On the third day, the stent is deflated and removed for the first time and disinfected with diluted sodium hypochlorite. Anti-swelling or heparin-based gels are applied on eventual haematomas.

After 4 days, the urethral catheter is removed, and the patient experiences urination for the first time. Now dilatations with rigid vaginal stents begin, and the patient is taught the correct manoeuvres for insertion and care. We usually adopt Amielle Comfort (Owen Mumford) vaginal dilators which have been designed for women experiencing vaginal discomfort and penetration problems from vaginism, dyspareunia, and gynaecological surgery.

The recommended position to insert into neovagina the lubricated dilators is to lie flat on the back with the knees bent and legs slightly apart. Alternatively, the patient can stand with one leg raised on a chair. Dilators can be washed with water and soap, and dried thoroughly ensuring all traces of soap have been removed before their insertion into the neovagina.

Psychosexual therapists teach how to do the following [18]:

- To control breathing.
- To relax the legs as much as possible.
- To gently ease the lubricated dilator in an upward and backward direction as deeply as is.comfortable.
- To leave the dilator in position for up to 5 min.

When a patient feels comfortable with using the smallest dilator, gradually move to the next size and so on. Moreover, during the first postoperative days, we suggest to use during the night the adjustable vaginal stent which allows a continuous dilation of the neovagina during the night hours.

In the first postoperative period, we suggest to repeat this procedure four to five times a day in a place that is comfortable and ensures her privacy. When no complication occurs, the patient can be discharged 5–6 days after surgery. When patients feel comfortable with inserting the larger dilators, no secretion is evident and no pain is referred, they may be ready to attempt penetrative sexual intercourse. In our experience, the timing of the first intercourse is 45–60 days after surgery.

23.10   Possible Side Effects and Complications

A frequent side effect is the development of haematoma of the labia of the neovagina which is particularly in presence of abundant skin and usually resolves spontaneously (Fig. 23.13).

If surgery lasts too much, BMI is high, and patient's legs are not well positioned during the

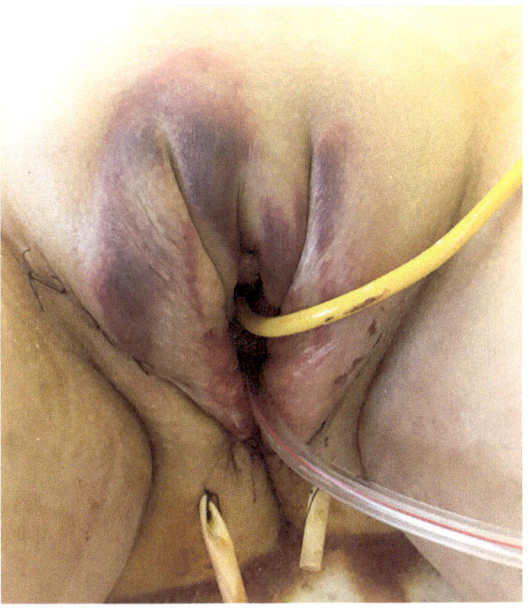

Fig. 23.13   Haematoma of the labia of the neovagina

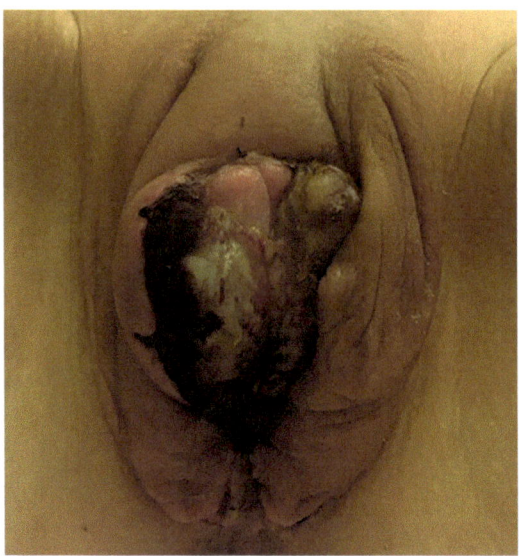

Fig. 23.14 Neourethral necrosis

operation, a leg muscular contusion may develop due to the prolonged lithotomy position during operation: this rare event requires fasciotomy of the peronaeorum communis fascia to be performed as soon as possible (4–6 h after the first intervention) [19].

In our experience, an important critical step is the preparation of the neurovascular dorsal penile bundles. Injury to the arteries or nerves may result in an impaired blood supply or reduced sensation of the clitoris.

Very rare is the eventuality of total necrosis of the neoclitoris (Fig. 23.14).

Another possible complication is neo-meatal stricture or substenosis. In our opinion, it is extremely important to widely spatulate the urethra and to suture the neo-meatus with separate stitches.

Other possible major complications include the following:

- Partial necrosis of the penile or scrotal flap.
- Bleeding from the urethra and the neoclitoris.
- Shortening or substenosis of the neovagina.

In case of partial or total prolapse of the neovagina, a second surgical treatment is necessary [20].

References

1. Belgrano E, Trombetta C, Repetto U, Pittaluga P, De Rose AF, Giuliani L. Pseudoermafroditismo maschile con persistenza delle strutture mulleriane: descrizione di un caso. Atti 58° Congr. S.I.U.-Roma, 25–28 settembre 1985. Acta Urol Ital. 1986;429–433.
2. Belgrano E, Repetto U, Trombetta C, Siracusano S, Bozzo W, Pittaluga P. Persistenza delle strutture mulleriane: descrizione di un caso. Rassegna Ital Chir Pediatr. 1986;28(2):120–3.
3. Trombetta C, Siracusano S, Gabriele M, Belgrano E. Hernia uteri inguinalis: un caso particolare di pseudoermafroditismo maschile. Atti 5° Corso Agg. Androl. di interesse chir.- Fiuggi Terme, 27–28 giugno 1988. Andrologia Chirurgica in Età Pediatrica. Acta Med Austriaca. 1989;1989:77–82.
4. Belgrano E, Trombetta C, Siracusano S, Desole S. Creazione di neovagina in due casi di pseudoermafroditismo. In: Atti del 63° Congr. S.I.U. (Società Italiana di Urologia)—Ancona, 9–12 Settembre 1990; 1990.
5. Trombetta C, Siracusano S, Desole S, Foddis G, Usai V, Belgrano E. Creazione di una neovagina in caso di pseudoermafroditismo: presentazione di due soluzioni tecniche. Atti 40° Convegno S.U.I.C.M.I.-Alghero, 23–25 Maggio 1991. Acta Urol Ital. 1992;(suppl. 5):231–234.
6. Belgrano E, Fabris B, Trombetta C. Il Transessualismo: identifi cazione di un percorso diag-nostico e terapeutico. Milano: E. Kurtis; 1999. p. 1–374.
7. Wierckx K, Elaut E, Declercq E, Heylens G, De Cuypere G, Taes Y, Kaufman JM, T'Sjoen G. Prevalence of cardiovascular disease and cancer during cross-sex hormone therapy in a large cohort of trans persons: a case–control study. Eur J Endocrinol. 2013;169(4):471–8. https://doi.org/10.1530/EJE-13-0493.
8. Van Kesteren PJ, Asscheman H, Megens JA, Gooren LJ. Mortality and morbidity in transsexual subjects treated with cross-sex hormones. Clin Endocrinol (Oxf). 1997;47:337–42.
9. Trombetta C, Buttazzi L, Liguori G, Belgrano E. Sex reassignment surgery: male-to-female transsexual operation. eUROtraining. In: International symposium on update on pelvic surgery. Genova, 5–7 Nov; 1998.
10. Trombetta C, Liguori G, Buttazzi L, Belgrano E. Surgical treatment of male-to-female transsexual patients: our experience. Urogynaecologia Int J. 1999;12(3):182–5.
11. Trombetta C, Liguori G, Bucci S, Salamè L, Garaffa G, Cova M, Belgrano E. Radiological evaluation of vaginal width and depth in male-to-female transsexuals by the use of magnetic resonance imaging. World J Urol. 2004;22(5):405–8.
12. Trombetta C, Liguori G, Buttazzi L, Bucci S, Belgrano E. Our technique for treatment of male-

to-female transsexual patients. Br J Urol Int. 2000;86:202.

13. Trombetta C, Liguori G, Benvenuto S, Petrovic M, Napoli R, Umari P, Rizzo M, Zordani A. Neourethroclitoroplasty according to Petrovic. Urologia. 2011;78(4):267–73.

14. Trombetta C, Liguori G, Buttazzi L, Bucci S, Belgrano E. Male-to-female sex reassignment surgery (SRS): urological technique. 100th AUA Orlando 25–30 Maggio 2002. J Urol. 2002;167(4 (suppl)):149. (abstract no 597).

15. Stanojevic DS, Djordjevic ML, Milosevic A, Sansalone S, Slavkovic Z, Ducic S, Vujovic S, Perovic SV, Belgrade Gender Dysphoria Team. Sacrospinous ligament fixation for neovaginal prolapse prevention in male-to-female surgery. Urology. 2007;70(4):767–71.

16. Rezwan N, Basit AA, Andrews H. Bilateral ureteric obstruction: an unusual complication of male to female gender reassignment surgery. BMJ Case Rep. 2014;BCR-204894. https://doi.org/10.1136/bcr-2014-204894.

17. Savoca G, Trombetta C, De Stefani S, Raber M, Siracusano S, Belgrano E. Creazione di neovagina: presentazione di due soluzioni tecniche. In: Acts 9° Congress. S.I.A.—Ancona, 14–16 Sept "Andrologia 1995". Bologna: Monduzzi Ed; 1995. p. 321–4.

18. Trombetta C, Liguori G, Bucci S, Belgrano E. Surgical therapy in transsexual patient: a multidisci-plinary approach. 18° congress of the European Association of Urology, Madrid, 12–15 March2003. Eur Urol. 2003;2(1):97.

19. Raza A, Byrne D, Townell N. Lower limb (well leg) compartment syndrome after urological pelvic surgery. J Urol. 2004;171:5–11.

20. Selvaggi G, Bellringer J. Gender reassignment surgery: an overview. Nat Rev Urol. 2011;8:274–82.

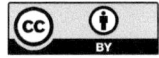

Gender Affirming Surgery: Assigned Female at Birth

Gennaro Selvaggi

24.1 Introduction

24.1.1 Definitions and Epidemiology

The acronym AFAB refers to those persons who have been 'Assigned Female at Birth'. AFAB persons who, later in life, do not identify as female, are said to present a condition named 'Gender Incongruence' (GI). They might identify as men, or as non-binary. Persons presenting the condition of GI might experience a Gender Dysphoria (GD), which is defined as the discomfort due to the mismatch between their anatomical characteristics and the gender in which they are self-identifying. Thus, patients with GD are requesting surgical procedure (s) in order to align one's body—mostly chest and genitals—to best match with one's identity. The final aim is to reduce one's dysphoria [1–4].

Epidemiological studies report a prevalence of AFAB persons with GD to range between 1:30,400 and 1:200,000 within the western population [5], and this number has increased in last decades [6]. Specifically, circa 75% of the AFAB persons with GI is identifying as male, while the rest 25% is identifying as non-binary [7, 8].

In this chapter, we present a summary of the surgical procedures as commonly requested by AFAB persons (trans men and non-binary) that are presenting GD.

24.1.2 Guidelines and Regulations

The *World Professional Association for Transgender Health* (WPATH) currently publishes a series of guidelines, which are named as Standards of Care (SOC), for patients presenting GI; in the SOC, eligibility criteria for surgery are presented. The last, and seventh version of the WPATH Standards of Care was published in 2011 [9, 10]. An updated version is expected anytime soon.

At the centre of the diagnostic process is the 'real life—experience'. During the 'real life—experience', patients are taking and living in the desired gender role full time for at least 1 year; during this period, patients are regularly followed by a gender counsellors and/or a mental health professional.

WPATH highlights that SOC are recommendations, and these should be adapted to patients' culture and to national laws. Finally, WPATH highlights that treatments paths should be individualized [9].

G. Selvaggi (✉)
Department of Plastic and Reconstructive Surgery, Institute of Clinical Sciences, The Sahlgrenska Academy, Sahlgrenska University Hospital, University of Gothenburg, Gothenburg, Sweden

© The Author(s) 2023
C. Bettocchi et al. (eds.), *Practical Clinical Andrology*,
https://doi.org/10.1007/978-3-031-11701-5_24

24.1.3 Aim of the Treatment

Based on a relatively wide scientific literature with *low level of evidence* (i.e., mostly consisting on small case series, few long-term follow-ups, and non-validated patients reported outcomes measurements [11]), the WPATH suggests to treat individuals with GD with a combined treatment, which is composed of psychotherapy, hormonal therapy, and surgery [9].

The specific aim of the surgery is to align one's body anatomy to one's gender identity. Thus, AFAB persons with GD might request chest-contouring mastectomy (CCM), hystero-ovariectomy, vaginectomy, penile shaft reconstruction, either with or without urethra reconstruction, scrotal reconstruction, testicle implants and, as final stage, erection implant [12]. Some patients might also ask for liposuction to flanks, hips and thighs; facial implants (to achieve a 'stronger'—thus more masculine—face); and pectoralis implants. It is unclear to which extent this series of procedures is reducing one's GD, or it is simply enhancing the individual self-esteem.

As said, the scientific literature is providing only limited evidence (mostly, level V of evidence: *expert opinions* [12, 13]) on what is the most appropriate treatment plan for each specific individual. Nevertheless, the literature is confirming that surgical treatment can help in reducing one's dysphoria, and in improving patients' quality of life [9]. In the author's own experience with more than 1000 patients, *regret* rate is very low (less than 1%, which is consistent with peer-expert surgeons).

In this chapter, we focus on technical details for CMM and genital surgery (metoidioplasty and phalloplasty). We do omit on technical details on procedures that are widely performed for other patients' groups as well, such as liposuction and lipofilling, and hystero-ovariectomy.

24.1.4 Standards of Care Specific Criteria for Chest-Contouring Mastectomy and Genital Surgery

As according to the seventh version if the WPATH Standards of Care [9]: surgeons are responsible for discussing with patients: the different surgical techniques available, and their advantages, disadvantages, limitations, risks, and complications; examples of successful and unsuccessful cases have to be shown. Specific criteria for CCM are as follows: one referral letter with diagnosis of GD, capacity to make a full-informed decision and to consent for the treatment, and age of majority; there is no need to be or have been on hormonal therapy for proceeding with CCM. Specific criteria for genital surgery are same as those for CCM, plus hormonal therapy is required for a minimum of 12 months as well as a 12-month period living in the identity-congruent gender role [9].

24.2 Chest-Contouring-Mastectomy

Nearly all trans men and many non-binary AFAB individuals might seek for CCM surgery; usually, the aim is to reduce GD and/or (isolated) breast dysphoria. The surgery mostly consists in (partial) removal of the breast glandular tissue and, often, reduction of the Nipple-Areola-Complex (NAC); liposuction can also be used to complete the chest contouring [14].

24.2.1 Surgical Planning

Several authors have described approaches to select the most appropriate surgical technique for CCM [14–18]. These approaches take into account patient readiness for surgery (confirmed by the mental health professional, usually at the times of the diagnosis); assessment of the breast anatomical characteristics (volume of breast tissues, ptosis, skin excess, and elasticity [15]); family history for breast disease, which is especially important in patients with genetic risks for breast cancer; and patient's wishes [14].

Specifically, if there is a family history for breast cancer (including BRCA genes), a specialist breast oncologist should be consulted for a prophylactic mastectomy.

The importance of one's wishes has been previously highlighted [14]: in dubious cases, as when the patient is presenting an average breast size without significant ptosis, the patient should decide whether to go for a concentric circular technique (in order to avoid horizontal scarring, but undergo multiple staged surgeries if necessary), or a free nipple graft technique (in order to avoid multiple surgeries, but accepting the long horizontal scarring). To date, no algorithm has been validated by an evidence-based science [14].

24.2.2 Surgical Techniques

Common surgical techniques for CCM are hereby presented; mostly, these techniques were originally described for cis men presenting with gynecomastia.

Semicircular Technique: This is used for small volume breast, and it leaves inconspicuous scar, which is located at the inferior border of the areola [19].

Concentric Circular: This is used for average size breast (variable, according to the authors, and anyway less than 300 cc). Two circles are drawn: the first outside the areola, and the second within the same areola; the skin between the circles is de-epithelialized, a dermo-glandular pedicle is harvested, and the breast is removed. Although with this technique long scars are avoided, there is an higher risk of bleeding if compared to the *amputation with free nipple graft technique*, and scar revisions are not uncommon [14, 20]. Pre-op and post-op result of this technique is shown in Figs. 24.1 and 24.2.

Amputation with Free Nipple Graft: This is used for ptotic, or large breasts.

The incision is positioned onto the inframammary fold, and the NAC is harvested as a graft and transplanted to a new position. This is a reliable technique, although the (low) risk of bad scarring and NAC necrosis, and the permanent presence of a long scar all over the chest wall [14, 21–23]. Pre-op and post-op result of this technique is shown is Figs. 24.3 and 24.4.

Technique Variations and Revisions Surgeries: Other less common techniques consist in breast reduction techniques with pedicled NAC flap

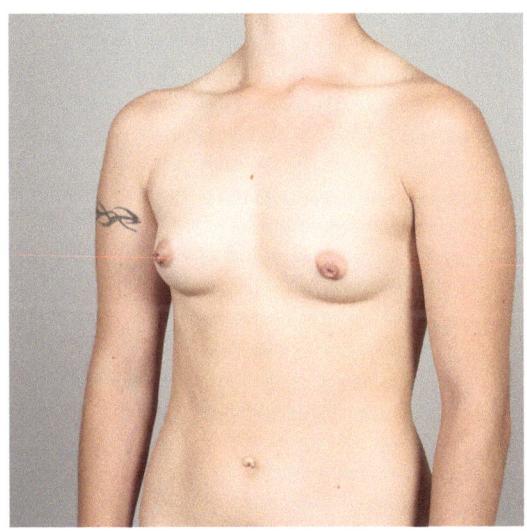

Fig. 24.1 Breast in trans man patient, with indication to concentric circular mastectomy

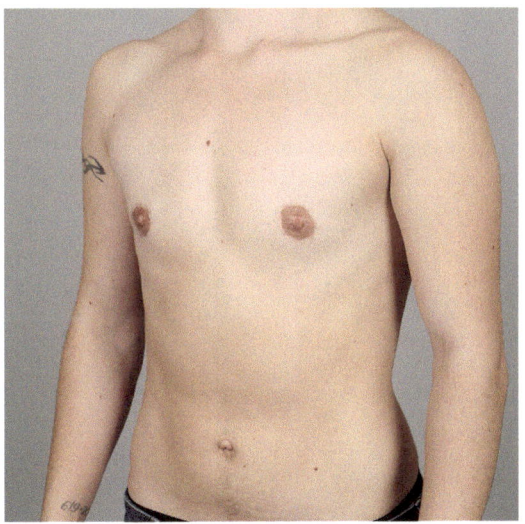

Fig. 24.2 Post-operative outcome following concentric circular mastectomy in patient from Fig. 24.1

(which are usually leaving extended scars) [14, 17, 19]; extended concentric circular techniques (scars are positioned horizontally, medially, and laterally to the circular peri-areolar scar; this technique is used today quite exclusively for secondary cases) [14–16]; liposuction (which is rarely used alone, but mostly in combination with other techniques or for revision surgery) [14–17]; lipofilling for revision surgeries [14–17]. In fact, fol-

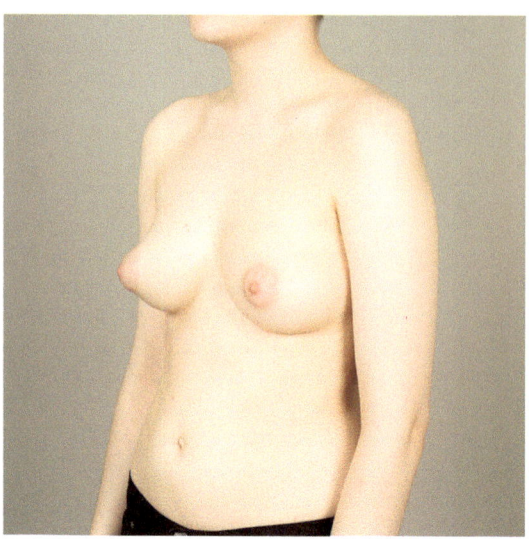

Fig. 24.3 Breast in trans man patient, with indication to amputation with free NAC graft mastectomy

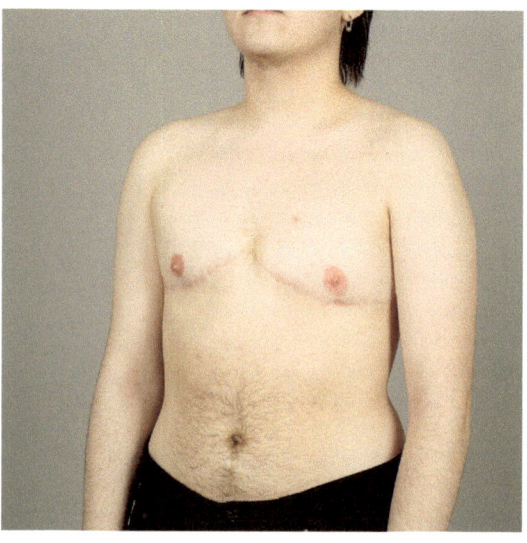

Fig. 24.4 Post-operative outcome following amputation with free NAC graft mastectomy in patient from Fig. 24.3

lowing the primary surgery, patients might still seek for reducing residual skin or breast tissue; better contouring the chest wall with fat grafting; revising scars; and reshaping or resizing the NAC. Usually, the revision rate is up to 25% [14].

In addition to the surgical techniques presented above, patients might also ask to reduce the nipple itself: techniques are various and none is standard.

24.2.3 Post-Operative Rehabilitation and Cancer Prevention

Post-operative care is easy: patients can return to full physical activities usually in 6 weeks following the surgery.

Complications are variable from 0% to 14% and consist in bleeding/hematoma, seroma, infection, wound dehiscence, hypertrophic/keloid scarring; asymmetrical shape of chest contour (i.e., asymmetrical distribution of the residual skin or breast tissue), asymmetrical size and/or position of the NAC; loss of tactile and erogenous sensitivity of NAC and breast skin; and NAC malposition and/or necrosis [14].

Regardless of the operative technique used, some small amount of breast tissue might be left in place voluntarily. In fact, small amount of breast tissue can be used to resemble the pectoralis muscle, or simply to create a larger chest size in people with higher BMI, thus helping for achieving a contour more proportionated to the rest of the upper body.

Finally, it is unclear to what extent CCM is reducing the risk of breast cancer; it is also unclear whether the testosterone therapy is preventing or, in selected cases, triggering the occurrence of breast cancer; thus, research is needed to draw evidence-based guidelines to recommend which patients should be followed up for prevention of breast cancer, and which radiological examination should be used.

24.3 Penis Reconstruction

Penis reconstruction has different goals, as according to patients' wishes.

Ideally, it could allow patient for urination while standing, to allow for sexual penetration, and it could create a penis which can be cosmetically acceptable and let the patient to pass in social situations; the ultimate goal is always to reduce one's GD.

The first surgery for penis reconstruction was performed by Bogoras in 1939 with bipedicled abdominal tubed flaps [24], and named *peniplas-*

Fig. 24.5 Penile prosthesis, usually used by trans men as packer

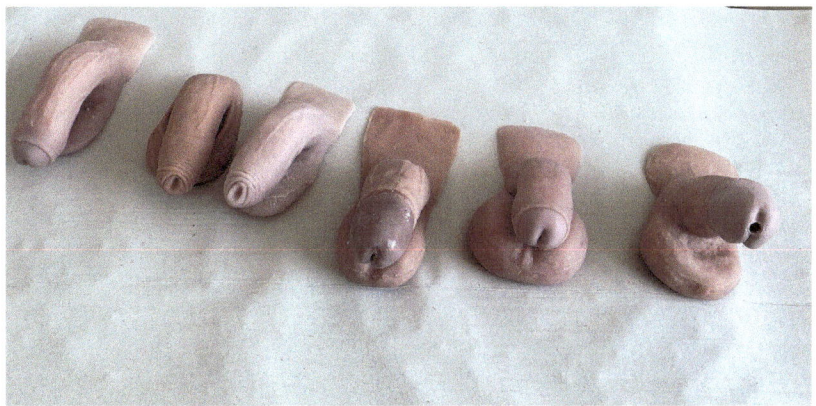

tica totalis; later, it was Sir Harold Gillies [25] who performed the first (multi-staged) phalloplasty to a trans man person, Dr. Gillon, in the UK in the 30's. Techniques for *phalloplasty* have evolved from local flaps (such as suprapubic and groin flaps), to microsurgical flaps (such as free radial forearm flap, fibula free flap, and latissimus dorsi flap). More recently, the anterolateral flap has been more commonly performed; combined flaps (e.g., anterolateral flap for penis reconstruction combined with radial forearm flap for urethra reconstruction) have been described, both for primary as well as for secondary cases.

As an alternative to phalloplasty, a *metoidioplasty* can be performed to elongate a clitoris to construct a penis of small size [26–28].

To date, not every trans man is keen to go through all the surgical steps leading to a full functioning penis. In fact, a non-surgical alternative is possible: many patients are seeking for an external prothesis shaped as a penis (Fig. 24.5), which is usually custom made of medical silicone by a specialized anaplastologist.

24.3.1   Surgical Planning

As to a previous publication from our group from Sahlgrenska University Hospital [8], patients' wishes are different, and one's identity is indicative for one's choice: non-binary AFAB persons are likely not to be interested in the ability for active penetrative sexual intercourses with a reconstructed penis, and they are likely to keep the vagina; on the other hand, binary trans men are likely to seek for a full-functioning penis (i.e., ability for urinating while standing, and for penetration) and for removal of the vagina; trans men are also requesting for the ejaculation function which—to date—has not been developed yet by surgeons. Common to all patients is to keep the original erogenous sensation (triggered from the clitoris), and possibly to have it triggered also from the reconstructed penis.

Thus, due to the many possible surgical approaches, the informative sessions and the decision-making process are key to the final success of the operation. Firstly, patients should be screened by a mental health professional for not presenting unrealistic expectations or a wishful thinking [29]; in fact, the psychologist takes account of patients' wishes and fears, and understands how meeting (or not) one's own goals shall impact one's GD. Secondly, patients are meeting the surgeon (s) and expressing specific priorities in merit to what they want to achieve with the surgery; at this time, the surgeon can examine the anatomy (size of clitoris, presence of adequate fat tissue at the arm and thighs, presence of hair, etc.) and discuss outcomes and risks of the various procedure; also, the surgeon clearly explain the limits of a specific procedure in relation to patient's own goal. Usually, after the first meeting with the surgeon, patients have to think over, rediscuss and, at a later time, decide which approach and surgical technique to take [9]. Table 24.1 shows questions and significant information necessary for the decision-making process.

Table 24.1 Questions and possible decisions when discussing surgical options with the surgeon

Questions	Significant information
Would you be happy with a small sized-penis? Would you be happy with a penis with small girth?	A metoidioplasty is creating a small-sized penis A radial forearm flap in a person with low to normal BMI is usually create a small girth penis
Do you want to keep sensation to your penis?	Metoidioplasty usually preserves one's erogenous sensation Local flap phalloplasties (groin and suprapubic flaps) usually do not bring sensation to the reconstructed penis Distant flaps (radial forearm, anterolateral thigh flap, and latissimus dorsi) are innervate, but nerve anastomosis has to be made in order for the penis to have erogenous and/or tactile sensations. Latissimus dorsi can also contract
Do you want to keep or remove the vagina? How important is to preserve it?	Many surgeons prefer to remove the vagina when reconstructing the urethra, since they might use part of its mucosa for urethra lengthening
Are you willing to accept a donor site morbidity (possibly unsightful donor area, surgical complications to the donor area, and stigmata)?	The donor site scar will always be noticeable. To achieve a large girth penis, a thinker flap needs to be used, thus the donor site will look more uneven with the surrounding tissues
How important is the ability for active sexual penetration with the reconstructed penis?	Metoidioplasty is usually not giving the ability for competent active sexual penetration Local flaps (suprapubic, groin) require erection implant. Erection implant means additional surgery, additional risks for complication (e.g., infection, extrusion), and eventually the need to substitute the erection implant in few years The important issue with these local flaps and erection implant is that these flaps do not bring in tactile sensation, thus the insertion of the implant is at very high risk for decubitus, sore formation, and implant extrusion in the future Latissimus dorsi usually gives the ability for competent active sexual penetration, when the patient is contracting the muscle which, at the same time, is becoming shorter Radial forearm flap and thigh flaps require an erection implant, which means additional surgery, additional risks for complication, and eventually the need to substitute the erection implant in few years Penetrative sexual intercourse could be painful
How important is to be able to void while standing? How important to avoid complication like urinary fistula, be obliged to have a urinary catheter or suprapubic catheter for long time?	Regardless whether going for metoidioplasty or phalloplasty, reconstruct the urinary channel means more extensive surgery, and very high risk for complications (e.g., urinary fistula and urinary stenosis), future check-ups (including urethroscopy), and corrective surgeries Regardless whether going for metoidioplasty or phalloplasty, the reconstructed urethra will present a U-shape, and it will be with difficulty to empty it completely by normal urination; thus, some leakage of residual urine is possible Residual urine might also mean higher risk for urinary infection If not urinary reconstruction is not successful, patient might end up with a permanent perineal urethrostomy
How important is to undergo a fast preparation to surgery? How important is to avoid multi-staged surgery? How important is to have a quick recovery and any type of adjustments following the surgery?	Preparation to metoidioplasty only requires testosterone (some surgeons are also advising a pumping system) to enlarge the clitoris as much as possible prior to the surgery Preparation to urethra reconstruction, as well as phalloplasties, usually requires epilation of the donor site Epilation should be total for the areas going to be used for urethra reconstruction, while areas going to be used for the penile shaft can be epilated following the surgery Preparation to free flaps might require additional radiological examinations Metoidioplasty without urethra reconstruction is the simplest technique Metoidioplasty with vaginectomy, urethra reconstruction, and insertion of testicle implants directly in the labia majora is a combination of procedure that can be performed all-in-one-stage
How important is to avoid recurrent visits to the hospital, recurrent operations, and various check-ups?	Techniques including urethroplasty usually are at higher risk for recurrent operations and/or post-op check-ups

Due to the multiple and specific goals of each person, there is no surgical technique that can be considered as the gold standard for penis reconstruction. In fact, many AFAB patients simply go for CCM, and they avoid any type of surgery to their genitals, while others might opt for a simple elongation of the clitoris to create a micropenis (metoidioplasty), or for a phalloplasty (with local or distant flaps). None of these surgical approaches and techniques has to be considered substandard, and no technique could be considered the ultimate one for penis reconstruction, regardless the complexity of some of these, and regardless the multiple functional outcomes achievable.

24.3.2 Surgical Techniques

General information on specific surgical techniques is hereby presented.

Either metoidioplasty or phalloplasty can be differently combined with urethra reconstruction, vaginoplasty, scrotoplasty, insertion of testicle, and erection implants. Table 24.2 is listing limits and benefits for the most common used and described techniques [26]. It must be stressed that, to date, scientific literature is not presenting high level of evidence manuscripts reporting on patient reported outcome measurements at long-term follow-up.

Table 24.2 Techniques for penis reconstruction in trans men

Surgical technique	Benefits	Limits
Metoidioplasty	Easy technique (no microsurgical skills required) Reduced risk for complications Recovery time quicker compared to free flap techniques	Tiny penis Hardly capable for sexual penetration Urinary complications possible
Radial forearm flap	Possible ability for sexual intercourse Possible ability for urination	Multiple stages Urinary tract problems Stiffener required for erection Donor-site morbidity RFF with bone component possibly abandoned
Anterolateral thigh flap	Possible ability for sexual intercourse Possible ability for urination	Multiple stages Often need to be combined with another flap for urinary tract reconstruction Stiffener required for erection Donor-site morbidity
Fibula flap	Possible ability for sexual intercourse Without needing for erection device	Multiple stages Need to be combined with another flap for urinary tract reconstruction Donor-site morbidity Possibly abandoned
Latissimus dorsi flap	Erection and penetration possible by contracting the muscle-penis	Multiple stages required for urinary tract reconstruction Erection and penetration function questionable Donor-site morbidity Sensitivity not reported
Suprapubic flap/groin flap	Local flap: Relatively easier surgery	Multiple stages required for penis and for urinary tract reconstruction Cosmetic appearance unsatisfactory Donor site morbidity (aesthetic) Sensation questionable Possibility to insert an erection implant in case of sensation?

24.3.2.1 Metoidioplasty

This surgical technique [26–28] is based on the procedures for correction of microphallus, have later described as metoidioplasty by Lebovic and Laub [30, 31], or clitoris-penoid by Eicher [32]. Urethral lengthening and surgical refinements were described by Hage [33] and Perovic [34].

Usually, this surgery is possible only in case of an hypertrophied clitoris following the hormonal (testosterone) therapy. Some patients are also using vacuum devices pre- and post-operatively; however, its effectiveness in enlarging the clitoris or the reconstructed penis has not been validated.

Nowadays, metoidioplasty can be performed with or without urethra reconstruction for urinary function, and with or without removal of the vaginal mucosa and closure of the cavity (vaginectomy).

For urethra reconstruction, surgeons might use vaginal flap, vaginal mucosa graft, local labia minora, or buccal mucosa graft; all combinations are possible. Whenever a urinary tract reconstruction is attempted, urinary complications such as fistulas, strictures, post-operative urinary infections, and urinary leakage (sometimes simple dribbling) are possible and not uncommon [12].

Patients might opt for testicle implants at the time of the primary operation, or later on. Patients might also opt to have a scrotal pouch reconstruction (using labia majora as according to the Hoebeke technique [35]) or to insert the implants directly into the labia majora (Fig. 24.6).

Compared to other techniques for phalloplasty, metoidioplasty has a shorter hospital stay, there is no additional donor site morbidity from other parts of the body, and it should keep erogenous sensitivity; also, half of the patients able to void whilst standing [33, 34, 36]. Downside is that the phallus created is short (with a mean of 5.7 cm—range 4–10 cm) [33]; finally, few patients are claiming to be able for penetrative sexual intercourse [28].

24.3.2.2 Phalloplasty

The penile shaft can be constructed with local flaps such as the supra-pubic flap or groin flap; free radial forearm flap (Fig. 24.7); pedicled antero-lateral thigh flap (rarely performed as a free flap) (Fig. 24.8); free latissimus dorsi flap. Although performed in the past, there are no recent reports of free fibula flap in the literature [26–28].

Phalloplasty can be performed: with or without urethra reconstruction for urinary function, and with or without removal of the vaginal mucosa and closure of the cavity (vaginectomy).

When a urethra reconstruction is attempted, the pars fixa of the urethra (from the original meatus to the base of the penis) is reconstructed as done for the metoidioplasty (i.e., by displacing the clitoris upward and using the labia minora, and eventually a small vaginal flap).

More options are possible for the reconstruction of the pars pendulans (penile urethra).

For penis reconstruction with local flap such as suprapubic and groin, vaginal epithelium graft and tubularized skin can be used; however, this technique is seldom able to reach the tip of the phallus [12, 37].

In case of a radial forearm free flap phalloplasty, the pars pendula is reconstructed rolling the flap as a tube-within-a-tube, with the ulnar part being the urethra; with an antero-lateral thigh flap, the urethra can be reconstructed by rolling the same flap as a tube-within-a-tube, but this is possible only if the flap is very thin;

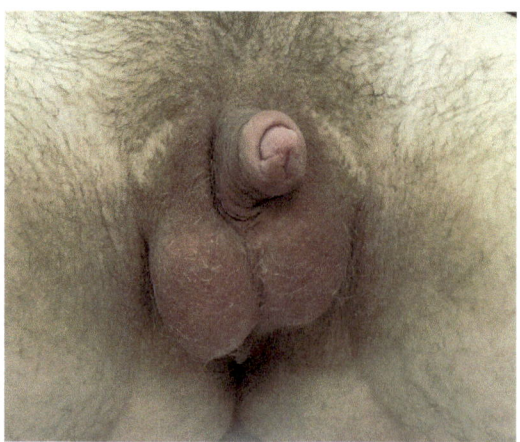

Fig. 24.6 Metoidioplasty with urethra reconstruction, vaginectomy, and testicle implant inserted directly into the labia majora

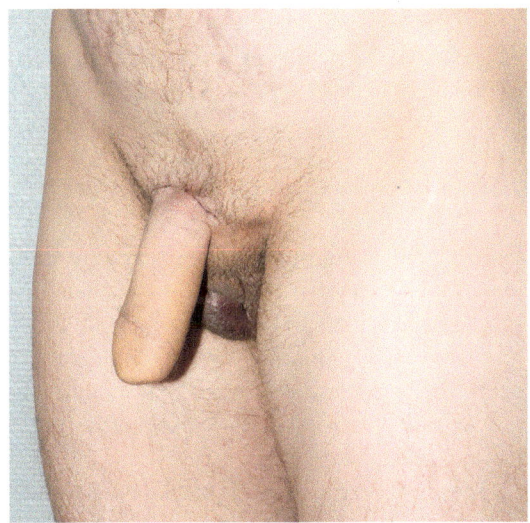

Fig. 24.7 Phalloplasty with free RFF, vaginectomy and scrotoplasty (according to the Hoebeke's technique). The urethra has been reconstructed rolling the fee RFF as a tube-within-a-tube. The patient also got testicle and erection implants (post-op result 1 week following testicle and erection implants)

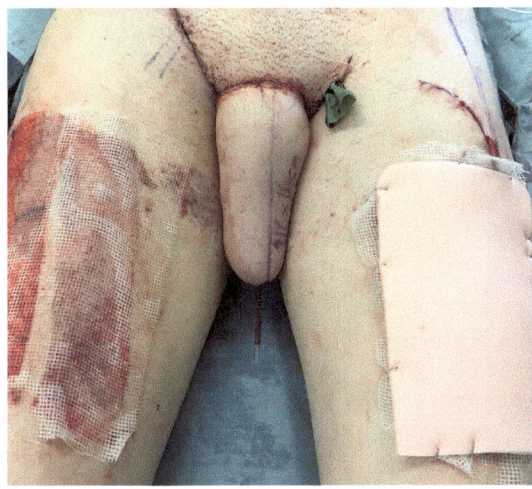

Fig. 24.8 This patient originally underwent metoidioplasty with urethra reconstruction; later, he has decided to go for phalloplasty. This figure is showing the phalloplasty with combined ALT flap for shaft reconstruction, free RFF for urethra reconstruction, vaginectomy, and scrotoplasty (according to the Hoebeke's technique). The patient is planned for glans reconstruction with the Norfolk's technique, testicle and erection implants, at a later stage

differently, the urethra has to be reconstructed with a free radial forearm flap, or with a superficial circumflex iliac artery perforator (SCIAP) flap. Pre-fabricating the urethra within the same flap has also been described when free RFF and ALT have been used for penile shaft construction.

As for metoidioplasty, whenever a urinary tract reconstruction is attempted, urinary complications (fistulas, strictures, post-operative urinary infections and urinary leakage or dribbling) are common. Thus, patients must be really motivated to undergo urethra reconstruction. Indeed, an unsuccessful attempt for urethra reconstruction can always be converted in a permanent urethral perineostomy, thus returning to a similar situation as to pre-operatively [12].

In order to provide the penis with erogenous sensation, the clitoris can be displaced at the base of the new phallus. Also, cutaneous nerves from flaps such as RFF and ALT can be connected to the dorsal nerves of the clitoris, and to the ilioinguinal nerve [12].

Finally, to shape the tip of the penis as glans and providing a coronal sulcus, the 'Norfolk' technique can be used [38], regardless the type of flap chosen for phalloplasty. The glans can later be tattooed.

Reconstructions of specific complications using flaps are partial and total necrosis; the risk for total necrosis for free flap reconstruction is up to 2%.

24.3.2.3 Vaginectomy

A submucosa vaginectomy can be performed, usually at the time of the metoidioplasty or phalloplasty. This consists in removing the mucosa of the vagina only. In order not to leave residual mucosa in place, gynaecologists usually recommend to remove the uterus prior to performing the vaginectomy.

Indeed, there are patients that want to preserve the vagina for keeping the ability for penetrative intercourse; also, there are patients that are not bothered by having the vagina, since it might not affect negatively once GD, thus they prefer not undergoing surgeries with lower priority.

24.3.2.4 Scrotoplasty and Testicle Implants

When reconstructing the scrotum, surgeons must plan for both reconstructing of the scrotal envelope and providing volume and internal shape which, in a cis man, is obtained by the presence of two testicles.

Thus, the easiest technique is to insert oval-shaped silicone implants (named 'testicle implants' by the manufacturers) directly into the labia majora. However, the result of this approach results in two separate pouches, which indeed can be joined together, usually in a second stage. However, this approach does not locate the testicle in the natural position, which is obtained only when the scrotum is presenting some degree of ptosis. Thus, Hoebeke [35] developed a technique consisting in harvesting and rotating (medially) two superiorly-based labia majora flaps. This technique achieves confer the scrotum ptosis and an anterior position. In a following stage, testicle implants can be inserted.

24.3.2.5 Erection Implants

When requested by the patient, an erection implant can be inserted. In order to prevent decubitus and extrusion of the implant, best is to insert it when the penile shaft has gained full tactile (or erogenous) sensation, which is usually happening around 1 year following the phalloplasty with nerve anastomosis.

Few literature is reporting on the use of erectile implants following penis reconstruction in trans men. Specifically, there are several complications associated with implant placement in the reconstructed penis, such as hematoma, infection, urinary fistulas and strictures, partial or total penis necrosis, as well as implant deformity [39–42].

Different implants have been used during the years, and these were originally manufactured for cis men with impotence, thus, these were planned for a different anatomy (corpora cavernosa vs. operated tissue) and to be, usually, in an older population group. Both malleable (Draphase, Spectra, Coloplast) and inflatable implants (Dynaflex, AMS, Coloplast) have been tested. Finally, erection implants specific for trans men post phalloplasty have been manufactured by

ZSI. Generally, up to 50% of the implants need to be explanted at 5 years follow-up, usually because of infection, extrusion, or pubic pain [39, 42].

24.3.3 Pre-Operative Preparations

Patients are requested to stop smoking completely 6 weeks prior to surgery, and their BMI should be less than 30.

Electrolysis epilation is fundamental for nearly every patient that have been planned for urethroplasty with any hair-bearing tissue, e.g., a radial forearm flap.

The epilation regimen might take 6–12 months, depending on the amount and type of hair follicles. Normally, patients undergo one epilation session every 3–4 weeks. Last epilation session should not be closer than 3 weeks to the surgery. Besides epilation to the tissue going to be urethra, the tissue to become penile shaft (such as the dorsal and radial part of the forearm in a full RFF penile reconstruction, or the thigh for an ALT flap) also needs to be epilated; still, this could be done successively to the surgery.

Patients are suspending the hormonal therapy 3–4 weeks prior to surgery, in order to reduce the risk for DVT. Seven to ten days before surgery, it is advised not to use any medication or food supplements affecting the coagulation system.

Patients start Clexane (5000 UI) the night before the surgery; this therapy is maintained until discharge. In the morning prior to surgery, patients receive one tablet of Bactrim forte as prophylaxis antibiotic.

24.3.3.1 Post-Operative Rehabilitation

Post-operative care is easier when urethra has not been reconstructed; although patients without urinary complications might return to full physical activities usually in 6 weeks following the surgery, the majority needs post-op urinary controls for dribbling/leakage of urine, and for possible urinary infections and stenosis in the future.

Since the surgery for penis reconstruction is usually multi-staged, the entire peri-operative period (from pre-op examinations to the completion of the last stage), can take up to 2 years or more.

Additionally, those who have undergone erectile implant placement might need to follow up, and eventually replace, the same erection implant.

24.3.3.2 Ongoing Researches

Recently, researches have been performed to bone-anchor the external prosthesis (named 'epithesis') by titanium screws, which can osteointegration into the pubic bones. Although first clinical cases have been described, this is still experimental: silicone penile epithesis prototypes need further development, and then, these prototypes need to be tested on a large scale of patients [43].

Also, after the first four successful cases of penis transplantation to cis man, research programs for penis transplantation to trans men have started and first manuscripts on surgical anatomy have been published [44–46].

Finally, many preclinical researches have been conducted on engineered urethra reconstruction: no applications in humans have been reported [47].

References

1. World Health Organization. ICD-11: classifying disease to map the way we live and die. Geneva: WHO; 2018. http://www.who.int/health-topics/international-classification-of-diseases. Accessed 21 Apr 2020.
2. World Health Organization. Manual of the international statistical classification of diseases, injuries, and causes of death. Tenth Revision. Geneva: WHO; 1992.
3. World Health Organization. International classification of diseases and related health problems—10th revision. Geneva: WHO; 2007.
4. American Psychiatric Association. Diagnostic and statistical manual of mental disorders. 5th ed. Washington: American Psychiatric Association; 2013.
5. De Cuypere G, Van Hemelrijck M, Michel A, et al. Prevalence and demography of transsexualism in Belgium. Eur Psychiatry. 2007;22(3):137–41.
6. Reed B, Rhodes S, Schofield P, Wylie K. Gender variance in the UK: prevalence, incidence, growth and geographic distribution. GIRES. 2009. http://www.gires.org.uk/assets/Medpro-Assets/GenderVarianceUK-report.pdf. Accessed 30 Sept 2021.
7. James SE, Herman JL, Rankin S, Keisling M, Mottet L, Anafi M. The report of the 2015 US transgender survey. Washington, DC: National Center for Transgender Equality; 2016.
8. Jacobsson J, Andreasson M, Kolby L, Elander A, Selvaggi G. Patients' priorities regarding female-to-male gender affirmation surgery of the genitalia—a pilot study of 47 patients in Sweden. J Sex Med. 2017;14(6):857–64.
9. WPATH. Standards of Care for the Health of Transsexual, Transgender, and Gender Nonconforming People, 7th Version. WPATH. 2011. http://www.wpath.org. Accessed 21 Apr 2020.
10. Selvaggi G, Dhejne C, Landen M, Elander A. The 2011 WPATH standards of care and penile reconstruction in female-to-male transsexual individuals. Ther Adv Urol. 2012;2012:581712.
11. Andreasson M, Georgas K, Elander A, Selvaggi G. Patient reported outcome measures used in gender confirmation surgery—a systematic review. Plast Reconstr Surg. 2018;141(4):1026–39.
12. Selvaggi G, Bellringer J. Gender reassignment surgery: an overview. Nat Rev Urol. 2011;8(5):274–82.
13. HTA-report Gender Affirmation Surgery for Gender Dysphoria—effects and risks. Accessed 19 Sept 2019.
14. Selvaggi G. Mastectomy in trans men. In: Cordova A, Innocenti A, Toia F, Tripoli M, editors. Plastic and cosmetic surgery of the male chest. Berlin: Springer; 2020.
15. Monstrey S, Selvaggi G, Ceulemans P, Van Landuyt K, Bowman C, Blondeel P, Hamdi M, De Cuypere G. Chest-wall contouring surgery in female-to-male transsexuals: a new algorithm. Plast Reconstr Surg. 2008;121:849–59.
16. Bjerrom Ahlin H, Elander A, Kolby L, Selvaggi G. Improved results after the implementation of the Ghent algorithm for subcutaneous mastectomy in female-to-male transsexuals. J Plast Surg Hand Surg. 2014;48(6):362–7.
17. Claes KEY, D' Arpa S, Monstrey S. Chest surgery for transgender and gender nonconforming individuals. Clin Plast Surg. 2018;45:369–80.
18. Top H, Balta S. Transsexual mastectomy: selection of appropriate technique according to breast characteristics. Balkan Med J. 2017;34:147–55.
19. Wolter A, Diedrichson J, Scholz T, Arens-Landwehr A, Liebau J. Sexual reassignment surgery in female-to-male transsexuals: an algorithm for subcutaneous mastectomy. JPRAS. 2015;68:184–91.
20. Davidson BA. Concentric circle operation for massive gynecomastia to excise the redundant skin. Plast Reconstr Surg. 1979;63(3):350–4.
21. Wray RC Jr, Hoopes JE, Davis GM. Correction of extreme gynaecomastia. Br J Plast Surg. 1974;27(1):39–41.
22. Eicher W. Transsexualism. Dtsch Krankenpflegez. 1992;45(3):183–7.
23. Lindsay WRN. Creation of a male chest in female transsexuals. Ann Plast Surg. 1979;3(1):39–46.
24. Bogoras N. Uber die volle plastische Wiederherstellung eines zum Koitus fahigen Penis (Peniplastica totalis). Zentralbl Chir. 1936;22:1271.

25. Gillies H, Millard RD Jr. Genitalia. In: The principles of art of plastic surgery. London: Butterworth; 1957. p. 368–88.

26. Selvaggi G, Bellringer J. Gender reassignment surgery: an overview. Nat Rev Urol. 2011;8(5):274–82. Epub 2011 Apr 12.

27. Selvaggi G, Elander A. Penile reconstruction/formation. Curr Opin Urol. 2008;18(6):589–97.

28. Salgado CJ, Monstrey SJ, Djordjevic ML, editors. Gender affirmation. Medical and surgical perspective. New York: Thieme Medical; 2017.

29. Selvaggi G, Giordano S. The role of mental health professionals in gender reassignment surgery: unjust discrimination or responsible care? Aesthetic Plast Surg. 2014;38(6):1177–83.

30. Laub DR, Laub DR II, Hentz VR. Penis construction in female-to-male transsexuals. In: Eicher W, Kubli F, Herms V, editors. Plastic surgery in the sexually handicapped. New York: Springer-Verlag; 1989. p. 113–28.

31. Lebovic GS, Laub D. Metoidioplasty. In: Ehrlich RM, Alter GJ, editors. Reconstructive and plastic surgery of the external genitalia: adult and pediatric. Philadelphia: WB Saunders; 1999. p. p355–60.

32. Eicher W. The inverted penis skin technique in male-to-female transsexuals. In: Eicher W, Kubli F, Herms V, editors. Plastic surgery in the sexually handicapped. Berlin: Springer-Verlag; 1989. p. 91–112.

33. Hage JJ. Metaidoioplasty: an alternative phalloplasty technique in transsexuals. Plast Reconstr Surg. 1996;97:161–7.

34. Perovic SV, Djordjevic ML. Metoidioplasty: a variant of phalloplasty in female transsexuals. BJU Int. 2003;92:981–5.

35. Selvaggi G, Hoebeke P, Ceulemans P, Hamdi M, Van Landuyt K, Blondeel P, De Cuypere G, Monstrey S. Scrotal reconstruction in female-to-male transsexuals: the novel scrotoplasty. Plast Reconstr Surg. 2009;123(6):1710–9.

36. Hage JJ, van Turnhout AA. Long-term of metaidoioplasty in 70 female-to-male transsexuals. Ann Plast Surg. 2006;57(3):312–6.

37. Bettocchi C, Ralph DJ, Pryor JP. Pedicled pubic phalloplasty in females with gender dysphoria. BJU Int. 2005;95(1):120–4.

38. Gilbert DA, Jordan GH, Devine CJ Jr, Winslow BH. Microsurgical forearm "cricket bat-transformer" phalloplasty. Plast Reconstr Surg. 1992;90(4):711–6.

39. Polchert M, Dick B, Raheem O. Narrative review of penile prosthetic implant technology and surgical results, including transgender patients. Transl Androl Urol. 2021;10(6):2629–47.

40. Hoebeke PB, Decaestecker K, Beysens M, et al. Erectile implants in female-to-male transsexuals: our experience in 129 patients. Eur Urol. 2010;57:334–40.

41. Falcone M, Garaffa G, Grillo A, et al. Outcomes of inflatable penile prosthesis insertion in 247 patients completing female to male gender reassignment surgery. BJU Int. 2018;121:139–44.

42. Blewniewski M, Ostrowski I, Pottek T, et al. Safety and efficacy outcomes of ZSI475 penile prosthesis. Urologia. 2017;84:98–101.

43. Selvaggi G, Branemark R, Elander A, Liden M, Stalfors J. Titanium-bone-anchored penile epithesis: pre-operative planning and immediate post-operative results. J Plast Surg Hand Surg. 2015;49(1):40–4.

44. Selvaggi G, Wesslen E, Elander A, Wroblewski P, Thorarinsson A, Olausson M. Penile transplantation in female-to-male sex reassignment surgery: a cadaveric study. BioMed Res Int. 2018;2018:6754030.

45. Tuffaha SH, Sacks JM, Shores JT, Brandacher G, Lee WP, Cooney DS, Redett RJ. Using the dorsal, cavernosal, and external pudendal arteries for penile transplantation: technical considerations and perfusion territories. Plast Reconstr Surg. 2014;134:111e–9e.

46. Selvaggi G, Manner K, Sakinis A, Olausson M. A pilot retrospective CT angio study of the internal pudendal arteries in male bodies, for the purpose of penis transplantation to trans men. J Plast Surg Hand Surg. 2021;19:1–6. Online ahead of print. https://doi.org/10.1080/2000656X.2021.1927058.

47. Saad S, Osman NI, Chapple CR. Tissue engineering: recent advances and review of clinical outcome for urethral strictures. Curr Opin Urol. 2021;31(5):498–503. https://doi.org/10.1097/MOU.0000000000000921.

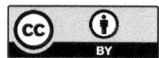

Sexual Pain Disorders, Vestibulodynia, and Recurrent Cystitis: The Evil Trio

A Clinical Conversation on the Uroandrological Perspective

Alessandra Graziottin and Elisa Maseroli

Abbreviations

AD	Arousal disorders
CIF	Clinical impact factor
DSM	Diagnostic and statistical manual of mental disorders
EcN	*E. coli* Nissle 1917
ED	Erectile dysfunction
FSD	Female sexual disorders
GPPPD	Genito-pelvic pain penetration disorder
GSM	Genitourinary syndrome of the menopause
HSSD	Hypoactive sexual desire disorder
IBS	Irritable bowel syndrome
ISSWSH	International Society for the Study of Women's Sexual Health
LUTS	Lower urinary tract symptoms
MSD	Male sexual disorders
NGF	Nerve growth factor
PCC	Post-coital cystitis
PEA	Palmitoylethanolamide
PID	Pelvic inflammatory disease
SPD	Sexual pain disorders
UPEC	Uropathogenic *E. coli*
UTI	Urinary tract infection
WHO	World Health Organization

A. Graziottin (✉)
Department of Obstetrics and Gynecology, University of Verona, Verona, Italy

Center of Gynecology and Medical Sexology, H. San Raffaele Resnati, Milan, Italy

Alessandra Graziottin Foundation for the Cure and Care of Pain in Women NPO, Milan, Italy
e-mail: direzione@studiograziottin.it

E. Maseroli
Andrology, Women's Endocrinology and Gender Incongruence Unit, Careggi University Hospital, Florence, Italy

The best general is not the one who gets one hundred victories in one hundred battles, but the one who overcomes the enemy without giving battle. He is the most skilled.
Know each other and themselves: victory without risks. Know the terrain and environmental conditions: victory on all fronts.—Sun-Tzu "The art of war", VI century B.C.

25.1 Introduction

The most skilled uroandrologists want to know more about female sexual disorders (FSD) to enrich their clinical practice and therapeutic efficacy. Physicians who have a more committed therapeutic relationship with their patients and longer follow-up periods have noted that urological complaints often coexist with FSD.

Recurrent cystitis, specifically post-coital cystitis, is often comorbid with two conditions: painful sexual intercourse ("sexual pain disorders" or "dyspareunia") and/or vaginal dryness. This trio is more frequent in young patients, and increasingly

© The Author(s) 2023
C. Bettocchi et al. (eds.), *Practical Clinical Andrology*,
https://doi.org/10.1007/978-3-031-11701-5_25

reported after menopause [1, 2]. In the background of these complaints, vestibulodynia/vulvar pain is the most frequently complained gynecological comorbidity in the premenopausal years [3].

After menopause, recurrent post-coital cystitis with the associated cluster of other urological, vaginal, and sexual symptoms is currently encompassed by the term "genitourinary syndrome of menopause" (GSM) every uroandrologist should become familiar with. The working definitions are summarized in the pertinent paragraphs [4, 5].

The goal of this chapter is to improve the clinicians' awareness and clinical outcomes of women affected by recurrent post-coital cystitis and associated FSDs, who are often treated with the minimalistic approach of repeated antibiotic treatment. Therefore, neglected FSDs and shared pathophysiological etiologies can contribute to maintaining the problem in the shadow of persistent diagnostic omissions. Specific attention will be devoted to discuss provoked vestibulodynia/vulvar pain and GSM in order to share a comprehensive vision enriched with therapeutic approaches that have proven effective in gynecological practice. A brief paragraph will be dedicated to the associated sexual comorbidities associated with GSM.

These conditions and their comorbidity with FSD will be analyzed here from a pragmatic clinical perspective, which is useful in a physicians' daily practice.

25.2 Sexual Pain-Related Disorders and Comorbid Lower Urinary Symptoms

25.2.1 Nosology and Current Definitions

The DSM-IV-TR includes two conditions related to sexual pain in women: dyspareunia, defined as genital and/or pelvic pain during sex, and vaginismus, referring to an involuntary spasm or tightening of the pelvic muscles [6]. In the DSM-5, the two disorders were collapsed into a single entity, emphasizing the multidimensional nature of genital pain and the common overlap between pain during intercourse and difficulties with penetration. This category, named genito-pelvic

pain/penetration disorder (GPPPD), was defined as persistent or recurrent difficulties with one or more of the following: (1) vaginal penetration during intercourse; (2) vulvovaginal or pelvic pain during vaginal intercourse or attempts at penetration; (3) fear or anxiety about vulvovaginal or pelvic pain in anticipation of, during, or as a result of vaginal penetration; and (4) tightening or tensing of the pelvic floor muscles during attempted vaginal penetration [7]. As for other FSDs, symptoms must be present for at least 6 months, causing significant distress.

In the ICD-11 Mortality and Morbidity Statistics, the World Health Working Group on Sexual Disorders and Sexual Health used the term "sexual pain-penetration disorder," which is "characterized by at least one of the following: (1) marked and persistent or recurrent difficulties with penetration, including due to involuntary tightening or tautness of the pelvic floor muscles during attempted penetration; (2) marked and persistent or recurrent vulvovaginal or pelvic pain during penetration; (3) marked and persistent or recurrent fear or anxiety about vulvovaginal or pelvic pain in anticipation of, during, or as a result of penetration" [8]. To diagnose a sexual pain-penetration disorder, the symptoms must not be entirely attributable to a medical condition (including insufficient vaginal lubrication) or a mental disorder, and they must be associated with clinically significant distress. Dyspareunia has been retained as a separate category and is defined as a "symptom caused by physical determinants," "characterized by recurrent genital pain or discomfort that occurs before, during, or after sexual intercourse, or superficial or deep vaginal penetration that is related to an identifiable physical cause, not including lack of lubrication" [8].

In 2014, the International Society for the Study of Women's Sexual Health (ISSWSH) and the North American Menopause Society introduced new terminology for vulvovaginal atrophy. The GSM includes but not limited to genital symptoms of dryness, burning, and irritation; sexual symptoms of lack of lubrication, discomfort or pain, and impaired function; and urinary symptoms of urgency, dysuria, and recurrent urinary tract infections (rUTI) [5].

In 2015, the nomenclature of other conditions related to sexual pain in women has been revised in a consensus document endorsed by the International Society for the Study of Vulvovaginal Disease, ISSWSH, and International Pelvic Pain Society [9]. Accordingly, persistent vulvar pain is defined as "Vulvar pain caused by a specific disorder: Infectious, Inflammatory, Neoplastic, Neurologic, Trauma, Iatrogenic, Hormonal deficiencies," and differentiated from Vulvodynia, defined as "vulvar pain of at least 3 months' duration, without a clear identifiable cause, which may have potential associated factors" [9]. Descriptors of vulvodynia are related to localization (localized: vestibulodynia or clitorodynia, generalized, or mixed), triggers (provoked, i.e., insertional and contact vs. spontaneous or mixed), onset (primary or secondary), and temporal patterns (intermittent, persistent, constant, immediate, and delayed) [9].

25.2.2 Methodology

Key concepts about sexual pain/penetration disorders are summarized, where pertinent, to set the scene of clinical considerations useful for the most appropriate comorbidity reading, and to finally potentiate clinical outcomes. The detailed definitions and characteristics of other FSDs are discussed in the pertinent chapter (Graziottin, Maseroli, and Vignozzi, FSD: a clinical perspective) of this book.

In this chapter, a concise pragmatic approach closer to a clinical conversation on these topics is discussed. When sophisticated definitions of FSD are involved, a simpler descriptive wording of the problem will also be used to ease conversations with patients and colleagues not specifically trained in sexual medicine.

25.2.3 Working Definitions in the Clinical Setting

Actors to be considered in the clinical setting include the following:

- **Recurrent cystitis**: An rUTI is defined as ≥2 episodes of UTI within 6 months or ≥3 episodes of UTI within 12 months with >10³ CFU/mL isolated [10].

In this article, the term "cystitis" is defined as follows:

1. Bladder infection that causes irritative voiding symptoms.
2. Non-infective bladder inflammation (often associated with pathogenic biofilms within the urothelial cell, with negative urine culture) [11].
3. Symptoms in the absence of overt bladder inflammation.

- **Recurrent post-coital cystitis**: complain of cystitis usually 24—72 h after intercourse. Most studies discuss recurrent cystitis in women, but only a few indicate the post-coital symptoms and signs of bladder infection.
- **Painful sexual intercourse or sexual pain/ penetration disorders or genito-pelvic pain penetration disorders (GPPPD)**.

Genito-pelvic pain penetration disorder is defined by the DSM-5 as persistent and recurrent difficulties with one or more of the following, as mentioned above:

1. Vaginal penetration during intercourse.
2. Vulvovaginal or pelvic pain during vaginal intercourse or attempts at penetration.
3. Fear of anxiety about vulvovaginal or pelvic pain in anticipation of, during, or as a result of vaginal penetration.
4. Tightening or tensing of the pelvic floor muscles during attempted vaginal penetration.

This complicated definition is difficult to use for patients and colleagues. Recent consensus and reviews suggest a more evidence-based description of FSDs with regard to DSM-5 [12]. In clinical conversation, the terminologies "**sexual pain**" or "**painful sexual intercourse**" are easier to understand. The term "sexual pain disorders" encompasses the following former clinical entities:

- **Dyspareunia**: recurrent or persistent genital pain associated with sexual intercourse, which causes personal distress.

- **Vaginismus**: recurrent or persistent involuntary spasm of the pelvic floor muscles, i.e., the levator ani surrounding the outer third of the vagina. This condition is associated with variable fear of intercourse that interferes with vaginal penetration and causes personal distress [13, 14].

Genitourinary syndrome of the menopause is a cluster of symptoms and signs associated with a reduction in estrogen, testosterone, and progesterone, causing the involution of the labia minora and majora, clitoris and cavernosal bodies, vestibule/vaginal introitus, vagina, urethra, bladder, and levator ani muscle [5]. It includes the following symptoms [15]:

- Vulvo-vaginal symptoms:
  - Dryness.
  - Burning sensation.
  - Itching.
  - Vaginal discharge.
- Urinary symptoms:
  - Urgency.
  - Dysuria.
  - Infections/recurrent cystitis.
- Sexual symptoms:
  - Lack of lubrication/vaginal dryness.
  - Coital pain.
  - Sexual dysfunctions.

In summary, among women of fertile age, one of the most likely etiologies of urinary symptoms is tightly connected to the causes of sexual and vulvar pain and hypertonus of the pelvic floor, while during menopause, urinary symptoms, as well as sexual dysfunction are commonly related to a decrease in the production of sexual hormones, which could lead to GSM.

Key Point When recurrent cystitis is reported, physicians should always ask if the woman has the following:

- Bladder symptoms or an overt cystitis 24–72 h after intercourse.
- Pain at the entrance of the vagina at the beginning of intercourse and/or burning pain after intercourse.

- Vaginal dryness.
- Post-menopausal vaginal, sexual, and/or urological symptoms.

25.2.4 Lower Urinary Tract Symptoms and Female Sexual Disorders: From Epidemiological Data to Clinical Meaning

Women present a high comorbidity between urological complaints, such as lower urinary tract symptoms (LUTS), specifically recurrent post-coital-cystitis (RPCC), and FSD [1, 3].

Data indicate a comorbidity of 60% between recurrent cystitis, provoked vestibulodynia/vulvodynia, and introital dyspareunia when the woman consulted a urologist because of bladder inflammation [1–3].

Comorbidity with recurrent cystitis was lower, but still elevated (37.4%), in the largest series of vulvar pain (1183 cases) published so far in the world. The consulted physician was a gynecologist, and the reported FSD comorbidities were sexual pain/introital dyspareunia (64.0%) and vaginal dryness (29.8%) (Table 25.1).

The comorbidities emerging from this Italian observational study indicate that every physician should go beyond the limited specialistic vision to broaden his/her pathophysiological understanding of recurrent cystitis with the understanding of other etiological factors. This may translate into more timely and effective treatment, reduced number of recurrences, and comprehensive improvement of associated comorbidities.

The significant comorbidity between LUTS and sexual pain with introital dyspareunia, and between LUTS and arousal disorders with vaginal dryness has been well described since the classic epidemiological study of Laumann et al., 1999 [16] (Table 25.2).

This significant association, also proven in this study, deserves further clinical consideration.

1. Lower urinary tract symptoms can be predictors of comorbid sexual pain disorder (SPD) and arousal disorder (AD). This supports the

Table 25.1 Vulvar pain, female sexual disorders, recurrent cystitis, and comorbidities

The leading complaints to ask during gynecological consultation are as follows:
- Vulvar pain (94.1%)
  Of these patients
    - 70.8% had spontaneous or provoked vestibulodynia
    - 23.3 had generalized vulvodynia [3]
- Comorbid FSDs (93.8%)
    - 64.0% had sexual pain disorders with introital dyspareunia
    - 29.8% had severe vaginal dryness due to inadequate arousal
The leading comorbidities emerging from clinical history and examination are as follows:
- Recurrent postcoital cystitis, present in 37.4% of patients
    - 19% recurrent cystitis
    - 17.9% postcoital cystitis
- Recurrent vulvovaginitis from *Candida* spp. was reported in 32% of the patients. This is worth noting because of the following:
    - Aggressive recurrent *Candida* infections are frequently triggered by repeated antibiotic treatments
    - Vulvar vestibulitis/provoked vestibulodynia has an aberrant immune allergic reaction to *Candida* antigens, at least in this subset of patients, and is one of the most powerful etiological triggers
- Gastrointestinal comorbidities (97.4%): Relevant and usually under-investigated in these patients
    - 28.0% had irritable bowel syndrome (IBS), more than three times the Italian national data
    - 23.5% had obstructive constipations, more than twice the national figures
    - 11.7% had painful bowel voiding (often comorbid with anorectal and/or pelvic endometriosis)
    - 10.7% had hemorrhoids
    - 10.7% suffered from abdominal pain
    - 10.1% complained of comorbid food allergies
- Hyperactive pelvic floor (87.2%): The tightened, retracted, and painful elevator ani contributes to the biomechanical etiology of vulvar pain, introital dyspareunia, poor genital arousal, and recurrent post-coital cystitis. To address this, an etiological common denominator of these conditions is mandatory
- Severe menstrual pain, comorbid with endometriosis in 11.7% of the study women, may contribute to chronic pelvic pain

Table 25.2 Latent classes of FSD by risk factors with focus on SPD and AD

Predictors	Sexual pain disorders	Arousal disorders
Lower urinary tract symptoms	7.61 (4.06–14.26)	4.02 (2.75–5.89)
Emotional problems or stress	1.82 (1.05–3.13)	4.65 (3.22–6.71)

Values shown are adjusted odds ratio (95% confidence interval) [16]

recommendation that uroandrologists should routinely investigate the presence of SPD and/or AD in female urological patients, at least when they complain of recurrent post-coital cystitis.

2. Emotional factors and/or stress can be powerful predictors of AD, independent of and/or associated with LUTS.

3. Recurrent or persistent LUTS can further worsen different emotional problems, including the following:

(a) Trait and state anxiety, including performance anxiety, as most of these women suffer from fear of experiencing sexual pain again and/or having another cystitis in the following days [17, 18].

(b) Performance anxiety, which triggers acute systemic and genital vasoconstriction. In women and men, it is a powerful and underdiagnosed co-factor of arousal disorders, contributing to inadequate/absent lubrication in women, and erectile dysfunction (ED), mostly maintenance ED in men [18].

(c) Depression, which further reduces sexual drive and may contribute to arousal disorders [19].

(d) Relational issues: attachment dynamics may deserve a psychodynamic evaluation when insecure attachment is in play. It potentiates anxiety, it is a predictor of FSD and male sexual disorders (MSD), as well proven in the study by Ciocca et al. (2015), and may impair the conscious and unconscious coping strategies of the couple [20].

(e) Contribute to MSD, particularly in aging men with impending ED.

Despite this evidence, the high comorbidity between LUTS and sexual pain disorders is still under-reported by women, under-diagnosed, and under-treated by physicians. This clinical neglect may become an under-appreciated maintenance factor in the LUTS the woman is trying to improve, in addition to the FSD persistence [21].

Therefore, the analysis of the shared pathophysiology that supports comorbidity is a prerequisite for designing well-tailored therapeutic strategies rooted in a comprehensive clinical vision.

25.2.5 FSD as Predisposing/ Precipitating Factors for MSD

In parallel, MSD, such as ED, may be a predisposing and precipitating factor in FSDs. The GPPPD [14], i.e., sexual pain disorders, including the former clinical entities of dyspareunia and vaginismus and/or a clinical condition now described as GSM, are among the most powerful and neglected co-factors of MSD, particularly for couples around the fifth decade or beyond. The GSM presents with comorbid gynecological, urological, and sexual symptoms, which are well known by uroandrologists.

A man with ED can be the "symptom carrier" and his partner the "symptom inducer," or co-inducer when she is affected by severe vaginal atrophy and dryness with acquired loss of sex drive and interest, and/or she complains of introital dyspareunia with a tightened pelvic floor, which makes penetration difficult or impossible.

Facts that support the analysis of these comorbidities are the shared pathophysiology between critical aspects of GPPPD and GSM, possibility of using topical (vaginal and vulvar) treatments that combine safety and efficacy with ease of prescription and follow-up over time, and the best outcomes physicians can offer to their patients

when both partners' sexual health is well considered in the clinical setting [22].

Finally, this was the most important clinical consideration. A closer collaboration between urologists and gynecologists that both trained in sexual medicine increases the possibility of building a consultation paradigm to be transmitted and taught to our junior colleagues and residents to increase their clinical competence in addressing sexual comorbidities and underlying medical conditions in both partners. This requires substantial committed change with two consistent rewards. First, a much more satisfying clinical outcome for the individual patient and couple, from the sexual health and relational points of view. Second, there is a great reward for the physician's clinical impact factor (CIF), which is potentiated by a more comprehensive and skilled clinical approach. Synergy with other health care professionals (gastroenterologists, psychiatrists, psychosexologists, physiotherapists, and midwives trained in pelvic floor rehabilitation) is appropriate when clinically indicated.

25.2.6 Epidemiology of Sexual Pain Disorders

Sexual pain is an extremely relevant issue, given its prevalence in the population. Several epidemiological studies have estimated that 11—21% of women complain of sexual pain during their lifetime. Data from our group agree with the literature, showing that 14% of patients aged between 20 and 70 years reported sexual pain.

25.2.7 Clinical Approach to Sexual Pain Disorders

The clinical history should focus on specific characteristics of GPPPD/sexual pain disorders, investigating if sexual pain the woman complains of is [12]:

- Lifelong vs. acquired.
- Generalized vs. situational.
- Mainly driven by biological factors, psychogenic factors, or both.
- Causing personal distress to the patient or not.

25.2.8 Etiological Complexity of Sexual Pain

Every kind of pain, as well as sexual pain, has three main contributing factors such as:

- **Biological factors**: in which pain reflects the severity of tissue inflammation and damage (neurological, mucocutaneous, anorectal, muscular, vascular, endocrine, and immunitary) [23–25]. Inflammation in the peripheral tissues and nervous system (neuroinflammation) is the common denominator of all medical conditions when pain is the leading symptom [26, 27].

Life in health means trillions of physiological inflammations have been successfully carried out by the body's immune system.

Physiologic inflammation is:

- **Resolving**, i.e., finalized to restore the tissue anatomic and functional integrity ("scarless," according to English speaking researchers; with "restitutio ad integrum," i.e., to restore full tissue integrity, according to Latin physicians) [28, 29]. Emerging data on resolvins and mechanisms used by nerves to resolve persisting pain highlight the need for an update in this critical part of gynecological, urological, and sexual disorders that cause pain in women [30].
- **Of limited intensity**, sufficient to complete the process.
- **Of short duration**, adequate to restore the tissue integrity.

Pathologic inflammation is progressively

- Non-resolving.
- Of chronic duration.
- Of variable intensity, which is likely to worsen if predisposing, precipitating, and/or maintenance factors remain undiagnosed and/or inadequately addressed [31].

To address the immunitary/inflammatory component of every kind of pain, including that originating from recurrent (post coital) cystitis, bladder pain syndromes, and sexual pain disorders is a key part of the treatment strategy.

- **Psychological factors**, such as coping strategies, psychosexual history, fear of pain and its meaning, body image and feelings, presence and severity of anxiety, depression, and/or other psychological/psychiatric conditions.
- **Contextual factors**, for example, quality of family support, socioeconomic level, working conditions, meaning of pain, relational, and couple issues.

Comorbidity between recurrent (post-coital) cystitis and FSD is maintained by persistent pathologic inflammation causing increasing tissue destruction and pain on one side, and progression of the intensity and number of comorbidities on the other.

Inflammation can be worsened by psychological and contextual factors through persistent activation of the corticotrophin-releasing pathway. To address pathologic inflammation, the common denominator of many comorbidities, the FSD first associated with recurrent cystitis is key if the goal of effective treatment is to be pursued.

25.3 Pathogenic Biofilms, in the Shadow of LUTS and Sexual Pain Disorders

A specific issue in recurrent cystitis and vulvovaginitis involves the so-called "pathogenic biofilms." They can be intracellular when urothelial cells are invaded by proliferating UPECs, leading to intracellular bacterial communities (IBCs), and less frequently, by other bacteria, intra- and extra-cellularly in the vaginal mucosa [11, 32, 33].

Pathogenic biofilms are important structures in the field of medicine. They explained this as follows [34, 35]:

- Incomplete or absent response to prolonged antibiotic therapy.
- Presence of comorbid forms of antibiotic-resistant infections.

- Increased bacterial resistance to immune effectors.
- Tendency of the infection to become chronic.

Mature biofilms are complex and dynamic biostructures that create a suitable environment for bacteria and other organisms to survive and persist in. This polymicrobial community is enclosed in a self-produced extracellular matrix that adheres to inert or living surfaces, such as mucosae. Therefore, the biofilm composition is as follows: matrix (85%) and microorganisms (15%) [36, 37]. Biofilms present a primitive form of circulation, allowing the flow of water and nutrients.

Most resident human microbiotas are normally organized in biofilms; for example, *Lactobacillus* spp., together with *Bifidobacterium* and *Saccharomyces* spp., sustain homeostasis of the vaginal environment [38, 39]. They are known to have extremely important functions, such as maintaining low pH (4.5), preventing invasion by other pathogens, aiding intracellular clearance, and restoring the integrity of the vaginal epithelium by inducing the formation of tight junctions between epithelial cells [40]. Therefore, probiotics are considered to be of primary importance in the modulation of genital and sexual health.

Dysbiosis can lead to the development of pathological biofilms in which harmful bacterial species, such as *Staphylococcus aureus*, *Enterobacteriaceae*, and *Candida* spp. proliferate. In 2008, the National Institute of Health estimated that up to 80% of bacterial infections affecting humans in Western countries were caused by pathogenic biofilms [41]. In the deepest part of the biofilm structure, a subpopulation of dormant cells or persister cells is found, which is thought to be responsible for resistance to antibiotics and immune effectors, and for the restoration of the bacterial load after failed antibiotic/antimycotic therapy [42–44]. In addition to being physically inaccessible to bactericidal substances, these semi-quiescent cells engage in active exchange of plasmids bearing antibiotic resistance genes (conjugation), thereby favoring the development of intra- and inter-species resistant strains [45]. In the bladder, pathogenic bio-films act as an endogenous reservoir of pathogens that lead to chronicization of infections and a persistent state of low-grade inflammation with periodic peaks that progressively damage the sophisticated structure of the bladder wall until it is replaced by scar tissue typical of interstitial cystitis.

Importantly, new evidence shows that pathogenic biofilms can be extracellular or intracellular when bacteria reside and proliferate, forming biofilm-like structures inside the cellular environment. These are particularly relevant in the field of urogynecology (e.g., uropathogenic *E. coli*—UPEC) [46], as they are recognized triggers of recurrent vaginitis and cystitis, which are well-known comorbidities associated with sexual pain. For example, UPEC enters a cycle of attachment, invasion, and intracellular replication with the latter stages protected from external antimicrobials. Intracellular bacterial communities exfoliate together with the epithelium in which they are hosted and enter a new phase of attachment and re-infection [33].

Vaginitis is caused by polymicrobial growth sessile syndrome and is characterized by changes in the proportions of predominant bacterial and fungal strains. Modifications of the vaginal ecosystem are linked not only to vaginitis but also to the development of recurrent cystitis. Indeed, it has been observed that women with recurrent cystitis have vaginal colonization of *E. coli* during the 14 days prior to symptomatic urinary tract disease; they display an inverse relationship between the number of *E. coli* and *lactobacilli*. Therefore, we may summarize that the majority of women with recurrent vaginitis and cystitis have a pathogenic intracellular UPEC biofilm in the bladder and/or a vaginal pathogenic intra- and extracellular biofilm [43, 47].

As anticipated in the previous sections, UTIs are clearly correlated (60%) with sexual pain in the form of provoked vestibulodynia, dyspareunia, or coital pain. Epidemiological data from Laumann et al. [48] linked sexual pain disorders to LUTS with an odd ratio of 7.61. Candidiasis is also an important infectious comorbidity of sexual pain, since it triggers provoked vestibulodynia and introital dyspareunia by inducing an aberrant local immune reaction in predisposed individuals [2].

Mast cells are the main local effector cells of vestibular inflammation [49–51]. When stimulated, mast cells degranulate pro-inflammatory cytokines and nerve growth factors in the higher layers of the mucosa, inducing the proliferation of free pain nerve terminals and mediating a tenfold increase in nociceptors [51–53]. Since infectious agents, such as bacteria, can directly activate nociceptors, a vicious circle is established in which bacteria activate neurons that modulate pain and inflammation, causing hyperalgesia [51, 54].

Key Point The shift of pain from acute, nociceptive to chronic and neuropathic pain is mediated by the persistence of the pain signal. Bacteria can activate pain neurons and fibers. For this reason, clinicians must pay significant attention to the disruption of microbiotas with aggressive antibiotic therapies, as it may inadvertently intensify pain perception and comorbidities while contributing to antibiotic resistance.

25.3.1 Clinical Approach to Recurrent *Post-Coital* Cystitis and Comorbid Vestibulodynia and Sexual Pain Disorders

Careful clinical history is the gold standard to effectively address comorbidities [3, 14, 31].

Specific questions useful in clinical uroandrologist practice include the following:

- "Many women with recurrent (post-coital) cystitis suffer from sexual pain at the entrance of the vagina when they have intercourse: do you have this problem as well?"
- "If yes, what did you first suffer from: recurrent cystitis or sexual pain? Or were they both present in your sexual experiences?"
- "If yes, did you suffer from these problems, recurrent cystitis and sexual pain, from the very beginning of your sexual life, or later on?"

- If later, in your opinion, which were the most relevant factors that triggered those problems: antibiotic courses, recurrent vulvovaginal *Candida* infections, genital surgery, vaginal delivery, gastrointestinal problems and/or bowel infections, partner change with bigger genital dimensions, excessive Kegel or yoga exercises.
- "Do you feel genital pain at the entrance of the vagina (vestibulodynia) or diffuse to the external genitalia (vulvodynia)?" [55]
- "If yes, is it spontaneous or triggered by intercourse, finger stimulations, trousers, or other factors?"
- "Do you suffer as well from bowel problems, IBS constipation, and food allergies?"
- "Did these bladder and sexual problems cause or worsen anxiety and depression or cause problems in your relationship?"

During the physical examination, further questions are key in mapping pain sites, reading carefully the natural history of the specific comorbidities involved to plan a structured multimodal approach [3, 14, 31].

Where does it hurt? Notably, the localization of sexual pain is the strongest predictor of the presence and type of biological etiology involved. The clinician can use a genital figure to map the pain sites to facilitate communication with the patient.

When did the vulvar pain began?

- When vulvar pain begins during childhood, it may be provoked by trauma. This could be an unintentional trauma, such as a fall in the playground or an intentional trauma, such as abuse or genital mutilation.
- If the pain begins after puberty, the most likely reason is the administration of antibiotic treatment, exacerbating *Candida* infections, which can contribute to the development of vestibulodynia.
- If the pain began during first intercourse, it might have been a case of vaginismus.
- If it started after undergoing treatment with a contraceptive pill, vaginal dryness and a hyperactive pelvic floor might be considered.

- If pain started after changing a partner, it could be due to the dimensions of the genitalia of the new partner.
- The pain could have started after delivery, with 23% of women declaring persistent dyspareunia up to 18 months after vaginal delivery.
- After menopause because of GSM.
- After medical treatment, including surgery and laser.
- After the onset of a neurological disease.

When does it hurt?
- During foreplay and before beginning intercourse, congestion due to genital arousal can amplify the burning feelings of the already inflamed vestibule.
- At the beginning of the intercourse, when penetration can provoke/worsen microabrasions of the vestibular mucosa, and if the hyperactive elevator ani squeezes and reduces the vaginal opening and/or vaginal dryness, it contributes to mucosal vulnerability.
- After intercourse, pain provoked by microabrasions and activation of the superficialized nerve pain fibers stimulates burning feelings that may last for hours or days after intercourse.

What are the associated symptoms?
Sexual pain can be exacerbated by multiple factors that deserve cross-expertise in gynecology, urology, coloproctology, and physiotherapy. The three main factors underlying sexual pain can be summarized as follows:

- Hyperactive pelvic floor disorders, predisposing to vestibular and urethral traumas during intercourse.
- Inflammation of genital and pelvic organs (vulva, bladder, bowel, etc.) and also systemic (e.g., brain).
- Altered sexual hormone levels (and sexual hormone receptors) in the blood and tissues, driving urethral, bladder, and genital trophism.

For this reason, clinicians must be trained in sexual medicine to carefully examine the genitals, vulva, and pelvic floor under static and dynamic conditions. Better if a multi-competent health team is established. The patient's examination includes the following [3, 14, 31]:

- **The vulva**: Swab tests reveal acute pain, usually at five and seven, when looking at the entrance of the vagina as a clock face. The swab test can also elicit burning pain at six, when sub-atrophic mucosa is present or at 12. The latter is more frequently associated with bladder symptoms, such as urethralgia and/or bladder pain and is more difficult to treat and resolve.
- **The vestibular area**: Redness can be observed in the vestibular region at five and seven when labia are pulled apart, indicating an inflamed vestibule that is the anatomic basis of provoked vestibulodynia, the former "vulvar vestibulitis," where wording well indicated the inflammatory etiology of the clinical picture.
- **The perineal region**: Clinicians should measure the perineal length. The patient might have displayed a retracted centrum tendineum because the hyperactive pelvic floor pushed the anus towards the vagina. During intercourse, the tightened pubococcygeus branch of the levator ani behaved like a sling. The force vectors pushed the erected penis against the urethra and bone. The resulting urethral biomechanical trauma can activate the IBCs of the uropathogenic *Escherichia coli*, contributing to the precipitation of acute urethritis and/or cystitis.
- **The perianal area**: Pay attention to anal comorbidities, thromboses, hemorrhoids, rhagades, and inflammation. Sentinel hemorrhoids could be present at 12 or in comorbidity with obstructive constipation, suggesting an "inverted command," with the elevator ani further contraction instead of relaxation when the command of bowel voiding is given.
- **Medium and deep vagina**: Examine the tension of the pelvic floor at the insertion of the spine when the examined fingers press on it. The patient might feel a localized myalgia, the so-called "tender point" when pain is limited to the site of pression, or a kind of irradiated pain to the pelvis or labia when a more inflammated, myalgic "trigger point" is pressed. Pay

attention to the non-metameric irradiation of pain described by the patient (e.g., deep in the pelvis and/or towards the outer genitals). The deep vagina must also be examined to test for deep dyspareunia, which might indicate endometriosis or pelvic inflammatory disease, PID [3, 14, 31]. Dyspareunia and endometriosis are frequently referred to as "the evil twins."

Comorbidities could also alert and help clinicians diagnose hyperactive pelvic floor conditions [3]. Symptoms include the following:

- **Intestinal symptoms** [3]:
  - Irritable bowel syndrome.
  - Obstructive constipation, particularly when life is long. Therefore, it is important to ask patients about their bowel habits.
  - Hemorrhoids, suggestive of inverted command of the pelvic floor muscles, besides intestinal cofactors.
  - Abdominal pain.
- **Food allergies**.
- **Dyspareunia**.
- **LUTS**, e.g., post-coital cystitis.
- **Recurrent candidiasis**.

25.3.2 Multimodal Treatment Strategy

Comorbidities between **recurrent postcoital cystitis, vestibulodynia/vulvar pain, and sexual pain/introital dyspareunia** must be addressed in parallel.

The multimodal therapy must be planned strategically.

- First, the issue of the **hyperactive pelvic floor** must be addressed in a timely manner at the first visit, paying attention to posterior and/or anterior triggers. Electromyography of the levator ani in women with hyperactive pelvic floor and sexual pain symptoms clearly shows anomalous electrical activity (no electric silence), particularly when the woman is asked to strain the levator ani. Thus, the pelvic floor must be relaxed by therapeutic interventions that include the following:

  - Physiotherapy and transcutaneous electrostimulation [14, 31].
  - Pharmacological therapy: Vaginal diazepam synergizes with physiotherapy to accelerate healing. Local off-label administration of diazepam is a recognized, strategic choice in multimodal treatment of sexual pain and other urinary comorbidities caused by non-relaxing pelvic floor, while limiting systemic effects. The intra-vaginal administration of 5 mg of diazepam before bedtime reduces the hyperactivity of the levator ani muscle, helping with the physiotherapy treatment of the biomechanical etiology of vulvodynia, sexual pain, and recurrent post-coital cystitis [56, 57].
  - Teaching and training of patients to use diaphragmatic breathing, leading to pelvic floor relaxation with appropriate exercises.
- Second, **inflammation** must be addressed using multimodal anti-inflammatory therapies [14, 31]. Scientific evidence shows that locoregional inflammation is sustained by upregulated mast cells in tissues, particularly near nerve fibers, which release granules of pro-inflammatory cytokines and nerve growth factor (NGF). These substances create an appropriate milieu for the proliferation of pain fibers that mediate nociceptive and neuropathic pain. Inflammation can be reduced by aiding the healing of nerve fibers with alphalipoic acid, palmitoylethanolamide (PEA), topical testosterone, amitriptyline, and gabapentin.
- Third, reducing the aggressiveness of *Escherichia coli* with:

  - **Prevention of pathogenic biofilms**: The presence of pathogenic biofilms is a common denominator that triggers comorbid recurrent cystitis and vaginitis in women, particularly when associated with sexual pain disorders. Therefore, the therapeutic goal is to deconstruct the biofilms, exposing the germs to endogenous and exogenous antimicrobial substances to clear the infection and allow tissue repair.

One of the main strategies to interfere with biofilm formation is to prevent the first stage of adhesion to the epithelia and to facilitate detachment and elimination in urine. In the case of UPEC, adhesion can be efficiently antagonized by D-mannose, a natural monosaccharide with high affinity for *E. coli* fimbriae FimH [58, 59].

D-mannose exists in an exogenous form; in fact, it is extracted from a variety of plants (mainly wood of larch and birch) and in an endogenous form on cell surfaces and in plasma, where it is used for glycoprotein biosynthesis. From a pharmacological point of view, it can be supplemented orally because it is not metabolized and 90% is excreted in urine [60]. Therefore, D-mannose can reach the urothelium, thereby intercepting and neutralizing the adhesion of *E. coli* and other fimbriated bacteria [61, 62]. When used topically in the vagina, it prevents vaginal infections and contributes to the regeneration of the extracellular matrix by acting on fibroblasts. Clinical studies have been performed in women with acute symptomatic or chronic UTIs. Women treated with D-mannose instead of antibiotics showed delayed recurrence of 200 vs. 52,7 days [63]. In summary, D-mannose is safe and can be used to prevent infections in a prophylaxis therapy of 1 g twice a day in combination with an alkalinizing agent, such as sodium bicarbonate 250 mg for 24 weeks–6 months. Its efficacy has been estimated to be comparable to 50 mg of daily nitrofurantoin, but with fewer adverse effects [63, 64]. Interestingly, D-mannose is also safe during pregnancy and breastfeeding, making it a viable therapeutic alternative to prevent/treat UTI-vulnerable patients with UTIs.

- The strategic use of probiotics, Sects. 25.3.3 and 25.3.4, as this key aspect deserves careful discussion.

- After menopause, it is essential to treat GSM with appropriate topical treatment with estrogens, testosterone, and/or prasterone to restore vulvovaginal and bladder trophism (Sect. 25.3.5).

25.3.3 Recurrent Cystitis and Sexual Pain: What Probiotics Have to Say

The management of recurrent cystitis is highly variable within and between countries [65]. The case definition and diagnosis are not clear, as clinical and biological factors and/or overall risk factors are not considered. This results in a monolithic approach, involving iterative antibiotic treatment courses, leading to the emergence of antimicrobial-resistant bacteria and significant side-effects [66]. The risk factors for an episode of cystitis are described in [67].

The evident and marked correlation between rUTI and intestinal microenvironment requires a shift in attention to the treatment of this district and to make some important considerations.

- Uropathogenic *Escherichia coli* is responsible for 85% of rUTIs, whereas 15% are caused by *Proteus mirabilis*, *Klebsiella*, *Enterobacter*, *Enterococcus faecalis*, and others. Therefore, *E. coli* is the most dangerous enemy [68, 69].
- The germ causing cystitis comes from the colon through two contamination routes: the "exogenous" route (germs may get backward to the bladder through the urethra, if the external genitalia are contaminated with feces) and the "endogenous" route (the passage of germs from the intestinal ecosystem through the disrupted colonic wall, inside the blood, and then to the bladder wall) [70].
- Despite the fact that antibiotics are the cornerstone and are included in the guidelines for UTI management, the wide, repeated, and sometimes inappropriate use of antibiotics has led to over a threefold increase in multidrug-resistant of *E. coli* [71]. Moreover, the use of antibiotics worsens intestinal dysbiosis, which is a predisposing factor for infection recurrence.
- Altered intestinal flora (dysbiosis) may lead to the overgrowth of *Enterobacteriaceae*, the causative agents of the majority of RUTIs.
- The IBS with the associated hyperactive mast-cells in the intestinal mucosa and increased passage (translocation) of intestinal germs through the intestinal cells (leaky

gut syndrome) is a key predisposing factor to rUTIs, frequently comorbid with the IBS itself [72, 73].

- Constipation, which tends to get worse with age and menopause, is another intestinal predisposing factor since it prolongs the contact time with toxins and allergens that impair the intestinal barrier and promotes the proliferation of pathogenic germs [74, 75].

In this chapter, the role of probiotics will be considered with comprehensive attention to different predisposing and precipitating factors of recurrent cystitis, sexual pain disorders, and vulvar pain discussed above, with a special focus on the role of bowel factors.

Since dysbiosis and disruption of intestinal balance are important in the onset of rUTI, the key intestinal interventions that should be implemented to prevent rUTI include the following:

- Bowel habits were normalized through an adequate nutritional program (preferably agreed with a nutrition specialist) and an increase in daily water intake [76].
- Fighting intestinal comorbidities (and predisposing factors), such as IBS and constipation.
- Use probiotics and prebiotics to help improve the colonic ecosystem [77].

25.3.4 Probiotics to Address Dysbiosis: Which Ones, When, and Why?

Probiotics are not all the same; each strain performs specific actions.

Knowing the specific characteristics of each strain and its interaction with the host is essential to establish a "targeted therapy" using the most appropriate probiotic.

When probiotics can help:

- **In association with antibiotic therapy**: Recurrent/prolonged antibiotic courses devastate the intestinal ecosystem, causing a reduction in biodiversity, lowering immune defenses, and creating ecological gaps that

favor the selection and proliferation of pathogenic germs [78, 79]. Antibiotic-induced dysbiosis is generalized and involves both the small intestine and colon. In this case, two approaches proved to be effective.

- _Saccharomyces boulardii,_ a yeast of tropical origin that is a fungus, is not affected by the action of antibiotics. Administered orally, it does not colonize and does not replace the intestinal flora, but transits by carrying out antimicrobial, anti-secretory, anti-toxin, and immunomodulatory activities [80].
- Symbiotics: These products, consisting of a combination of probiotics (preferably multi-strain) and prebiotics, have shown that if administered in association with antibiotics, they are able to counteract the general dysbiosis generated by the drug, preventing all related side effects. Symbiotics, therefore, act as "intestinal protectors," counteracting the proliferation of pathogenic germs and selection of resistant strains [81, 82].
- **For IBS patients**: A recent meta-analysis summarized the effects of probiotics in the treatment of IBS [83]. This paper underlines that probiotics bring significant, albeit partial, benefits in the therapy of IBS (especially on global symptoms), although at the moment, it is not clear which species/strains are the most effective. The therapeutic choice of periodic changes in probiotic strains is considered appropriate for restoring, respecting, and maintaining the biodiversity of the bowel microbiota.
- **To fight constipation**: Adults with functional constipation have significantly decreased numbers of Bifidobacteria and _Lactobacilli_ in stool samples, as well as higher breath methane, compared to control subjects [84, 85].

Probiotics appear to have beneficial effects on chronic idiopathic constipation, and a recent meta-analysis suggested that probiotic supplementation is moderately efficacious in decreasing intestinal transit times compared with the control [83], which has been attributed to the capacity of probiotics to alter the

GI microflora, improve intestinal motility, and alter biochemical factors. These properties have been observed in *Lactobacillus* and *Bifidobacterium* species, and several traits of **Bifidobacterium animalis subsp. lactis HN019** (HN019) have been studied with regard to its probiotic activity, such as its identity, safety, antipathogenic effects, immune enhancement, and intestinal colonization [86].

The end products of bacterial fermentation can also affect gut motility. In particular, lactic acid and SCFA produced by the fermentation of soluble fibers, such as **inulin** (prebiotics) reduce colonic pH, promote intestinal contractility, and reactivate the propulsive activity of the colon [87, 88].

Furthermore, the supernatant from *Escherichia coli* **Nissle 1917** increased the maximal tension forces of smooth muscle from the human colon in an in vitro study, although blockage of enteric nerves abolished these effects, suggesting that *E. coli Nissle* may potentially influence contractility by direct stimulation of smooth muscle cells. This effect was not attributed to fermentation end products, such as SCFAs, but to other unidentified contractility-enhancing agents [89].

- **To enhance the immune system**: The gut-associated lymphoid tissue (GALT) represents about 80% of the immune system of our organism and is strongly influenced by the intestinal microbiota. Probiotics in general, and some *lactobacilli* strains in particular, have an immunostimulatory action that guarantees the correct and effective activation of our body's defenses.
- **To restore intestinal barrier**: Microbiota dysbiosis can impair the epithelial barrier, leading to the so-called "leaky gut," allowing the intestinal content to be in contact with the host periphery potentially inducing inflammatory responses. Many probiotics may exert a protective effect on barrier function, which is achieved by preventing the colonization of pathogens, interacting directly with host enterocytes, and metabolizing undigested carbohydrates to short-chain fatty acids. New

commensal species are being isolated and used for therapeutic purposes, as so-called next-generation probiotics, alongside *Lactobacilli* and *Bifidobacteria*, which have a long history of use as probiotics. Among these new probiotics, *Akkermansia muciniphila* was found to have a positive effect on intestinal integrity and restoration of the mucus layer thickness. Unfortunately, *A. muciniphila* is a strictly anaerobic Gram-negative strain; therefore, it is very difficult to produce and market on a large scale [90].

A peculiar case in the management of recurrent cystitis is that of *Escherichia coli* **Nissle 1917 (EcN)**, a Gram-negative strain isolated in 1917 by Prof. Alfred Nissle, from whom it took its name. Although this bacterium belongs to the *E. coli* family, it is absolutely safe and shows interesting beneficial activities for which it should be considered a "probiotic drug."

The strain-specific effects of EcN are as follows:

1. **Antimicrobial effect**: According to its genotypic and phenotypic characteristics, EcN is the only one able to directly counteract pathogenic strains of *E. coli* by competing with them for nutrients and colonization of the mucosa [91, 92]. Interestingly, antibacterial action is also carried out directly through the production of microcins, and indirectly by stimulating the release of defensins by the colonic epithelium, both substances with bactericidal activity [93, 94]. Additionally, several randomized clinical studies have shown that EcN is effective in reducing the severity of rotavirus diarrhea and modulating viral immunity [95].

2. **Strengthening of the intestinal barrier**: EcN increases the expression of tight junction proteins (ZO1, ZO2, and occludin), restoring the integrity and permeability of the intestinal barrier disrupted by infections and/or inflammation [96]. The consequence for clinical practice is that the EcN strain allows to counteract the "leaky gut syndrome"; thus, effectively blocking bacterial translocation [97].

This can reduce the vulnerability to UPEC infections in the vagina and bladder and reduce the critical comorbidity between bowel disorders and vulvar pain, leading to the etiology of associated sexual pain.

3. **Anti-inflammatory and analgesic action**: By a direct cross-talk with the intestinal epithelium cells, EcN stimulates the production of anti-inflammatory cytokine IL-10 and inhibits the synthesis and release of proinflammatory cytokines (IL-12, IL2, IL-5, IL4, TNF-α, and IFN-γ) and prostaglandin E2 (PGE2) [98, 99]. Furthermore, EcN produces an analgesic lipopeptide capable of crossing the epithelial barrier and inhibiting the activation of nociceptors in sensory neurons [100]. These features result in an anti-inflammatory power comparable to that of a drug (mesalazine), which is essential for reducing the latent chronic inflammatory state, with mast cell proliferation and hyperstimulation of pain sensory neurons caused by chronic recurrence and often with a high frequency of infections. Therefore, the EcN could actively contribute to reducing visceral pain associated with RC and IBS, but related as well to vulvodynia and chronic pelvic pain [101, 102].

Finally, the EcN is a safe product that does not contain any pathogenic factors, does not produce enterotoxins, and does not confer resistance to antibiotics. The EcN has been used for more than 100 years in adults, children, and pregnant women.

25.3.5 Role of Topical Sexual Hormones to Address Cystitis Associated with GSM

The post-menopausal phase of women's life is characterized by a decrease in the production of sexual hormones [14, 31, 103–105]. Testosterone and dehydroepiandrosterone mediate essential aspects of women's health; they peak around 20 years of age and then decrease progressively [105].

At the time of physiologic menopause, women lose, on average, 50% of their testosterone, and 60–70% of their DHEA. Testosterone loss reached 80% in bilateral ovariectomy. The estradiol and progesterone levels disappeared after menopause. Androgenic loss dramatically potentiates the negative effects of estrogen and progesterone. Androgens are far more represented in women's body than estradiol (with the exception of pregnancy) TAB Lobo, 1999 Courtesy of Rogerio Lobo, 2000. Women's genital organs, urethra, bladder, and pelvic floor muscles are extremely rich in testosterone receptors that modulate different aspects of tissue health [106–108].

The loss of sexual hormones increases the vulnerability of the bladder trigonus, urethra, vestibulum, and vagina to biomechanical trauma during intercourse. The vestibular and vaginal mucosae and urethral urothelium are progressively weakened and made thin by inflammation triggered by menopausal hormone loss, aging, and the intracellular pathogenic biofilm themselves.

This vulnerability is potentiated by the presence of an intact pelvic floor (typical of nulliparous women or women who delivered by cesarean sections) [14, 31, 55]. After menopause, the elevator ani muscle fibers progressively shorten and are replaced by collagen fibers of poor quality. This further reduces the diameter of the vaginal entrance diameter, causing vestibular mucosal microabrasions, local inflammation with a hyperactive pelvic floor, and sexual pain at the beginning of vaginal penetration.

Systemic effect of hormone deficiency leads to hallmark microbiological manifestations, such as dysbiosis of the bowel and vaginal microbiota, with increased vulnerability to colonization from colonic germs and pathogenic biofilm formation, predisposing to vaginal, urinary, and sexual pathologies.

Genital pain is a powerful reflex inhibitor of genital arousal and of vaginal lubrication, in a vicious circle. This worsens the defensive hyperactivity of the pelvic floor while increasing the vulnerability of the vestibule, vagina, and urethra to microabrasions, secondary to biomechanical trauma, which is further amplified by the loss of sexual hormones and reduced/absent lubrication.

During vaginal penetration, the tightened pubococcygeus muscle pushes the erected penis against the urethra and pubic symphysis. This causes biomechanical trauma of the urethra and triggers the multiplication and aggressiveness of intracellular pathogenic biofilms, which are more severe in cases of severe vaginal atrophy and hyperactive pelvic floor.

Strategies to reduce GSM aim to improve urogenital trophism and vaginal lubrication while reducing introital sexual pain and post-coital-cystitis/urethralgia [22]. These include, but are not limited to, different hormonal therapies administered directly to the vulva and vagina.

- Topical vaginal estrogens (estradiol, estriol, and promestriene) that significantly improve vaginal and urethral trophism, vaginal microbiota, vessel responsiveness, and vaginal lubrication while reducing genital dryness and vaginal dysbiosis.
- Topical vaginal prasterone (TVP), a synthetic DHEA, has been approved worldwide [109–114]. Its trophic impact, limited to vaginal/urethral tissues, could be of special interest to uroandrologists. The ovules, applied in the vagina every night, every other night, according to the severity of the atrophy, at bedtime, significantly improve lubrication while decreasing the introital and bladder/urethral inflammation and sexual pain [109].
- Topical vulvar and vaginal testosterone of vegetal origin. Increasing evidence indicates the powerful impact of testosterone on women's health [115, 116].
- Specifically, in contrasting many aspects of GSM. Ambivalences and "unproven concerns" have prevented specific recommendations on its use, with the exception of the therapy of hypoactive sexual desire disorders [116–119]. However, off-label use is increasing worldwide, given the positive feedback women report to their physicians. Topical testosterone cream improves vulvovaginal trophism. It improves the responsiveness of vaginal nitrergic fibers (1/3). The other two-thirds are vipergic fibers and require estradiol as a permitting factor. Application of the

woman's finger to the upper part of the vagina improves trophism of the urethra corpus spongiosum (equivalent to the male). When well engorged and congested, the urethral corpus spongiosum behaves as a dynamic "air bag" that protects the urethra from further biomechanical trauma at penetration, thereby reducing the biomechanical component of recurrent post-coital cystitis. In the clinical setting, androgens are increasingly considered powerful therapeutic agents for the treatment of GSM and associated comorbidities [120].

- As a useful prohormone in women to restore age-related loss and associated symptoms that contribute to the systemic and urogenital effects of testosterone loss, DHEA is increasingly appreciated [121, 122].

The uroandrologist can recommend topical hormonal treatment to post-menopausal women using different approaches, including:

- Refer the patient to a gynecologist, possibly working in a sexual medicine team or at least well-trained in sexual medicine.
- To personally treat the patient and prescribe different hormonal options. It is mandatory to have a recent mammography, pelvic ultrasonography, and a paper smear to exclude potential lesions that contraindicate the treatment and require immediate attention to potentiate the woman's confidence and outcomes.

Targeted antibiotics should be used in selected cases of severe hemorrhagic cystitis and/or in patients who do not respond to the above-mentioned first-line preventive treatment. New paradigms and specific urological therapies are to be decided on the individual patient.

25.4 Conclusions

Sexual pain/penetration disorders are often comorbid with spontaneous or provoked vestibulodynia and recurrent and/or post-coital cystitis. The accurate diagnosis of common etiopathological denominators can provide uroandrologists the opportunity to address and treat recurrent cystitis and associated comorbidities with a more timely and effective multimodal strategy.

Key management points include relaxation of the hyperactive pelvic floor, which is responsible for the biomechanical etiology of introital sexual pain, associated vestibulodynia, and post-coital cystitis. Physiotherapy, electromyographic biofeedback, and vaginal diazepam can progressively reduce pelvic floor hyperactivity with progressive reduction of sexual pain, vestibulodynia, and comorbid post-coital cystitis.

Active prevention of *Escherichia coli* aggressiveness through modulation of pathogenic biofilms is essential. D-mannose is increasingly used because of its biomechanical action, which is useful in long-term treatments without causing resistance. Owing to its safety profile, it can be used during pregnancy and breastfeeding.

A competent use of probiotics can modulate intestinal and vaginal dysbiosis; thus, reducing the predisposing role of gastrointestinal factors in the pathophysiology of recurrent cystitis and vestibulodynia/vulvar. Among the many available probiotics, EcN has the best documented evidence of a specific role in fighting against UPEC. However, changing the choice of probiotics over time is key to maintaining the biodiversity of bowel and vaginal microbiota.

After menopause, the topical use of sexual hormones (estrogen, prasterone, and testosterone) can effectively address GSM and the associated pathophysiological factors contributing to sexual pain and recurrent cystitis.

With a strategic vision, the comorbidity between sexual pain-penetration disorders, vulvar pain, and recurrent cystitis can be more effectively addressed. This translates into better outcomes in the urological, gynecological, and sexual domains with higher satisfaction among women, couples, and caring uroandrologists.

References

1. Boeri L, Capogrosso P, Ventimiglia E, Scano R, Graziottin A, Dehò F, Montanari E, Montorsi F, Salonia A. Six out of ten women with recurrent urinary tract infections complain of distressful sexual dysfunction—a case-control study. Sci Rep. 2017;7:44380. https://doi.org/10.1038/srep44380.

2. Salonia A, Clementi MC, Graziottin A, Nappi RE, Castiglione F, Ferrari M, Capitanio U, Damiano R, Montorsi F. Secondary provoked vestibulodynia in sexually active women with uncomplicated recurrent urinary tract infections. J Sex Med. 2013;10:2265–73.

3. Graziottin A, Murina F, Gambini D, Taraborrelli S, Gardella B, Campo M. Vulvar pain: the revealing scenario of leading comorbidities in 1183 cases. Eur J Obstet Gynecol Reprod Biol. 2020;252:50–5.

4. Mili N, Paschou SA, Armeni A, Georgopoulos N, Goulis DG, Lambrinoudaki I. Genitourinary syndrome of menopause: a systematic review on prevalence and treatment. Menopause. 2021;28:706–16.

5. Portman DJ, Gass MLS, Kingsberg S, et al. Genitourinary syndrome of menopause: new terminology for vulvovaginal atrophy from the international society for the study of women's sexual health and the north American menopause society. J Sex Med. 2014;11:2865–72.

6. American Psychiatric Association. Diagnostic and statistical manual of mental disorders. 4th ed. Arlington, VA: American Psychiatric Association; 2000.

7. American Psychiatric Association. Diagnostic and statistical manual of mental disorders. 5th ed. Arlington, VA: American Psychiatric Association; 2013.

8. World Health Organization (WHO). International statistical classification of diseases and related health problems. 11th ed. Geneva: WHO; 2019.

9. Bornstein J, Goldstein AT, Stockdale CK, Bergeron S, Pukall C, Zolnoun D, Coady D. 2015 ISSVD, ISSWSH and IPPS consensus terminology and classification of persistent vulvar pain and vulvodynia. Obstet Gynecol. 2016;127:745–51.

10. McKertich K, Hanegbi U. Recurrent UTIs and cystitis symptoms in women. Aust J Gen Pract. 2021;50:199–205.

11. Anderson GG, Dodson KW, Hooton TM, Hultgren SJ. Intracellular bacterial communities of uropathogenic Escherichia coli in urinary tract pathogenesis. Trends Microbiol. 2004;12:424–30.

12. Parish SJ, Cottler-Casanova S, Clayton AH, McCabe MP, Coleman E, Reed GM. The evolution of the female sexual disorder/dysfunction definitions, nomenclature, and classifications: a review of DSM, ICSM, ISSWSH, and ICD. Sex Med Rev. 2021;9:36–56.

13. Burri A, Hilpert P, Williams F. Pain catastrophizing, fear of pain, and depression and their association with female sexual pain. J Sex Med. 2020;17:279–88.

14. Graziottin A, Gambini D. Evaluation of genitopelvic pain penetration disorder. In: The textbook of clinical sexual medicine. Cham: Springer; 2017. p. 289–304.

15. Palacios S. Androgens and female sexual function. Maturitas. 2007;57:61–5.
16. Laumann EO, Paik A, Rosen RC. Sexual dysfunction in the United States: prevalence and predictors. JAMA. 1999;281:537–44.
17. Knowles KA, Olatunji BO. Specificity of trait anxiety in anxiety and depression: meta-analysis of the state-trait anxiety inventory. Clin Psychol Rev. 2020;82:101928. https://doi.org/10.1016/j.cpr.2020.101928.
18. Pyke RE. Sexual performance anxiety. J Sex Med. 2020;8:183–90.
19. Basson R, Gilks T. Women's sexual dysfunction associated with psychiatric disorders and their treatment. Women Health. 2018;14:1745506518762664. https://doi.org/10.1177/1745506518762664.
20. Ciocca G, Limoncin E, Di Tommaso S, et al. Attachment styles and sexual dysfunctions: a case-control study of female and male sexuality. Int J Impot Res. 2015;27:81–5.
21. Kagan R, Kellogg-Spadt S, Parish SJ. Practical treatment considerations in the management of genitourinary syndrome of menopause. Drugs Aging. 2019;36:897–908.
22. Faubion SS, Kingsberg SA, Clark AL, et al. The 2020 genitourinary syndrome of menopause position statement of the North American Menopause Society. Menopause. 2020;27:976–92.
23. Orr N, Wahl K, Joannou A, Hartmann D, Valle L, Yong P, Babb C, Kramer CW, Kellogg-Spadt S, Renzelli-Cain RI. Deep dyspareunia: review of pathophysiology and proposed future research priorities. Sex Med Rev. 2020;8:3–17.
24. Van Lankveld JJDM, Granot M, Weijmar Schultz WCM, Binik YM, Wesselmann U, Pukall CF, Bohm-Starke N, Achtrari C. Women's sexual pain disorders. J Sex Med. 2010;7:615–31.
25. Kao A, Binik YM, Kapuscinski A, Khalifé S. Dyspareunia in postmenopausal women: a critical review. Pain Res Manag. 2008;13:243–54.
26. Benatti C, Blom MCJ, Rigillo G, Alboni S, Zizzi F, Torta R, Brunello N, Tascedda F. Disease-induced neuroinflammation and depression. CNS Neurol Disord-Drug Targets. 2016;15:414–33.
27. Soriano A, Andy U, Hassani D, Whitmore K, Harvie H, Malykhina AP, Arya L. Relationship of bladder pain with clinical and urinary markers of neuroinflammation in women with urinary urgency without urinary incontinence. Female Pelvic Med Reconstr Surg. 2021;27:E418–22.
28. Saito-Sasaki N, Sawada Y, Nakamura M. Maresin-1 and inflammatory disease. Int J Mol Sci. 2022;23(3):1367. https://doi.org/10.3390/ijms23031367.
29. Abdolmaleki F, Kovanen PT, Mardani R, Gheibi-hayat SM, Bo S, Sahebkar A. Resolvins: emerging players in autoimmune and inflammatory diseases. Clin Rev Allergy Immunol. 2020;58:82–91.
30. van der Vlist M, Raoof R, Willemen HLDM, et al. Macrophages transfer mitochondria to sensory neurons to resolve inflammatory pain. Neuron. 2022;110:613–626.e9.
31. Graziottin A, Gambini D, Bertolasi L. Genital and sexual pain in women. In: Vodusek D, Boller F, editors. Neurology of sexual and bladder disorders: handbook of clinical neurology, vol. 130. 3rd ed. Amsterdam: Elsevier; 2015. p. 395–412.
32. Harriott MM, Lilly EA, Rodriguez TE, Fidel PL, Noverr MC. Candida albicans forms biofilms on the vaginal mucosa. Microbiology. 2010;156:3635–44.
33. Rosen DA, Hooton TM, Stamm WE, Humphrey PA, Hultgren SJ. Detection of intracellular bacterial communities in human urinary tract infection. PLoS Med. 2007;4:1949–58.
34. Hall CW, Mah TF. Molecular mechanisms of biofilm-based antibiotic resistance and tolerance in pathogenic bacteria. FEMS Microbiol Rev. 2017;41:276–301.
35. Vuotto C, Longo F, Pascolini C, Donelli G, Balice MP, Libori MF, Tiracchia V, Salvia A, Varaldo PE. Biofilm formation and antibiotic resistance in Klebsiella pneumoniae urinary strains. J Appl Microbiol. 2017;123:1003–18.
36. McCrate OA, Zhou X, Reichhardt C, Cegelski L. Sum of the parts: composition and architecture of the bacterial extracellular matrix. J Mol Biol. 2013;425:4286–94.
37. Hobley L, Harkins C, MacPhee CE, Stanley-Wall NR. Giving structure to the biofilm matrix: an overview of individual strategies and emerging common themes. FEMS Microbiol Rev. 2015;39:649.
38. Freitas AC, Hill JE. Quantification, isolation and characterization of Bifidobacterium from the vaginal microbiomes of reproductive aged women. Anaerobe. 2017;47:145–56.
39. Donders GGG, Bellen G, Ruban KS. Abnormal vaginal microbioma is associated with severity of localized provoked vulvodynia. Role of aerobic vaginitis and Candida in the pathogenesis of vulvodynia. Eur J Clin Microbiol Infect Dis. 2018;37:1679–85.
40. Godha K, Tucker KM, Biehl C, Archer DF, Mirkin S. Human vaginal pH and microbiota: an update. Gynecol Endocrinol. 2018;34:451–5.
41. Jamal M, Ahmad W, Andleeb S, Jalil F, Imran M, Nawaz MA, Hussain T, Ali M, Rafiq M, Kamil MA. Bacterial biofilm and associated infections. J Chin Med Assoc. 2018;81:7–11.
42. Fisher RA, Gollan B, Helaine S. Persistent bacterial infections and persister cells. Nat Rev Microbiol. 2017;15:453–64.
43. Graziottin A, Zanello RP, D'Errico G. Cistiti e vaginiti recidivanti: ruolo dei biofilm e delle persister cells. Dalla fisiopatologia a nuove strategie terapeutiche. Minerva Ginecol. 2014;66:497–512.
44. Paraje MG. Persist and triumph: persistent cells in microbial biofilm. Rev Argent Microbiol. 2018;50:231–3.
45. Stalder T, Top E. Plasmid transfer in biofilms: a perspective on limitations and opportunities. NPJ Biofilms Microbiomes. 2016;2:16022.

46. Mirzaei R, Mohammadzadeh R, Sholeh M, et al. The importance of intracellular bacterial biofilm in infectious diseases. Microb Pathog. 2020;147:104393. https://doi.org/10.1016/j.micpath.2020.104393.

47. Graziottin A, Zanello PP. Pathogenic biofilms: their role in recurrent cystitis and vaginitis (with focus on D-mannose as a new prophylactic strategy). In: Studd J, Seang LT, Chervenak FA, editors. Current progress in obstetrics and gynaecology, vol. 3. 2nd ed. Mumbai: Kothari Medical; 2015. p. 218–38.

48. Laumann EO, Paik A, Rosen RC. Sexual dysfunction in the United States. JAMA. 1999;281:537.

49. Halperin R, Zehavi S, Vaknin Z, Ben-Ami I, Pansky M, Schneider D. The major histopathologic characteristics in the vulvar Vestibulitis syndrome. Gynecol Obstet Invest. 2005;59:75–9.

50. Papoutsis D, Haefner HK, Crum CP, Opipari AW, Reed BD. Vestibular mast cell density in vulvodynia: a case-controlled study. J Low Genit Tract Dis. 2016;20:275–9.

51. Bornstein J, Goldschmid N, Sabo E. Hyperinnervation and mast cell activation may be used as histopathologic diagnostic criteria for vulvar vestibulitis. Gynecol Obstet Invest. 2004;58:171–8.

52. Bohm-Starke N, Hilliges M, Falconer C, Rylander E. Neurochemical characterization of the vestibular nerves in women with vulvar vestibulitis syndrome. Gynecol Obstet Invest. 1999;48:270–5.

53. Bohm-Starke N, Hilliges M, Falconer C, Rylander E. Increased intraepithelial innervation in women with vulvar Vestibulitis syndrome. Gynecol Obstet Invest. 1998;46:256–60.

54. Bohm-Starke N, Falconer C, Rylander E, Hilliges M. The expression of cyclooxygenase 2 and inducible nitric oxide synthase indicates no active inflammation in vulvar vestibulitis. Acta Obstet Gynecol Scand. 2001;80:638–44.

55. Graziottin A, Murina F. Vulvar pain: from childhood to old age. 1st ed. Berlin: Springer Nature; 2017.

56. Crisp CC, Vaccaro CM, Estanol MV, Oakley SH, Kleeman SD, Fellner AN, Pauls RN. Intra-vaginal diazepam for high-tone pelvic floor dysfunction: a randomized placebo-controlled trial. Int Urogynecol J. 2013;24:1915–23.

57. Murina F, Felice R, Di Francesco S, Oneda S. Vaginal diazepam plus transcutaneous electrical nerve stimulation to treat vestibulodynia: a randomized controlled trial. Eur J Obstet Gynecol Reprod Biol. 2018;228:148–53.

58. Kyriakides R, Jones P, Somani BK. Role of D-mannose in the prevention of recurrent urinary tract infections: evidence from a systematic review of the literature. Eur Urol Focus. 2021;7:1166–9.

59. Lenger SM, Bradley MS, Thomas DA, Bertolet MH, Lowder JL, Sutcliffe S. D-mannose vs other agents for recurrent urinary tract infection prevention in adult women: a systematic review and meta-analysis. Am J Obstet Gynecol. 2020;223:265.e1–265.e13.

60. Sharma V, Freeze HH. Mannose efflux from the cells: a potential source of mannose in blood. J Biol Chem. 2011;286:10193–200.

61. Denda M. Effects of topical application of aqueous solutions of hexoses on epidermal permeability barrier recovery rate after barrier disruption. Exp Dermatol. 2011;20:943–4.

62. Sharon N. Carbohydrates as future anti-adhesion drugs for infectious diseases. Biochim Biophys Acta. 2006;1760:527–37.

63. Porru D, Parmigiani A, Tinelli C, et al. Oral D-mannose in recurrent urinary tract infections in women: a pilot study. J Clin Urol. 2014;7:208–13.

64. Kranjčec B, Papeš D, Altarac S. D-mannose powder for prophylaxis of recurrent urinary tract infections in women: a randomized clinical trial. World J Urol. 2014;32:79–84.

65. Haslund JMQ, Rosborg Dinesen M, Sternhagen Nielsen AB, Llor C, Bjerrum L. Different recommendations for empiric first-choice antibiotic treatment of uncomplicated urinary tract infections in Europe. Scand J Prim Health Care. 2013;31:235–40.

66. Julien A. Recurrent cystisis: no medicine preventive means. Prog Urol. 2017;27:823–30.

67. Ben Hadj Messaoud S, Demonchy E, Mondain V. Recurring cystitis: how can we do our best to help patients help themselves? Antibiotics. 2022;11:269.

68. Hannan TJ, Mysorekar IU, Hung CS, Isaacson-Schmid ML, Hultgren SJ. Early severe inflammatory responses to uropathogenic E. coli predispose to chronic and recurrent urinary tract infection. PLoS Pathog. 2010;6:29–30.

69. Mulvey MA, Schilling JD, Hultgren SJ. Establishment of a persistent Escherichia coli reservoir during the acute phase of a bladder infection. Infect Immun. 2001;69:4572–9.

70. Graziottin A. Recurrent cystitis after intercourse: why the gynaecologist has a say. In: Studd J, Seang LT, Chervenak FA, editors. Current progress in obstetrics and gynaecology, vol. Vol. 2. Mumbai: TreeLife Media; 2014. p. 319–36.

71. Laxminarayan R, Duse A, Wattal C, et al. Antibiotic resistance-the need for global solutions. Lancet Infect Dis. 2013;13:1057–98.

72. Donskey CJ. The role of die intestinal tract as a reservoir and source for transmission of nosocomial pathogens. Clin Infect Dis. 2004;39:219–26.

73. Rescigno M. The intestinal epithelial barrier in the control of homeostasis and immunity. Trends Immunol. 2011;32:256–64.

74. Grundy L, Brierley SM. Cross-organ sensitization between the colon and bladder: to pee or not to pee? Am J Physiol Gastrointest Liver Physiol. 2018;314:G301–8.

75. Kaplan SA, Dmochowski R, Cash BD, Kopp ZS, Berriman SJ, Khullar V. Systematic review of the relationship between bladder and bowel function: implications for patient management. Int J Clin Pract. 2013;67:205–16.

76. Shaughnessy AF. Increased water intake decreases UTI recurrence in women. Am Fam Physician. 2019;99(6):Online. PMID: 30874417

77. Gerritsen J, Smidt H, Rijkers GT, De Vos WM. Intestinal microbiota in human health and

disease: the impact of probiotics. Genes Nutr. 2011;6:209–40.

78. Lange K, Buerger M, Stallmach A, Bruns T. Effects of antibiotics on gut microbiota. Dig Dis. 2016;34:260–8.

79. Vangay P, Ward T, Gerber JS, Knights D. Antibiotics, pediatric dysbiosis, and disease. Cell Host Microbe. 2015;17:553–64.

80. Szajewska H, Kołodziej M. Systematic review with meta-analysis: saccharomyces boulardii in the prevention of antibiotic-associated diarrhoea. Aliment Pharmacol Ther. 2015;42:793–801.

81. Mekonnen SA, Merenstein D, Fraser CM, Marco ML. Molecular mechanisms of probiotic prevention of antibiotic-associated diarrhea. Curr Opin Biotechnol. 2020;61:226–34.

82. De Bortoli N, Leonardi G, Ciancia E, et al. Helicobacter pylori eradication: a randomized prospective study of triple therapy versus triple therapy plus lactoferrin and probiotics. Am J Gastroenterol. 2007;102:951–6.

83. Ford AC, Quigley EMM, Lacy BE, Lembo AJ, Saito YA, Schiller LR, Soffer EE, Spiegel BMR, Moayyedi P. Efficacy of prebiotics, probiotics, and synbiotics in irritable bowel syndrome and chronic idiopathic constipation: systematic review and meta-analysis. Am J Gastroenterol. 2014;109:1547–62.

84. Dimidi E, Christodoulides S, Scott SM, Whelan K. Mechanisms of action of probiotics and the gastrointestinal microbiota on gut motility and constipation. Adv Nutr. 2017;8:484–94.

85. Barichella M, Pacchetti C, Bolliri C, et al. Probiotics and prebiotic fiber for constipation associated with Parkinson disease. Neurology. 2016;87:1274–80.

86. Sanders ME. Summary of probiotic activities of Bifidobacterium lactis HN019. J Clin Gastroenterol. 2006;40:776–83.

87. Marteau P, Jacobs H, Cazaubiel M, Signoret C, Prevel JM, Housez B. Effects of chicory inulin in constipated elderly people: a double-blind controlled trial. Int J Food Sci Nutr. 2011;62:164–70.

88. Agostoni C, Berni Canani R, Fairweather-Tait S, et al. Scientific opinion on the substantiation of a health claim related to "native chicory inulin" and maintenance of normal defecation by increasing stool frequency pursuant to article 13.5 of regulation (EC) no 1924/2006. EFSA J. 2015;13:3951.

89. Bär F, Von Koschitzky H, Roblick U, Bruch HP, Schulze L, Sonnenborn U, Böttner M, Wedel T. Cell-free supernatants of Escherichia coli Nissle 1917 modulate human colonic motility: evidence from an in vitro organ bath study. Neurogastroenterol Motil. 2009;21(5):559–66. https://doi.org/10.1111/j.1365-2982.2008.01258.x.

90. Hiippala K, Jouhten H, Ronkainen A, Hartikainen A, Kainulainen V, Jalanka J, Satokari R. The potential of gut commensals in reinforcing intestinal barrier function and alleviating inflammation. Nutrients. 2018;10(8):988. https://doi.org/10.3390/nu10080988.

91. Reissbrodt R, Hammes WP, Dal Bello F, Prager R, Fruth A, Hantke K, Rakin A, Starcic-Erjavec M, Williams PH. Inhibition of growth of Shiga toxin-producing Escherichia coli by nonpathogenic Escherichia coli. FEMS Microbiol Lett. 2009;290:62–9.

92. Leatham MP, Banerjee S, Autieri SM, Mercado-Lubo R, Conway T, Cohen PS. Precolonized human commensal Escherichia coli strains serve as a barrier to E. coli O157:H7 growth in the streptomycin-treated mouse intestine. Infect Immun. 2009;77:2876–86.

93. Kleta S, Nordhoff M, Tedin K, Wieler LH, Kolenda R, Oswald S, Oelschlaeger TA, Bleiß W, Schierack P. Role of F1C fimbriae, flagella, and secreted bacterial components in the inhibitory effect of probiotic Escherichia coli Nissle 1917 on atypical enteropathogenic E. coli infection. Infect Immun. 2014;82:1801–12.

94. Schlee M, Wehkamp J, Altenhoefer A, Oelschlaeger TA, Stange EF, Fellermann K. Induction of human β-defensin 2 by the probiotic Escherichia coli Nissle 1917 is mediated through flagellin. Infect Immun. 2007;75:2399–407.

95. Henker J, Laass M, Blokhin BM, Bolbot YK, Maydannik VG, Elze M, Wolff C, Schulze J. The probiotic Escherichia coli strain Nissle 1917 (EcN) stops acute diarrhoea in infants and toddlers. Eur J Pediatr. 2007;166:311–8.

96. Barbaro MR, Fuschi D, Cremon C, Carapelle M, Dino P, Marcellini MM, Dothel G, De Ponti F, Stanghellini V, Barbara G. Escherichia coli Nissle 1917 restores epithelial permeability alterations induced by irritable bowel syndrome mediators. Neurogastroenterol Motil. 2018:e13388. https://doi.org/10.1111/nmo.13388.

97. Ukena SN, Singh A, Dringenberg U, et al. Probiotic Escherichia coli Nissle 1917 inhibits leaky gut by enhancing mucosal integrity. PLoS One. 2007;2:1308.

98. Helwig U, Lammers KM, Rizzello F, et al. Lactobacilli, bifidobacteria and E. coli nissle induce pro- and anti-inflammatory cytokines in peripheral blood mononuclear cells. World J Gastroenterol. 2006;12:5978–86.

99. Otte JM, Mahjurian-Namari R, Brand S, Werner I, Schmidt WE, Schmitz F. Probiotics regulate the expression of COX-2 in intestinal epithelial cells. Nutr Cancer. 2009;61:103–13.

100. Pérez-Berezo T, Pujo J, Martin P, et al. Identification of an analgesic lipopeptide produced by the probiotic Escherichia coli strain Nissle. Nat Commun. 2017;8(1):1314. https://doi.org/10.1038/s41467-017-01403-9.

101. Chalmers KJ, Madden VJ, Hutchinson MR, Moseley GL. Local and systemic inflammation in localized, provoked Vestibulodynia. Obstet Gynecol. 2016;128:337–47.

102. Graziottin A, Skaper SD, Fusco M. Mast cells in chronic inflammation, pelvic pain and depression in women. Gynecol Endocrinol. 2014;30:472–7.

103. Bianchi VE, Bresciani E, Meanti R, Rizzi L, Omeljaniuk RJ, Torsello A. The role of androgens in women's health and wellbeing. Pharmacol Res. 2021;171:105758. https://doi.org/10.1016/J.PHRS.2021.105758.

104. Davis SR, Wahlin-Jacobsen S. Testosterone in women-the clinical significance. Lancet Diabetes Endocrinol. 2015;3(12):980–92. https://doi.org/10.1016/S2213-8587(15)00284-3.

105. Davison SL, Bell R, Donath S, Montalto JG, Davis SR. Androgen levels in adult females: changes with age, menopause, and oophorectomy. J Clin Endocrinol Metab. 2005;90:3847–53.

106. Mason DM, Friedensohn S, Weber CR, Jordi C, Wagner B, Meng S, Gainza P, Correia B, Reddy ST. Deep learning enables therapeutic antibody optimization in mammalian cells by deciphering high-dimensional protein sequence space. bioRxiv. 2019:617860.

107. Palacios S. Expression of androgen receptors in the structures of vulvovaginal tissue. Menopause. 2020;27(11):1336–42. https://doi.org/10.1097/GME.0000000000001587.

108. Reddy RA, Cortessis V, Dancz C, Klutke J, Stanczyk FZ. Role of sex steroid hormones in pelvic organ prolapse. Menopause. 2020;27:941–51.

109. Labrie F, Bélanger A, Cusan L, Candas B. Physiological changes in dehydroepiandrosterone are not reflected by serum levels of active androgens and estrogens but of their metabolites: intracrinology. J Clin Endocrinol Metab. 1997;82(8):2403–9. https://doi.org/10.1210/jcem.82.8.4161.

110. Labrie F, Archer D, Bouchard C, et al. Serum steroid levels during 12-week intravaginal dehydroepiandrosterone administration. Menopause. 2009;16:897–906.

111. Labrie F, Martel C. A low dose (6.5 mg) of intravaginal DHEA permits a strictly local action while maintaining all serum estrogens or androgens as well as their metabolites within normal values. Horm Mol Biol Clin Invest. 2017;29:39–60.

112. Archer DF, Labrie F, Bouchard C, et al. Treatment of pain at sexual activity (dyspareunia) with intra-vaginal dehydroepiandrosterone (prasterone). Menopause. 2015;22:950–63.

113. Labrie F, Archer DF, Koltun W, et al. Efficacy of intravaginal dehydroepiandrosterone (DHEA) on moderate to severe dyspareunia and vaginal dryness, symptoms of vulvovaginal atrophy, and of the genitourinary syndrome of menopause. Menopause. 2016;23:243–56.

114. Portman DJ, Labrie F, Archer DF, et al. Lack of effect of intravaginal dehydroepiandrosterone (DHEA, prasterone) on the endometrium in postmenopausal women. Menopause. 2015;22:1289–95.

115. Davis SR. Androgen therapy in women, beyond libido. Climacteric. 2013;16(Suppl 1):18–24. https://doi.org/10.3109/13697137.2013.801736.

116. Hubayter Z, Simon JA. Testosterone therapy for sexual dysfunction in postmenopausal women. Climacteric. 2008;11(3):181–91. https://doi.org/10.1080/13697130802162822.

117. Rowen TS, Davis SR, Parish S, Simon J, Vignozzi L. Methodological challenges in studying testosterone therapies for hypoactive sexual desire disorder in women. J Sex Med. 2020;17(4):585–94. https://doi.org/10.1016/j.jsxm.2019.12.013.

118. Krapf JM, Simon JA. The role of testosterone in the management of hypoactive sexual desire disorder in postmenopausal women. Maturitas. 2009;63(3):213–9. https://doi.org/10.1016/j.maturitas.2009.04.008.

119. Johansen N, Lindén Hirschberg A, Moen MH. The role of testosterone in menopausal hormone treatment. What is the evidence? Acta Obstet Gynecol Scand. 2020;99:966–9.

120. Maseroli E, Vignozzi L. Testosterone and vaginal function. Sex Med Rev. 2020;8:379–92.

121. Huang K, Cai HL, Bao JP, Wu LD. Dehydroepiandrosterone and age-related musculoskeletal diseases: connections and therapeutic implications. Ageing Res Rev. 2020;62:101132.

122. Tang J, Chen L-R, Chen K-H. The utilization of Dehydroepiandrosterone as a sexual hormone precursor in premenopausal and postmenopausal women: an overview. Pharmaceuticals (Basel). 2021;15(1):46. https://doi.org/10.3390/ph15010046.

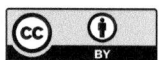